Simulation Scenarios for Nursing Educators

Suzanne Hetzel Campbell, PhD, RN, WHNP-BC, IBCLC, graduated with her BS and MS in nursing from the University of Connecticut, and her PhD in nursing from the University of Rhode Island. She obtained her post-master's certificate as a women's health nurse practitioner from Boston College. At the writing of the first edition of this book, she was associate professor, associate dean for academic programs, and project director for the Fairfield University School of Nursing Robin Kanarek Learning Resource Center. She taught at Fairfield University from 2000 to 2012. Her increasing interest in web-enhanced learning and simulation-based pedagogy has led to publications and workshops on these topics; she uses her own experience to empower nursing faculty. Dr. Campbell was a board member and faculty liaison for the School of Nursing Advisory Board at Fairfield from 2008 to 2011, and she oversaw a $1.06 million 5-year project, which included building renovation, classroom upgrades, faculty development, and integration of simulation throughout the nursing curriculum. In June 2011, Dr. Campbell became interim dean at Fairfield University School of Nursing for the academic year 2011 to 2012. In this role, she hired a new lab director, continued simulation research, and worked with the administration to support plans for an interdisciplinary health science building, incorporating arts and sciences, business, engineering, graduate education, and applied professions. As described by some of the authors in this book, these plans for an integrative health science building and an interdisciplinary focus at Fairfield University have been realized with the support of visionary leadership, a supportive advisory board, and hard-working faculty.

In July 2012, Dr. Campbell was appointed director of the School of Nursing at the University of British Columbia (UBC), Vancouver, British Columbia, Canada, where her vision for interprofessional education incorporating the use of simulation and a global approach to health care professional education is being realized. Her global outreach in the use of simulation has included work on a health communication instrument with colleagues from Fairfield and UBC, which was tested internationally and won the Best Research Paper Award in 2015 in the International Nursing Association for Clinical Simulation and Learning's (INACSL) *Clinical Simulation in Nursing* journal. In British Columbia, she has been part of research teams looking at communication modules for safe patient handover curriculums and is presently testing a Global Interprofessional Therapeutic Communication Scale (GITCS©). In addition to U.S. and Canadian international presentations, Dr. Campbell has presented on simulation in Hong Kong, Brazil, Shanghai, and Chile, and is collaborating with colleagues in Australia and South Africa. She is excited to bring an international perspective to the third edition of this text, with colleagues from several countries representing the universal use of simulation for nursing and health professional education.

Karen M. Daley, PhD, RN, graduated from Villanova University with a BS in nursing, from Troy State University with an MS in nursing, and from Rutgers—the State University of New Jersey with a PhD in nursing. At Western Connecticut State University, Dr. Daley spearheaded the implementation of human patient simulation throughout the curriculum and is primarily responsible for the acquisition of SimMan technology, the expansion and development of the nursing labs and the Nursing Resource Center, and the upgrade of resources for the nursing labs. As the chair of the Learning Resources Committee, she acquired additional lab space for an additional SimMan lab, an assessment lab, a technology classroom, and a pediatrics/obstetrics area. A new intensive care unit lab opened in the fall of 2008, funded by a federal initiative.

In June 2011, Dr. Daley became the dean of the College of Health Professions at Davenport University in Grand Rapids, Michigan. She now oversees the Allied Health, Health Information Management, Occupational Therapy, and Nursing programs. Davenport's simulation facilities are state of the art, with four simulation labs on four campuses. In May 2012, Dr. Daley realized her dream of having multidisciplinary health students embedded in a mass disaster drill simulation. Her primary focus is implementing simulation in interprofessional teams and the integration of telehealth simulations across all programs. In this work, she continues to work to integrate simulation throughout nursing and the health curriculum; to facilitate faculty training in simulation-focused learning experiences in their classes; and to encourage the use of simulation for education, training, and to enhance interprofessional education, communication, and teamwork.

Simulation Scenarios for Nursing Educators

Making It Real

Third Edition

Suzanne Hetzel Campbell, PhD, RN, WHNP-BC, IBCLC

Karen M. Daley, PhD, RN

Editors

SPRINGER PUBLISHING COMPANY

Springer Publishing Company, LLC
11 West 42nd Street
New York, NY 10036
www.springerpub.com

Acquisitions Editor: Joseph Morita
Senior Production Editor: Kris Parrish
Compositor: Newgen KnowledgeWorks

ISBN: 978-0-8261-1936-0
ebook ISBN: 978-0-8261-1939-1

17 18 19 20 21/ 5 4 3 2 1

The author and the publisher of this work have made every effort to use sources believed to be reliable to provide information that is accurate and compatible with the standards generally accepted at the time of publication. Because medical science is continually advancing, our knowledge base continues to expand. Therefore, as new information becomes available, changes in procedures become necessary. We recommend that the reader always consult current research and specific institutional policies before performing any clinical procedure. The author and publisher shall not be liable for any special, consequential, or exemplary damages resulting, in whole or in part, from the readers' use of, or reliance on, the information contained in this book. The publisher has no responsibility for the persistence or accuracy of URLs for external or third-party Internet websites referred to in this publication and does not guarantee that any content on such websites is, or will remain, accurate or appropriate.

Library of Congress Cataloging-in-Publication Data
Names: Campbell, Suzanne Hetzel, editor. | Daley, Karen M., editor.
Title: Simulation scenarios for nursing educators : making it real / Suzanne Hetzel Campbell,
   Karen M. Daley, editors.
Other titles: Simulation scenarios for nurse educators.
Description: Third edition. | New York, NY : Springer Publishing Company,
   LLC, [2018] | Preceded by Simulation scenarios for nurse educators /
   Suzanne Hetzel Campbell, Karen M. Daley. 2nd ed. c2013. | Includes
   bibliographical references and index.
Identifiers: LCCN 2017029015 | ISBN 9780826119360 (pbk.) | ISBN 9780826119391 (ebook)
Subjects: | MESH: Education, Nursing—methods | Patient Simulation | Curriculum
Classification: LCC RT73 | NLM WY 18 | DDC 610.73071/1—dc23
LC record available at https://lccn.loc.gov/2017029015

Contact us to receive discount rates on bulk purchases.
We can also customize our books to meet your needs.
For more information please contact: sales@springerpub.com

Printed in the United States of America by Gasch Printing.

This book is dedicated to all those who have helped along the way. To our husbands and families who never stop believing, supporting, and inspiring us: You are the wings upon which we soar. We also dedicate this book to all nursing faculty, without whom none of this would be possible, and to our colleagues and the administrators at our respective universities who have helped pave the way, moved mountains, and given full support to integrating simulation within the nursing curriculum. To nursing students at all levels: Excellence in nursing is not just a goal; it is a journey. Simulation can help take you there.

CONTENTS

PART I: SETTING THE FOUNDATION FOR SIMULATION

PART II: INNOVATIVE NURSING SCENARIOS IN DIVERSE SETTINGS FOR DIVERSE STUDENTS

A. Specialty Undergraduate Nursing: Medical–Surgical

PART IV: THE SIMULATION JOURNEY CONTINUES

CONTRIBUTORS

Darin Abbey, RN
CISCL Director
Adjunct Associate Professor
University of Victoria School of Nursing
Clinical Instructor, University of British
  Columbia
Island Medical Program
Victoria, British Columbia, Canada

Lynn Allchin, PhD, CHPN, CNE, RN
Triage Staff Nurse
Ambulatory Gynecologic Oncology
Hartford HealthCare
Hartford, Connecticut

Natalia Del Angelo Aredes, PhD, RN
Faculty
School of Nursing of Ribeirão Preto
University of São Paulo
Ribeirão Preto, São Paulo, Brazil

Heather Jane Bader, MSN, RN
Patient Care Nurse Manager
Lawrence and Memorial Hospital
New London, Connecticut

**Jeanine Beasley, EdD, OTR/L, CHT,
  FAOTA**
Professor
Occupational Science and Therapy
  Department
Grand Valley State University
Grand Rapids, Michigan

**Audrey M. Beauvais, DNP,
  MSN, MBA, RN, CNL**
Associate Dean and Associate Professor
Marion Peckham Egan School of Nursing
  and Health Studies
Fairfield University
Fairfield, Connecticut

Kimberly Bilskey, BSN, RN, MICN
Clinical Education Specialist,
  Critical Care
Valley Children's Hospital
Madera, California

Jeff Bishop, MD, FRCPC
Clinical Assistant Professor
University of British Columbia
Island Medical Program
Victoria, British Columbia, Canada

Andrew Booth, DHEd, PA-C
Chair
Physician Assistant Studies Department
Grand Valley State University
Allendale, Michigan

Leonie Rose Bovino, PhD, RN, CEN
Assistant Professor
Quinnipiac University
School of Nursing
Hamden, Connecticut

Dennis J. Brown, MPH, PA-C, DFAAPA
Clinical Assistant Professor of Physician
  Assistant Studies
Quinnipiac University
Hamden, Connecticut

Gloria Brummer, DNP, RN, CNE, CEN
Associate Professor
St. John's College of Nursing
Springfield, Illinois

**Carolynn Spera Bruno, PhD, APRN,
  CNS, FNP-C**
Clinical Assistant Professor of Nursing
New York University
Rory Meyers College of Nursing
New York, New York

Kellie Bryant, DNP, WHNP, CHSE
Executive Director of Simulation
Columbia University
New York, New York

Julie A. Bulson, DNP, MPA, RN, NE-BC
Director
Emergency Preparedness
Spectrum Health
Grand Rapids, Michigan

Lillian Campbell, PhD
Assistant Professor of English
Helen Way Klingler College of Arts and
   Sciences
Marquette University
Milwaukee, Wisconsin

**Suzanne Hetzel Campbell, PhD, RN,
   WHNP-BC, IBCLC**
Associate Professor, Director (2012–2017)
School of Nursing, Faculty of Applied
   Science
The University of British Columbia
Vancouver, British Columbia, Canada

**Mary Ann Cantrell, PhD, RN,
   CNE, FAAN**
Professor
College of Nursing
Villanova University
Villanova, Pennsylvania

Emma Carrick, RN, BN, RSCN
Clinical Nurse Educator
Island Health
Clinical Instructor
University of British Columbia
Island Medical Program
Victoria, British Columbia, Canada

**Leslie Catron, MAED, BSN, RN,
   FAHCEP, CHSE**
Clinical Education Specialist
Simulation Coordinator
Valley Children's Hospital
Madera, California

Pamela Causton, MN, RN
Associate Professor
Faculty of Health Sciences
University of the Fraser Valley
Chilliwack, British Columbia, Canada

Sek-ying Chair, RN, MBA, PhD
Director and Professor
The Nethersole School of Nursing
Faculty of Medicine
The Chinese University of Hong Kong
Shatin, N.T., Hong Kong

Ka-ming Chow, RN, RM, DN
Assistant Professor
Bachelor of Nursing Programme Director
The Nethersole School of Nursing
Faculty of Medicine
The Chinese University of Hong Kong
Shatin, N.T., Hong Kong

Rita M. Coggins, MSN, RN, CHSE
Assistant Director of Concepts
   Integration Laboratories
College of Nursing
East Carolina University
Greenville, North Carolina

Mary S. Cook, DNP, RN, CNS, CNE
Clinical Associate Professor of Nursing
Byers School of Nursing
Walsh University
North Canton, Ohio

Mary Ann Cordeau, PhD, RN
Associate Professor
School of Nursing
Quinnipiac University
Hamden, Connecticut

Karen M. Daley, PhD, RN
Dean, Associate Professor
College of Health Professions
Davenport University
Grand Rapids, Michigan

Julie de Salaberry, RN, MSN(c)
Director, Maternal Newborn Programs
Neonatal Intensive Care and Neonatal
    Follow-Up
BC Women's Hospital and Health Center
Vancouver, British Columbia, Canada

Margaret Devoest, PharmD
Professor, Pharmacy Practice
College of Pharmacy
Ferris State University
Big Rapids, Michigan

Ranjit K. Dhari, RN, BN, MSN
Lecturer
School of Nursing
University of British Columbia
Vancouver, British Columbia, Canada

Desiree A. Díaz, PhD, RN-BC,
    CNE, CHSE-A
Assistant Professor
College of Nursing
University of Central Florida
Orlando, Florida

Meredith Dodge, MSN, RN
Assistant Clinical Professor
School of Nursing
University of Connecticut
Storrs, Connecticut

Brian Farrell, MD, CCFP(EM)
Clinical Assistant Professor
Department of Emergency Medicine
University of British Columbia
Victoria, British Columbia, Canada

Sharon R. Flinn, PhD, OTR/L,
    CHT, FAOTA
Associate Professor (retired)
Master of Occupational Therapy Program
College of Health Professions
Davenport University
Grand Rapids, Michigan

Luciana Mara Monti Fonseca, PhD, RN
Associate Professor
College of Nursing
University of São Paulo at
    Ribeirão Preto
Ribeirão Preto, São Paulo, Brazil

Doris French, MSN, RN,
    CNOR, NE-BC
Simulation Special Projects
Grand Valley State University
Allendale, Michigan

Barbara Glynn, DNP, RN-BC
Assistant Professor
School of Nursing
Quinnipiac University
North Haven, Connecticut

Sandra Goldsworthy, PhD, RN,
    CNCC(C), CMSN(C)
Associate Dean
Teaching Learning and Technology
Associate Professor
Research Professorship in
    Simulation
Faculty of Nursing
University of Calgary
Calgary, Alberta, Canada

Robin S. Goodrich, EdD, RN
Campus President
Chamberlain College of Nursing
North Brunswick, New Jersey

Kathleen A. Gordon, MSN, RN, CNS,
    CNE, CHSE
Simulation Lab Coordinator
Assistant Professor
Aultman College of Nursing and Health
    Sciences
Canton, Ohio

Margaret B. Gray, DNP, MSN, RN-BC
Assistant Professor of Nursing
School of Nursing
Quinnipiac University
North Haven, Connecticut

Tania Grgurich, DHSc RT(R)(M)(CT) ARRT
Clinical Associate Professor of Diagnostic Imaging
Quinnipiac University
School of Health Sciences
Hamden, Connecticut

Sheila C. Grossman, PhD, APRN, FNP-BC, FAAN
Professor of Nursing & Coordinator of FNP Track
Director, Evaluation, Faculty Scholarship & Mentoring
Marion Peckham Egan School of Nursing and Health Studies
Fairfield University
Fairfield, Connecticut

Wendy A. Hall, RN, PhD
Professor
University of British Columbia
School of Nursing
Vancouver, British Columbia, Canada

Jennifer L. Herbst, JD, M. Bioethics, LLM
Professor of Law and Medical Sciences
Quinnipiac University School of Law
Frank H. Netter MD School of Medicine
Hamden, Connecticut

Melissa Holland, RN, BSN, MSc Clin Ed
Nurse Clinician, Island Health
Sessional Instructor, University of Victoria
Victoria, British Columbia, Canada

Cathryn Jackson, RN, MSN
Senior Instructor
Coordinator Simulation Lab
University of British Columbia
School of Nursing
Vancouver, British Columbia, Canada

Suzan Kardong-Edgren, PhD, RN, ANEF, CHSE, FSSH, FAAN
Professor and Director of the Rise Center
Robert Morris University
Moon, Pennsylvania

Christine Kasinskas, MS, DPT
Clinical Assistant Professor of Physical Therapy
Quinnipiac University
North Haven, Connecticut

Anne Kent, RN, BSN, MSN
Associate Professor
University of British Columbia
Abbotsford, British Columbia, Canada

Alison Kris, RN, PhD
Associate Professor of Nursing
Fairfield University
Marion Peckham Egan School of Nursing and Health Studies
Fairfield, Connecticut

Shannon Krolikowski, MSN, RN
Associate Chair
College of Health Professions/Nursing
Davenport University
Midland, Michigan

Joan Esper Kuhnly, DNP, NNP-BC, APRN, IBCLC, CNE
Associate Professor
University of Connecticut
Storrs, Connecticut

Jared M. Kutzin, DNP, MS, MPH, RN, FSSH
Associate Dean
Harriet Rothkopf Heilbrunn School of Nursing
Long Island University
Brooklyn, New York

Jean W. Lange, RN, PhD, FAAN
Founding Dean and Professor
Quinnipiac University
School of Nursing
Hamden, Connecticut

Beth Latimer, DNP, APRN, GNP-BC
Clinical Assistant Professor
Rory Meyers College of Nursing
New York University
New York, New York

Theresa L. Leto, DHS, MOT, OTR/L
Associate Professor
Occupational Therapy Program
College of Health Professions
Davenport University
Grand Rapids, Michigan

Meghan A. Lewis, MA, ATC, LAT
Assistant Clinical Professor/Clinical Coordinator
Department of Athletic Training and Sports Medicine
Quinnipiac University
Hamden, Connecticut

Jenna A. LoGiudice, PhD, CNM, RN
Assistant Professor
Marion Peckham Egan School of Nursing and Health Studies; and
Program Director
DNP Nurse MidwiferyProgram
Fairfield University
Fairfield, Connecticut

Anna Macdonald, PhD
Manager
Center of Interprofessional Clinical Simulation Learning
Vancouver Island Health Authority
Victoria, British Columbia, Canada

Maura MacPhee, RN, PhD
Professor
University of British Columbia
School of Nursing
Vancouver, British Columbia, Canada

Diana R. Mager, DNP, RN-BC
Associate Professor
Marion Peckham Egan School of Nursing and Health Studies
Fairfield University
Fairfield, Connecticut

Bette Mariani, PhD, RN, ANEF
Associate Professor of Nursing
Villanova University
College of Nursing
Villanova, Pennsylvania

Colleen H. Meakim, MSN, RN, CHSE, ANEF
Director
Simulation and Learning Resource Center
Villanova University College of Nursing
Villanova, Pennsylvania

Rose Milano, RN, BSN, MS, DNP, ACNP-BC
Trauma Nurse Practitioner
Assistant Professor, School of Nursing
Adult-Gerontology Acute Care Nurse Practitioner Program
Assistant Professor, School of Medicine
Department of Surgery, Division of Trauma, Critical Care, Acute Care Surgery
Oregon Health & Science University
Portland, Oregon

Nancy A. Moriber, PhD, CRNA, APRN
Program Director
Fairfield University and Bridgeport
    Hospital Nurse Anesthesia Program; and
Assistant Professor
Marion Peckham Egan School of Nursing
    and Health Studies
Fairfield University
Fairfield, Connecticut

Laura Mutrie, MSW, LCSW
Clinical Assistant Professor of Social Work
Quinnipiac University
School of Health Sciences, Social Work
North Haven, Connecticut

Karen M. Myrick, DNP, APRN,
    FNP-BC, ANP-BC
Associate Professor of Nursing
Quinnipiac University
School of Nursing
North Haven, Connecticut

Julie L. Polanic, MSN, RN, CNL
Nursing Faculty
College of Health Professions
Davenport University
Grand Rapids, Michigan

Lillian A. Rafeldt, MA, RN, CNE
Professor of Nursing
Three Rivers Community College
Norwich, Connecticut

Kathryn M. Reynolds, MSN, RN, PNP
Clinical Assistant Professor
Villanova University
College of Nursing
Villanova, Pennsylvania

Catherine Napoli Rice, RN, BSN,
    MSN, EdD
Professor
Western Connecticut State University
Danbury, Connecticut

Anka Roberto, DNP,
    PMHNP-BC, APRN
Visiting Assistant Professor, Director of
    Simulation
Fairfield University
Fairfield, Connecticut

Leland J. Rockstraw, PhD, RN
Associate Clinical Professor
Drexel University
College of Nursing and Health
    Professions
Philadelphia, Pennsylvania

Darlene Rogers, BSN, RN
Simulation Coordinator
Quinnipiac University
School of Nursing
Hamden, Connecticut

Maureen M. Ryan, RN, BN, MN, PhD
Assistant Teaching Professor
Clinical Simulation(s) Coordinator
School of Nursing
University of Victoria
Victoria, British Columbia, Canada

Carol R. Sando, RN, PhD, CNE
Associate Professor
Delaware State University
Department of Nursing
Dover, Delaware

Samantha Scanlon, RN BSN
Simulation Coordinator
Grand Valley State University
Allendale, Michigan

Joyce M. Shea, DNSc, APRN,
    PMHCNS-BC
Associate Dean and Associate Professor
Marion Peckham Egan School of Nursing
    and Health Studies
Fairfield University
Fairfield, Connecticut

Michael J. Shoemaker, DPT, PhD
Board-Certified Geriatric Clinical Specialist
Associate Professor of Physical Therapy
Grand Valley State University
Grand Rapids, Michigan

Suzanne C. Smeltzer, EdD, RN,
  ANEF, FAAN
Professor and Director
Center for Nursing Research
Villanova University College of Nursing
Villanova, Pennsylvania

Monica P. Sousa, EdD, ACNS-BC, APRN
Associate Professor
Western Connecticut State University
Danbury, Connecticut

Joshua Squiers, PhD, ACNP-BC,
  AGACNP-BC, FCCM
Assistant Professor of Nursing
Oregon Health & Science University,
  School of Nursing
Director of the Acute Care Nurse
  Practitioner Program
Assistant Professor of Anesthesiology
Oregon Health & Science University,
  School of Medicine
Division of Cardiac and Surgical
  Subspecialty Critical Care
Portland, Oregon

Lee-Anne Stephen, MN, RN
Associate Professor
Faculty of Health Sciences
University of the Fraser Valley
Chilliwack, British Columbia, Canada

Geraldine Jacobus Terry, MD, MSN, RN
Assistant Professor and Course
  Coordinator for IPE
Integrated Team Care
Kirkhof College of Nursing
Grand Valley State University
Grand Rapids, Michigan

Suzanne Turner, MSN, RN
Nursing Laboratory Coordinator
Three Rivers Community College
Norwich, Connecticut

Philip Van Lente, MD
Associate Professor
College of Human Medicine
Michigan State University
East Lansing, Michigan

Tracy Van Oss, DHSc, MPH, OTR/L,
  FAOTA
Clinical Associate Professor of
  Occupational Therapy
Quinnipiac University
School of Health Sciences
North Haven, Connecticut

Rebecca J. Ventura, MSN, RN,
  RMA(AMT)
Assistant Professor
Associate Department Chair/Program
  Director
College of Health Professions
Davenport University
Grand Rapids, Michigan

Linda H. Warren, EdD, RN,
  MSN, CCRN
Associate Professor
Department of Nursing
Western Connecticut State
  University
Danbury, Connecticut

Dawna Williams, RN, MN
Associate Professor
Faculty of Health
  Sciences
University of the Fraser Valley
Chilliwack, British Columbia,
  Canada

FOREWORD

We have come a long way in the 4 years since the previous edition of the book. Over the past few years, in the world of clinical simulations, the pedagogy, adoption, and the science have escalated. We have a lot more to do, but we are on the right path. This book, *Simulation Scenarios for Nursing Educators: Making It Real*, is a must-buy book, particularly if you are getting started in creating and integrating clinical simulations in your nursing program. Living up to the goals and outcomes of the first and second editions, the authors have continued to develop and refine more step-by-step guidelines for nursing faculty. These guidelines enable faculty to design, develop, and implement clinical simulation scenarios in diverse settings, with diverse patients, and for different levels of students, from the novice in a fundamentals course to the student in a senior-level critical care or capstone course, to a nurse practitioner in a graduate program.

The authors have done a wonderful job of providing clinical scenarios on major health disruption topics that any nursing student would need to experience from prelicensure to graduate to doctorate. Each chapter that focuses on the clinical simulation scenario contains essential elements such as the scenario objectives, prescenario checklists, an implementation plan, evaluation criteria, debriefing guidelines, and considerations for running the scenario in the future. What more would educators want?

The organization of the book is in four main categories: (a) setting the foundation, (b) innovative nursing scenarios in diverse settings for diverse students, (c) interdisciplinary and interprofessional scenarios, and (d) simulation journey. These continue to provide information to all levels of nurse educators, from novices to those experienced in the simulation world. The authors set the stage with the first section of the book by outlining foundational points, including the groundwork around simulation theories and frameworks to help guide the educator in this area of pedagogy.

Unique to this book, and what sets it apart from other books on simulations and clinical scenarios, are the personal experiences, local and global, that the authors bring to the chapters. The authors' passion, enthusiasm, and inspiration are truly reflected and demonstrated in each chapter. Authors talk about lessons learned, teaching strategies, and in-depth research and exploration of their topics. This book is an excellent guide for nursing faculty just getting started with simulations and is a validation for faculty who are already using this pedagogy.

Whether you are beginning on the simulation journey or just want to refine and add more to the area of clinical simulations in your own nursing program or school, you will find ideas to foster your own teaching practices that can enhance students' learning. The authors have included their experiences on how to develop a simulation center and approaches to developing faculty for simulations to debriefing and evaluation, as well as final words of wisdom on the future of simulations. The book is comprehensive, resourceful, and a gift for nurse educators embarking on the development and implementation of clinical simulations.

Key highlights in the book include the practice application of how to develop, implement, and evaluate clinical simulations in a nursing program. The authors make understanding simulation pedagogy an easy and exciting journey; one that educators will want to try to embrace even when there is hesitation and uncertainty. Other key topics include the richness of providing knowledge, strategies, and recommendations on how to implement simulations in different types of course or clinical settings. For example, if you are in doubt about how simulations can be incorporated in a primary care setting, one chapter provides ideas, scenario objectives, and examples of how the simulation pedagogy can be used in this type of environment. The entire spectrum of courses, from fundamentals, health assessment, and medical–surgical nursing courses, to more complex levels, such as trauma resuscitation, are discussed, with authors providing specific examples, simulation scenarios that include patient information, simulation objectives, preparation lists, and other information on all necessary components to develop and implement the simulation successfully. Various chapters address the diverse patient population, including geriatric, pediatric, trauma, obstetric, and community-based patients, in terms of simulations that can be designed and implemented in those contexts. Finally, Chapter 55 offers a scholarly perspective on how to publish your own work in this area of pedagogy and scholarship.

Experiential learning, such as we demonstrate through clinical simulations, is the future for preparing nurses to transition into the health care arena to provide safe, competent care. As the National Council of State Boards of Nursing's (NCSBN) large, multisite, national simulation study demonstrated (Hayden, Smiley, Alexander, Kardong-Edgren, & Jeffries, 2014), the evidence is there. When student learning occurred through clinical simulations, used as a substitute for real clinical time, overall, there was a positive impact on helping students bridge the gap from theory to practice as evidenced by the research. We no longer need to ask whether simulations work, but rather to ask how we can best implement and immerse our learners in realistic clinical scenarios in safe, nonthreatening environments that prepare them to provide quality, safe patient care. As nursing leaders embrace the future of nursing education recommendations as outlined by the Institute of Medicine (2011), this book provides educators the knowledge, skills, and tools to prepare for educational reform to manage the shortage of clinical learning experiences, the lack of clinical sites, shortage of nurse educators, and the need to better prepare students for clinical decision making in a complex health care environment. This book provides practical solutions to transform clinical education. The creativity and innovation demonstrated by the authors in this third edition provide a wonderful continued journey to meeting these challenges.

Pamela R. Jeffries, PhD, RN, FAAN, ANEF
Professor, Dean
George Washington University School of Nursing
Washington, DC

REFERENCES

Hayden, J. K., Smiley, R. A., Alexander, M., Kardong-Edgren, S., & Jeffries, P. R. (2014). The NCSBN National Simulation Study: A longitudinal, randomized, controlled study replacing clinical hours with simulation in prelicensure nursing education. *Journal of Nursing Regulation, 5*(2), C1–S64.

Institute of Medicine. (2011). *The future of nursing education: Leading change, advancing health*. Washington, DC: National Academies Press.

PREFACE

Nursing education is situated in a unique moment in time. In what has been called the *perfect storm* (Hinshaw, 2008), a faculty shortage has collided with a nursing shortage, and the two have resulted in challenges for nursing educators. In addition, new generations of tech-savvy nursing students are before us in our classrooms. In the face of this challenge, nursing educators have the opportunity to create a new paradigm for teaching that reflects students' need for interactive technology. Throughout history, nurses have always responded to crises with creativity and innovation, and the same is true today. By complementing our traditional teaching with simulation, we, as educators, are addressing our need to do more with less. In making simulation *real*, we can deliver our teaching in an engaging yet effective manner, thereby transforming nursing education through a simulation-based pedagogy.

It has been fascinating to observe the breadth and depth of interest in the first two editions of our text. With one editor living internationally and having contact with people from around the globe, the distinction of this third edition is the incorporation of an international perspective, a stronger section on interprofessional simulation, and authors from other disciplines outside nursing. These additions can be found in shared scenarios from Hong Kong (Chapter 15); chapters revised to include a Canadian and Brazilian context (Chapters 4, 5, 6, and 20); examples from several Canadian schools of nursing; and interdisciplinary authors from medicine, occupational therapy, physio/physical therapy, social work, allied health, and English.

This book is divided into four parts. Part I provides an introduction to simulation-focused pedagogy with an explanation and updates on the Framework for Simulation Learning in Nursing Education©. Following that is an overview of the integration of simulation into nursing curricula; an examination of teaching and assessing health communication in a simulated environment; options for building a learning resource center, including audiovisual capabilities; and the description of innovative approaches to simulation-based faculty development. New to the section, a chapter on integrating disability into nursing education with standardized patients and the use of IV simulations has been added.

Part II presents a collection of 27 exemplars, including 10 brand-new simulation scenarios for this edition and significant revisions to the others, such as addition of the INACSL Best Practice Standards: Simulation^SM (International Nursing Association for Clinical Simulation in Learning [INACSL], 2016) and updated evidence-based practice guidelines. These chapters contain increasingly complex scenarios in multiple clinical areas and testimonies of practicing faculty in a variety of settings at different levels of nursing education. Part II is divided into five key areas of specialty undergraduate nursing: (a) medical–surgical; (b) obstetric and pediatric; (c) older adult; (d) thematic scenarios on cultural humility, Quality and Safety Education in Nursing, and mental health; and (e) advanced practice nurses.

The following template has been used for the chapters in Part II:

A. Discussion of implementation of simulation-based pedagogy in each contributor's individualized teaching
B. Description of educational materials available in your teaching area and relative to your specialty
C. Specific objectives for simulation utilization within a specific course and the overall program
D. Introduction of scenario to include setting the scene, technology used, objectives, and description of participants [setting the scene and technology used; objectives; description of participants]
E. Description of the running of the scenario

F. Presentation of completed template [title; focus area; scenario description; pre-scenario set-up checklist; patient data form; evaluative criteria].

G. Debriefing guidelines.

H. Suggestions/key features to replicate or improve.

I. Recommendations for further use.

J. Discussion of simulation-based pedagogy and how this new technology has contributed to improved student outcomes.

k. Expert recommendations and words of wisdom.

l. Evaluation of best practice standards and use of credentialed simulation faculty.

References
Further Readings

In this edition, because of the increased use of simulation for interdisciplinary and interprofessional education, we have dedicated Part III to 16 scenarios with this focus; 10 are brand new. These scenarios capture many of the key themes in nursing, including ethics, spirituality, palliative care, communication, and cultural humility. They are meant to show nursing faculty that simulation development and incorporation into the curriculum are both feasible and fun. The book provides concrete information about the use of simulation in a variety of programs, courses, and schools with flexible simulator uses, including static and live actors, and low-, medium-, and high-fidelity human patient simulators (HPSs). These practical applications are for individuals who are interested in taking first steps toward incorporating simulation or for those who have begun but want to expand beyond a typical medical–surgical, intensive care, and trauma focus. INACSL's Standards of Practice: Simulation Glossary (2016) describes skill development and clinical judgment that fits with this book's goal to encourage the development of critical thinking, clinical reasoning, and clinical judgment, as well as to develop caring, competent, and safe practitioners who demonstrate psychomotor skills and problem-solving capabilities that lead to safe, excellent, reflective practice. Hints for suspending disbelief and "making it *real*" for students and faculty are incorporated throughout the book.

Part IV explores the continuing simulation journey in nursing education. Given the continued work of the coeditors with the chapter authors and faculty in their own institutions, the framework of simulation learning was updated and placed in Chapter 2 of this book to provide better context for our readers. For this new edition, the role of certification in simulation for nursing education has been updated to incorporate the changing landscape. In addition, a model for "writing across the curriculum" that focuses on how to write like a nurse in clinical simulation environments has been added by an English professor well versed in nursing simulation. Support for publishing your simulation work is provided by the editor of *Clinical Simulation in Nursing*, Suzan Kardong-Edgren. Lastly, Chapter 56 details the evolution of simulation and its integration in nursing curriculum and practice since the publication of the first edition of this book.

A template for creating scenarios is provided throughout the book, including the following:

*   Student preparation materials, such as suggested readings, skills necessary for scenario enactment, and websites with more information, based on INACSL Best Practice Standards: Simulation (INACSL, 2016)
*   Forms to enhance the realness of the scenario, such as patient data forms, patient medication forms, and assessment tools (or websites, where they can be acquired) and table exemplars for setting the scene and scenario implementation
*   Checklists, such as health communication checklists to use in the creation of scenarios, evaluation criteria checklists for assessing student performance in scenarios, and debriefing guidelines

The intent is to provide faculty with a strong foundation to be able to run multiple scenarios in a variety of clinical specialties geared at different learning levels and with different learning objectives, providing opportunities to match the scenario to essential documents (American Association of Colleges of Nursing [AACN], 2008, 2011) and competencies [e.g., NCLEX-RN® test plan (NCSBN, 2015)].

It seems only fitting that the second edition was released after the 101st birthday of "Mrs. Chase"—the soft, lightweight doll that had hand-painted, raised facial features and included stitched jointed hips, knees, elbows, and shoulders, who was both flexible and durable (Herrmann, 2008). In 1911, this first manikin arrived at the Hartford Hospital Training School for Nurses at the request of "Miss A. Lauder Sutherland, an 1891 graduate of Toronto General Hospital who was then the superintendent of nurses and the principal of the Hartford (CT) Hospital Training School for Nurses (1905–1918)" (Herrmann, 2008, p. 53).

Today, upon the release of this third edition, nurse educators mature in their use of simulation, transition from flexible/durable manikins to wireless environments, virtual simulations, and virtual reality, while evaluating the impact of simulation on patient care, safety, and quality of care as well as the return on investment. We've come a long way in 100 years!

This long-awaited book provides *real* life stories of faculty in the trenches providing the light at the end of the tunnel to the sometimes challenging, but always worthwhile, journey of simulation integration!

Suzanne Hetzel Campbell
Karen M. Daley

REFERENCES

American Association of Colleges of Nursing. (2008). *The essentials of baccalaureate education for professional nursing practice.* Washington, DC: Author. Retrieved from http://www.aacn.nche.edu/education-resources/BaccEssentials08.pdf

American Association of Colleges of Nursing. (2011, March 21). *The essentials of master's education in nursing.* Washington, DC: Author. Retrieved from http://www.aacn.nche.edu/education-resources/MastersEssentials11.pdf

Herrmann, E. K. (2008). *Remembering Mrs. Chase. Before there were smart hospitals and Sim-Men, there was "Mrs. Chase"* (pp. 52–55). Brooklyn, NY: NSNA. Retrieved from http://www.nsna.org/Portals/0/Skins/NSNA/pdf/Imprint_FebMar08_Feat_MrsChase.pdf

Hinshaw, A. S. (2008). Navigating the perfect storm: Balancing a culture of safety with workforce challenges. *Nursing Research, 57*(1S), S4–S10.

International Nursing Association for Clinical Simulation and Learning. (2016). Standards of best practice: Simulation. *Clinical Simulation in Nursing, 12,* S48–S50. doi:10.1016/j.ecns.2016.10.001

National Council of State Boards of Nursing. (2015). *NCLEX-RN examination: Test plan for the National Council Licensure Examination for Registered Nurses.* Retrieved from https://www.ncsbn.org/RN_Test_Plan_2016_Final.pdf

ACKNOWLEDGMENTS

To all those who contributed time and effort in creating their scenarios for this book, we thank you from the bottom of our hearts for sharing your knowledge and expertise in describing your challenges and victories using simulation. There are numerous individuals who provided support. In grateful recognition we name a few at Fairfield University: the administration, especially Dean Jeanne Novotny, whose vision for the school has been an inspiration; Laboratory Director Diana R. Mager, whose expertise in organizing, running, and overseeing the lab made this all possible; colleague and Codirector Phil Greiner, whose insight in so many areas has led to this greater vision; the School of Nursing Advisory Board, without whom this project would not have come to fruition, especially the chair, Nancy Lynch, whose guidance and tireless perseverance have led to marvelous outcomes; major donor Robin Kanarek, whose passion for nursing provides endless encouragement; Media Department Manager Kirk Anderson, who is always just a phone call away; the Center for Academic Excellence, especially Larry Miners, whose support for faculty development has been key to our progress; and the Computing and Network Services departments, as well as the students who have patiently worked with us throughout the years.

At Western Connecticut State University, grateful thanks are extended to the faculty and staff as well as the Learning Resources Committee, which truly did all the work supporting simulation; and to the Western Connecticut State University class of 2008, who inspired and created the student-generated senior scenarios.

Thanks to the nursing faculty of Davenport University, who have realized the dream of state-of-the-art simulation facilities as a standard, not just a remote goal; and to our visionary president, Dr. Pappas, and the provost, Dr. Rinker, who led the way. This vision has allowed us to grow and spread our wings with state-of-the-art simulation facilities for all programs. Most important, thanks is expressed to the amazing faculty, staff, and students of Davenport's College of Health Professions, who inspire us every day to be our best.

Sincere appreciation to the University of British Columbia in providing support and the colleagues in the School of Nursing and other health disciplines who share their passion for simulation and innovative teaching pedagogy. Gratitude as well to the many colleagues in the province of British Columbia and throughout Canada who have continued to share their knowledge and expertise. Finally, thanks to colleagues internationally who inspire us to continue reaching and dreaming for new ways of educating the next generation.

Suzanne is grateful for the opportunity to be on the global stage, which has convinced her of the utility of simulation, regardless of language and cultural differences, to teach the foundational "art of nursing."

The names have changed over the years but we express our help and gratitude to the unnamed influencers of our careers, our passion for nursing, and the use of simulation in education.

Specifically for this third edition, we would like to acknowledge the work of student Paramdeep Nahal, who assisted two very busy administrators in staying on task and coordinating 56 chapters and more than 100 authors. Without her dedicated and precise work, we would not have been able to complete this edition in a timely manner with the level of attention to detail and flow that we have accomplished.

So many have helped us, wiped our weary brows, and made sure we were able to march on. We cannot possibly name them all.

PART I

Setting the Foundation for Simulation

CHAPTER 1

Simulation-Focused Pedagogy for Nursing Education

Suzanne Hetzel Campbell and Karen M. Daley

THE CHALLENGE OF TEACHING IN THE 21ST CENTURY

This book is written on the basis of our personal experiences with audiences of nursing faculty regionally, nationally, and internationally who have expressed frustration, consternation, anxiety, and bewilderment about "where to start" with simulation, especially with human patient simulators (HPSs). We have been privileged to be present at the start of simulation, with the inherent frustration of explaining to administration and fellow faculty the potential and vision that this innovative learning experience can provide for nursing students.

It is our hope that the simulation scenarios and other valuable information included in this text provide nurse educators with a place to start—a template for the creation of their own broad and relevant experiences in the classroom and in clinical settings. It is paramount that we share our passion for the process and our strong belief that all faculty can contribute, at whatever level of simulation, to this process. Yes, there are gaps and challenges expressed in the literature; yes, faculty struggles to meet the new demands of this technology within the realm of faculty shortages and workload. Yet, the potential benefits to faculty and students are clear, especially by enhancing critical thinking beyond protocol and critical pathways. Often, it is an astute, expert nurse who, in noting subtle changes in a patient, enacts the kind of care that saves the patient's life. Nurses are the front-line providers of care.

Simulation is presented by allowing for reflection on all aspects of care. The built-in debriefing period, which encourages reflection on thoughts, actions, and outcomes, also leads to better transfer of knowledge to practice and more versatile thinking processes for future application individually, in groups, and across interprofessional teams with a focus on patient-centered care. In addition, the faculty role of mentor and facilitator in this process combines faculty expertise with student innovation. It is a learning process for all, which improves methods of teaching and learning overall.

ROLE OF SIMULATION IN NURSING EDUCATION

So many changes have occurred since the first edition of this book. The scenarios and information have been shared globally and Dr. Campbell's Academia.edu website, which contains some of the text has been viewed 4,558 times and downloaded 302 times since 2012. One of the biggest changes for simulation in nursing is that the International Nursing Association for Clinical Simulation and Learning (INACSL) has taken the lead in defining best practices, referenced as INACSL Standards of Best Practice: Simulation^{SM} (INACSL, 2013/2016) and which includes: Standard I: Terminology

(Meakim et al., 2013), Standard II: Professional Integrity of Participants (Gloe et al., 2013), Standard III: Participant Objectives (Lioce et al., 2013), Standard IV: Facilitation (Franklin et al., 2013), Standard V: Facilitator (Boese et al., 2013), Standard VI: The Debriefing Process (Decker et al., 2013), Standard VII: Participant Assessment and Evaluation (Sando et al., 2013), Standard VIII: Interprofessional Education (Decker et al., 2015), and Standard IX: Simulation Design (Lioce et al., 2015). During the writing, these standards were updated and can be found on the INACSL website (INACSL, 2013/2016). Dr. Campbell was invited to review the revisions and give input as an individual contributor. Other areas promising an increasing consistency in simulation programs include the NCSBN's *Simulation Guidelines for Prelicensure Nursing Program* (Alexander et al., 2015), while Cheng and colleagues (2016) have consolidated the reporting guidelines for health simulation research by extending the Consolidated Standards of Reporting Trials (CONSORT) and STrengthening the Reporting of OBservational studies in Epidemiology (STROBE) statements. The intention of these guidelines and best practices is not to squelch the innovative potential that nursing faculty bring to simulation, but rather to provide credibility in reporting the effect of simulation in nursing education and research. As the coeditors know well, nursing faculty are often teaching "on the fly." Although it is helpful to have standards and guidelines, we don't want to underestimate the refreshing expertise nurses bring that encourages creativity and innovation in nursing faculty. In hindsight, the chapter template and scenarios provided in the first edition of this text actually took into consideration most of the areas that are today identified as best practices.

Initially, many nurse educators and researchers were at the forefront in recognizing simulation as a valuable tool for gaining knowledge (Alinier, Hunt, & Gordon, 2003; Childs & Sepples, 2006; Henneman & Cunningham, 2005; Jeffries, 2005; Roberts & McGowan, 2004). Although beyond our wildest dreams and expectations, considerable research, including multiple systematic reviews, integrated reviews of the literature, and carefully designed randomized-controlled studies (Adamson, 2015; Keers, Williams, Cooke, Walsh, & Ashcroft, 2014), are now setting the standard for high-level research in simulation, demonstrating the impact of this innovative method of teaching. In addition, the scholarship of teaching and learning has gained increased respect as the importance of demonstrating the efficacy of various methods of teaching to transfer knowledge and change behavior was recognized. This is especially important in the clinically based application of nursing science. Finally, the incorporation of interprofessional simulations for team training and patient safety are recognized as equally important and need to be considered in every nursing education program (Malt, 2015).

The availability of high-fidelity technology at a reasonable cost, and the availability of funds to purchase this equipment, has resulted in its widespread acquisition across the globe. Although some faculty have reported to us that, on delivery, these HPSs may remain in a box, unused. Other faculty, who have had the benefit of preassembly and attending 1- to 2-day workshops, need encouragement and inspiration to fully implement simulation within their individual courses and throughout their curriculum. When attending simulation conferences, it appears that everyone is incorporating and using simulation (or has bought the equipment). But when you talk to faculty, they are confused, overwhelmed, and frustrated with trying to write and implement scenarios into their individual courses.

One only needs to watch a group of students in a simulation to fully appreciate its teaching and learning potentialities at hand. After all, simulation prompts positive results. Although initially, the research for assessment and evaluation for nursing education fell behind the medical literature, currently, evidence exists that simulation results in better outcomes and improved performance (Cook et al., 2011, 2013), and more reliable and valid instruments are available for use to test and incorporate simulation (Kardong-Edgren, Adamson, & Fitzgerald, 2010), including this repository of instruments used in simulation research: www.inacsl.org/i4a/pages/index .cfm?pageID=3496. Early on, in a study of the use of clinical laboratories in Victoria, Australia (with site visits, interviews, and curricula review), researchers found that use of the laboratories was based on past experience, tradition, and resources rather than evidence (Wellard, Woolf, & Gleeson, 2007). Research on simulation in nursing is ongoing, and has matured to the stage where new meta-analyses and reviews of the literature continue to support the use of simulation for the education of health professionals. Early in this research trajectory, the benefits of simulation were well documented by the National League for Nursing (NLN)/Laerdal simulation study

(Jeffries & Rizolo, 2006), and current evidence has suggested that substituting simulation for clinical practice results in similar outcomes to traditional education for prelicensure nursing students (Hayden, Smiley, Alexander, Kardong-Edgren, & Jeffries, 2014).

On a broader level, an administration's procurement of the money for providing the necessary resources (faculty development, equipment purchase, building renovations, faculty time, etc.) does not transfer immediately into less faculty workload. In contrast, it often requires more investment of time and resources up front to get to the "work smarter, not harder" phase. One strategy has been to assign already overburdened lab directors with the "task" of incorporating simulation for faculty. Whether in static modules as testing before entering clinical, skill-based task training, or endpoint competency testing, the actual development and running of the scenarios is parceled out to lab staff, information technology personnel, and others. As this process may not directly involve faculty, their valuable educational and clinical expertise is more often overlooked. Another strategy allows for individual faculty to initiate simulation within their own teaching load in single courses. Faculty find this process time-consuming and complex when starting without the help or guidance of those more experienced in simulation (Nehring & Lashley, 2004). Currently, to meet this faculty knowledge gap, simulation training and/or certification has become more commonplace, for example, through the Society for Simulation in Health Care (ssih.org/certification). In addition, multiple workshops are available through conferences (www.inacsl.org), and nursing programs are including courses and certificates in advanced innovative educational methodologies, including simulation. See Chapter 54 for more information about simulation certification and accreditation.

We feel that simulation offers an innovative approach that complements and easily integrates into the existing nursing curricula, addressing the needs of a new generation of nurses and a society with increasingly complex health care needs. In order to fully appreciate the incorporation of simulation and the driving forces behind this movement, one needs to recognize that the challenges include understanding issues facing nursing education, the influence of technology on theoretical and conceptual aspects of nursing education, learning in the digital culture, and the challenge of suspending disbelief to make simulations real. In order for a transfer of knowledge to occur, the student's role in the simulation needs to be as authentic as possible.

Some of the issues facing nursing education include the increased acuity level of patients, the nursing faculty and staff shortages, limited clinical sites, and the shifting role of the nurse. Quality and safety of patient care have become a major societal focus driving the increased accountability of nursing faculty and students to provide safe, effective, knowledgeable nurses who can function in a highly complex health care environment. Nurses are expected to demonstrate leadership skills in the coordination of patient care and safety, and even in the role of overseeing interprofessional teams that provide multifaceted care. Increasingly, nurses are expected to use their knowledge to transform health care delivery. Simulation provides an environment for the teaching and learning of interprofessional collaboration through scenarios embedded with communication, safety, delegation, critical thinking, and other important nursing program outcomes where novice nursing students can practice in a safe environment (Berndt, 2014; Fisher & King, 2013; Haskvitz & Koop, 2004; Jeffries, 2005; Jose & Dufrene, 2014; Keers et al., 2014; Radhakrishnan, Roche, & Cunningham, 2007; Zhang, Thompson, & Miller, 2011). Finally, the challenge of assessment and evaluation of student performance can go beyond skill-based assessment to include nontechnical skills, such as communication and conflict resolution, as well as more summative processes such as student growth over time, development of critical thinking, and socialization into professional nursing practice.

THEORETICAL AND CONCEPTUAL ISSUES
IN NURSING EDUCATION

When viewed as a learning tool, simulation aligns well with the theoretical and conceptual foundations of nursing education. Models and frameworks have been proposed and used to help conceptualize the role of simulation in nursing education. One such model describes a simulation protocol that was formulated by the University of Maryland School of Nursing (Larew, Lessans, Spunt, Foster, & Covington, 2006). This protocol, based on the work of Benner (1984), uses a cue-based system with escalating prompts to move students through recognition to assessment to intervention to problem resolution. Recommendations to highlight one problem at a time, allowing the scenarios to be student directed with time for processing in the pacing of the scenario, laid the foundation for further development of simulation frameworks. Jeffries and Rodgers (2007) proposed a theoretical framework for simulation from "insights gained from theoretical and empirical literature" (p. 22) on simulation in nursing and related disciplines. This eclectic approach to formulating simulation frameworks provides the basis for a holistic, flexible, and multifaceted method of integrating simulation into nursing education.

In addition to those seminal works cited earlier (Jeffries & Rodgers, 2007; Larew et al., 2006), we have considered the work of Tanner (2006) in our conceptualization of simulation. Tanner's model of clinical judgment is relevant in simulation because a large part of it involves clinical judgment and decision making. His description of aspects of the process includes noticing, interpreting, responding, and reflecting. This model emphasizes expectations of the situation that may be implicit or explicit. A particular emphasis on reflection finds support in the recent literature, which highlights reflection as an essential element in the improvement of clinical reasoning (Tanner, 2006). In simulation, an equivalent concept is debriefing, which should include Tanner's reflection-on-action as a synthesis of experiential knowledge resulting in the formulation of best practices. In a clinical situation, nursing students often observe and are unable to enact interventions independently. In simulation, reflection on interventions can result in a second try in a safe environment, where improved outcomes are immediately evident.

Fink (2003), another driving force in our simulation-focused pedagogy, discussed the creation of significant learning experiences. On the basis of education research, he has compiled six major dimensions to "formulate significant learning goals" (p. 75). In considering these learning goals, we have identified areas that demonstrate how simulation complements nursing education to meet program goals and outcomes. For example, the goals include (a) foundational knowledge (nursing content), (b) application (enactment of the scenario allows for use of knowledge and skills in a safe environment), (c) integration (synthesizing the science of nursing with knowledge from all disciplines—in conjunction with critical thinking, this dimension incorporates decision making and priority setting), (d) human dimension (interacting with themselves and others to form a view of who they are as nursing professionals, including opportunities for collaboration), (e) caring (the art of nursing), and (f) learning how to learn (empowering students for professional lifelong learning). The debriefing component of simulation pedagogy allows for an integration of all six major dimensions of Fink's learning goals.

Of interest in simulation is social ecological theory (Stokols, 1996). This framework examines individual experiences and culture brought to social situations and how they impact behavioral outcomes. The social determinants of health (Wilkinson & Marmot, 2003), developed by the World Health Organization's European division in the 1990s, incorporate social ecological theory and continue to be imbedded as a foundation for *Healthy People 2020* (U.S. Department of Health and Human Services, 2000). These theoretical cores should be directly linked to simulations as they are being developed.

For example, a common challenge for nurses working in inpatient environments is the decontextualization of the patient. By this, we mean that care is being provided without an understanding of the social and physical environment or the behavioral motivators related to health of the individual patient. The result can be that patient teaching and other nursing activities done in the institution do not match the reality of the patient's home environment. In home health care, nurses often need to reteach the patient and/or caregiver to fit the care plan to the resources available.

In simulation, not only is the context of the patient important, but educators must consider the cultural predispositions that students bring into the learning environment, which may affect behavior and the outcome of the scenario. The same is almost true within the culture of a nursing floor or unit. Clinical judgments made may be influenced by these multiple factors and need to be considered in the culturally sensitive care of real patients. In addition, simulations can be manipulated such that the patients being cared for have a variety of cultural backgrounds, needs (including special needs of patients with disabilities or chronic and/or terminal diseases), experiences, and diverse social and environmental support systems. Including these factors enhances the simulation and learning experience for students and increases the "realness" of the scenario.

Related nursing concepts in simulation are *vigilance* and *failure to rescue*. As nursing educators, vigilance is one of the most important yet difficult concepts to teach to nursing students (Almerud, Alapack, Fridlund, & Ekebergh, 2007; Jacobs, Apatov, & Glei, 2007; Meyer & Lavin, 2005). Although introduced early in assessment courses, the evolution of vigilance as an essential function of a nurse is amenable to practice and refinement during simulation. Once taught in this setting, students become aware of the value of maintaining vigilance in actual health care settings. A consequence of failed vigilance is failure to rescue. Although unethical to practice in the clinical setting, a student who experiences failure to rescue in a simulation can follow through with reflective debriefing, reformulate a plan, carry out the new plan, and then successfully maintain vigilance. Students have reported, "never forgetting" the opportunity to "redo." Once again, this experience adds to the development of the student's vision of the impact of maintaining excellence in nursing care.

From the student's perspective, there have been reports that conceptualizing the scenario through the lens of the nursing process while in the midst of a simulation is extremely helpful in producing positive outcomes. It has been frequently observed in our teaching that students, in the excitement of enacting a scenario, jump past focused assessments and begin performing interventions without data to support their decisions. Gentle coaching and reminders by the instructors alleviate this tendency.

In theorizing about technology in simulation, one may want to consider that, beyond technological fidelity, there are actually three levels of fidelity: environmental, equipment, and psychological (Fritz, Gray, & Flanagan, 2007).

- **Environmental fidelity***:* "The realism of the environment in which the simulation takes place" (Fritz et al., 2007, p. 2).
- **Equipment fidelity***:* "Hardware and/or software realism of the simulator" (Fritz et al., 2007, p. 2).
- **Psychological fidelity***:* "The degree to which the trainee perceives the simulation to be a believable representation of the reality it is duplicating" (Fritz et al., 2007, p. 2).

In nursing, we have incorporated these fidelities by making simulation as real as possible—a suspension of disbelief—so that the student interacts and participates more fully. The way space is structured to look and feel like a clinical unit, with necessary equipment, sets the scene for the simulation. In addition, events need to flow smoothly (e.g., responses from "patients" and "families") so that the student acknowledges his or her role in meeting patient needs.

There are three goals or levels of enacting a reality-based simulation:

1. **For students**: The simulation must be believable. They must take on the role of the "nurse" and feel the responsibility for the care, assessment, and delegation necessary to meet the needs of this "real" patient. If the patient takes a turn for the worse, can students believe that their actions (or inactions) may lead to an adverse outcome for the patient (maybe even death)? In reality, we would not want them to have a life-threatening experience with a real patient in clinical; however, simulation provides a safe environment to learn skills necessary for the prevention of adverse outcomes. It is necessary to "suspend reality" and allow the students to embrace their role and act confidently with the necessary clinical reasoning to accomplish their objectives. The debriefing component of the simulation is much richer if the students self-reflect from a perspective that their actions and decisions really made a difference in the outcome of care.

2. **For faculty**: Simulation must also be believable for faculty in the sense that they can accomplish this and meet their educational goals via simulation; it is feasible, possible, and fun.

From learning theory and brain theory, faculty are encouraging the use of the right and left brain, which has been demonstrated to better embed the experience, and make the substance of what is learned more accessible or easily retrieved for use in future, varied, patient encounters (Seigel, 2007). Faculty need to feel supported in their integration and use of simulation in their courses and they need to receive the resources necessary (time, equipment, information technology [IT] support) to effectively accomplish their goals.

3. **Translation into practice**: Tapping into an emotional or psychological component for the students when learning has been demonstrated to improve memory and allow for better information retrieval. Knowledge stored is more accessible and easily tapped for use in practice in a variety of situations. Students use a synthesis of past experiences to pool best practices into actual practice.

LEARNING IN THE DIGITAL CULTURE

Technology in nursing education is here to stay. Today's students learn and study in the digital culture into which they were born. Multitasking is not an issue and, in fact, seems to be the way student brains are wired. Teaching to this group, whose attention span may be less than 10 to 15 minutes, requires new and innovative approaches other than the didactic. Repetition and visual, auditory, and kinesthetic stimulation in an environment in which students can move and interact while learning provide the variety of stimuli needed.

Of course, simulation also is one method to supplement didactic teaching. As such, educator expertise is essential when incorporating simulation. It requires background knowledge of the curriculum and the ability to assess where students should be, what they are capable of, and how nursing graduates from the program function in the workforce. To provide optimal student learning experiences, changes in educational practices need to be incorporated with pedagogical principles, which in turn guide the development and implementation of simulation activities and the integration of technology (Jeffries, 2005). Simulation provides another avenue for achieving these outcome objectives. The importance of the integration of, exposure to, and mastery of technology has been confirmed and included in the revision of *The Essentials of Baccalaureate Education for Professional Nursing Practice* (American Association of Colleges of Nursing [AACN], 2008). For its part, the NLN (2003) challenges nursing to "reconceptualize reform in nursing education" by encouraging innovative teaching practices (p. 3). For this third edition, a global perspective of nursing education competencies has been considered and is noted where available.

Simulated patients allow for standardized learning experiences. Scenarios designed by nursing educators provide for focused learning with prescribed outcomes. Student performance can be measured and documented across groups at specific points of time in important focus areas of the curriculum. Results of these measurements can be used for assessment and evaluation of progress toward curricular goals and program outcomes.

Murray, Grant, Howarth, and Leigh (2008) discussed the use of simulation for teaching and learning to support practice learning and stated that, "simulation is a strategy to enhance clinical competence" (pp. 5–6). It is used as a supplement to clinical preparation or for clinical remediation, and provides opportunities for students to practice clinical skills and interactions outside the actual patient setting. Kuiper, Heinrich, Matthias, Graham, and Kotwall (2008) concurred, stating that the results of their study show that evidence "supports the use of simulation as a source of remediation for students with clinical challenges and for an enhancement of didactic content" (p. 12). Simulation has also been shown to increase the confidence of students in a low-anxiety setting before clinical experiences (Murray et al., 2008). A recent integrative review from 17 studies reported a similar positive effect of simulation on student confidence (Boling & Hardin-Pierce, 2016), whereas Kardong-Edgren (2013) warns about how the concept of self-efficacy is used and measured in simulation education.

Simulation contributes to the development of a reflective practitioner who demonstrates better decision-making skills and superior problem-solving skills by using more creative thinking (Carter, Creedy, & Sidebotham, 2016; Edwards, Hawker, Carrier, & Rees, 2015; Eppich & Cheng, 2015; Murray et al., 2008; Rauen, 2004). Unique to simulation exercises is the debriefing period, which allows for reflection on the effectiveness of interventions and processing of alternate theories for improving outcomes. Debriefing allows for reintegration of theory, evaluation of best practice, and an opportunity to learn about error management (Rudolph, Simon, Dufresne, & Raemer, 2006). This area has been well researched since the last edition and a best practice standard has been developed (Decker et al., 2013; Dreifuerst, 2012).

We are situated in a unique time period in which the ability to use simulation fits with the issues of growing nursing faculty shortages and limited resources for student admission to programs, as well as those related to clinical or agency use. In addition, safety and quality-of-care issues increase the importance of student education in situations in which they can feel safe in providing care and transform an observational experience into a hands-on simulated learning experience.

As aptly put by Starkweather and Kardong-Edgren (2008), "The best outcomes with simulation occur when it is integrated across a curriculum, creating a challenge for academic nursing administrators, curriculum committees and faculty members who are struggling with how to incorporate simulation into, rather than on top of, already crowded curricular agendas" (p. 2). However, one must start at the beginning, and simulation often begins with one faculty member in one course. Part I of this book explores the integration of simulation within a curriculum, outlining a framework of simulation learning created by the coeditors of this book; a review of health communication; innovative approaches to faculty development, including interprofessional facilitation; building a learning resource center; the use of audiovisual solutions; patients with unique needs; and specific skills. In order to meet the needs of nurse educators who are looking for help with designing and implementing simulation, we have written and collected scenarios currently in use by seasoned faculty. It is our hope that the exemplars in Part II fuel and encourage those who are enthusiastic about integrating simulation within their nursing programs. Given the focus on interprofessional education, Part III of this third edition focuses on interdisciplinary and interprofessional scenarios with rich diversity to meet the needs of today's nursing programs. Finally, Part IV of this book explores future directions for simulation in nursing education, including information on how to write in clinical simulations and publish your work, as well as differentiating certification and accreditation for the evaluation of your professional development needs.

CONCLUSION

Although we initially believed that the "perfect storm" was near and the survival of the profession of nursing and the outcome of health care were at risk, we recognize that it has now arrived. We are weathering through this perfect storm, but the storm persists. What is encouraging to us is that much of what was outlined in this chapter in the first edition has been strengthened by empirical data, supporting theories, and tested interventions. One such theoretical framework that was outlined in our first edition is expanded in the next chapter. In addition, best practice standards now support how we have developed, outlined, and structured this book for sharing the knowledge and expertise we have gained over the years. We strongly believe that simulation-focused pedagogy holds many rewards, but working through the challenges and the need for extra resources to incorporate it awaits us. Infusing our passion for the process and our love of teaching and learning is the goal of this book. If we can help even one faculty member enhance teaching to incorporate these ideas for interactive learning that engages and excites students, then our mission is complete.

REFERENCES

American Association of Colleges of Nursing. (2008). *The essentials of baccalaureate education for professional nursing practice*. Washington, DC: Author. Retrieved from http://www.aacnnursing.org/Portals/42/Publications/BaccEssentials08.pdf

Adamson, K. (2015). A systematic review of the literature related to the NLN/Jeffries simulation framework. *Nursing Education Perspectives, 36*(5), 281–291.

Alexander, M., Durham, C. F., Hooper, J. I., Jeffries, P. R., Goldman, N., Kardong-Edgren, S. S.,...Tillman, C. (2015). NCSBN simulation guidelines for prelicensure nursing programs. *Journal of Nursing Regulation, 6*(3), 39–42. doi:10.1016/S2155-8256(15)30783-3

Alinier, G., Hunt, W. B., & Gordon, R. (2004). Determining the value of simulation in nurse education: Study design and initial results. *Nurse Education in Practice, 4*(3), 200–207.

Almerud, S., Alapack, R. J., Fridlund, B., & Ekebergh, M. (2007). Of vigilance and invisibility—Being a patient in a technologically intense environment. *Nursing in Critical Care, 12*(3), 151–158.

Benner, P. (1984). *From novice to expert: Excellence and power in clinical nursing practice*. Menlo Park, CA: Addison Wesley.

Berndt, J. (2014). Patient safety and simulation in prelicensure nursing education: An integrative review. *Teaching & Learning in Nursing, 9*(1), 16–22. doi:10.1016/j.teln.2013.09.001

Boese, T., Cato, M., Gonzalez, L., Jones, A., Kennedy, K., Reese, C.,...Borum, J. C. (2013). INACSL standards of best practice: Simulation standard V: Facilitator. *Clinical Simulation in Nursing, 9*(6S), S22–S25.

Boling, B., & Hardin-Pierce, M. (2016). The effect of high-fidelity simulation on knowledge and confidence in critical care training: An integrative review. *Nurse Education in Practice, 16*(1), 287–293.

Carter, A. G., Creedy, D. K., & Sidebotham, M. (2016). Efficacy of teaching methods used to develop critical thinking in nursing and midwifery undergraduate students: A systematic review of the literature. *Nurse Education Today, 40*, 209–218.

Cheng, A., Kessler, D., Mackinnon, R., Chang, T. P., Nadkarni, V. M., Hunt, E. A.,...International Network for Simulation-based Pediatric Innovation, Research, and Education (INSPIRE) Reporting Guidelines Investigators. (2016). Reporting guidelines for health care simulation research: Extensions to the CONSORT and STROBE statements. *Advances in Simulation, 25*(1), 1–13. doi:10.1186/s41077-016-0025-y

Childs, J. C., & Sepples, S. B. (2006). Lessons learned from a complex patient care scenario. *Nursing Education Perspectives, 27*(3), 154–158.

Cook, D. A., Hamstra, S. J., Brydges, R., Zendejas, B., Szostek, J. H., Wang, A. T.,...Hatala, R. (2013). Comparative effectiveness of instructional design features in simulation-based education: Systematic review and meta-analysis. *Medical Teacher, 35*(1), e867–e898.

Cook, D. A., Hatala, R., Brydges, R., Zendejas, B., Szostek, J. H., Wang, A. T.,...Hamstra, S. J. (2011). Technology-enhanced simulation for health professions education: A systematic review and meta-analysis. *Journal of the American Medical Association, 306*(9), 978–988.

Decker, S. I., Anderson, M., Boese, T., Epps, C., McCarthy, J., Motola, I.,...Lioce, L. (2015). Standards of best practice: Simulation standard VIII: Simulation-enhanced interprofessional education (Sim-IPE). *Clinical Simulation in Nursing, 11*(6), 293–297.

Decker, S. I., Fey, M., Sideras, S., Caballero, S., Rockstraw, L., Boese, T.,...Borum, J. C. (2013). INACSL standards of best practice: Simulation standard VI: The debriefing process. *Clinical Simulation in Nursing, 9*(Suppl. 6), S26–S29. doi:10.1016/j.ecns.2013.04.008

Dreifuerst, K. T. (2012). Using debriefing for meaningful learning to foster development of clinical reasoning in simulation. *Journal of Nursing Education, 51*(6), 326–333.

Edwards, D., Hawker, C., Carrier, J., & Rees, C. (2015). A systematic review of the effectiveness of strategies and interventions to improve the transition from student to newly qualified nurse. *International Journal of Nursing Studies, 52*(7), 1254–1268.

Eppich, W., & Cheng, A. (2015). Promoting excellence and reflective learning in simulation (PEARLS): Development and rationale for a blended approach to health care simulation debriefing. *Simulation in Healthcare, 10*(2), 106–115.

Fink, L. D. (2003). *Creating significant learning experiences: An integrated approach to designing college courses.* San Francisco, CA: Jossey-Bass.

Fink, L. D. (2013). *Creating significant learning experiences, revised and updated.* San Francisco, CA: Jossey-Bass.

Fisher, D., & King, L. (2013). An integrative literature review on preparing nursing students through simulation to recognize and respond to the deteriorating patient. *Journal of Advanced Nursing, 69*(11), 2375–2388.

Franklin, A. E., Boese, T., Gloe, D., Lioce, L., Decker, S., Sando, C. R.,…Borum, J. C. (2013). INACSL standards of best practice: Simulation standard IV: Facilitation. *Clinical Simulation in Nursing, 9*(6S), S19–S21.

Fritz, P. Z., Gray, T., & Flanagan, B. (2007). Review of mannequin-based high-fidelity simulation in emergency medicine. *Emergency Medicine Australasia, 20*(1), 1–9.

Gloe, D., Sando, C. R., Franklin, A. E., Boese, T., Decker, S., Lioce, L.,…Borum, J. C. (2013). INACSL standards of best practice: Simulation standard II: Professional Integrity of Participant(s). *Clinical Simulation in Nursing, 9*(6S), S12–S14.

Haskvitz, L. M., & Koop, E. C. (2004). Students struggling in clinical? A new role for the patient simulator. *Journal of Nursing Education, 43*(4), 181–184.

Hayden, J. K., Smiley, R. A., Alexander, M., Kardong-Edgren, S., & Jeffries, P. R. (2014). The NCSBN National Simulation Study: A longitudinal, randomized, controlled study replacing clinical hours with simulation in prelicensure nursing education. *Journal of Nursing Regulation, 5*(2), C1–C64.

Henneman, E. A., & Cunningham, H. (2005). Using clinical simulation to teach patient safety in an acute/critical care nursing course. *Nurse Educator, 30*, 172.

International Nursing Association for Clinical Simulation and Learning. (2013, updated 2016). INACSL standards of best practice: Simulation. Retrieved from http://www.inacsl.org/i4a/pages/index .cfm?pageid=3407

Jacobs, J. L., Apatov, N., & Glei, M. (2007). Increasing vigilance on the medical/surgical floor to improve patient safety. *Journal of Advanced Nursing, 57*(5), 472–481.

Jeffries, P. R. (2005). A framework for designing, implementing, and evaluating simulations used as teaching strategies in nursing. *Nursing Education Perspectives, 26*(2), 96–103.

Jeffries, P. R. (2007). *Simulation in nursing education.* New York, NY: National League for Nurses.

Jeffries, P. R., & Rizollo, M. A. (2006). Designing and implementing models for the innovative use of simulation to teach nursing care of ill adults and children: A national, multi-site, multi-method study. In P. Jeffries (Ed.), *Simulation in nursing education* (pp. 145–159). New York, NY: National League for Nurses.

Jeffries, P. R., & Rodgers, K. J. (2007). Theoretical framework for simulation design. In P. Jeffries (Ed.), *Simulation in nursing education* (pp. 21–33). New York, NY: National League for Nurses.

Jose, M. M., & Dufrene, C. (2014). Educational competencies and technologies for disaster preparedness in undergraduate nursing education: An integrative review. *Nurse Education Today, 34*(4), 543–551.

Kardong-Edgren, S. (2013). Bandura's self-efficacy theory: Something is missing. *Clinical Simulation in Nursing, 9*(9), e327–e328. doi:10.1016/j.ecns.2013.07.001

Kardong-Edgren, S., Adamson, K. A., & Fitzgerald, C. (2010). A review of currently published evaluation instruments for human patient simulation. *Clinical Simulation in Nursing, 6*(1), e25–e35. Retrieved from https://www.researchgate.net/profile/Suzie_Kardong-Edgren/publication/238153705_A_ Review_of_Currently_Published_Evaluation_Instruments_for_Human_Patient_Simulation/ links/54fb5c0f0cf20700c5e70bf7.pdf

Keers, R. N., Williams, S. D., Cooke, J., Walsh, T., & Ashcroft, D. M. (2014). Impact of interventions designed to reduce medication administration errors in hospitals: A systematic review. *Drug Safety, 37*(5), 317–332.

Kuiper, R. A., Heinrich, C., Matthias, A., Graham, M. J., & Kotwall, L. B. (2008). Debriefing with the OPT model of clinical reasoning during high-fidelity simulation. *International Journal of Nursing Education Scholarship, 17*(5), 1–14.

Larew, C., Lessans, S., Spunt, D., Foster, D., & Covington, B. G. (2006). Application of Benner's theory in an interactive simulation. *Nursing Education Perspectives, 27*(1), 16–21.

Lioce, L., Meakim, C. H., Fey, M. K., Chmil, J. V., Mariani, B., & Alinier, G. (2015). INACSL standards of best practice: Simulation standard IX: Simulation design. *Clinical Simulation in Nursing, 11*(6), 309–315.

Lioce, L., Reed, C. C., Lemon, D., King, M. A., Martinez, P. A., Franklin, A. E.,...Borum, J. C. (2013). INACSL standards of best practice: Simulation standard III: Participant objectives. *Clinical Simulation in Nursing, 9*(6S), S15–S18.

Malt, G. (2015). Cochrane review brief: Interprofessional education: Effects on professional practice and healthcare outcomes. *Online Journal of Issues in Nursing, 20*(2). doi:10.3912/OJIN.Vol20No2CRBCol02.

Meakim, C., Boese, T., Decker, S., Franklin, A. E., Gloe, D., Lioce, L.,...Borum, J. C. (2013). INACSL standards of best practice: Simulation standard I: Terminology. *Clinical Simulation in Nursing, 9*(6S), S3–S11.

Meyer, G., & Lavin, M. A. (2005). Vigilance: The essence of nursing. *Online Journal of Issues in Nursing, 10*(1). doi:10.3912/OJIN.Vol10No03PPT01

Murray, C., Grant, M. J., Howarth, M. L., & Leigh, J. (2008). The use of simulation as a teaching and learning approach to support practice learning. *Nurse Education in Practice, 8*(1), 5–8.

National League for Nursing. (2003). Position statement: Innovation in nursing education: A call to reform. Retrieved from www.nln.org/aboutnln/PositionStatements/innovation.htm

Nehring, W. M., & Lashley, F. R. (2004). Current use and opinions regarding human patient simulators in nursing education: An international survey. *Nursing Education Perspectives, 25*(5), 244–248.

Radhakrishnan, K., Roche, J. P., & Cunningham, H. (2007). Measuring clinical practice parameters with human patient simulation: A pilot study. *International Journal of Nursing Education Scholarship, 4*, Article 8. doi:10.2202/1548-923X.1307

Rauen, C. A. (2004). Simulation as a teaching strategy for nursing education and orientation in cardiac surgery. *Critical Care Nurse, 24*(3), 46–51.

Roberts, S. W., & McGowan, R. J. (2004). The effectiveness of infant simulations. *Adolescence, 39*(155), 475–487.

Rudolph, J. W., Simon, R., Dufresne, R. L., & Raemer, D. B. (2006). There's no such thing as "nonjudgmental" debriefing: A theory and method for debriefing with good judgment. *Simulation in Healthcare: Journal of the Society for Simulation in Healthcare, 1*, 49–55. doi:10.1097/01266021-200600110-00006

Sando, C. R., Coggins, R. M., Meakim, C., Franklin, A. E., Gloe, D., Boese, T.,...Borum, J. C. (2013). Standards of best practice: Simulation standard VII: Participant assessment and evaluation. *Clinical Simulation in Nursing, 9*(6S), S30–S32.

Seigel, D. (2007). *The mindful brain: Reflection and attunement in the cultivation of well-being.* New York, NY: W. W. Norton.

Starkweather, A. R., & Kardong-Edgren, S. (2008). Diffusion of innovation: Embedding simulation into nursing curricula. *International Journal of Nursing Education Scholarship, 5*, Article 13. doi:10.2202/1548-923X.1567

Stokols, D. (1996). Translating social ecological theory into guidelines for community health promotion. *American Journal of Health Promotion, 10*, 282–298.

Tanner, C. A. (2006). Changing times, evolving issues: The faculty shortage, accelerated programs, and simulation. *Journal of Nursing Education, 45*(3), 99–100.

U.S. Department of Health and Human Services. (2000). *With understanding and improving health and objectives for improving health: Healthy People 2010.* Washington, DC: U.S. Government Printing Office.

Wellard, S. J., Woolf, R., & Gleeson, L. (2007). Exploring the use of clinical laboratories in undergraduate nursing programs in regional Australia. *International Journal of Nursing Education Scholarship, 4*(1), 1–11.

Wilkinson, R., & Marmot, M. (2003). *Social determinants of health: The solid facts* (2nd ed.). Copenhagen, Denmark: World Health Organization.

Zhang, C., Thompson, S., & Miller, C. (2011). A review of simulation-based interprofessional education. *Clinical Simulation in Nursing, 7*(4), e117–e126.

CHAPTER 2

Framework for Simulation Learning in Nursing Education

Karen M. Daley and Suzanne Hetzel Campbell

As stated in the previous chapter, we believe a simulation-focused pedagogy of learning brings together an eclectic combination of learning, ecological, and nursing theory. As a result, we proposed the following framework in the first edition, rooted in the research on simulation, based on our experiences in teaching within a simulation-focused pedagogy, and combined with a collective synthesis of the experiences of the contributors to this book. The following framework outlines the components underlying our perception of simulated learning for nursing education (Figure 2.1; Daley & Campbell, 2008).

As stated in Chapter 1, Jeffries and Rogers (2007) have presented the Nursing Education Simulation Framework, which takes into account what is known about learning and cognition for the design of simulations. Since then, Jeffries's framework has been identified as a middle range theory, and is now referred to as the *NLN Jeffries Simulation Theory* (Jeffries, 2015a, 2015b). Additional guidelines are now also available from National Council of State Boards of Nursing (NCSBN) for Prelicensure Nursing Programs (Alexander et al., 2015). The Framework for Simulation Learning in Nursing Education presented in this text represents a student-centered approach to learning through simulation-focused pedagogy for integration throughout the nursing curriculum. This learning takes into consideration the desired outcomes for nursing students and practitioners (including safety, excellence, and reflective practice) at varied levels and presents an additional conceptualization of making simulation *real* for nursing education.

Guided by ecological theory, it is important to assess what the learner brings to learning (Stokols, 1996). Students come to the academic setting with a preset combination of individual experiences and culture as a lens through which learning experiences are viewed. Think, for example, how a nursing student approaches learning after having cared for a dying family member as compared with a student without that experience. Using ecological theory, when considering a student's personal culture, including race, ethnicity, gender, sexual identity, age, disability, geographic location, and socioeconomic status (Office of Disease Prevention and Health Promotion, 2016), and the possibility of varied health belief customs, learning can be approached in different traditional methods. Students come to nursing from varied educational backgrounds (traditional undergraduate students, second-degree students, and adult learners) and cultural and life experiences, creating a challenge for the educators to create a stimulating learning experience. In working with this diverse student population, in addition to the previously identified factors, one must also take into account the digital culture in which they live and experience learning, and move through it to reach a state of readiness for learning.

The central portion of the framework reflects the students' interaction with nursing education. Set within the context of any nursing program's standard accreditation and regulation competencies are three broad goals and learning outcomes, which are consistently identified. Nursing students are expected to: think critically, communicate effectively, and intervene therapeutically.

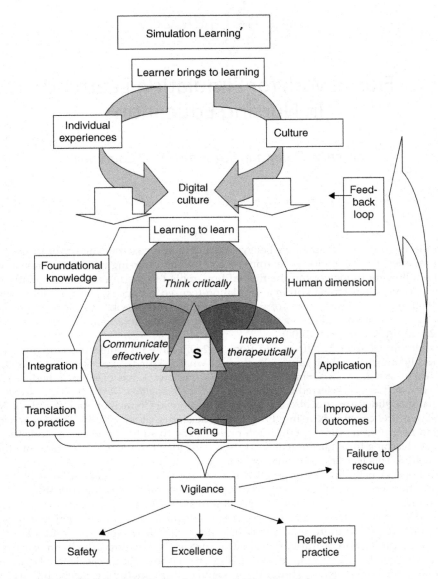

Figure 2.1   Framework for Simulation Learning in Nursing Education.

S, simulation.

Source: Adapted from Daley and Campbell (2008).

These learning outcomes are represented in Figure 2.1 by the three circles that are overlapped by the triangle, representing simulation. Simulation as a teaching tool meets all three broad goals demonstrating the rationale and importance of integrating simulation throughout the curriculum. Allowing the students to practice in a simulated real-life situation (in real time) requires that they use critical thinking and clinical reasoning skills. By using these skills the students are able to decide on interventions that cause immediate responses in the patient (human patient simulator or standardized patient). The debriefing period allows for an evaluation of whether those interventions were effective or therapeutic, which helps students become reflective practitioners. Performing the scenarios in conjunction with classmates enhances their use of communication, delegation, and teamwork skills. The power of simulation lies in its ability to target these learning outcomes in an engaging and interactive manner beyond the didactic approach, which leads to better outcomes and more sustainable learning.

The triangle shape itself in the framework in Figure 2.1 depicts the three fidelities discussed by Fritz, Gray, and Flanagan (2007) that contribute to making the simulation as realistic as possible: equipment fidelity, environmental fidelity, and psychological fidelity. These fidelities provide the foundation for suspension of reality that is crucial to the success of the simulation experience. Paramount to any simulation is the debriefing period in which reflection on action can take place in order to set the groundwork, and over time reinforce the formation of a reflective practitioner (Tanner, 2006).

When teaching a student within this framework, it is important to consider Fink's (2003) six dimensions: learning to learn, foundational knowledge, the human dimension, integration, application, and caring. Represented by the hexagon in the center of Figure 2.1, these dimensions provide a support structure around which simulations can be planned and carried out. The faculty create more significant learning experiences, set the stage for an increased transfer of knowledge, and enhance the interactive component of their teaching by considering these dimensions.

As students move through a curriculum combining simulation and these pedagogical principles, the ultimate outcome is a student who learns vigilance. As an aspect of the overall concept of surveillance, nursing has focused on vigilance because of the literature on quality outcomes (Almerud, Alapack, Fridlund, & Ekebergh, 2007; Jacobs, Apatov, & Glei, 2007; Meyer & Lavin, 2005). Once mastered, vigilance results in improved safety, excellence in nursing care, and reflective practice that addresses the patient's needs holistically. In addition, it creates a reflective practitioner who strives for lifelong learning, personal improvement, and enhanced satisfaction with his or her career (Blum et al., 2004; Haller et al., 2008; Shapiro et al., 2004; Sweeney, Warren, Gardner, Rojek, & Lindquist, 2014).

Considering the nursing shortage and issues of retention among nurses, modeling this critical thinking, clinical reasoning, and reflective practice to help students recognize their passion for nursing could have long-term effects. Mastering vigilance—recognizing when patients need immediate and effective intervention—takes time and practice. In those instances when vigilance is not mastered, simulation learning provides a safe feedback loop back through the learning experience, allowing the student (or practitioner) another chance at mastery. The overall process works toward translation of knowledge to practice and improved outcomes for the student and program, as represented at the bottom portion of Figure 2.1. In addition, the quality of practitioners is enhanced, which translates to safer care, as well as more satisfied, caring, and reflective practitioners who continue to have the ability to transform the profession of nursing. The framework brings together a caring person who, through the mastery of vigilance, reflects the three outcomes of safety, excellence, and reflective practice. Safety represents overriding concern for positive outcomes related to nursing care (e.g., no falls, pressure ulcers, or infection). Excellence in nursing is based on standards of care, quality outcomes, and evidence-based practice. Finally, reflective practice supports our conception of the caring professional who uses critical thinking, clinical reasoning, clinical judgment, and reflective debriefing in his or her daily practice (Jones, Reese, & Shelton, 2014; Kaakinen & Arwood, 2009).

Since the publication of the second edition of this text, the International Nursing Association for Clinical Simulation and Learning (INACSL) Best Practice Standards: Simulation (INACSL, 2013/2016), NCSBN multisite study (Hayden, Smiley, Alexander, Kardong-Edgren, & Jeffries, 2014), and guidelines (Alexander et al., 2015) have all been published. Much work has been done. Jeffries continues to guide simulation nurse educators in formulating high-quality simulations and providing priorities for the future to test our assumptions in the efficacy of nursing simulation (Jeffries, 2015a, 2015b). The American Association of Colleges of Nursing (AACN) BSN Essentials (AACN, 2008) recognized the importance of simulation experience to augment clinical learning and as a complement to direct care opportunities, predicting that over time evidence might emerge regarding the substitution of simulation for patient experiences within a proper balance (p. 34).

When evaluating the relevance of the framework to current practice and research, several updates and insights are appropriate. Ecological theory (Stokols, 1996) continues to provide an opportunity to examine the ecosystem in which learning occurs and provides a window into the complexities of the environment in which learners learn. Fink (2013) has expanded his conceptualization of creating significant learning experiences and these standards remain relevant in simulation in nursing education. The reflective thinking of a reflective practitioner is now included in research-based standards and guidelines for debriefing that are being tested (Decker et al., 2013; Dreifuerst, 2009, 2012; Shinnick, Woo, Horwich, & Steadman, 2011). The research in nursing on vigilance through simulation continues and includes studies on the deteriorating patients in failure-to-rescue scenarios and crisis resource management (Blum et al., 2004; Cooper et al., 2010; Endacott et al., 2012; Fisher & King, 2013; Haller et al., 2008; Kelly, Forber, Conlon, Roche, & Stasa, 2014; Liaw, Scherpbier, Klainin-Yobas, & Rethans, 2011; Merriman, Stayt, & Ricketts, 2014). Similarly, research has explored the assessment and evaluation of communication, both practitioner to patient (Campbell, Pagano, O'Shea, Connery, & Caron, 2013; O'Shea, Pagano, Campbell, & Caso, 2013; Pagano et al., 2015), and during patient handovers (Enlow, Shanks, Guhde, & Perkins, 2010; Fay-Hillier, Regan, & Gallagher Gordon, 2012; Härgestam, Lindkvist, Brulin, Jacobsson, & Hultin, 2013; Hill & Marcellus, 2015). Chapter 4 discusses teaching and evaluation of communication with simulation. The outcomes remain the same as illustrated by the framework, but we have more research substantiating these results in simulation education.

Kolb (1984) contributes to our understanding of simulation in nursing education and has recently provided new insights. Research is beginning to show that although debriefing is often the most significant experience in a simulation experience, creating a feedback loop or a "redo," as depicted in the framework, solidifies the simulation experience as a significant learning moment that may be more transferable to actual patient care. In applying Kolb's theory of experiential learning, simulations have included the first three essential stages of the theory: concrete experience, reflective observation, and abstract conceptualization, which fit well with prebriefing, participating in a simulation, and debriefing. The fourth stage of active experimentation may need to be considered and would allow students to return to the scenario to try again or "re-do" to allow a full integration of theory to practice, transforming learning into "new ways of thinking and new behaviors" (Lisko & O'Dell, 2010). Including a session to return to the side of the HPS and try again may prove beneficial. Although many simulations end before that step, we recommend extending the simulation experience to include this fourth stage and may provide the answer to the question: Is simulation transferable to actual performance of the student and professional nurse?

How far we have come in so little time! Challenges still exist, such as assessment, evaluation, and the wise use of resources for simulation-focused pedagogy. It is our hope that our work, the work of our contributors, and our framework assist in moving nurse educators along in their journey to integrate simulation throughout their nursing curriculum. Go forth and simulate! Faculty, students, administration, and, most important, our patients reap the benefits! The depth, breadth, and value of this book continues to be in the stories told, the ideas shared, and the variety of teaching scenarios now available to all.

REFERENCES

Alexander, M., Durham, C. F., Hooper, J. I., Jeffries, P. R., Goldman, N., Kardong-Edgren, S. S., . . . Tillman, C. (2015). NCSBN simulation guidelines for prelicensure nursing programs. *Journal of Nursing Regulation, 6*(3), 39–42. doi:10.1016/S2155-8256(15)30783-3

Almerud, S., Alapack, R. J., Fridlund, B., & Ekebergh, M. (2007). Of vigilance and invisibility—Being a patient in technologically intense environments. *Nursing in Critical Care, 12*(3), 151–158.

American Association of Colleges of Nursing. (2008). *The essentials of baccalaureate education for professional nursing practice*. Washington, DC: Author. Retrieved from http://www.aacnnursing.org/Portals/42/Publications/BaccEssentials08.pdf

Blum, R. H., Raemer, D. B., Carroll, J. S., Sunder, N., Felstein, D. M., & Cooper, J. B. (2004). Crisis resource management training for an anaesthesia faculty: A new approach to continuing education. *Medical Education, 38*(1), 45–55.

Campbell, S. H., Pagano, M., O'Shea, E. R., Connery, C., & Caron, C. (2013). Development of the Health Communication Assessment Tool: Enhancing relationships, empowerment, and power-sharing skills. *Clinical Simulation in Nursing, 9*(11), e543–e550. doi:10.1016/j.ecns.2013.04.016

Cooper, S., Kinsman, L., Buykx, P., McConnell-Henry, T., Endacott, R., & Scholes, J. (2010). Managing the deteriorating patient in a simulated environment: Nursing students' knowledge, skill and situation awareness. *Journal of Clinical Nursing, 19*(15–16), 2309–2318.

Daley, K., & Campbell, S. H. (2008). *Framework for simulation learning in nursing education.* Working paper, Fairfield University School of Nursing, Fairfield, CT.

Decker, S., Fey, M., Sideras, S., Caballero, S., Rockstraw, L., Boese, T., . . . Borum, J. C. (2013). Standards of best practice: Simulation Standard VI: The debriefing process. *Clinical Simulation in Nursing, 9*(6), S26–S29. doi:10.1016/j.ecns.2013.04.008

Dreifuerst, K. T. (2009). The essentials of debriefing in simulation learning: A concept analysis. *Nursing Education Perspectives, 30*(2), 109–114.

Dreifuerst, K. T. (2012). Using debriefing for meaningful learning to foster development of clinical reasoning in simulation. *Journal of Nursing Education, 51*(6), 326–333.

Endacott, R., Scholes, J., Cooper, S., McConnell-Henry, T., Porter, J., Missen, K., . . . Champion, R. (2012). Identifying patient deterioration: Using simulation and reflective interviewing to examine decision making skills in a rural hospital. *International Journal of Nursing Studies, 49*(6), 710–717.

Enlow, M., Shanks, L., Guhde, J., & Perkins, M. (2010). Incorporating interprofessional communication skills (ISBARR) into an undergraduate nursing curriculum. *Nurse Educator, 35*(4), 176–180.

Fay-Hillier, T. M., Regan, R. V., & Gallagher Gordon, M. (2012). Communication and patient safety in simulation for mental health nursing education. *Issues in Mental Health Nursing, 33*(11), 718–726.

Fink, L. D. (2003). *Creating significant learning experiences: An integrated approach to designing college courses.* San Francisco, CA: Jossey-Bass.

Fink, L. D. (2013). *Creating significant learning experiences, revised and updated.* San Francisco, CA: Jossey-Bass.

Fisher, D., & King, L. (2013). An integrative literature review on preparing nursing students through simulation to recognize and respond to the deteriorating patient. *Journal of Advanced Nursing, 69*(11), 2375–2388.

Fritz, P. Z., Gray, T., & Flanagan, B. (2008). Review of mannequin-based high-fidelity simulation in emergency medicine. *Emergency Medicine Australasia, 20*(1), 1–9.

Haller, G., Garnerin, P., Morales, M. A., Pfister, R., Berner, M., Irion, O., . . . Kern, C. (2008). Effect of crew resource management training in a multidisciplinary obstetrical setting. *International Journal for Quality in Health Care, 20*(4), 254–263.

Härgestam, M., Lindkvist, M., Brulin, C., Jacobsson, M., & Hultin, M. (2013). Communication in interdisciplinary teams: Exploring closed-loop communication during in situ trauma team training. *BMJ Open, 3*(10), e003525. doi:10.1136/bmjopen-2013-003525

Hayden, J. K., Smiley, R. A., Alexander, M., Kardong-Edgren, S., & Jeffries, P. R. (2014). The NCSBN national simulation study: A longitudinal, randomized, controlled study replacing clinical hours with simulation in prelicensure nursing education. *Journal of Nursing Regulation, 5*(2), S1–S64.

Hill, W., & Marcellus, L. (2015, June). *IDRAW—Interactive handover: What should I be worried about? Quality measurement in ICU: A feasibility study and knowledge translation.* Paper presented at the BC-PSQC Quality Forum 2015, Vancouver, British Columbia. Retrieved from http://www.slideshare.net/bcpsqc/grouse-f6-what-should-i-be-worried-about-wrae-hill

International Nursing Association for Clinical Simulation and Learning. (2013, updated 2016). INACSL standards of best practice: Simulation. Retrieved from https://www.inacsl.org/i4a/pages/index.cfm?pageid=3407

Jacobs, J. L., Apatov, N., & Glei, M. (2007). Increasing vigilance on the medical/surgical floor to improve patient safety. *Journal of Advanced Nursing, 57*(5), 472–481.

Jeffries, P. R. (2015a). Reflections on clinical simulation: The past, present, and future. *Nursing Education Perspectives, 36*(5), 278–279.

Jeffries, P. R. (2015b). Signs of maturity: Simulations are growing and getting more attention. *Nursing Education Perspectives, 36*(6), 358–359.

Jeffries, P. R., & Rogers, K. J. (2007). Theoretical framework for simulation design. In P. R. Jeffries (Ed.), *Simulation in nursing education* (pp. 21–33). New York, NY: National League for Nurses.

Jones, A. L., Reese, C. E., & Shelton, D. P. (2014). NLN/Jeffries simulation framework state of the science project: The teacher construct. *Clinical Simulation in Nursing, 10*(7), 353–362. doi:10.1016/j.ecns.2013.10.008

Kaakinen, J., & Arwood, E. (2009). Systematic review of nursing simulation literature for use of learning theory. *International Journal of Nursing Education Scholarship, 6,* Article 16. doi:10.2202/1548-923X.1688

Kelly, M. A., Forber, J., Conlon, L., Roche, M., & Stasa, H. (2014). Empowering the registered nurses of tomorrow: Students' perspectives of a simulation experience for recognising and managing a deteriorating patient. *Nurse Education Today, 34*(5), 724–729.

Kolb, D. A. (1984). *Experiential learning: Experience as the source of learning and development.* Englewood Cliffs, NJ: Prentice Hall.

Liaw, S. Y., Scherpbier, A., Klainin-Yobas, P., & Rethans, J. J. (2011). Rescuing A Patient In Deteriorating Situations (RAPIDS): An evaluation tool for assessing simulation performance on clinical deterioration. *Resuscitation, 82*(11), 1434–1439.

Lisko, S. A., & O'Dell, V. (2010). Integration of theory and practice: Experiential learning theory and nursing education. *Nursing Education Perspectives, 31*(2), 106–108.

Merriman, C. D., Stayt, L. C., & Ricketts, B. (2014). Didactic methods to teach undergraduate adult nursing students to recognize and assess the deteriorating patient. *Clinical Simulations in Nursing, 10*(3), e119–e127.

Meyer, G., & Lavin, M. A. (2005). Vigilance: The essence of nursing. *Online Journal of Issues in Nursing, 10*(1). doi:10.3912/OJIN.Vol10No03PPT01

Office of Disease Prevention and Health Promotion. (n.d.). Leading health indicators development and framework. In *Healthy People 2020.* Retrieved from https://www.healthypeople.gov/2020/leading-health-indicators/Leading-Health-Indicators-Development-and-Framework

O'Shea, E. R., Pagano, M., Campbell, S. H., & Caso, G. (2013). A descriptive analysis of nursing student communication behaviors. *Clinical Simulation in Nursing, 9*(1), e5–e12. doi:10.1016/j.ecns.2011.05.013

Pagano, M. P., O'Shea, E. R., Campbell, S. H., Currie, L. M., Chamberlin, E., & Pates, C. A. (2015). Validating the Health Communication Assessment Tool (HCAT). *Clinical Simulation in Nursing, 11,* 402–410. doi: 10.1016/j.ecns.2015.06.001

Shapiro, M. J., Morey, J. C., Small, S. D., Langford, V., Kaylor, C. J., Jagminas, L., ... Jay, G. D. (2004). Simulation based teamwork training for emergency department staff: Does it improve clinical team performance when added to an existing didactic teamwork curriculum? *Quality & Safety in Health Care, 13*(6), 417–421.

Shinnick, M. A., Woo, M., Horwich, T. B., & Steadman, R. (2011). Debriefing: The most important component in simulation? *Clinical Simulation in Nursing, 7*(3), e105–e111. doi:10.1016/j.ecns.2010.11.005

Stokols, D. (1996). Translating social ecological theory into guidelines for community health promotion. *American Journal of Health Promotion, 10*(4), 282–298.

Sweeney, L. A., Warren, O., Gardner, L., Rojek, A., & Lindquist, D. G. (2014). A simulation-based training program improves emergency department staff communication. *American Journal of Medical Quality, 29*(2), 115–123.

Tanner, C. A. (2006). Thinking like a nurse: A research-based model of clinical judgment in nursing. *Journal of Nursing Education, 45*(6), 204–211.

CHAPTER 3

Integrating Simulation-Focused
Pedagogy Into Curriculum

Karen M. Daley and Suzanne Hetzel Campbell

This chapter describes how simulation fits the needs for 21st-century nursing education. Aspects that are covered include the changing needs for nursing education in a technologically complex environment, how to succeed when incorporating simulation, the importance of the faculty role in embedding simulation throughout the nursing curriculum, meeting the challenges of clinical placement, and specific challenges and benefits to integrating simulation into the curriculum with an evidence-based practice focus.

SIMULATION: THE MISSING PIECE

Historically, education at all levels has emphasized critical thinking as a standard. Students now arrive on campus with the basic skills to learn through critical thinking. However, distinct to this generation of learners is the ability to use and adapt readily to the rapid technological advances seen since the turn of the century. Although they primarily use this technology as a source of entertainment and creativity, these students often arrive knowing more about technology than their teachers and expecting nontraditional teaching methods that incorporate technology at every turn. As always, the challenge on college campuses is for faculty to stay abreast, if not ahead of, a typical undergraduate's technology-laden learning needs in addition to facilitating the higher level of critical thinking expected of college graduates. Simulation provides the missing piece for nursing education through harnessing each student's enthusiasm for technology into an interactive and valuable learning experience in which to engage in critical thinking (Radhakrishnan, Roche, & Cunningham, 2007).

The past 20 years have seen major advancements in technology available in nursing education, and most faculty and nursing programs have recognized the need for incorporating technology into the way they are teaching. Technology-equipped classrooms are the norm, enabled to have the capability to use streamlined video, have in-classroom web access, and use web-based learning platforms in each class. Students are also encouraged to "Google." Virtual hospitals have appeared online, interactive nursing case studies are readily available, and we now have the ability to stream actual patient data in real time into remote classrooms for analysis. In addition, high-technology products have become available for students to learn nursing in lifelike patient encounters. Most recent, with the creation of high-fidelity human patient simulators (HPSs), there is an opportunity to take simulation to a higher interactive level within the bounds of practice and safety before actual patient interactions. This technology is within reach of most nursing programs from the traditionally basic level to the most cutting edge.

However, navigating the simulation maze, obtaining and renovating space, and, most important, obtaining faculty buy-in and promoting ownership of simulation within the curriculum have not proved to be a smooth transition. At present, the need for more complicated scenarios has evolved as patients have become sicker and staff nurses have been required to provide more complex care. Nursing faculty who are feeling the responsibility of arriving at hospitals with competently trained students have identified the need to practice complex care before clinical experiences. Simulation meets this need.

The traditional approach to the use of simulation in nursing curricula is to develop independent modules that students must complete and be assessed on before entering the clinical areas. Traditionally, low-fidelity simulations on static manikins have been delivered by lab personnel under the direction of faculty. These scenarios are easily set up, require low-maintenance materials, and allow for easy evaluation. These methods have a long history of proven success in task training and may or may not involve individual nursing faculty input. However, task-based modules, such as catheterization, do not require the same level of complexity, critical thinking, communication, and use of nursing skills as a scenario that integrates all these areas.

In contrast, the simulations provided in this book come from competent clinical and seasoned faculty members who have been actively integrating simulation into every course taught. This feature brings a new level of curricular sophistication and provides an example for others on how the methods they are using to teach already can be incorporated with a simulation-focused pedagogy. Throughout the text, the term *simulation-focused pedagogy* is used to describe a method of using simulation and scenarios to integrate content and multiple concepts in all areas of nursing care to provide an interactive environment by which students are held accountable to use the information they are learning. Simulation integrates theoretical didactic components with critical thinking to enact nursing behaviors in a safe, efficient, ethical manner or as an end-point (capstone) measure of competencies. Although assimilating simulation-focused pedagogy has become a worthy and essential curricular goal, most nursing educators have struggled to find ways to integrate simulation throughout each program's curriculum.

Early literature had emphasized purely medical and surgical uses for simulation; however, we feel strongly that simulation crosses all clinical areas of nursing curricula and is applicable in all areas. All faculty members are capable of being involved in the development, implementation, and evaluation of scenarios to meet their curricular goals. The scenarios presented provide a wide breadth of simulation scenarios for all levels of undergraduate and graduate nursing curricula, as well as new interprofessional scenarios.

ESSENTIAL TOOL KIT FOR SUCCESS: PERSISTENCE, VISION, AND PATIENCE

Many of us have arrived at simulation in one of these two ways: (a) as a dream for how things should be done with little or no financing or (b) as a well-financed initiative with no schematics for implementation of something designated as the "simulation lab." However, as one arrives at simulation, the realization occurs quickly that its implementation is a daunting task. Many levels arise for implementation, and hidden costs and factors are continually discovered. Yet, once implemented, the results are amazing.

Our joint experience is that persistence in pursuing the implementation of simulation is invaluable. One faculty member described this as a "dogged" and an unrelenting pursuit! Whether the vision has been dictated or created individually, it is this vision that helps to navigate the many obstacles and to meet the challenges that arise head on. Patiently reiterating the need, returning to key people to explain the rationale and vision, and writing and rewriting plans and strategies have been required throughout the experience. Key to this persistence have been the support, encouragement, and faith of the faculty.

FACULTY FACTOR

Building a foundation for the integration of simulation throughout the curriculum must take into account the faculty factor. Although most who are leading the way for the integration of simulation are comfortable with the technology, many nursing faculty groups reflect varying levels of technology training and usage of technology in their classes. High-fidelity simulation requires more than a basic understanding of computers. Most simulation companies who were initially willing to train faculty as needed are now charging for this service, necessitating a "train the trainers" type of initiative. This often forces a decision to find an expert or two who, in addition to a usual faculty load, is also responsible for training the entire faculty on how to use the simulators—a very daunting task. Finding time for individual or group training is essential but can be difficult to manage given the faculty shortages and already-busy workload of nursing faculty. As not all nursing programs have lab personnel, often individual faculty must be trained to run their own simulations. However, promoting ownership and individual buy-in within a faculty member's program or course and group simulation initiatives often eases the transition to integrating simulation into individual courses. Given the atmosphere of academic freedom, some strategies to encourage and inspire hesitant faculty may include inviting them to observe a scenario or role-play one of the parts; having an "open door" policy for interested faculty to discuss their ideas, outline templates, and receive coaching in simulation; retreats to strategize about methods to embed simulation and technology throughout the curriculum; and innovative ideas for faculty professional development (see Chapter 4).

If an enthusiastic early adopter is identified, it is imperative that faculty who are novices in simulation have the opportunity to feel supported in exploring innovative teaching models that incorporate state-of-the-art simulation. A junior colleague of ours has shared the following:

> As educators providing instruction via high-tech simulation, we can provide today's students with a safe and controlled environment in which to learn. What became increasingly apparent to me in my first experience as a clinical coordinator at a highly respected (simulation and learning) laboratory was what we were providing our students and what we were practicing in our department were two different concepts. Despite having a "Safe Zone" sticker on my office door for students to know they would be free from bullying, discrimination, and shaming while in my office, the same could not be said for how my departmental colleagues were treating each other. *Simulation shaming* is a term to explain the environment created within the department that disrupts the ability to provide the best experience for our students. Within my own department, it amazed me how destructive this practice can be, not only to the staff itself but to the ability to provide the highest quality of instruction to the students. This caused those part-time staff members to feel as though their contributions were not as important as those who were addressed professionally and therefore (the staff) were less likely to contribute. In institutions where *simulation shaming* is both practiced and unimpeded, an environment is created that not only circumvents accountability but has the potential to marginalize valuable opportunities for our students. One could argue that if we expect our students to be accountable for their performance, respect the differences of both colleagues and patients, and speak kindly, we must expect the same from ourselves. (C. Kraft, personal communication, November 12, 2016)

For instance, we worry that junior faculty and lab staff's contribution to simulation may not be represented in authorship—we need to ensure that junior faculty are supported and recognized in their contributions and inspired to continue to develop their simulation and teaching expertise. As a discipline, we are known for "eating our young," which has been conceptualized as vertical violence and bullying, and we recognize this as one of the many concerns in retaining nurses in practice and education. We can no longer tolerate this behavior, given the shortages we are facing and the intellect wasted. As the use of simulation accelerates, we ask all nursing educators to maintain the highest levels of professional integrity and face their fears to support new ways of thinking, teaching, and practicing this profession we love (International Nursing Association for Clinical Simulation and Learning [INACSL], 2016).

CLINICAL EXPERIENCE VERSUS SIMULATION

The need for simulated nursing experiences has been reinforced by the scarcity of clinical placement sites. Program enrollments have increased the large numbers of students needing clinical experiences and a nursing shortage that requires adequate staffing to handle students has created stress for both academic institutions and hospitals alike. This situation has sparked much discussion about how much clinical time should be replaced with simulation or whether simulation should ever replace clinical time at all. Although most nursing programs are de- ciding this issue individually, each program has required hours for program completion by individual state boards of nursing and in Canada, by provincial Colleges of Nurse Regulators. In one state, a brainstorming session of the statewide deans and directors was held early in this new era of simulation and, in general, it was suggested that no more than 10% of clinical time would be used for simulation. Other states have made arrangements for incorporating simu- lation into calculated clinical time. The National Council of State Boards of Nursing (NCSBN) position paper of 2005 reported that boards addressed two major issues: (a) the increased use of technology for nursing education clinical experiences and (b) the use of clinical sites and learning centers. Although nursing education experiences should represent the full life span with actual patients, they may include innovative teaching strategies that complement clin- ical, like simulation, but should not entirely replace clinical. In reality, with practice time in the simulation lab, students may enter the clinical sites at a higher cognitive and skill level with increased confidence, and therefore get more out of the experience (Bremner, Aduddell, Bennett, & VanGeest, 2006; Murray, Grant, Howarth, & Leigh, 2008; NCSBN, 2005; Nehring, 2008). This finding was supported by a study conducted by the NCSBN and results were released in 2014, stating:

> It was found that up to 50 percent simulation was effectively substituted for traditional clinical experience in all core courses across the prelicensure nursing curriculum under conditions com- parable to those described in the study. Additionally, the use of up to 50 percent simulation did not affect NCLEX pass rates. (Hayden, Smiley, Alexander, Kardong-Edgren, & Jeffries, 2014, p. S38)

These findings confirm the validity of the efficacy of substituting simulation for clinical time in well-chosen educational experiences (Hayden et al., 2014).

A frequently used method of integrating simulation as a complement to clinical experience is doing simulations early in the semester. Nursing faculty are often unfamiliar with a new group of students and need to assess their competency level before placing them with actual patients. The use of simulated scenarios can help prepare students for the higher level of patient care required in a new semester. Faculty can then move forward into the semester having assessed strengths, weaknesses, and areas in need of improvement.

Another method of implementing simulation within a semester is transforming what cur- rently exists in the form of weekly task-oriented modules to simulation scenarios. Traditionally used to demonstrate competency on one static task, simulations transform a static task into an engaging and realistic patient interaction involving communication, safety precautions, and the need to react to changing physiologic conditions. In addition, when hospitals have the available resources (e.g., high-fidelity HPSs), clinical faculty may choose to incorporate a simulation into a postconference session to share an important learning experience with the whole group, reinforce important aspects of care, and debrief to assist the students in recognizing alternative scenarios for providing care and assessing and evaluating patient reaction to the plan of care and actual nursing interventions.

Simulation has also been used for clinical remediation when a student is struggling in clinical (Bremner et al., 2006; Haskvitz & Koop, 2004; Kuiper, Heinrich, Matthias, Graham, & Kotwall, 2008). A student can be assigned time in the lab with a simulator to reprocess a difficult clinical situation, to practice a skill that she or he was unable to perform in clinical, and/or to recreate an actual patient situation that a student needs to process more slowly in order to understand. Providing an opportunity in which students can process in a safe environment often increases a student's confidence in actual patient interactions. From an assessment standpoint, if a student is not safe and not meeting the objectives in clinical, simulation can help both the faculty and student pinpoint deficits in critical thinking and decision making.

Faculties have also found simulations to be useful as an end-point assessment of knowledge learned. Simulation testing can be used at the close of the semester as a final competency assessment or as a program assessment before graduation. Hospitals have now begun testing minimum competencies of both new graduates and new hires using simulators and scenarios. End-point simulation testing has better prepared new graduates for this challenge.

FORMAL CURRICULAR CHANGE VERSUS INTEGRATION INTO THE EXISTING CURRICULUM

We have heard many faculty members discuss the fact that adding simulation would require a major and formal change in their program curriculum. We respectfully disagree. Simulation is, simply, a learning tool. We have been using simulation since the practice of teaching nursing began. We used each other in nursing school to learn our assessments, practiced static skills on static manikins, and gave injections to oranges. Certainly, computerized simulation is at a different level, but we have found that, other than adding or rewording some course objectives or retooling a practice module to a technology-enhanced module, there has not been a need to rewrite the curriculum. In addition, we now see graduate-level courses on technology-based learning that may include simulation. Most programs have been able to seamlessly add simulation as a within-course learning experience.

ESTABLISHING THE FIT ACROSS THE CURRICULUM

The goal of simulation has been to enhance critical thinking and decision making at all levels of a nursing curriculum through realistic interactions with a simulated patient. Simulation can be implemented in every course, although some aspects of this implementation depend on the availability of faculty who are able to join in the scenario (possibly running the simulation equipment, being a disconcerted family member, or even being the voice of the patient). At a second-year or program-entry level, uses for simulation include physical assessment within the first medical–surgical course and in studying pharmacology. In learning physical assessment, students can use simulation to assess body sounds, locate landmarks, and run and rerun system assessments as needed for enhancing learning. In a lower level medical–surgical course, students can interact with the simulated patient before meeting patients and practice communication techniques. An instructor may decide to introduce a difficult patient scenario to a novice nursing student so that strategies for success can be practiced before meeting an actual challenging patient. Simulation has been used in teaching pharmacology to bring home the seriousness of prioritizing a patient's safety in medication administration (Seropian, Dillman, Lasater, & Gavilanes, 2007). Using a high-fidelity HPS, an instructor has the capacity to show real-time effects of a medication as it is administered. Within a scenario, the instructor can show the positive effects as well as the side effects of certain medications, while demonstrating the physiologic impact of that medication in specific disease categories.

In midlevel curriculum or at the third-year level, simulation can be used in the application of the nursing process throughout the life span. Simulation scenarios can be developed in chronic and acute medical–surgical care, family care, care of mother and baby, pediatrics, geriatrics, home care, and psychiatric care. These scenarios can be tailored to involve multiple students and faculty enacting various family and professional roles in order to demonstrate the complexity of holistic care.

At the senior level, simulation is effective in teaching the application of the nursing process in complex and emergency nursing care (Childs & Sepples, 2006; Comer, 2005). Although it is impractical and unethical to wait until an actual patient situation becomes an emergency, student responses to emergency and life-threatening scenarios can be assessed through the use of simulation. These scenarios can be run or programmed to have multiple outcomes depending on the students' actions within the scenario. Many dispute the ethics of letting a simulator flatline in a scenario, simulations that test a student's knowledge in resuscitation, either alone or in a team, have been reported to be important learning experiences for students who are able to practice their first code on a simulated patient. Although students verbalize disappointment when the outcome is not positive, they are very enthusiastic about running and rerunning the scenario until a positive outcome is achieved. This experience is unique to the high-fidelity simulators. In contrast, if a positive outcome is not achieved, students are provided the opportunity to practice good communication skills with family members and broach topics of organ donation, spirituality, and proper protocol for pronouncement of death and management of the body. Even though these are perceived as challenging situations to enact, graduates often identify such situations as areas in which they wish there had been more instruction while in nursing school so that they would be properly prepared for their real-life experiences as a nurse.

Although most scenarios are generated by faculty for use in their own courses, simulations have also been developed by students, as suggested by Larew, Lessans, Spunt, Foster, and Covington (2006). At all levels of the curriculum, students can be encouraged to use actual patient data to build their own scenario for their own learning as well as for demonstration purposes for the class (see Chapter 44 for an example of student-generated senior scenarios). One university professor is using student-developed studies in the pediatric clinical rotation. As it is often challenging to find high-acuity pediatric patients on a consistent basis in any clinical setting, this professor instructs the students to generate a complex scenario as a replacement or supplement to actual patients cared for. Students then demonstrate for the class and submit a paper summary for grading. The person who specializes in simulation works with the students to familiarize them with the medium-fidelity HPS as part of the project, but learning the ins and outs of running the technology is part of the learning experience.

As another example, in a women's health course, students in groups are responsible for presenting specific case scenarios on key areas, such as ectopic pregnancy and preterm labor. They are given some basic guidelines of information but are responsible for researching the clinical condition, identifying the nurse's role, and coming up with an appropriate care plan. This method can involve role play or the use of simulated patients, and their peers are more engaged when involved in this style of interactive learning. From here, the faculty goes on to incorporate content-appropriate material and reinforce the important points that all the students can relate back to with the benefit of a concrete "scenario."

EVIDENCE-BASED PRACTICE

An essential component to integrating simulation throughout the curriculum is the inclusion of evidence-based practice. Scenarios should include reference lists of research studies and standards of care used (Childs, Sepples, & Chambers, 2007). The students should also have access to resources before, during, and after simulations, for finding additional information needed to complete or understand the scenario. Just as is true in nursing care of real patients, students should be using only the latest research in the implementation of care on the simulated patient. Students may be asked in advance to pull standards of care and research before simulations. They may have access to the web through the classroom computer or a tablet. In addition, many programs have set up simulation websites for use by the students and faculty in learning more about the simulation process and for quick access to important websites as references. For faculty, it is helpful if a scenario references the National Council Licensure Examination for Registered Nurses (NCLEX-RN®) test plan categories (NCSBN, 2015) and/or accreditation bodies, such as the American Association of Colleges of Nursing (AACN; 2008, 2011) and its Essentials documents and current revisions, for curricular reference points.

As mentioned in Chapter 1, INACSL *Standards of Best Practice: Simulation* (2013) added Standard VIII: Interprofessional Education (Decker et al., 2015). Health care professional programs are including competencies for accreditation and regulation and expecting students to learn together. Simulation provides a unique opportunity for interprofessional education and practice and demonstrated enhanced learning and skill performance, and research supports its usefulness (Bambini, Washburn, & Perkins, 2009; Koo, Idzik, Hammersla, & Windemuth, 2013; Murphy, Curtis, & McCloughen, 2016; Watts et al., 2014). Chapter 5 of this book incorporates an innovative approach to faculty development for interprofessional simulation and Part III includes 16 scenarios for interprofessional education.

BENEFITS ACROSS THE CURRICULUM

The benefits of integrating simulation throughout the curriculum are immediately evident: students respond enthusiastically to the technology but, more important, are able to accurately diagnose and intervene in nursing problems beyond faculty expectations. Because of the breadth of programming of the medium- and high-fidelity HPSs, faculty no longer have to search for actual patients with all heart, lung, and abdominal problems and abnormal sounds. This allows for the recognition of an assessment factor already learned before actual patient care, significantly increasing the likelihood of accurate assessment while caring for actual patients. In addition, students can be exposed to more conditions in a more controlled environment at a more rapid pace. Simulation takes on a life of its own, thus becoming "real" to the students.

In conclusion, this chapter has emphasized the importance of integrating a simulation-focused pedagogy throughout the curriculum to best meet the needs of your program. In order to help with curriculum mapping using scenarios in this text, the authors of the scenarios have been asked to identify the objectives, competencies, and/or essentials that are accomplished by their scenario. Given that the NCLEX-RN exam is the licensing exam in both the United States and Canada, some authors have also included information to map the scenario by the NCLEX-RN exam test plan, wherever feasible (NCSBN, 2015). Our goal with this text was to incorporate the expertise of nursing faculty, practitioners, and interprofessional colleagues to provide as much information as possible for the smooth integration of simulation and experiential learning in nursing programs around the globe.

REFERENCES

American Association of Colleges of Nursing. (2008). *The essentials of baccalaureate education for professional nursing practice*. Washington, DC: Author. Retrieved from http://www.aacnnursing.org/Portals/42/Publications/BaccEssentials08.pdf

American Association of Colleges of Nursing. (2011). *The essentials of master's education in nursing for professional nursing practice*. Washington, DC: Author. Retrieved from http://www.aacnnursing.org/Portals/42/Publications/MastersEssentials11.pdf

Bambini, D., Washburn, J., & Perkins, R. (2009). Outcomes of clinical simulation for novice nursing students: Communication, confidence, clinical judgment. *Nursing Education Perspectives, 30*(2), 79–82.

Bremner, M. N., Aduddell, K., Bennett, D. N., & VanGeest, J. B. (2006). The use of human patient simulators: Best practices with novice nursing students. *Nurse Educator, 31*(4), 170–174.

Childs, J. C., & Sepples, S. B. (2006). Lessons learned from a complex patient care scenario. *Nursing Education Perspectives, 27*(3), 154–158.

Childs, J. C., Sepples, S. B., & Chambers, K. (2007). Designing simulation for nursing education. In P. Jeffries (Ed.), *Simulation in nursing education* (pp. 35–58). New York, NY: National League for Nurses.

Comer, S. K. (2005). Patient care simulations: Role playing to enhance clinical understanding. *Nursing Education Perspectives, 26*(6), 357–361.

Decker, S. I., Anderson, M., Boese, T., Epps, C., McCarthy, J., Motola, I., … Lioce, L. (2015). Standards of best practice: Simulation standard VIII: Simulation-enhanced interprofessional education (Sim-IPE). *Clinical Simulation in Nursing, 11*(6), 293–297.

Haskvitz, L. M., & Koop, E. C. (2004). Students struggling in clinical? A new role for the patient simulator. *Journal of Nursing Education, 43*(4), 181–184.

Hayden, J. K., Smiley, R. A., Alexander, M., Kardong-Edgren, S., & Jeffries, P. R. (2014). The NCSBN National Simulation Study: A longitudinal, randomized, controlled study replacing clinical hours with simulation in prelicensure nursing education. *Journal of Nursing Regulation, 5*(2), S1–S64.

International Nursing Association for Clinical Simulation and Learning. (2013). Standards of best practice: Simulation standard VIII: Simulation-enhanced interprofessional education (Sim-IPE). *Clinical Simulation in Nursing, 11*(6), 293–297.

International Nursing Association for Clinical Simulation and Learning. (2016). Standards of best practice: Simulation: Professional INTEGRITY. *Clinical Simulation in Nursing, 12,* S30–S33. doi:10.1016/j.ecns.2016.09.010

Koo, L. W., Idzik, S. R., Hammersla, M. B., & Windemuth, B. F. (2013). Developing standardized patient clinical simulations to apply concepts of interdisciplinary collaboration. *Journal of Nursing Education, 52*(12), 705–708.

Kuiper, R. A., Heinrich, C., Matthias, A., Graham, M. J., & Kotwall, L. B. (2008). Debriefing with the OPT model of clinical reasoning during high-fidelity patient simulation. *International Journal of Nursing Education Scholarship, 17*(5), 1–14.

Larew, C., Lessans, S., Spunt, D., Foster, D., & Covington, B. G. (2006). Innovations in clinical simulation: Application of Benner's theory in an interactive patient care simulation. *Nursing Education Perspectives, 27*(1), 16–21.

Murphy, M., Curtis, K., & McCloughen, A. (2016). What is the impact of multidisciplinary team simulation training on team performance and efficiency of patient care? An integrative review. *Australasian Emergency Nursing Journal, 19*(1), 44–53.

Murray, C., Grant, M. J., Howarth, M. L., & Leigh, J. (2008). The use of simulation as a teaching and learning approach to support practice learning. *Nurse Education in Practice, 8*(1), 5–8.

National Council of State Boards of Nursing. (2005). Clinical instruction in prelicensure nursing programs. Retrieved from https://www.ncsbn.org/Final_Clinical_Instr_Pre_Nsg_programs.pdf

National Council of State Boards of Nursing. (2015). NCLEX-RN examination: Test plan for the National Council Licensure Examination for Registered Nurses. Retrieved from https://www.ncsbn.org/RN_Test_Plan_2016_Final.pdf

Nehring, W. M. (2008). U.S. boards of nursing and the use of high-fidelity patient simulators in nursing education. *Journal of Professional Nursing, 24*(2), 109–117.

Radhakrishnan, K., Roche, J. P., & Cunningham, H. (2007). Measuring clinical practice parameters with human patient simulation: A pilot study. *International Journal of Nursing Education Scholarship, 4,* Article 8. doi:10.2202/1548-923X.1307

Seropian, M., Dillman, D., Lasater, K., & Gavilanes, J. (2007). Mannequin-based simulation to reinforce pharmacology concepts. *Simulation in Healthcare, 2*(4), 218–223.

Watts, P., Langston, S. B., Brown, M., Prince, C., Belle, A., Skipper, M. W.,…Moss, J. (2014). Interprofessional education: A multi-patient, team-based intensive care unit simulation. *Clinical Simulation in Nursing, 10*(10), 521–528. doi:10.1016/j.ecns.2014.05.004

CHAPTER 4

Teaching and Evaluating Therapeutic Communication in Simulated Scenarios

Suzanne Hetzel Campbell, Natalia Del Angelo Aredes, and Ranjit K. Dhari

Communication is the foundation for all interpersonal relationships and involves an authentic presence and facilitative style that indicates one's interest in and care for another. In health care, an interaction between health care professionals and patients is called *therapeutic communication* and is operationally defined as "aims to enhance the patient's comfort, safety, trust, or health and well-being" ("Therapeutic communication," 2017). When therapeutic communication is done well, patients are comforted, feel safe, and develop a sense of trust in health care professionals. This contributes to improved health or sense of well-being and a safe environment with improved quality of care. Communication is necessary to build trustworthy and therapeutic relationships.

In looking for frameworks that resonate with the importance of communication, the language within the American Academy Colleges of Nursing BSN and MSN Essentials refers to communication within leadership, advocacy, telehealth, and interprofessional areas (American Association of Colleges of Nursing [AACN], 2008, 2011) and there is an acknowledgment of the importance of communication as a critical skill to be practiced and learned as part of professional nursing. However, the Canadian Code of Ethics for Registered Nurses holds references to communication in both ethical responsibilities 2 and 3 under A. Providing Safe, Compassionate, Competent, and Ethical Care:

2. Nurses engage in *compassionate care through their speech and body language* and through their efforts to understand and care about others' health-care needs.

3. Nurses *build trustworthy relationships* as the foundation of *meaningful communication*, recognizing that building these relationships involves a conscious effort. Such relationships are critical to understanding people's needs and concerns. (CNA, 2008, p. 8)

One of the main competencies health professionals are expected to master is therapeutic communication; regulators look for it in ethical codes of conduct and accrediting bodies evaluate curriculum and education looking for evidence of students' mastery of communication, both with patients and interprofessionally. Competency in communication is an expectation of all health professionals.

Studies have suggested that communication may have direct and/or indirect effects on patients' health, such that when patients receive clinicians' support and clear explanations about treatment, they establish trust and better understand the next steps. This open communication facilitates the follow-up process and positively affects the health outcomes. Through effective communication, health teams work together with the patient to recognize patients' needs and devise a suitable plan to meet those needs (Leonard, Graham, & Bonacum, 2004). Misconceptions can be identified and clarified, accommodating patients' varying health literacy needs, leading to power sharing in decision making and improving self-maintenance of patient health (Siminoff et al., 2011; Street, Makoul, Arora, & Epstein, 2013).

The World Health Organization (WHO) has outlined a framework for action on interprofessional education (Interprofessional Education Collaboration [IPEC], 2011; WHO, 2010) and encourages practitioners coming together in team-training exercises. The simulation environment provides an opportunity to bring together health professionals from varying backgrounds to allow for the development of leaders and promotion of ethical behaviors as they gain a perspective on each other's roles and scopes of practice, and an opportunity to foster professional attitudes. In addition, these simulated scenarios provide a practice arena for both technical and nontechnical skills, such as communication strategies, and research demonstrates that this method of teaching can affect the quality and safety of patient care (Commission, 2010; Cooper et al., 2012; Institute of Medicine [IOM], 2001).

Other researchers have identified a connection between miscommunication and adverse events or errors in clinical practice, which affects the quality of care (Fay-Hillier, Regan, & Gallagher Gordon, 2012). In order to minimize miscommunication, a variety of strategies and tools have been used from other disciplines with good outcomes. Nevertheless, these strategies are often limited to communication among health professionals rather than communication between health professionals and their patients. One example is the SBAR acronym purported to improve communication in urgent situations by incorporating the following aspects in the report or handover: situation, background, assessment, and recommendation (Clancy, 2008; Institute for Healthcare Improvement [IHI], 2016; Thomas, Bertram, & Johnson, 2009). Another tool for communication among health professionals is iDRAW, which aims to define a pattern of information to be exchanged between health professionals in nonurgent handover situations by incorporating an interactive component and its acronym; iDRAW, stands for: i = identify patient and most responsible practitioner (MRP), D = diagnosis/current problems, R = recent changes (e.g., up to date vitals), A = anticipated changes (in next few hours), and W = what to watch for (Hill, 2013; Hill & Marcellus, 2015). Finally, TeamSTEPPS® has been used for interdisciplinary team-based communication (Weaver et al., 2010; Zhang, Miller, Volkman, Meza, & Jones, 2015).

In the past two editions of this text, this chapter has outlined the usefulness of simulation for the teaching, assessment, and evaluation of health communication for practitioner–patient, practitioner–practitioner, and team communication (O'Shea, Pagano, Campbell, & Caso, 2013; Pagano & Greiner, 2013). This new chapter provides an overview of methods to assess and evaluate therapeutic communication by health care professionals with patients. The focus of this chapter is on the education, assessment, and evaluation of health communication skills to improve health outcomes (Bhui et al., 2015) through patient-centered care (Epstein & Street, 2007) with the use of simulation. It provides a brief introduction of the development of a new Global Interprofessional Therapeutic Communication Scale (GITCS©) and subsequent development of train-the-trainer videos for health professions educators. Many researchers and health professions educators have invested their time and resources into enhancing therapeutic communication through the use of innovative teaching and learning models, such as simulation. Their goal is to prepare health professionals in their ongoing development of therapeutic communication or relationship techniques that will create a high-quality and safe health care system that truly serves the populations in need. Ultimately, these techniques can improve patients' experiences within the health care system—increasing patients' understanding to maintain well-being, providing a more satisfactory interaction so patients are partners in determining their treatment and plan of care, and removing accessibility barriers, such as cultural and health literacy factors, that may create a less-than-optimal experience.

Communication skills are widely recognized as a desirable "nontechnical" skill for nurses (Lai, 2016). Mental health nurses have provided leadership in studying therapeutic communication with standardized patients (SPs; Doolen, Giddings, Johnson, de Nathan, & Badia, 2014), yet communication is a core competency for all nursing disciplines as well as all health professionals: physicians, nurses, nutritionists, physiotherapists, psychologists, social workers, and so on. Health care providers are in direct contact with patients and their families and communicate in team-based situations continuously, such that communication in the health care context is a main issue reflecting on quality and safety, especially in areas such as the emergency room or operating room (Shapiro et al., 2004; Theilen et al., 2013; Weaver et al., 2010). Therefore, enhancing our ability to educate prelicensure and practicing clinicians by developing methods, education tools, and evaluation or assessment capabilities is crucial.

REVIEW OF LITERATURE: INSTRUMENTS TO SUPPORT TEACHING AND EVALUATION OF HEALTH PROFESSIONAL STUDENTS' HEALTH COMMUNICATION

In order to provide effective education in communication skills for health care professionals, it is necessary to move beyond conceptualization to feasible methods of implementation and measurement. Table 4.1 provides a review of the literature representing instruments that have been developed and validated to support teaching or evaluation in health communication. This recognizes the scarce resources presently available, similar to findings from a previous study (Caron et al., 2013). In addition, the International Nursing Association for Clinical Simulation and Learning (INACSL) has identified the gap in reliable and valid instruments or scales for testing, research, and evaluation in simulation, and has created a Repository of Instruments Used in Simulation Research (INACSL, 2015; Kardong-Edgren, Adamson, & Fitzgerald, 2010).

These instruments have been used to teach and evaluate therapeutic communication skills in health professionals, mostly physicians and nurses. The instruments identify important elements of therapeutic communication and include both positive and negative behaviors that influence the interaction, as well as concepts related to relationship building. Each instrument examined is attempting to systematize and measure the concept of therapeutic communication and in so doing brings to the forefront consistent themes and behaviors. These instruments all have strengths for the context in which they were used, but a global scale, adapted for different cultural contexts and translated into different languages specific to health care professional and patient communication, does not yet exist.

When considering something as simple as introductions, differences among cultures abound. For example, in certain cultures, patients may not make direct eye contact while communicating with a health care provider, which can sometimes be perceived as the patient being disinterested or disengaged; however, the patient may be quietly reflecting or might not be comfortable holding the gaze of someone of another gender. In the health care setting, a smile with eye contact is the most common and socially acceptable greeting during an introduction between health care professionals and patients. In North America, a handshake is perceived, for the majority, as a respectful and appropriate introductory greeting. Individuals from South Asian cultures would perceive a nod with no touching at all to be more respectful. In Brazil, although a handshake may be an appropriate greeting, it is perceived to be very formal and generally associated with a business environment. Apart from introductions, the health care planning process also presents a plethora of cultural differences. For example, in some cultures, it is the family who helps to devise the plan especially if the patient is living in an extended family household or the patient relies on family members to help interpret and navigate the health care system. Simulation provides a risk-free opportunity for students to learn about therapeutic communication in a culturally safe manner.

Because of globalization, nurses find themselves caring for diverse people from a variety of countries with social, cultural, and religious differences and whose interaction and expectation of health care professionals may vary widely as well. Navigating care requires advanced communication skills and a solid foundation in health care professional curriculum with an opportunity to practice, receive feedback, and reflect on best practices. Simulation is well suited for this type of experiential learning.

Therefore, after an attempt to translate one of the instruments in Table 4.1, a decision was made to start from scratch with an international team and create an instrument that would be

Table 4.1	Instruments Used to Measure Health-Professional Students' Health Communication[a]		
Instrument/Authors	**Purpose**	**Communication Elements**	**Observation**
SCCAP (Siminoff Communication Content and Affect Program; Siminoff et al., 2011)	Codify situations of communication in health	Positive behavior: reassurance, clarification, and offer of service Negative behavior: threatening, indifference, and disparaging	Therapeutic communication is composed of purpose, care logistics, disease and treatment, medical history, psychosocial aspects, and prognosis
OSCAR (Objective, Structured Communication Assessment of Residents; Caron et al., 2013)	Teach communication skills among residents and medical students	These 13 items include a nonjudgmental attitude with patients, explanation of jargon, consulting the patient to guide decision making and an emphasis on organization and time management	Categories: relationship development, case goals, and overall organization and time management. The teacher or instructor can score the resident as unsatisfactory, proficient, advanced, and outstanding in each category, except for introduction, which is either yes/no
T-Com-Skill Scale (Baumann, Baumann, Le Bihan, & Chau, 2008)	Measure patients' perception of medical doctors' therapeutic communication skills	This 15-item list includes: completeness of information given, attention to patient's difficulties during treatment, adequate use of words according to patient's health literacy and more	This 9-item Likert scale (from 0—never to 9—always) strongly emphasizes the medical consultation and weakly includes aspects regarding empathy, power sharing, and holistic approach
HCAT (Health Communication Assessment Tool; Pagano et al., 2015)	Teach communication skills to nursing students in U.S. context (application in simulation strategy)	This has 22 items encompassing both verbal and nonverbal communication, introductions, respectful behaviors during interaction, and holistic approach beyond biological factors. Constructs included: Empathetic; Introduction; Trust Building; Patient/Family Education; and Power-sharing behaviors.	The instructor rates on a 5-point Likert scale (ranging from 1—strongly disagree to 5—strongly agree, with 3—unsure); through observation of a communication scene. Five factors explained 57% of the variance, Cronbach's $\alpha = 0.89$
Competency Assessment Tool for Therapeutic Communication (National Education Framework Cancer Nursing; Aranda & Yates, 2009)	Measure communication skills of specialist cancer nurses	Includes learning aspect of therapeutic communication, concern with patient privacy and input, verbal and nonverbal skills, empathy, and multidisciplinary perspective	Focuses on domains of professional practice, critical thinking and analysis, provision and coordination of care, and collaborative therapeutic practice Items scored from 0 to 2, resulting in ranges of performance levels: competent (established as nurse specialist), competent (beginning as nurse specialist), and not yet competent

[a] As this chapter focuses on student–patient interactions, patient handover instruments, such as those mentioned earlier, SBAR, iDRAW, and Team STEPPS™, are purposefully not covered in this table.

globally adaptable, reflective of a broad range of interprofessional health care professionals, and useful in academic and clinical environments. For this reason, the GITCS was developed (Campbell & Aredes, 2017).

GITCS DEVELOPMENT

Attempting to use one of the other communication scales proved to be very ineffective because of poor interrater reliability and difficulty translating the scales in an international environment. This led to the authors going back to examine theory and skills from mental health on "therapeutic communication." Based on empirical knowledge from years of practicing and teaching nursing and with input from interprofessional and international colleagues from many disciplines, a 45-item scale was developed and was used in a pilot study with nine nursing faculty from seven schools in a province in Canada to evaluate student nurse communication during a simulated scenario with either a human patient simulator (HPS) or an SP. Two expert panels reviewed the items and identified constructs for each of these items (Campbell & Aredes, 2017).

This scale developed items categorized according to active listening, empathy, empowerment, verbal and nonverbal communication, rapport and trust building, barriers, and cultural boundaries, among others. The goal was to create an instrument capable of supporting faculty, students, and health professionals in learning and assessing appropriate actions to establish and maintain therapeutic communication in an international environment. The hope is that the use of GITCS will allow teachers and facilitators to identify individuals' strengths and weaknesses easily during active learning experiences, such as simulations or interactions with patients in clinical practicums (students) or work activities (health professionals).

A recent study (Lum, Dowedoff, & Englander, 2016) stated the importance of training immigrant nurses in therapeutic communication, considering the differences in the process of nursing education and work in practice amid various countries, in addition to changes in the cultural context and, sometimes, language. Although the study arose in Canada, we believe that, given globalization, this discussion is relevant in many countries and the researchers' findings for a need to strengthen therapeutic communication in nursing courses and strengthen self-assessment among nurses about their knowledge in communication resonates with what we have experienced.

GITCS was developed and is being validated in Canada. Validity and reliability will be tested using an international and interprofessional sample of health care professional educators who use simulation for education. A multicenter research project in a province in Canada will also test its reliability and validity across sites, level of students, and varied simulation and clinical experiences. In addition, it will be translated into French, Portuguese, Spanish, Mandarin, and Punjabi, in collaboration with colleagues in Quebec, Brazil, Chile, Hong Kong, and India, respectively. Other validation in countries where English is the main language will be possible, including the United Kingdom, Ireland, Australia, United States, and other areas with interested participants. The scale will be appropriate for use in simulated and clinical environments, with prelicensure or seasoned clinicians.

LIGHTS, CAMERA, AND ACTION

To set up a train-the-trainer opportunity for health care professions faculty and in order to validate the GITCS, videos were developed demonstrating interactions between an RN and a patient during a home care visit. Therefore, it was possible to test the items' application over the same interaction presented in three different ways: overall therapeutic communication with good behaviors, overall nontherapeutic communication with poor behaviors, and mixed communication combining both good and poor behaviors.

Because of the complexity of clinical settings, we chose to film the videos in a structured environment using a trained actor and public health nurse faculty with decades of experience. The scenario involved a visit by a public health RN to an older adult at her home and was roughly scripted based on Chapter 24 in the second edition of this text (Mager, 2012).

The videos provided a level of consistency for train-the-trainer education and validation of the instruments' reliability. In addition, the videos match teaching needs by allowing for pausing, rewinding, forwarding, and replaying anytime depending on the students' needs. Other studies have shown positive results using videos of simulation for teaching and evaluating therapeutic communication in health care (Hammer, Fox, & Hampton, 2014).

FILMING: THE CHALLENGES OF PRODUCING AN EDUCATIONAL VIDEO

In preparation for the production of videos for train-the-trainer education, the authors used a scenario from the second edition of this text (Mager, 2012), home care of a patient with elevated blood sugars, to create a script with three modules that became three separate videos. As mentioned previously, the goal was to create modules demonstrating good, bad, and mixed therapeutic communication. The intention in creating the videos was to be able to portray sufficiently different interactions that would demonstrate good and poor therapeutic communication behaviors.

Lessons learned in creating these videos included that it would have been helpful for more of a rehearsal process before filming the videos. Scheduling conflicts meant that the faculty member was unable to meet the crew or the actress before the filming process began. In hindsight, it is important to have time allotted for the actors to meet and practice with the director's guidance. A suggestion would be to consider including the actors in the development of the script, the production meetings, allowing ample time for discussion and questions so that they have a clear understanding of the video and its purpose. This would enhance the development of such tools and create a more beneficial learning process for all involved. When the faculty member and actress finally met, they became comfortable with each other and briefly practiced the scenarios before the filming began.

As a faculty member acting the RN role, the scenario of overall therapeutic communication with good behavior was easy to memorize and act out during production. However, it was challenging and difficult to act out the patient scenario with overall nontherapeutic communication with bad behaviors. It had become second nature to always conduct communication with patients using excellent therapeutic communication skills so that when prompted to act out scenes with bad behavior, it was challenging to speak. This made it difficult to follow the script, which was incumbent to demonstrating bad communication and meeting the goal of the video. In future, recognizing that a seasoned and expert nurse may face more challenges with the poor behavior video, we would have scheduled more time for filming that portion. We also recommend that it would have been better to film this more difficult scenario first.

These videos provided nurse educators concrete examples of good and poor behaviors and allowed for an opportunity to reflect on therapeutic communication. This opportunity for reflection allowed discussion of strategies for improved communication and methods to develop trust and rapport while being respectful and actively listening to the client's needs. Finally, videotaped examples allowed for moving at the individual's own pace of learning and helped to connect effective communication techniques to actual clinical practice, which can encourage students to think of examples of when communication with a patient went particularly well or particularly poorly.

In the area of instrument development, video recording can also be used as a strategy to educate faculty about the instrument's features and uses, and can allow for beginning interrater reliability testing and enhancement.

EVALUATING THERAPEUTIC COMMUNICATION THROUGH SIMULATION

Creative and experimental strategies for learning and the adoption of more participative learning theories, in the student's point of view, have increased alongside technology and innovation (Hammer et al., 2014). The use of simulation in teaching therapeutic health communication is successful when students are able to project themselves into a "real situation," experiment with different approaches, debrief with a group, and know they are in a controlled environment that allows for error without life-threatening adverse events. Many studies have reported simulation use as a strategy to teach communication in the health arena and have identified favorable results (Caron et al., 2013; Fay-Hillier et al., 2012; Fejzic & Barker, 2015; Kameg, Howard, Clochesy, Mitchell, & Suresky, 2010; Strada, Vegni, & Lamiani, 2016); and as such, simulation is a valuable ally of health communication skills improvement.

When running a simulation, faculty are encouraged to observe the dynamic interaction critically by using a tool to assess various areas of therapeutic communication and positive or negative interactions. After the scenario is complete there is time to use debriefing questions to discuss with students their perception of their performance and identify what they felt good about and areas where they believe they can do better.

Learning about health communication is an important activity even for experienced professionals. One research study used simulation to train health professionals from diverse backgrounds to communicate with their patients around the topic of sexuality. Even with a mean of 11 years of experience in the clinical practice field, the participants, physicians, nurses, and psychosocial professionals consistently reported acquiring new strategies of communication to not only approach the sexuality subject, but also to explore patients' health concerns related to sexuality. The researchers emphasized the importance of communication and relational skills, and appreciated the interactivity allowed through simulation as a pedagogical approach (Strada et al., 2016).

Simulation promotes engaging experiences of learning for adults (students, health professionals, and even professors, in the perspective of continuous learning). It naturally arouses curiosity and inquiry, providing a rich environment to develop critical thinking, clinical reasoning, and self-reflection (Hammer et al., 2014). Faculty and students observe that they like this form of "hands-on" activity and found, even if they were the observer and member of the debriefing group, they felt they had better knowledge about the team and experienced greater satisfaction in the method of learning (Fay-Hillier et al., 2012; Fejzic & Barker, 2015; Strada et al., 2016).

Studies that combined health communication skills training and simulation did have differences in preference related to the use of actors—SPs over HPSs, even with high-fidelity HPSs. Researchers stated that sometimes it is hard to interact properly with an HPS because it does not manifest nonverbal signs (Kameg, Mitchell, Clochesy, Howard, & Suresky, 2009), which are considered important in communication. In this regard, it is important to consider what is being accomplished and how you will teach and evaluate health communication skills through simulation whether the "patient" is an HPS or an SP.

Debriefing is the core of simulation as it is the moment for reflection, concept rebuilding based on simulated actions, and exchange of information with colleagues and teachers or facilitators (Decker et al., 2013). After the simulation scenario, it is crucial to discuss the effectiveness of communication with students identifying what went well and what might be improved to enhance the relationship between the health professional and the patient and their families to provide patient-centered care. Considering that most clinical experiences do not allow for clinical faculty to observe every interaction or provide feedback for students about their communication skills, simulation provides a feasible venue to build skills to mastering therapeutic communication.

FUTURE OF THERAPEUTIC COMMUNICATION

Based on our academic and clinical practice in Canada, the United States of America, and Brazil, we conclude that checklists or instruments support the debriefing process to provide useful feedback to students or health professionals, to identify completed performance, and facilitate the follow-up of skills improvement throughout the course. However, we are still lacking a robust, valid, and reliable tool to measure outcomes in health communication between professionals and patients and families, in both global and interprofessional scenarios. The researchers who used simulation to teach communication did not have this type of instrument, because they usually developed their own to conduct research or approached self-efficacy techniques to present data. Still, all of them stated that this lack of a standard measurement tool is a limitation and suggested one should be developed for future research and that it would be best to use validated instruments (Fay-Hillier et al., 2012; Fejzic & Barker, 2015; Hammer et al., 2014; Kameg et al., 2010; Kawamura, Mylopoulos, Orsino, Jimenez, & McNaughton, 2016).

Given the complexity of a faculty's role, it is important to establish a way to evaluate health communication globally. Faculty members are responsible for complex evaluations during a simulation, including clinical reasoning, critical thinking, as well as cognitive and procedural knowledge. Therefore, a valid, reliable, and simple instrument to measure student performance would be a valuable asset.

Broadly, the flexibility simulation provided is an incentive for teachers to offer engaging learning in therapeutic communication skills training that is aligned with learning objectives and patient-centered care. This chapter describes some of the instruments and scales available today as well as an innovative new method for validating an instrument that will also be used in a train-the-trainer fashion globally.

REFERENCES

American Association of Colleges of Nursing. (2008). *The essentials of baccalaureate education for professional nursing practice.* Washington, DC: Author. Retrieved from http://www.aacnnursing.org/Portals/42/Publications/BaccEssentials08.pdf

American Association of Colleges of Nursing. (2011). *The essentials of master's education in nursing.* Washington, DC: Author. Retrieved from http://www.aacnnursing.org/Portals/42/Publications/MastersEssentials11.pdf

Aranda, S., & Yates, P. (2009). *A national professional development framework for cancer nursing* (2nd ed.). Canberra, Australia: The National Cancer Nursing Education Project (EdCaN), Cancer Australia.

Baumann, M., Baumann, C., LeBihan, E., & Chau, N. (2008). How patients perceive the therapeutic communications skills of their general practitioners, and how that perception affects adherence: Use of the TCom-skill GP scale in a specific geographical area. *BMC Health Services Research, 8,* 244–253.

Bhui, K. S., Aslam, R. W., Palinski, A., McCabe, R., Johnson, M. R., Weich, S., … Szczepura, A. (2015). Interventions to improve therapeutic communications between Black and minority ethnic patients and professionals in psychiatric services: Systematic review. *British Journal of Psychiatry: The Journal of Mental Science, 207*(2), 95–103.

Campbell, S. H., & Aredes, N. D. A. (2017, June 21). *Reliability and validity of the global interprofessional therapeutic communication scale (GITCS©).* Paper Presentation at INACSL International Annual Conference, Washington, DC, USA.

Canadian Nurses Association. (2008). Code of ethics for registered nurses. Retrieved from https://www.cna-aiic.ca/~/media/cna/page-content/pdf-fr/code-of-ethics-for-registered-nurses.pdf?la=en

Caron, A., Perzynski, A., Thomas, C., Saade, J. Y., McFarlane, M., & Becker, J. (2013). Development of the objective, structured communication assessment of residents (OSCAR) tool for measuring communication skills with patients. *Journal of Graduate Medical Education, 5*(4), 570–575.

Clancy, C. M. (2008). The importance of simulation: Preventing hand-off mistakes. *Association of peri-Operative Registered Nurses Journal, 88*(4), 625–627.

Commission, J. (2010). 2010 national patient safety goals. Retrieved from www.jointcommission.org/standards_information/npsgs.aspx

Cooper, S., Beauchamp, A., Bogossian, F., Bucknall, T., Cant, R., Devries, B.,...Young, S. (2012). Managing patient deterioration: A protocol for enhancing undergraduate nursing students' competence through web-based simulation and feedback techniques. *BioMed Central Nursing, 11*(1), 18.

Decker, S., Fey, M., Sideras, S., Caballero, S., Rockstraw, L., Boese, T.,...Borum, J. C. (2013). Standards of best practice: Simulation standard VI: The debriefing process. *Clinical Simulation in Nursing, 9*(6), S26–S29. doi:10.1016/j.ecns.2013.04.008

Doolen, J., Giddings, M., Johnson, M., de Nathan, G. G., & Badia, L. O. (2014). An evaluation of mental health simulation with standardized patients. *International Journal of Nursing Education Scholarship, 11*(1), 1–8. doi:10.1515/ijnes-2013-0075

Epstein, R. M., & Street, J. R. (2007). *A framework for patient-centered communication in cancer care: Promoting healing and reducing suffering.* Bethesda, MD: National Cancer Institute.

Fay-Hillier, T. M., Regan, R. V., & Gallagher Gordon, M. (2012). Communication and patient safety in simulation for mental health nursing education. *Issues in Mental Health Nursing, 33*(11), 718–726.

Fejzic, J., & Barker, M. (2015). Implementing simulated learning modules to improve students' pharmacy practice skills and professionalism. *Pharmacy Practice, 13*(3), 583. doi:10.18549/PharmPract.2015.03.583

Hammer, M., Fox, S., & Hampton, M. D. (2014). Use of a therapeutic communication simulation model in pre-licensure psychiatric mental health nursing: Enhancing strengths and transforming challenges. *Nursing and Health, 2*(1), 1–8. doi:10.13189/nh.2014.020101

Hill, W. (Producer). (2013). *Interior Health—"Transfer of Accountability"—Interactive handover* [Video]. Retrieved from https://www.youtube.com/watch?v=GSHcub4K-uk

Hill, W., & Marcellus, L. (2015, February). *IDRAW—Interactive handover: What should I be worried about? Quality measurement in ICU. A feasibility study and knowledge translation.* Paper presented at the BC-PSQC Quality Forum 2015, Vancouver, British Columbia. Retrieved from http://www.slideshare.net/bcpsqc/grouse-f6-what-should-i-be-worried-about-wrae-hill

Institute for Healthcare Improvement. (2016). SBAR toolkit. Retrieved from http://www.ihi.org/resources/pages/tools/sbartoolkit.aspx

Institute of Medicine. (2001). *For the committee on quality of health in America. To err is human: Building a safer health system.* Washington, DC: National Academies Press.

International Nursing Association for Clinical Simulation and Learning. (2015). Repository of instruments used in simulation research. Retrieved from http://www.inacsl.org/i4a/pages/index.cfm?pageID=3496

Interprofessional Education Collaboration. (2011). *Core competencies for interprofessional collaborative practice: Report of an expert panel.* Washington, DC: Author.

Kameg, K., Howard, V. M., Clochesy, J., Mitchell, A. M., & Suresky, J. M. (2010). The impact of high fidelity human simulation on self-efficacy of communication skills. *Issues in Mental Health Nursing, 31*(5), 315–323.

Kameg, K., Mitchell, A. M., Clochesy, J., Howard, V. M., & Suresky, J. (2009). Communication and human patient simulation in psychiatric nursing. *Issues in Mental Health Nursing, 30*(8), 503–508.

Kardong-Edgren, S., Adamson, K. A., & Fitzgerald, C. (2010). A review of currently published evaluation instruments for human patient simulation *Clinical Simulation in Nursing, 6*(1), e25–e35. doi:10.1016/j.ecns.2009.08.0004

Kawamura, A., Mylopoulos, M., Orsino, A., Jimenez, E., & McNaughton, N. (2016). Promoting the development of adaptive expertise: Exploring a simulation model for sharing a diagnosis of autism with parents. *Academic Medicine, 91*(11), 1576–1581.

Lai, C.-Y. (2016). Training nursing students' communication skills with online video peer assessment. *Computers & Education, 97,* 21–30. doi:10.1016/j.compedu.2016.02.017

Leonard, M., Graham, S., & Bonacum, D. (2004). The human factor: The critical importance of effective teamwork and communication in providing safe care. *Quality & Safety in Health Care, 13*(Suppl. 1), i85–i90.

Lum, L., Dowedoff, P., & Englander, K. (2016). Internationally educated nurses' reflections on nursing communication in Canada. *International Nursing Review, 63*(3), 344–351.

Mager, D. M. (2012). Home care patient with elevated blood sugars. In S. H. Campbell & K. M. Daley (Ed.), *Simulation scenarios for nursing educators: Making it real* (2nd ed., pp. 253–262). New York, NY: Springer Publishing.

Mosby's Medical Dictionary, 8th edition. (2009). Retrieved from http://medical-dictionary.thefree dictionary.com/therapeutic+communication

O'Shea, E., Pagano, M., Campbell, S. H., & Caso, G. (2013). A descriptive analysis of nursing student communication behaviors. *Clinical Simulation in Nursing, 9*(1), e5–e12.

Pagano, M., & Greiner, P. A. (2013). Enhancing communication skills through simulations. In S. H. Campbell & K. M. Daley (Ed.), *Simulation scenarios for nursing educators: Making it real* (2nd ed., pp. 17–23). New York, NY: Springer Publishing.

Pagano, M. P., O'Shea, E. R., Campbell, S. H., Currie, L. M., Chamberlin, E., & Pates, C. A. (2015). Validating the health communication assessment tool (HCAT). *Clinical Simulation in Nursing, 11*(9), 402–410.

Shapiro, M. J., Morey, J. C., Small, S. D., Langford, V., Kaylor, C. J., Jagminas, L., ...Jay, G. D. (2004). Simulation based teamwork training for emergency department staff: Does it improve clinical team performance when added to an existing didactic teamwork curriculum? *Quality & Safety in Health Care, 13*(6), 417–421.

Siminoff, L. A., Rogers, H. L., Waller, A. C., Harris-Haywood, S., Esptein, R. M., Carrio, F. B., ...Longo, D. R. (2011). The advantages and challenges of unannounced standardized patient methodology to assess healthcare communication. *Patient Education and Counseling, 82*(3), 318–324.

Strada, I., Vegni, E., & Lamiani, G. (2016). Talking with patients about sex: Results of an interprofessional simulation-based training for clinicians. *Internal and Emergency Medicine, 11*(6), 859–866.

Street, R. L., Jr., Makoul, G., Arora, N. K., & Epstein, R. M. (2013). How does communication heal? Pathways linking clinician-patient communication to health outcomes. *Patient Education and Counseling, 74*(3), 295–301. doi:10.1016/j.pec.2008.11.015

Theilen, U., Leonard, P., Jones, P., Ardill, R., Weitz, J., Agrawal, D., & Simpson, D. (2013). Regular in situ simulation training of paediatric medical emergency team improves hospital response to deteriorating patients. *Resuscitation, 84*(2), 218–222.

Therapeutic communication. (2017). *Taber's cyclopedic medical dictionary* (23rd ed.). Philadelphia, PA: F. A. Davis.

Thomas, C. M., Bertram, E., & Johnson, D. (2009). The SBAR communication technique: Teaching nursing students professional communication skills. *Nurse Educator, 34*(4), 176–180.

Weaver, S. J., Rosen, M. A., DiazGranados, D., Lazzara, E. H., Lyons, R., Salas, E., ...King, H. B. (2010). Does teamwork improve performance in the operating room? A multilevel evaluation. *Joint Commission Journal on Quality and Patient Safety, 36*(3), 133–142.

World Health Organization. (2010). Framework for action on interprofessional education and collaborative care. Retrieved from http://www.who.int/hrh/resources/framework_action/en

Zhang, C., Miller, C., Volkman, K., Meza, J., & Jones, K. (2015). Evaluation of the team performance observation tool with targeted behavioral markers in simulation-based interprofessional education. *Journal of Interprofessional Care, 29*(3), 202–208.

CHAPTER 5

Innovative Approaches to Simulation-Based Faculty Development

Suzanne Hetzel Campbell, Maura MacPhee, and Maureen M. Ryan

The demands for meeting the needs of 21st-century students, especially in the health professions, are increasing exponentially. A method of using technology, simulation, has been recognized as a valuable tool for the development of critical thinking and clinical reasoning and competence in nursing students (Adamson, 2015; Cant & Cooper, 2010; Carter, Creedy, & Sidebotham, 2016; Chau et al., 2001; Dreifuerst, 2012; Fero et al., 2010; Hayden, Smiley, Alexander, Kardong-Edgren, & Jeffries, 2014; Jeffries, 2005; Nehring, Lashley, & Ellis, 2002; Peteani, 2004; Rauen, 2004). Although students tend to favor the use of simulation in teaching (Gillan, Jeong, & van der Riet, 2014), the faculty can be resistant to this complex teaching methodology recognizing the investment in time and resources and the learning curve it involves (Nehring & Lashley, 2004). Even so, it is feasible to increase faculty capacity in the use of simulation without negative impacts on faculty work life or student outcomes (Richardson, Goldsamt, Simmons, Gilmartin, & Jeffries, 2014). Because of the high costs associated with the use of patient simulators in nursing education (Harlow & Sportsman, 2007; Metcalfe, Hall, & Carpenter, 2007), care must be taken in the planning, implementation, and evaluation of simulation-based programs and in the preparation of faculty for its integration and use.

As mentioned in Chapter 3, faculty buy-in is of the utmost importance in a successful integration of simulation and technology into the nursing curriculum. With all the advances in education and technology, nursing faculty can feel overwhelmed with the increasing expectations. They need time to integrate these new teaching tools and receive assistance with the actual process. The chapter in the second edition of this text described the "faculty learning community" that was created at Fairfield University School of Nursing—it was novel at the time and the facilitator for that group helped write the chapter (Shea, Campbell, & Miners, 2013). In this edition, this chapter outlines some innovative methods for developing faculty and even interprofessional opportunities for increasing the use, effectiveness, and excitement of simulation pedagogy in health care professional education. Examples from two universities in British Columbia (BC), Canada, will be provided as well as a global perspective of the "state of faculty development."

Traditionally, faculty who are early adopters and take on the initiative of incorporating simulation into their courses may at best receive course release time to revise a course on their own. Usually, it is another "expected addition" to the faculty role. The equipment is purchased, a lab director oversees its use, and faculty are expected to work this out. To provide optimum student learning experiences, changes in educational practices need to be incorporated with pedagogic principles, which in turn guide the development and implementation of simulation activities and the integration of technology (Jeffries, 2005). Faculty need to be given the opportunity to reflect on connections between simulation and (a) their individual teaching philosophy and (b) the attainment of student competency in core areas.

With the many changes occurring in the health care delivery system, it is important to develop resilience in the nursing faculty so that they can feel confident in their ability to educate the next generation of learners. As one of the authors and editors of this book, I have had the privilege of traveling around the globe and meeting colleagues from nursing and a multitude of disciplines who are struggling with similar challenges—the need to educate more health professionals with fewer resources and fewer faculty. Socializing students into the profession of nursing, helping them gain the foundational knowledge they need, yet be able to apply it in real time to constantly changing situations is the goal and passion of nursing faculty. Using creative teaching methods and experiential learning allows for that transition and growth, and often faculty and students come to find that it helps them dig deeper and learn more. In planning for simulation, I have seen many schools with good intentions order all the equipment and not take into consideration the faculty development needed to learn to use it and the pedagogy needed to integrate it into the curriculum. The university administration has recognized the need for "flipped classrooms," flexible and experiential learning, yet may not recognize the commitment needed to make it happen. Learning to integrate technology and new learning styles into one's teaching requires time, guidance, and support. The rest of this chapter introduces two different ways of moving forward with innovative methods to develop health professional faculty in their ability to integrate technology, experiential learning, and be excited in their role. We hope the insights provide you with ideas for your own programs.

OVERVIEW OF FACULTY DEVELOPMENT AT THE UNIVERSITY OF BRITISH COLUMBIA SCHOOL OF NURSING—MAURA MACPHEE

In 2013, the University of British Columbia (UBC) began a campus-wide flexible learning initiative to enhance educational outcomes for students by enabling more flexible access to learning and improving teaching effectiveness through new learning models. Flexible learning encompasses pedagogical and logistical flexibility in higher education, typically facilitated by technology (Arfield, Hodgkinson, Smith, & Wade, 2013). Pedagogical flexibility includes flexible delivery, interaction, and media instruction; and logistical flexibility refers to flexibility of location, time, and pace of learning. Flexible learning approaches address the needs of diverse learners, and these approaches optimize the use of faculty time, expertise, and available resources (e.g., simulation lab space).

The faculty at the School of Nursing received a UBC Teaching and Learning Enhancement Fund (TLEF) award to facilitate flexible learning goal attainment, beginning with transformation of the undergraduate curriculum. We began by focusing on our practice-based education courses. A project team of undergraduate faculty members worked with two dedicated course and curriculum design experts from the UBC Centre of Teaching and Learning Technology (CTLT). With the TLEF award, we also hired a project manager to help us develop a 3-year project plan, timeline, budget, and evaluation strategies.

The overarching purpose for our TLEF award was to create an integrated learning model encompassing each component of our practice-based courses. Before the award, we had notable problems or "disconnects" between the theory and practice components of these courses. Our students learned about concepts in large lecture classes and often failed to have timely follow-through in the simulation lab and in practice. Our intention, therefore, was to use flexible learning strategies to make better linkages among existing course components, and to introduce flipped or blended learning to our curriculum.

Our integrated flexible learning model:

Online learning → active case-based learning → simulation → practice

The project team held a number of CTLT-led workshops to introduce nursing faculty to pedagogical and technological concepts associated with flexible learning. The purpose of these sessions was to better engage faculty in a community of teaching and learning, and to create a real institutional commitment to flexible learning. These sessions were particularly popular with our practice-based faculty and clinical instructors.

The TLEF award was also used to purchase a license for 1 year of unlimited use of an online nursing education resource for self-directed learning. The resource consists of "Master Educator" modules that demonstrate educational strategies and techniques. Faculty members could register via email and view and complete the online modules in their own time. Our Professional Practice Team, a faculty-led team of our clinical instructors, established regular sessions to view the modules together, and they developed a number of applications for preclinical student briefings, "teachable moments" during the clinical experience, and postclinical debriefing. Module content was also used to enhance orientation for new clinical instructors.

During the first year of our TLEF award, the project team focused on integration of online, modularized delivery of theory content within our six practice-based courses. These courses are:

- Foundations of Professional Practice (6 credits)
- Introduction to Professional Practice for Adults/Older Adults (8 credits)
- Professional Nursing Practice for Childbearing Women, Infants, and Their Families (6 credits)
- Professional Nursing Practice for Children and Their Families (6 credits)
- Professional Nursing Practice for Adults Living With Mental Illness and Their Families (6 credits)
- Professional Nursing Practice With Communities and Populations (6 credits) and
- Professional Nursing Practice With Adults/Old Adults and Their Families (6 credits).

Our first-year goal was to convert or "flip" approximately one third of traditional classroom seat time. Flipped classrooms offer pedagogical and logistical flexibility, and well-designed online learning can set the stage for more active engagement of students in class, in simulation labs, and in practice (McLaughlin et al., 2014; O'Flaherty & Phillips, 2015).

Faculty "champions" from the practice-based courses worked closely with our CTLT design experts to identify content in their curriculum that could be converted to online modules. To avoid the "talking head" phenomenon, CTLT experts taught the faculty how to create short, engaging modules with embedded questions. Case-based learning activities were developed to link online module prework to classroom dialogue and small-group work.

The next phase of our project is focused on linkages between online or in-class learning, simulation lab learning, and experiential learning in practice settings. The CTLT experts have helped us ensure that our redesigned curricular content and delivery will facilitate students' transformative learning experiences—and better induce a sense of thinking like a nurse (Benner, Sutphen, Leonard, & Day, 2009; Mezirow & Taylor, 2011).

Not surprising, our successes have depended on professional development and mentoring support for our clinical and tenured faculty. The constant evolution of new educational technology can challenge all of us. Release time and expert facilitation (e.g., CTLT) is needed to thoroughly engage faculty in the hard work of redesign, particularly the uptake of new technology. We are currently piloting commercially packaged online products to augment our own, faculty-designed modules. We would like to totally replace textbooks with online learning resources for students. Our project team hosted faculty sessions to preview new products with different vendors. We agreed to pilot two online products, and we committed some of our TLEF award to purchase the license for these products. We wanted to ensure a "fit" between our student–faculty needs and these products. Students, therefore, were not expected to purchase the program during the pilot phase. In both instances, these online products are United States' based. We were able to successfully adapt or "Canadianize" one product for our curriculum, and we are using the product in our introductory course for adult or older adult care. Students view online patient–nurse vignettes and complete group assignments in an online discussion forum. Although there was initial pushback from students, the second iteration of this course has gone more smoothly. We discovered that it was essential to engage with students right away, providing an overview of our flexible learning model. Including students as partners in the redesign process has helped us win over their skepticism.

With respect to the simulation lab and practice components of our model, we are limited by our physical space. We have been seeking out agreements with our practice partners to use their simulation space. We recently acquired another grant to develop a practice–academic collaboration for student–nurse simulation education. We codeveloped a range of simulation exercises (low to high fidelity) with nurse educators from nearby health care organizations. Our faculty also provided simulation training workshops for these nurse educators. Our faculty members have access to these sites' simulation labs during students' postclinical conference time. Our goal was to codevelop and corun simulations in practice sites for students and nursing staff, but we have had numerous scheduling challenges.

Evaluation strategies include annual student surveys and focus groups. We are tracking deliverables according to our project plan and timeline. Some of our key outcome indicators include the percentage of flipped content per course as well as the numbers of newly developed online modules, case scenarios, simulations, and pre-and postclinical briefing and/or debriefing packets. We are also determining whether there are explicit linkages among components of our model, based on course syllabus reviews by our Undergraduate Programs Committee. We have a number of research projects underway that are related to our flexible learning initiative. One collaborative research project is with Queensland University of Technology. We are developing screening tools for simulation lab and practice to assess students' clinical reasoning skills, based on a model by Levett-Jones and colleagues (2010).

In closing, one of the most notable outcomes of this initiative has been a culture shift among faculty with respect to pedagogical innovation. *Flexible learning* is a common term among faculty members, and use of online learning resources and simulation are becoming integral components of curriculum delivery. Students' resistance has been replaced by their desire to participate in more simulations. In fact, they are urging us to explore the new world of virtual simulation.

OVERVIEW OF FACULTY DEVELOPMENT AT THE UNIVERSITY OF VICTORIA: THE INTERPROFESSIONAL SIMULATION EDUCATOR PATHWAY—MAUREEN RYAN

In contemporary health care dialogues about health professional graduates, educators often hear that despite the best efforts of universities to ensure that their graduates are "practice ready," employers' call attention to a lack of job readiness. We suggest that one area of job readiness that is difficult for health professional students to learn during their education program concerns the executive skills necessary for teamwork (e.g., understanding roles, team communication, shared decision making) particularly in urgent patient care situations. Our collective experiences as clinical educators lead us to believe that health professional students do not have access to repeated, effective "hands-on training" in teamwork during their prelicensure education as a result of challenges associated in clinical placements. In other words, we question whether effective teamwork is consistently role-modeled in practice. As a result, our prelicensure students may have few executive skills in either leading or being part of collaborative team efforts that lead to safe and evidence-informed patient care on entry to the workforce. There is a call to attention to this problem in preparing health care professionals for interprofessional teamwork from the health care industry (Kohn, Corrigan, & Donaldson, 2000), and from Canada's National Steering Committee on Patient Safety (2002). We believe that waiting until students graduate and are on the job is almost too late for true effectiveness of team-based interprofessional education.

We believe that there should be a coherent and integrated interprofessional education (IPE) component of prelicensure education that places the patient in the center of focus. Such a program can provide opportunities for students from at least three different health professional education programs to work collaboratively on patient care teams on matters of mutual clinical concern. The benefits of an IPE program approach to teaching and learning about teamwork includes improving those professional practices and, as a result, patient outcomes (Vyas, McCulloh, Dyer,

Gregory, & Higbee, 2012; Zwarenstein, Goldman, & Reeves, 2009). Moreover, we suggest that if interprofessional student teams receive the necessary knowledge and practice before prelicensure examinations, they are better prepared for the realities of patient care practices (e.g., teamwork) in health care or "job ready" (Zwarenstein, Reeves, & Perrier, 2005).

Our collective experiences as simulation educators and our turn to literature informs us that simulation-based training is at the leading edge for teaching critical assessment; interprofessional team communication; and clinical judgment, reasoning, and reflective skills necessary for safe and effective patient care (Schwartz, Fernandez, Kouyoumijian, Jones, & Compton, 2007; Steadman et al., 2006; Ten Eyck, Tews, & Ballster, 2009). Concurrently, we acknowledge that one of the cited challenges in implementing effective and sustainable interprofessional education programs is faculty development (Gilbert, 2005; Steinert, 2005). Similarly, faculty development is required for implementing simulation education programs (Hallmark, 2015; McGaghie, Issenberg, Petrusa, & Scalese, 2010). However, the challenge that lay before us was how to develop simulation education for facilitators that would address the interprofessional competencies called for to prepare health professional prelicensure students for entry to practice, and, at the same time, honor the diversity of disciplinary perspectives. In the following paragraphs, we share the process that we have undertaken to design and implement an interprofessional simulation facilitator education pathway as a necessary first step to preparing for interprofessional education of health professional students and employees. We will begin by describing our context of simulation education practice at the Center for Interprofessional Clinical Simulation Learning (CICSL) at the Royal Jubilee Hospital, Victoria, BC, Canada. We share the framework that we used to unify our academic and clinical simulation educators and the ways in which we are currently evaluating the effectiveness of our program elements.

Interprofessional Simulation Education Context

In 2011, a provincial initiative through the Ministry of Advanced Education and Technology commenced that served to guide the advancement of patient simulation Centres on Vancouver Island. At the core of this movement was the ideal of cross-organizational collaboration. As a result of this initiative, a simulation center in Victoria was envisioned and the development was led by deans and Health Authority executive directors from three partner organizations (University of Victoria School of Nursing, UBC Island Medical Program, and the Vancouver Island Health Authority). A Governance Committee was formed to oversee the building and organizational structuring of what would be known as the *CICSL*. At the same time, a curriculum-working group (CWG) was formed with a faculty lead from the School of Nursing and the Island Medical Program and a lead from the Professional Practice Office at the Island Health Authority. The work of the CWG was to demonstrate within its respective curriculum or professional practice committees how patient simulation would be used. In addition, the CWG members were trained as simulation trainers through a certificate program at the Centre for Excellence in Simulation Education and Innovation (CESEI), Vancouver, Canada, with a view of creating a community of practice in simulation education through a train-the-trainer approach to simulation educator development.

The CICSL pioneers a simulation teaching and learning center with three key stakeholders: Vancouver Island Health Authority, UBC's Island Medical Program, and the University of Victoria's School of Nursing. Indeed, the mission of CICSL is to:

- Provide a sustainable, safe, and supportive learning environment
- Foster interprofessional and interinstitutional collaboration
- Improve simulation education through evidence-informed practice

The CICSL opened in September 2015 with four simulation laboratories, a debrief room, two observation rooms, three clinical skills rooms, and a videoconference space. We also had the data collected from disciplinary and interprofessional pilot projects through the work of the CWG, which we believed would inform our next directions in operationalizing simulation education in Victoria. What we had learned by 2014 is that our respective students were embracing simulation learning events and demanding more and more opportunities. At the same time, our faculty and clinical educators were telling us that faculty development opportunities were necessary; this was important to note, because our educators were not fully comfortable teaching and learning in a simulation environment. Thus, how could we introduce yet more content in the form of interprofessional simulations when our educators were not yet fully comfortable teaching within their own professional context?

Interprofessional Simulation Educator Pathway

The idea of faculty development commonly refers to those activities and programs designed to improve instruction. As such, historically, the individual faculty member's development in teaching and learning has been at the forefront. Recently, the notion of faculty learning communities has emerged, suggesting that teaching and learning development goes beyond the individual's self-reflection to group thinking based on the engagement with a valued teaching and learning method (e.g., simulation and/or interprofessional education in simulation). Amundsen and colleagues (2005) outline four conceptual categories to faculty development: skill focus, method focus, process focus, and discipline focus. Moreover, there are differences in the expectation of the individual instructor in each of the previously listed four categories, that is, the difference between developing a skill, integrating a method into your own teaching approach, understanding the processes of self-reflection that contribute to pedagogical growth in teaching communities, and recognizing the values and assumptions about the development of knowledge and learning within your discipline. With this understanding of a faculty development framework, we recognized that development in simulation education would be two-fold. First, our educators would need to learn the skills and methods of simulation education within their own discipline. Within their own curricula, they would need to establish a level of comfort with the role of simulation educator. We believed that when a comfort level with skills and method was reached, faculty would be open to look at processes of simulation education, such as the pedagogical shifts associated with interprofessional education and the move outside of disciplinary thinking to embrace the multiple ways in which patient care is understood in an interdisciplinary team. We also learned from our readings on interprofessional education that role clarity was an important construct in interprofessional collaboration. Simply, until the learner understands, embraces, and feels comfortable executing the role offered through early education experiences (e.g., year 1 and 2 in nursing education) they will struggle in a team setting, focusing on their individual learning needs, and not fully able to self-reflect on the interprofessional collaboration.

Currently, faculty and clinical leadership have developed an introduction to facilitating simulation programs at the CICSL. All simulation educators receive introductory workshops and are signed off as having the basic knowledge and skill in simulation education necessary for teaching. The first workshop is cotaught by a member of their faculty or institution alongside a technologist, who provides information on how to operate the equipment and what resources are available in the center. The second workshop or other education materials are offered within their institution. For example, in nursing a simulation education community of practice exists in which instructors receive opportunities to engage with simulation pedagogy as it is understood within the undergraduate nursing curriculum. They have the opportunity to devise a simulation education development plan setting their own individualized goals and meeting the objectives of their role as set forth by the School of Nursing. Thus, from the instructor comes a goal to engage in collaborative learning across disciplines with a view to interprofessional education. In the next section, we describe the interprofessional development currently in place at the CICSL.

The Interprofessional Simulation Educator Pathway follows the tenets of the National Interprofessional Competency Framework (NICF) developed by the Canadian Interprofessional

Health Collaborative (Bainbridge, Nasmith, Orchard, & Wood, 2010; Canadian Interprofessional Health Collaborative [CIHC], 2007, 2010). The framework describes six domains of practice that highlight the knowledge, skills, attitudes, and values essential to interprofessional collaboration. Within each domain are a set of competencies that may be used as an educative guide for prelicensure students and an assessment of competency in the transition to practice. These domains are:

1. Role clarification
2. Team functioning
3. Patient/client/family/community-centered care
4. Collaborative leadership
5. Interprofessional communication
6. Interprofessional conflict resolution

A full tutorial of domains, competencies, and the quality indicators within each domain goes beyond the scope of this chapter. You may wish to visit www.cihc.ca/files/CIHC_IPCompetencies_Feb1210.pdf for a full introduction to this framework.

Our intent in developing the pathway is to increase the number of faculty or clinician interprofessional simulation facilitators, and, as a result, the number of interprofessional simulation-based educational opportunities for students or employees of the three partner organizations. We believe that the achievement of this goal will contribute to a sustainable community of practice in interprofessional simulation education. To achieve this goal, we have outlined three phases of development for faculty.

Phase I

Participants will work through UBC's online module series "Interprofessional Collaboration on the Run" (www.ipcontherun.ca). This online learning resource provides an overview of concepts and principles related to interprofessional collaborative practice. Each module is based on one of the domains identified in the NICF described in the previous paragraphs, and has a self-assessment component built into the content. This self-assessment introduces the participants to the strengths they may already have in their knowledge and skill of interprofessional collaborative practices. In addition, they can outline their own individual learning needs to ready them for Phase II of the pathway. Each module takes about 30 minutes to complete.

Phase II

Expert simulation facilitators from academia and nursing, medicine, and allied health professions will facilitate hands-on application of the CIHC competencies using simulation-based learning events for health professional educators in education and practice facilities. The 4-hour learning event provides opportunities for participants to apply knowledge and practice skill in debriefing interprofessional competencies. The development of case scenarios will be informed by our practice leads, who will recount those areas in clinical practice in which interprofessional collaboration is needed and often missing.

Phase III

Our intent in this phase is to evaluate our pathway. We compare and contrast the knowledge, skills, and attitudes of simulation facilitators and student learners about the CIHC Interprofessional Competencies and the benefit of interprofessional education opportunities before and following the implementation of Phase I and Phase II. Data collected will measure the participant's baseline and predicted increase in knowledge, skills, and attitudes related to the use of IPE competencies. Moreover, we have established local evidence to inform ongoing support for IPE simulation education sessions, and we believe, inform and sustain an interprofessional collaboration community of practice.

CONCLUSION

This chapter has outlined some innovative ways of incorporating faculty professional development in the use of simulation and innovative technology to enhance teaching of nursing students and other health professionals. Managing faculty angst while they consider new methods of teaching to enhance their teaching effectiveness requires looking for creative ways to move forward and incorporating simulation so that it fits faculties' personal teaching philosophy and style. The increased growth in the nontraditional student population in nursing and students' demand for more use of technology in the classroom to prepare them for health care practice arenas means that faculty need to develop new strategies. Identifying faculty champions, leaders who can role-model and share ideas as well as support faculty in a collaborative and nonthreatening manner is key to the success of integrating simulation and new technologies into the classroom, lab, and clinical sites. Providing faculty the necessary resources is important for success and educating the next generation of nursing faculty in this technology is paramount.

REFERENCES

Adamson, K. (2015). A systematic review of the literature related to the NLN/Jeffries simulation framework. *Nursing Education Perspectives, 36*(5), 281–291.

Amundsen, C., Abrami, P., McAlpine, L., Weston, C., Krbavac, M., Mundy, A., & Wilson, M. (2005, April 11). *The what and why of faculty development in higher education: An in-depth review of the literature.* Paper presented at the American Education Research Association, Montreal, QC, Canada. Retrieved from https://convention2.allacademic.com/one/aera/aera05/index.php?click_key=1&cmd=Multi+Search+Load+Person&people_id=185918&PHPSESSID=b2fpor2113pb94bi0u1b8m1i04

Arfield, J., Hodgkinson, K., Smith, A., & Wade, W. (2013). *Flexible learning in higher education.* New York, NY: Routledge.

Bainbridge, L., Nasmith, L., Orchard, C. & Wood, V. (2010). Competencies for interprofessional collaboration. *Journal of Physical Therapy Education, 24*(1), 6–11.

Benner, P., Sutphen, M., Leonard, V., & Day, L. (2009). *Educating nurses: A call for radical transformation* (Vol. 15). San Francisco, CA: Jossey-Bass.

Canadian Interprofessional Health Collaborative. (2007). Interprofessional education and core competencies: Literature review. Retrieved from http://www.cihc.ca/files/publications/CIHC_IPE-LitReview_May07.pdf

Canadian Interprofessional Health Collaborative. (2010). A national interprofessional competency framework. Retrieved from https://www.cihc.ca/files/CIHC_IPCompetencies_Feb1210.pdf

Cant, R. P., & Cooper, S. J. (2010). Simulation-based learning in nurse education: Systematic review. *Journal of Advanced Nursing, 66*(1), 3–15.

Carter, A. G., Creedy, D. K., & Sidebotham, M. (2016). Efficacy of teaching methods used to develop critical thinking in nursing and midwifery undergraduate students: A systematic review of the literature. *Nurse Education Today, 40,* 209–218.

Chau, J. P., Chang, A. M., Lee, I. F., Ip, W. Y., Lee, D. T., & Wootton, Y. (2001). Effects of using videotaped vignettes on enhancing students' critical thinking ability in a baccalaureate nursing programme. *Journal of Advanced Nursing, 36*(1), 112–119.

Dreifuerst, K. T. (2012). Using debriefing for meaningful learning to foster development of clinical reasoning in simulation. *Journal of Nursing Education, 51*(6), 326–333.

Fero, L. J., O'Donnell, J. M., Zullo, T. G., Dabbs, A. D., Kitutu, J., Samosky, J. T., & Hoffman, L. A. (2010). Critical thinking skills in nursing students: Comparison of simulation-based performance with metrics. *Journal of Advanced Nursing, 66*(10), 2182–2193.

Gilbert, J. H. (2005). Interprofessional learning and higher education structural barriers. *Journal of Interprofessional Care, 19*(Suppl. 1), 87–106.

Gillan, P. C., Jeong, S., & van der Riet, P. J. (2014). End of life care simulation: A review of the literature. *Nurse Education Today, 34*(5), 766–774.

Hallmark, B. F. (2015). Faculty development in simulation education. *Nursing Clinics of North America, 50*(2), 389–397.

Harlow, K. C., & Sportsman, S. (2007). An economic analysis of patient simulators clinical training in nursing education. *Nursing Economic$, 25*(1), 24–29, 3.

Hayden, J. K., Smiley, R. A., Alexander, M., Kardong-Edgren, S., & Jeffries, P. R. (2014). The NCSBN national simulation study: A longitudinal, randomized, controlled study replacing clinical hours with simulation in prelicensure nursing education. *Journal of Nursing Regulation, 5*(2), S1–S64.

Jeffries, P. R. (2005). A framework for designing, implementing, and evaluating simulations used as teaching strategies in nursing. *Nursing Education Perspectives, 26*(2), 96–103.

Kohn, L., Corrigan, J., & Donaldson, M. (Eds.). (2000). *To err is human: Building a safer health system.* Washington, DC: Institute of Medicine, Committee on Quality of Health Care in America.

Levett-Jones, T., Hoffman, K., Dempsey, J., Jeong, S. Y., Noble, D., Norton, C. A., . . . Hickey, N. (2010). The "five rights" of clinical reasoning: An educational model to enhance nursing students' ability to identify and manage clinically "at risk" patients. *Nurse Education Today, 30*(6), 515–520.

McGaghie, W. C., Issenberg, S. B., Petrusa, E. R., & Scalese, R. J. (2010). A critical review of simulation-based medical education research: 2003-2009. *Medical Education, 44*(1), 50–63.

McLaughlin, J. E., Roth, M. T., Glatt, D. M., Gharkholonarehe, N., Davidson, C. A., Griffin, L. M., . . . Mumper, R. J. (2014). The flipped classroom: A course redesign to foster learning and engagement in a health professions school. *Academic Medicine, 89*(2), 236–243.

Metcalfe, S. E., Hall, V. P., & Carpenter, A. (2007). Promoting collaboration in nursing education: The development of a regional simulation laboratory. *Journal of Professional Nursing, 23*(3), 180–183.

Mezirow, J., & Taylor, E. W. (2011). *Transformative learning in practice: Insights from community, workplace, and higher education.* San Francisco, CA: Jossey-Bass.

National Steering Committee on Patient Safety. (2002). *Building a safer system: A national integrated strategy for improving patient safety in Canadian health care.* Ottawa, Canada: Author.

Nehring, W. M., & Lashley, F. R. (2004). Current use and opinions regarding human patient simulators in nursing education: An international survey. *Nursing Education Perspectives, 25*(5), 244–248.

Nehring, W. M., Lashley, F. R., & Ellis, W. E. (2002). Critical incident nursing management: Using human patient simulators. *Nursing Education Perspectives, 23*(3), 128–132.

O'Flaherty, J., & Phillips, C. (2015). The use of flipped classrooms in higher education: A scoping review. *Internet and Higher Education, 25*, 85–95. doi: 10.1016/j.iheduc.2015.02.002

Peteani, L. A. (2004). Enhancing clinical practice and education with high-fidelity human patient simulators. *Nurse Educator, 29*(1), 25–30.

Rauen, C. A. (2004). Simulation as a teaching strategy for nursing education and orientation in cardiac surgery. *Critical Care Nurse, 24*(3), 46–51.

Richardson, H., Goldsamt, L. A., Simmons, J., Gilmartin, M., & Jeffries, P. R. (2014). Increasing faculty capacity: Findings from an evaluation of simulation clinical teaching. *Nursing Education Perspectives, 35*(5), 308–314.

Schwartz, L. R., Fernandez, R., Kouyoumjian, S. R., Jones, K. A., & Compton, S. (2007). A randomized comparison trial of case-based learning versus human patient simulation in medical student education. *Academic Emergency Medicine, 14*(2), 130–137.

Shea, J. M., Campbell, S. H., & Miners, L. (2013). Faculty learning communities: An innovative approach to faculty development. In S. H. Campbell & K. M. Daley (Eds.), *Simulation scenarios for nursing educators: Making it real* (2nd ed., pp. 25–31). New York, NY: Springer Publishing.

Steadman, R. H., Coates, W. C., Huang, Y. M., Matevosian, R., Larmon, B. R., McCullough, L., & Ariel, D. (2006). Simulation-based training is superior to problem-based learning for the acquisition of critical assessment and management skills. *Critical Care Medicine, 34*(1), 151–157.

Steinert, Y. (2005). Learning together to teach together: Interprofessional education and faculty development. *Journal of Interprofessional Care, 19*(Suppl. 1), 60–75.

Ten Eyck, R. P., Tews, M., & Ballester, J. M. (2009). Improved medical student satisfaction and test performance with a simulation-based emergency medicine curriculum: A randomized controlled trial. *Annals of Emergency Medicine, 54*(5), 684–691.

Vyas, D., McCulloh, R., Dyer, C., Gregory, G., & Higbee, D. (2012). An interprofessional course using human patient simulation to teach patient safety and teamwork skills. *American Journal of Pharmaceutical Education, 76*(4), 71. doi:10.5688/ajpe76471

Zwarenstein, M., Goldman, J., & Reeves, S. (2009). Interprofessional collaboration: Effects of practice-based interventions on professional practice and healthcare outcomes. *Cochrane Database of Systematic Reviews, 2009*(3), CD000072. doi:10.1002/14651858CD000072.pub2

Zwarenstein, M., Reeves, S., & Perrier, L. (2005). Effectiveness of pre-licensure interprofessional education and post-licensure collaborative interventions. *Journal of Interprofessional Care, 19*(Suppl. 1), 148–165.

FURTHER READING

BC's Practice Education Committee. (2013). Advancing teamwork in health care: A guide and toolkit for building capacity and facilitating interprofessional collaborative practice and education. Retrieved from http://www.dal.ca/content/dam/dalhousie/pdf/healthprofessions/Interprofessional%20 Health%20Education/BCAHC%20-%20IPE%20Building%20Guide%20-%20January%202013-1.pdf

Mirriahi, N., Alonzo, D., & Fox, B. (2015). A blended learning framework for curriculum design and professional development. *Research in Learning Technology, 23*, 1–14. doi: 10.3402/rlt.v23.28451

CHAPTER 6

Building and Maintaining a Learning Resource Center

Karen M. Daley, Suzanne Hetzel Campbell, Diana R. Mager, and Cathryn Jackson

Traditionally, nursing programs have taught and practiced technical skills in a "nursing lab." As time has passed and technology has evolved, these labs have expanded to include computer stations, web access, and computer-based learning platforms for skill acquisition. Today, nursing labs often contain all the resources needed for teaching and learning nursing skills through integrated processes that include mock-ups of a hospital. In addition, the technology in the nurse's practice setting is growing and expanding at an exponential rate. Computers are used for fully computerized charting and for interfacing with all departments and personnel. For many hospitals, test results and orders are delivered via computer. In addition, many nursing stations—once essential as a place for nursing documentation—have been replaced with individual workstations on wheels, called *WOWs,* for each nurse for each shift. Each clinical placement for the student presents faculty and students with technologic challenges that change every semester; new computerized equipment and care systems abound. It has become essential that any nursing lab, frequently called a *learning resource center,* includes the latest state-of-the-art equipment for patient care as well as patient care delivery systems. It is no longer adequate for students to just show up and perform basic nursing tasks; it is essential for students to become an active part of the simulated learning environment in order to learn.

To that end, nursing programs are finding that the traditional lab is inadequate to meet the needs of today's students. Technology has become a necessary means to support, deliver, and evaluate nursing competencies. Skill-based education is still essential and can be delivered through static and computerized learning modules. However, preparation of students for a complex health care environment requires that students are educated not only in skills, but also in communication, safety, and collaborative care. Varied levels of technology assist in this endeavor. Whether static, low fidelity, medium fidelity, or high fidelity, all should be available to assist students in meeting learning objectives.

ENVISIONING A CENTER

Many programs have worked diligently to expand, room by room, from a nursing lab to a learning resource center. These centers include simulation labs, static skill labs, resource libraries with nursing references, and, ideally, a computer lab. Several programs have benefited from large grants that allowed architectural design and construction of the ideal environment. In either case, creating a vision and a plan are essential. Other schools have creatively used available space to alter the methods with which they provide simulation education. However, no amount of planning guarantees a smooth transition from lab to center.

The needs of a program shift quickly with enrollment changes, which challenges simulation practice space and classroom use. As enrollment increases and expansion of program courses extend into summer and intersession time periods, lab spaces need to be easily accessible to meet the needs of a variety of courses. The flexibility of the space is of utmost importance. The objective of providing a multifaceted learning experience must be the foundation of any learning resource center endeavor.

The vision for the center should not be a one-person quest; although, often that is exactly how the journey starts. Faculty buy-in is crucial! Otherwise, the human patient simulators (HPSs) may become nothing more than "very expensive paperweights" (J. Novotny, 2008, personal communication). Communicating the need campus-wide is an additional challenge. Just as no man is an island, no department exists alone. Many departments will be involved in the successful implementation of a learning resource center.

When considering the needs of the faculty, students, and curriculum, envisioning the center requires outlining areas of importance. These areas include space issues, equipment needs, technology, support personnel (lab, information technology [IT], and students), funding, and faculty development. One way of prioritizing these needs is to create a "wish list" to help identify what is realistic, given situational factors.

When creating a wish list, consider dividing it into the following sections:

- **Grand wish list:** Things you would get if you had unlimited funds.
- **Desired wish list:** Items that the faculty specifically request for courses.
- **Realistic wish list:** Items that match the actual funding and budget for purchase-order development based on a prioritization of the grand and desired wish lists.

Space issues, lab layouts and consideration of needs, and flexibility of space may include the following:

- Furniture that is easily mobile (stackable, rolling)
- Storage units for equipment and other resources
- Computer technology to meet multiple needs including wireless and cloud capabilities to capture and replay learning interactions
- Interchangeable classrooms for lecture, computer-assisted instruction, small-group interaction, health assessment, technical skill performance, group presentation, and simulation scenarios.

LEARNING RESOURCE ROOM AND OPERATING ROOM CENTER ESSENTIALS FOR SIMULATION LEARNING

No two nursing labs or learning resource centers are ever the same. When conceptualizing your center, important considerations include the following:

- Available space (e.g., is it shared with other university programs?)
- Large lab room versus multiple smaller rooms or areas
- Determination of the number of specialty rooms or areas, such as medical–surgical, intensive care unit (ICU), operating room (OR), pediatrics, women's health, home care, long-term care
- The relevance of lab needs to the present nursing curriculum (e.g., how many classes at a time will need the space, at what points in the semester, and during what time frames)

- Incorporation of other components or threads, such as communication, palliative care, leadership, delegation, and documentation
- Specific equipment needs
- A vision that incorporates input from faculty, administration, and students—buy-in is crucial at all levels
- Availability of lab personnel to assist with setting up and running the scenario
- Use of volunteers to role-play (visual and performing arts students, members of the AARP, retired doctors and nurses, health communication faculty or majors, other students and faculty)
- Faculty resources for curriculum development and planning (Center for Academic Excellence, Scholarship of Teaching and Learning Centers)
- Use of other departments and colleagues on campus, such as Business to help with the development of a plan for sustainability
- IT and media support

Early in the process of developing a center, one HPS may be used for multiple purposes, but over time, we have found it best to designate specialty areas in order to focus on specific learning experiences. Setting up simulation labs so that the specialty-specific simulation area is self-contained may be preferable (e.g., a pediatric area should have all pediatric equipment needed for scenarios and teaching). Should the rooms be separated by larger distances (e.g., separate buildings), one might find it necessary to duplicate equipment for both areas. Ideally, the simulation area should be a classroom-size area with a cart or cabinets that have room for all necessary equipment. If possible, having a classroom nearby with projection capability to record and project real-time scenario enactment from the simulation rooms would be ideal. In this situation, the larger classroom could function as a learning environment to allow the knowledge transfer from simulation to the classroom and, eventually, from the classroom to hands-on care. In a separate venue, the participants in the simulation need time for debriefing of the scenario during which a small group can sit to discuss specifics about its role and how things might go differently.

In addition, having a resource area, where copies of textbooks and references are available so that students can readily access the information needed to meet their learning goals during the simulation, is helpful. Often, when students have an opportunity to "redo," this reference area facilitates the processing of an unsuccessful scenario. Students can search for solutions on site and use the computers available.

Props that enhance the "realness" of the scenario are helpful as well, such as stretchers; charts; a crash cart; a defibrillator; EKG machine; and intravenous (IV) solutions, lines, and machines. The room or area should feel *real* as much as possible to enhance the authenticity of the scenario. Students should feel less like they are "playing pretend" and more like this simulation could really be happening. Of course, once the simulation starts, it often takes on a life of its own. In order to further enhance the realness, the setup needs to be efficient. The key to successful scenarios is to be able to set up quickly and dress the HPS for success with wounds, a Foley catheter and IV, medications, a chart, and equipment nearby. One idea is to put together grab and-go packets or plastic bins for each scenario so that assembly and takedown time are minimal. The packets or bins should be nearby in a cabinet or treatment-type cart for easy portability. Technical materials, such as video and sound equipment and various computers, should not be noticeable. Many programs use control rooms with a one-way mirror or have the scenario controller behind a curtain. However, with the addition of the personal digital assistant and now tablet remote access on some HPSs, the person controlling the scenario can be nearby or in the scene making rapid click-and-go adjustments to the scenario as it progresses.

Considering the high expense of these medium- and high-fidelity HPSs, having a plan for downtime usage becomes important as time passes. Often, HPS use is somewhat seasonal depending on course rotations, so making the most of using the HPS is key. Partnering with outside agencies for staff training, updating skills, accreditation standards, and/or new staff competency training allows collaboration with local key groups. Using the simulation lab as an income-generating entity during low usage times is always a possibility, as is donating use of the facility to agencies that have gone above and beyond accommodating student placements. Also, in the summer months, the simulation labs and learning resource center can be used for accelerated programs, graduate courses, and continuing education programs.

KAREN'S FIRST STORY: WESTERN CONNECTICUT STATE UNIVERSITY

At Western Connecticut State University (WCSU), our first lab expansion involved many individuals, from the dean to the chair of university computing, to maintenance, purchasing, and accounts payable, just to name a few. The second expansion involved the president, purchasing, multiple assistants and secretaries, and university computing technicians as well as several faculty members. Phase III of this expansion project resulted from a federal nursing initiative (U.S. Department of Education, 2008) negotiated by the university provost, and we needed many departments' help to renovate a space and to set up and maintain a lab. With a drastic increase in enrollment, expanding access to all levels of simulation is the primary goal. Having one or two people leading the way who have good relationships with all departments will facilitate the progress of the project, but an entire team working together during the implementation helps. Resources needed include working with Laerdal Create-a-Lab® and the university architect to develop the final layout. Often, there is no time for a new building, so making the most of the space you have, using fresh paint and minor renovations (e.g., removing old cabinets, replacing countertops), and rewiring for equipment is best when time is of the essence. Labs may need to be set up during times when classes are not in session, such as the summer months. Although having a vision is crucial, be open to other ideas to get what is needed, even if it may look very different from the initial picture in your mind.

Dollars, Donations, and Finances

Funding new resource centers and expansion projects is costly and challenging. Most facilities have written multiple grant applications and met with various successes and failures. Securing money from many sources is often necessary. It may take several months to years to secure adequate funding. In the case of WCSU, the simulation journey began to take shape after 2 years of grant writing. Three entities came together to finance the first HPS: the vice president of academic affairs; the dean's office; and the director of university computing, whose generosity provided the bulk of the money. Within 2 years, a new simulator and space were needed to provide more access to simulation. The timing was perfect, because a new science building on campus left the old building empty. With the backing of the university president, a five-room astronomy suite was designated as the new lab, and with cleaning, renovation, and electrical work, the space was made usable for us. Because the new science building was being finished, we had contractors on campus doing other work, so they were able to help with our renovations. In addition, another grant came in that year from which funds for equipment were secured. The lab was ready for the fall semester. Much more work was needed to upgrade the lab over time, but the space is an excellent area for an assessment lab, a simulation room, a seminar room, a pediatric lab, a classroom space with Internet access, and a resource room.

Individual faculty members have secured small grants for simulation projects, with funds for equipment embedded in the grant. This money was used to set up individual stations for each HPS. A crash cart or treatment cart works best to store the equipment needed for simulations. Each high-fidelity HPS began by residing in a hospital bed. These beds made it difficult to move the HPS. Stretchers work best to make the HPS movable. Some faculty have taken the HPS "on the road" by using wheelchairs. There are anecdotal reports that one HPS made it to graduation and made a speech. The more movable, the better for taking to class and doing mock codes in interesting places. Hospitals may donate minimally broken stretchers that are too dangerous for patients but are fine for an HPS.

Faculties have also secured summer curriculum funds in order to have focused time for scenario writing and setup. In addition, faculty have used faculty funds to attend training conferences, obtain time release for research studies using the new simulation equipment, and encourage colleagues to get outside training. In addition, it was necessary to train the university technology staff to help with upgrades and troubleshooting.

Of course, the best-case scenario is when a very large grant or donation is secured to cover all aspects of a learning resource center.

KAREN'S DAVENPORT UNIVERSITY SIMULATION EXPERIENCE

In June 2011, I had the privilege of joining Davenport University's College of Health Professions as the dean. This college was in the process of building three state-of-the-art simulation labs on three different campuses. When I arrived, the Grand Rapids lab was complete and awaiting some updated simulators. Within days of my arrival, I was asked to give approval for the plans for a newly constructed lab in Midland, Michigan, that was to be fully stocked and ready to start when the students arrived. By the fall of 2011 we held a ribbon-cutting ceremony for that Midland campus. At the same time, renovation of a fundamentals lab into a simulation lab was in progress in Warren, Michigan. We held the ribbon cutting for that lab in spring 2012.

Each lab contains a fundamentals area and a simulation lab complete with a control room and access to a computer lab. Each lab was fully funded by the university. Davenport's visionary president, Dr. Pappas, set a goal that every campus that had nursing programs would be outfitted with a state-of-the-art simulation lab. With the support of the provost, Dr. Rinker, we were able to achieve this goal. From that endeavor, we have secured additional funding from donors who became interested in purchasing the most updated equipment. This spring, Laerdal SimMoms® arrived on each campus. We have since witnessed several "births." Simulation expenses are now part of the yearly budget process on each campus. It is indeed exciting to have the full support of the administration as we move forward. As we built a new campus, we were able to equip it with a higher level of simulation labs available for the nursing students and health profession students.

Unique to Davenport is the role of the simulation, clinical, and lab coordinator. Each campus has a full-time faculty member in this role. These faculty members receive release time for this role (although not nearly enough). These coordinators work together to set the simulation goals for all four campuses and programs. Each orders supplies and facilitates scheduling of simulation experiences. Each will attend Drexel's Simulation Certification program within the next year to reaffirm their role as simulation experts.

For me (Karen), this is the realization of a dream that all students have access to the highest level of simulation experiences as a given, not as an additional educational experience. At the ribbon cutting, students spoke highly of the versatility of the simulation experiences and how simulation helped them achieve educational goals. In an excerpt from a speech by a Davenport student given at the Warren ribbon cutting, Jonne Toliver stated:

> It is very important in my learning experience to make a connection between theory concepts and clinical practice. This is the place where clinical thinking skills are built. In a simulation, you will be surprised how much knowledge you have retained because you have got the chance to experience it in some form or another. This is the place where mistakes are made, not because I don't understand the material, but because this is my first real-life experience seeing a condition. After the first encounter, I have baseline knowledge about what to expect if I ever see that again. This is the place where anxiety and fear come to the surface because of inexperience, but I am relieved to know in the back of my mind that this is a controlled environment that I have the opportunity to learn without any pressure. This is the place [where] I can get feedback from my

instructors, because when I reach a professional level I am the one that is responsible. This is the time for me to make safe adjustments to my technique before entering my career.
The transition from experiencing a lab with minimal variability to a simulation lab with infinite possibilities is a true accomplishment for Davenport University. Technology is an entity that surrounds us and this nursing lab implements the use of something that nurses use every day (J. Toliver, personal communication, April 23, 2012).

As is evident in Jonne's speech, although we set out believing that simulation would assist the students to learn nursing, it is the students who know the full value and make all of our simulation journeys worthwhile, no matter how we get there!

DIANA AND SUZANNE'S STORY: FAIRFIELD UNIVERSITY SCHOOL OF NURSING

For the Fairfield University School of Nursing (SON), the vision for the integration of simulation-focused learning developed over time and required support from a variety of individuals and groups. As is sometimes the case when the stars align and all the right pieces fall into place, we were fortunate to have that happen for us. In early 2005, there was a decentralizing of the development office at the university, which led to the SON receiving a designated development officer—the foundation relation officer. At about the same time, a nursing student graduated after working her senior year in the nursing lab and, at the pinning ceremony, handed the dean a check for $40,000 to purchase an HPS. Finally, a friend of the SON set up a Distinguished Lecturer Series and challenged the school to "plan for its future." The direct relationship with the development office, in addition to the formation of the Distinguished Lecturer Series, led to the formation of a SON Advisory Board (Appel, Campbell, Lynch, & Novotny, 2007). The nursing faculty worked on a vision and project plan for the learning resource center, with the core of the project being to recognize the gaps in present nursing education and the benefits of simulation-focused pedagogy.

Administrative support from the academic vice president, dean of the SON, and foundation relations officer led to the development of the 5-year Learning Resource Center Project (2006–2012), with Suzanne as the project director and Diana as the director of the Robin Kanarek Learning Resource Center (LRC). Diana's role was key to the integration of the project, as were nursing faculty input and enthusiasm. A university-wide committee was formed to get feedback and to gather ideas in all areas, including upgrading classrooms, adding new technology, purchasing simulation equipment, educating faculty and students in the use of the new equipment, using students for role-playing during scenarios, using health communication specialists, gaining input for development of scenarios, and requesting interdisciplinary guidance. Key to this vision was a plan specific to faculty development for this paradigm shift.

In addition, the university was going through changes, with a new president after 25 years as well as the development of the Center for Academic Excellence. The Center provided university-wide support to promote the development of best practices in the scholarship of teaching and learning. Faculty and staff, including input from media and IT departments, provided support and buy-in for the new project. In less than 3 years, the SON Advisory Board raised $1.06 million for the 5-year LRC project.

From the project's initial conception in 2005, the facility renovation was completed in the summer of 2006. Two simulation rooms were created with control from a central, double-sided mirrored room placed in between them, and within the university, the spaces became designated as exclusive for SON use. These rooms were converted into specialty areas (an intensive care and an OR) and three larger SON classrooms were renovated with state-of-the-art technology, wireless systems, and faculty computer consoles and audiovisual capabilities. The larger classrooms were remotely connected to the simulation rooms so that groups of students could observe classmates interacting during scenarios. In addition, two of the larger classrooms were equipped with the capability to record the class with live streaming of the audio, video, and PowerPoint slides available on the Internet. They were used to include students in class who were studying abroad, to prerecord nursing courses if a faculty member was at a conference, and to work with faculty in other countries by presenting and sharing content.

From Then, Until Now

Over the years, simulation-based pedagogy has been incorporated much more fully into Fairfield's nursing curriculum. To that end, a director of simulation was hired in 2015, and now works collaboratively with the LRC director. Not only have most faculty members attended simulation workshops and developed course and content-specific scenarios, but six faculty are pursuing certification via the Certification in Healthcare Simulation Education (CHSE) examination. Additionally, the school is seeking accreditation as a simulation center through the Society for Simulation in Healthcare, an organization with an interprofessional focus.

In 2016, the Fairfield University SON was named "The Marion Peckham Egan School of Nursing and Health Studies" and a new building broke ground in early spring 2016. Currently under construction, the new building will house state-of-the-art simulation areas, including three high-fidelity simulation rooms with corresponding control rooms and an integrated audiovisual capturing system, two operation rooms, a medication room, mental health interview rooms, health assessment and skills laboratories, and separate spaces for debriefing.

Since 2009, when the first edition of this book was published, many positive changes have occurred at Fairfield University. Government grants have allowed for equipment, IT assistance, and curriculum integration of simulation in the graduate program. A grant from the Health Resources and Services Administration (HRSA) had learning objectives to (P) Promote *Healthy People 2010* and *Healthy People 2020*, (R) Reflect on practice, (A) Acquire advanced practice registered nurses (APRN) skills, (T) Treat vulnerable diverse elders, (I) Intervene with maximal outcomes for older adults, (C) Communicate best practices in gerontology, and (E) Educate elders/ families (PRACTICE). This project addressed the preparation of advanced practice nurses to improve their assessment and management expertise in a primary care setting when working with diverse older adults through the use of simulation. An additional HRSA grant for the Comprehensive Anesthesia Training Through Simulation Project followed and allowed for a state-of-the-art anesthesia simulation laboratory to be built, and, with the new building, it will be expanded to several rooms in an operating suite. Our generous donors and friends of the Egan School have allowed us to embark on a fabulous new endeavor and we are exhilarated to begin using our future simulation and teaching spaces.

THE UNIVERSITY OF BRITISH COLUMBIA SCHOOL OF NURSING PERSPECTIVE, VANCOUVER, BC, CANADA

Leadership and Vision

When the LRC was first established in the University of British Columbia (UBC) School of Nursing in the 1980s, it was state of the art and fortunate to have leadership that identified the need for an LRC coordinator and dedicated staff; that commitment has continued. The leadership included seeing the LRC as a resource, a place for faculty development and student learning, and the vision to include a means of sustainability—paid staff and personnel. Within the UBC SON context, the LRC has expanded to work with faculty, including clinical instructors, and has been able to leverage the work accomplished there in proposals to the dean, university, and province for subsequent funding to build and support the necessary resources. Over time, the increasing complexity of nursing education with the commitment to transition the LRC to increase innovation and the use of technology, such as simulation models, has meant an increased need for faculty development, staff capacity building, and purchasing and maintenance of more highly complex systems. In addition, as a school with a long history of research and scholarship, known for its leadership within Canada and the world, and situated within a research-intensive globally recognized university, UBC School of Nursing leads with its expertise in curricular pedagogy and innovation and looks carefully at the integration of new methods of teaching.

The Canadian and provincial context in British Columbia is worth reflecting on for a moment. Nursing education is funded through the provincial government, Ministry of Health (120 bachelor of science in nursing [BSN] seats and 15 nurse practitioner [NP] seats) and subsidized by the university and faculty. With increasing costs of living (especially in Vancouver, BC) and faculty or staff salary increases yet decreasing provincial and national support, ongoing sustainment of equipment, staffing, and new technologies is a challenge. In addition in Canada, health care is provincially funded and more connections between the health authorities (regional systems governing acute, primary, and community care) and secondary education around health professional development and capacity building will require persistence within the professional collaborations to do it well. For example, in the health authorities, there are challenges as to who "owns" the simulation rooms (UBC Faculty of Medicine) and the equipment (health authority), and it is challenging to identify allocation of resources (time, space, staff) and coordination of events that are respectful of everyone's needs. Careful planning and identification of who is involved in the development, objective setting, facilitating, and debriefing of simulations, in labs or in situ, is imperative and it is key to have nurses on committees doing this planning. Several provincial groups support simulation in health professional education, such as the Simulation Technology Working Group (STWG) and the BC lab educators, who began as nursing faculty and staff but are broadening to include educators in the health authorities as well. These groups are exploring opportunities to coordinate the efforts, needs assessment, and tracking of different centers in the province. A centralized Provincial Simulation Committee, a group of simulation champions in the province came together monthly to create opportunities to connect and explore the interconnections of simulation and simulation resources across the educational institutions and health authorities.

Collaboration with practice partners and other schools of nursing in the province is a key goal, as well as is working with the community partners to share resources. At UBC, the health disciplines are situated in a research-intensive university in a publically funded system, so some of the ways we leverage funding is through our scholarship of teaching and learning. The original funding for purchase of HPSs came from the Teaching and Learning Enhancement Fund (TLEF), which was awarded to support the capacity of the school of nursing to implement the pedagogy of simulation. Subsequent TLEF's expanded this scholarship by working with practice partners in the health authorities. The goal is to continue to model this for future benefit. As you will find repeated throughout this book, there is an interest in the use of simulation for interprofessional education. Because the UBC School of Nursing is one of 18 in the province, many of the other schools of nursing have received provincial support to build state-of-the-art LRCs. In contrast, at UBC the majority of other health professions are based only at UBC (17 health disciplines), including medicine, pharmaceutical sciences, dentistry, physiotherapy, occupational therapy, and the like. As we focus on interprofessional education provincially, the UBC School of Nursing can be a leader bringing together multiple groups at UBC, the Health Authorities, as well as other universities and allied health groups. We recognize the need to go beyond individual schools to seek out opportunities for collaboration to further research, share resources, provide interprofessional learning, and enhance the caliber of practitioners to improve patient health and well-being.

Recognizing that the evolution of simulation and its integration into the nursing curriculum requires more than technicians—it needs faculty with expertise in supervising students—train-the-trainer models of incorporating faculty engagement have been implemented. Nurses have the expertise and capacity to be leaders in simulation pedagogy, without specific mandates from the Ministry of Health and Medicine, which tend to focus on acute care, trauma, and high-stake situations. UBC School of Nursing is reaching out to demonstrate what nursing brings to the table of interprofessional education, both in academe and the practice sites, including the use of standards; integration into pedagogy; the development, facilitation, and debriefing of scenarios that reflect the complex and holistic nature of patient health and well-being. Nursing also brings skill to team building and nontechnical skill development and pedagogically has been using an experiential approach to teaching for decades. Examples of the UBC School of Nursing interprofessional education (IPE) involvement over the past 5 years have included: integrated simulation with UBC Health (17 health disciplines on campus); medication reconciliation, including pharmacy, medical, and nursing students (RN and NP); participation in the UBC Health Connect—students from the 17 health professional programs are brought together for a 2-hour period in class sizes of 40 and put in interdisciplinary groups of six to eight to manage a case and reflect on preclass videos/ situations. In addition, a full-semester program in which a group of interdisciplinary students follows a "health mentor" through experience with chronic illness and interface with the health system also allows IPE. These opportunities bring students together and encourage interprofessional knowledge and understanding, allowing students to demonstrate respectful communication, learn about each other's roles in interactive scenarios, and participate in team-building exercises like the Health Care team challenge.

Lessons learned from building and developing basic lab facilities for the LRC at the UBC School of Nursing and continuing to meet the needs of educating our nursing students are that there are many players and making strategic alliances and connections that fit the mandate of the school continues to be a priority. Focusing on our strategic goals (e.g., research, practice–academic collaboratives, sharing resources to leverage facilities and resources and personnel) and recognizing the possibility that they could overlap helps us to stay on track. Since immigrating to Canada, Suzanne has seen many similarities with needs where she emigrated from for adequate use of simulation, experiential learning, and new technology. There is still the need for curriculum integration, faculty development, and turning our learning centers into innovative simulation centers that embrace new technology and new ways of learning. The UBC School of Nursing has built itself up from within, identified operations that work, and applied for TLEF and endowment funds for faculty development (see Chapter 5 for description at UBC). In the meantime, health authorities have built simulation centers that are beginning to increase in use. Our strength has been focusing on things that could make the difference as to whether we have the best space and identifying the right mix of staff and expertise for positive learning experiences. Collaborating around resources and research—to demonstrate the efficacy of the use of simulation—helps us to use it in the most effective way. There is still a need to examine the translation of knowledge to the behavior in clinical practice and for safe high-quality patient outcomes that enhance patient health and well-being. We continue to evolve and do not lose sight of the vision of why we are doing what we are doing. There are wonderful opportunities for growth; the UBC School of Nursing is situated to take a global perspective on the looming shortage of health professionals and faculty, the complex nature of health professional education and continuing professional development, and the complex environment with multiple players. Prioritizing and focusing on what can be accomplished and managed within our own context while providing support to colleagues and recognizing there are no quick and easy solutions—even as we use some specific strategies—allows us to continue to move forward. The traditional learning center needs to come together with the complexity of the practice environment it mirrors.

MAINTENANCE AND UPDATING/UPGRADING: CHALLENGE OF CONTINUOUS FUNDING

Of course, the good news is that simulation within a learning resource center can quickly become a well-used learning tool. This technology is often sought after by students picking colleges, matriculated students needing practice, and remediation and community agencies interested in the simulation for staff training and professional development. The bad news is that even the best HPS will need occasional maintenance and upgrading. When planning a learning resource center with simulation, it is wise to plan for the technology help you will need to maintain the HPS. At WCSU, a few staff in the University Computing department were interested, intrigued, and therefore very helpful whenever a technology issue arose. However, with our level of simulation expanding to what will be four high-fidelity HPSs, University Computing is currently working to hire a nursing department technologist who will be responsible for all the technology. Many programs have talented lab assistants who are very helpful with the simulation but need technological help when it comes to upgrades and maintenance. I (Karen) have been known to say repeatedly, "I have my PhD in nursing, not computers!" That being said, I have enjoyed the challenge of learning the technologic aspect of simulation, but not all faculty share my enthusiasm. In addition, there are the challenges of ordering replacement supplies and the inevitable crash of one of the HPSs who drowns in a simulated blood transfusion that springs a leak or a rogue intravenous line that infuses into the bed and not the HPS. In those cases, and to address the inevitable technology issues, purchasing a maintenance plan and extended warranties and securing replacement HPSs is wise. Most simulator companies will have those options available at purchase. Funding those yearly costs can be a challenge and should be planned for when building and planning a learning resource center. Ideally, as is true at WCSU, the *very* generous director of University Computing picks up those costs every year. At Davenport University, these expenses are budgeted in each campus's yearly budget.

At Fairfield University, maintenance and warranty plans have been purchased. One of the unanticipated extra expenses had to do with rewiring for the new HPS model. Initially, the HPS was wired to connect to the control room so that a microphone in that room could switch back and forth and the instructor's voice could come from the room (with directions for students) or from the HPS (with responses from the patient to the students' questions). With the advent of new technology that directly connected the HPS to a touch-screen monitor, rewiring was necessary and has caused many headaches. Even newer HPSs will incorporate wireless technology, although with the concrete used in our 1970s nursing building, it is possible that wireless technology may not work from the control room to the simulation rooms. Some of these expenses are just not easily anticipated, and future planning for the inevitable is prudent.

The newer grants being processed and funded at Fairfield University include these expenses for IT support, lab support to run the scenarios, and technology upgrades. This adds additional administrative work to the faculty receiving the grants and needs to be carefully considered in their workload and future assignments. Other challenges include changes that occur at the university level, including but not restricted to changes in the course management system vendors, incorporation of university-wide portfolios as the portals to student learning, and continuous upgrading of classroom and faculty technologies (e.g., computers) to keep pace with the technologic advancements. Sometimes, learning to work with what you have, recognizing its potential, and visualizing how it fits in your curriculum are key, without thinking you have to have the newest and the most up-to-date materials. Purchasing the newest things on the market is a risky and time-consuming endeavor as shown in Table 6.1.

CONCLUSION

We recognize the variety of programs, needs, and resources for each school of nursing. The complex factors of a university's strategic plans and missions, administrative support, outside funding opportunities, and the like are beyond the breadth and depth of this book. However, we hope that through sharing our stories, we have given you some insight into potential problems that may arise as well as ways to best meet the challenges associated with this paradigm shift. Throughout this book, other authors have shared their stories about how they are using simulation, the type of environment in which it is used, and what needs specific to their disciplines are most helpful for the successful integration of simulation.

Change is never easy, and finding a champion to lead faculty, students, administration, and staff down this path makes a big difference in how a learning resource center is perceived and how likely it is to succeed. The take-home message is this: Persist, go slowly, think outside the box, and garner the support of those around you to create a vision of how things will work best for you, your faculty, your university, and your students. But, most important, *have fun!* Share your stories. Laugh, learn, and embrace the process. The potential for growth is limitless. Good luck!

Table 6.1	Key Points for Consideration in Building/Renovating Simulation Labs	
	Fairfield University	**Western Connecticut State University**
Funding sources	Private funds State funds—specific grants Applied for federal funds	Multiple grants from university, state, and federal funds
Initial conceptualization	Conceptualized and funded first, grand wish list compiled, and consultant used for initial lab layout	Conceptualized first, followed by several rounds of small funding
Acquiring physical space	*Phase I*: Planned renovation of classroom space into large simulation area. Reclaimed areas within the School of Nursing. Includes advanced nursing care/ICU equipment and an OR area. Also, designation of existing lab space to simulation space specific for ICU, obstetrics, and home health. Basic upgrades to all spaces, including paint, window treatments, and lighting. *Phase II*: Expansion of obstetric facilities to include labor and delivery, postpartum, newborn nursery, and neonatal ICU with state grant funds (Connecticut Health and Education Facilities Authority, 2007). *Phase III*: Upgrade clinic setting for NP students (HRSA, 2010–2013). *Phase IV*: Upgrade OR area for nurse anesthetist student use with federal grant funds (HRSA, 2011–2014).	*Phase I*: Begins with a small simulation area designated in existing lab. *Phase II*: Five-room suite space acquired, room-by-room renovations, and flexible use of space. Resource rooms added over time to each area. *Phase III*: Area on another campus designed and renovated with separate simulation room adjacent to a new traditional lab. *Phase IV*: New space acquired and renovated for advanced nursing care/ICU (U.S. Department of Education, 2008).
Technology	Acquire three high-fidelity HPSs; one of medium-fidelity obstetric HPS; one each of medium-fidelity adult, child, and infant HPS; and static task trainers. Develop a large state-of-the-art controller room that can view both simulation rooms with video, audio, and projection capabilities. Enhance a large auditorium with Media-Site Live capability for live streaming audio/video of classes and simulations.	Acquire four high-fidelity HPSs; one medium-fidelity pediatric simulator, three static manikins and task trainers. Create a one scenario controller station, PDA scenario controllers on all other HPS.
Actual facility space	All simulation equipment is housed in one building in adjacent rooms.	Simulation facilities housed in three separate buildings and on two campuses.

(continued)

Table 6.1	Key Points for Consideration in Building/Renovating Simulation Labs	
	Fairfield University	**Western Connecticut State University**
Personnel	Diana Mager, Director; Robin Kanarek, Learning Resource Center. Suzanne Hetzel Campbell, Project Director	No lab assistant. Simulations run by individual instructors. Staffed with work-study students who open the lab for student practice.
	Work-study students staff the lab during semesters for student practice. Instructors run their own scenarios with assistance from directors, other faculty, and each other.	Load credit for maintaining lab and resources given to Learning Resources Committee chair or faculty who provide lab instruction and remediation.
	Acquired a part-time technology assistant and lab assistant as part of state grant for fiscal year 2008–2009.	Acquired a technology assistant for maintaining simulators in fall 2008.
Continuous funding	The initial vision of the project outlined a 4-year timeline; a budget was developed to incorporate all aspects: building and classroom renovation, equipment purchasing, faculty development, and assessment and evaluation.	Information Technology department of the university partially funded initial purchase of first HPS.
		Going forward, the Information Technology department has taken on responsibility of managing maintenance and warranty contracts, supervising the computers and computer technology necessary to run simulators, and providing technology assistance as needed.
Faculty development	HPS training and workshops provided by HPS company; faculty attendance and presentation at national and regional simulation and education conferences funded through faculty development funds.	HPS training and workshops provided by HPS company; individualized faculty-to-faculty training and small-group training as needed. New faculty training as requested by the Learning Resources Committee chair and current high-level faculty users.
	Faculty workshops for scenario writing, electronic medical record integration, and curriculum redesign held on campus throughout the semester. Small stipend for faculty participation.	Faculty use faculty development and travel funds to attend training and seminars on simulation.
	Individual Faculty Learning Community in place in 2007–2008, with subsequent course redesign and project development (see Chapter 4).	
	Individualized training as needed.	
	Support from University Center for Academic Excellence.	
	Full-day-and-a-half retreat planned for fall 2008 for curriculum development and technology integration for all School of Nursing faculty	

Assessment and evaluation	Five-year assessment plan is in place. Outside assessment team hired, university assessment director involved, baseline data gathered on all four cohorts of students in year 1 (2007–2008) in the form of surveys, focus groups, and student work and artifacts (including reflections). Other methods for program assessment will include the following: ERI scores on RN-Assess tests, NCLEX® pass rates, alumni survey data, and employer survey data as well as university-wide assessment tests. More specifically for individual class projects, faculty are assessing student work and reflection to determine effects of the new teaching paradigm.	Currently in Year 1 of full assessment plan after a 3-year development phase. The evaluation of simulation is embedded throughout the curriculum by documenting the overall program outcomes. Continued evaluation of the effects of simulation will be carried out by examining NCLEX® pass rates, pretesting and posttesting in the capstone course, and graduate and employer surveys. Simulation helps us to address all program outcomes, specifically, thinking critically, communicating effectively, and performing nursing interventions appropriate to the practice role.

ERI, Educational Resources, Inc.; HPS, human patient simulator; HRSA, Health Resources and Services Administration; ICU, intensive care unit; NCLEX, National Council Licensure Exam; OR, operating room; PDA, personal digital assistant.

REFERENCES

Appel, N., Campbell, S. H., Lynch, N., & Novotny, J. M. (2007). Creating effective advisory boards for schools of nursing. *Journal of Professional Nursing, 23*(6), 343–350.

Connecticut Health and Education Facilities Authority. (2007). *Award: $99,999 women's health simulation expansion project.*

Health Resources and Services Administration. (2010–2013). *HRSA 10–171. P.R.A.C.T.I.C.E: Geriatric diversity training for advance nursing education.*

Health Resources and Services Administration. (2011–2014). *Comprehensive Anesthesia Training Through Simulation (CATTS) project.*

Healthy People 2020. (n.d.). Leading health indicators development and framework. Retrieved from https://www.healthypeople.gov/2020/leading-health-indicators/Leading-Health-Indicators-Development-and-Framework

U.S. Department of Education. (2008). *CSUS initiative to improve the capacity and preparation of the nursing workforce.*

CHAPTER 7

Lights, Camera, Action! The Process of Evaluating, Acquiring, and Implementing an Audiovisual Capturing Solution to Enhance Learning

Colleen H. Meakim and Leland J. Rockstraw

The process of integrating an audio or visual capture solution is daunting at best; from developing a full knowledge base of the audiovisual process and product solutions (software and hardware) to understanding the needs of your faculty, students, staff, and institution. Getting it "right" will increase the effective installation and implementation of audiovisual equipment in your health care simulation center. This chapter introduces key components of audiovisual software and hardware; helps you ascertain the correct audiovisual product for your center; determines equipment and control room placement; explores key concepts regarding the incorporation of audiovisual usage among faculty, students, and other users; and offers ideas for policies and procedures to encourage usage of the equipment and optimize learning in the simulation environment.

THE PROCESS FOR DETERMINING AN AUDIO OR VISUAL CAPTURING SOLUTION

Deciding on the "right" audiovisual product for any institution involves a great deal of preparation by health care simulation center personal. Self-education, surrounding yourself with experts in audiovisual solutions, visiting other simulation centers, and talking with others currently using audio or visual systems will assist in the planning process, as well as enhance decision making. The following section introduces some common terms, provides a contextual understanding of audiovisual software and hardware, and includes a discussion of how this equipment will impact both primary users (simulation center staff) and end users (faculty and participants).

Simulation includes multiple modes, including partial task trainers, standardized patient (SP) actors, and high-fidelity computerized patient simulators (Jeffries, 2012). Although any nursing program would be prudent to plan for and purchase an audiovisual software solution for initial and future use of all forms of nursing simulation, including expansion into standardized patient examination room suites; for the purposes of this chapter, the design of simulation sites with audiovisual capturing solutions will primarily focus on the use of high-fidelity computerized patient simulators. Adaptations of this model can be made for suites using standardized patient rooms.

Initial steps in determining the right audiovisual capturing solution should begin with surveying the end users, including nursing faculty or staff development personnel, curriculum or staff development committee members, administrators, other key stakeholders, and simulation staff. This survey should seek to collect information regarding the proposed use of simulation, explore potential program growth, as well as identify projected student enrollment or usage by a department. Questions for personnel should include:

1. What are the plans to use simulation within the curriculum or in the staff development competency program?
2. What is the plan of the location of simulation activities? Will simulation take place in simulation labs only, wirelessly within classrooms, or in-situ on nursing units?
3. Will viewing of videos take place only in the simulation labs or virtually anywhere?
4. Will student population or health care staff size stay consistent or is growth planned?
5. How will the college or department use video captures for student or staff usage?

This information will assist with understanding how your program will require the software to perform or support the faculty, students, staff, and research efforts.

Design can include simple audiovisual capturing software to a more advanced solution, which will allow for the following: (a) design, storage, and management of simulation case scenarios; (b) camera movement during capture; (c) real-time documentation of participant performance; (d) faculty, participant, and/or staff access to videos (both live and archived); and (e) an ability to provide reports. An additional software consideration is the ease of use of the audiovisual software integration with computerized patient simulator(s) software to allow for immediate access for debriefing as well as comparing students' performance while visualizing key vital signs.

Health care professionals are asked to investigate, select, and integrate equipment and software with little to no knowledge or understanding of the technology in general as well as what the programs have to offer. It is vital to understand all key components of a potential audiovisual package in order to make the best decision for your program. The next section will introduce key components of audiovisual solutions that will help to navigate through all the options that are currently available.

Understanding Key Components of Audio/Visual Solutions

An understanding of the mission, plans, growth, and use of simulation within the nursing program will allow for planning and purchasing of the right software, thus meeting the initial needs as well as allowing for future growth and expansion. The use of technology in nursing simulation audiovisual software should assist the end user in the efficient running of equipment as well as decrease the time and efforts of the simulation staff in administrative functions. This automation allows the simulation staff to manage simulation equipment allowing for a reduced workload of programming, recording, and creating videos for review. The audiovisual simulation software "solution" can be sold as an all-in-one package or à la carte, allowing for selection of different components such as:

1. Administration of all key aspects of the software
2. Management of the different level users
3. Case configuration
4. Recording
5. Easy accessibility for users
6. Some form of assessment (data collection and scoring).

Table 7.1 identifies key aspects of audiovisual software solutions.

Table 7.1	Simulation Audiovisual Solution Software Key Aspects
Feature	**Specific Functions of the Feature**
Software administration	- Templates for cases, surveys, and assessments - Ability to create and maintain separate programs within the software - Manage emails, individual and program profiles
User management	- Create and manage users (faculty, students, staff, SPs, etc.) - Develop different levels of access to software and accessibility of videos - Bulk uploading of data (such as users, contact information) - Password access - Capability to send reminders - Task assignments (e.g., ability to assign assessment capabilities to a user level)
Case configuration	- Case creation and management - Case categorization - Document storage (labs, nursing reports, provider orders, etc.) - Electronic medical record capabilities
Recording(s)	- Ability to configure cameras to record automatically - Manual camera operations, which includes camera movement and last-minute camera changes - Provide live feeds for remote viewing from another location - Ability to search for a recording via participant name versus scenario versus date/time stamp
Accessibility	- Local network (within the simulation center) versus local domain (within the institution such as university campus) versus World Wide Web - Bandwidth requirements (discussion with your institutional networking department will ensure streaming of video) - File conversion time (time needed to access video following recording for debriefing) - Indexing abilities (assignment of departmental faculty, case, SPs, course specific) - Individual permissions (e.g., student permission to view individual videos to incorporate inclusive date and times)
Assessment	- Assessment items (measurable actions/competency or skill of participants or SPs; these items would include measurable performance behaviors, such as introducing one's self, good eye contact, asking health history questions, medication administration performance, and so on - Report generation (types of report, student specific vs. scenario specific vs. competency or skill)
Survey	-Opportunity to survey users pre/post simulation for testing, feedback, and so on.

SP, standardized patients.

VENDOR SELECTION

Understanding the process of investigating and selecting an audiovisual software solution vendor is critical because the search process is potentially the beginning of an association that could evolve into a service relationship before, during, and after the purchase. Identification of the project goals, followed by a call for proposals from vendors, can begin the official process. The call for proposals should ensure that only qualified vendors apply, allow for technology-specific comparisons, and place the responsibility of providing hardware and software information on the vendor. Time spent in developing and placing important questions specific to the audiovisual capturing solution within the call for proposals will assist in streamlining the process and avoid rework later in the process. Interviewing potential vendors during the call for proposals is an additional strategy that would be beneficial in the selection of an audiovisual solution partner. Additional comparative information regarding services of vendors can be gained during this interview process (Ness, 2006).

The cost of a fully integrated simulation product can be very costly and warrants a systemic process or due diligence. In an article titled, "Do the Due Diligence," Kevin Oakes (2004) suggests steps to take in determining the right vendor for an e-learning solution. These include investigating the vendor (is the company private or public), understanding sales tactics, and making site visits. Oakes suggests that companies that are traded publicly have transparent financial information available through a variety of resources, which would enable the user to understand the stability of and the potential for the company to be around to provide service after the sale. Educating yourself in understanding sales is helpful so you do not fall into the trap of sales tactics that create fear, uncertainty, and doubt (FUD) about the sales agent's competition. An informed buyer asks for the facts and/or documents to back up any proposal and also asks the vendor to support or defend these documents. The third phase includes what Oakes calls "hit(ting) the road" or making a site visit to the vendor's home office (2004, p. 16). These visits to the vendor's company will allow for gauging the atmosphere of the environment as well as the customer service of the employees. Incorporating these three approaches allows for a better understanding of any audiovisual solution vendor's stability and potential for creating a long-term positive relationship (Oakes, 2004).

With the initial understanding of the stability of a technological audiovisual solution vendor, a deeper investigation of understanding the services, sales, and support can begin. NPower Network (2011) reviews the process of technology vendor selection and suggests the following seven-step process or model before making a purchase. These steps include:

1. Assessing the viability (Is this purchase feasible/practical for my organization?)
2. Collecting requirements (What is necessary for my organization related to this product?)
3. Understanding the organization's requirements and options (What options are available to support the needs of the organization?)
4. Evaluating vendor options (Which of these companies may offer the product(s) that are the best fit for my organization?)
5. Selecting a vendor (Which price, components of the product, and ongoing contracts are reasonable and viable for my organization?)
6. Implementing the technology (Does the vendor have a history of delivering of the goods and services promised?)
7. Supporting and maintaining the purchased technology (How does the organization maintain this process/program and support it? [NPower Network, 2011]).

This article is a must read by any simulation staff making the decision to purchase an audiovisual software solution in that it provides a step-by-step "how to" from a technological perspective. Many health care personnel are intimidated by the need to make decisions regarding these technological resources. The author offers a readable/understandable article with a variety of very helpful suggestions and considerations to use during the vendor selection process. He includes exploration of a budget, including a potential variance; professional staff's ability to learn, use, and incorporate the new technology; sustainability of the new technology; ascertaining the return on investment and tips for the decision-making process (NPower Network, 2011).

Creating an evaluation matrix regarding different software solution vendors will assist in making the right purchase for your nursing simulation program. Include aspects such as software features, technology elements, quality of the product, costs (initial as well as maintenance), vendor company stability, general impressions, support provided during vendor selection, product installation and placement time frame, training, and technical support, and whatever other options relate to your program. All of these factors placed in a matrix will provide an opportunity for comparisons and assist in decision making (NPower Network, 2011).

During the authors' vendor selection, a comparison was made of existing audiovisual vendors by Rockstraw in early 2006 and by Meakim in 2007/2008 and again in 2013/2014. Exhibit 7.1 shows the vendor selection comparison checklist that was used during our programs' evaluations.

Exhibit 7.1 Audiovisual Solution Selection Comparisons Checklist			
	Vendor A	**Vendor B**	**Vendor C**
Physical location of vendor (this may affect timeliness of installation process and repairs)			
Number of year's vendor has been in existence (may lend insight as to stability of company and experience level of employees)			
List of previous institutions/universities using vendor (these references will allow for investigation of customer satisfaction as well as what would or would not be helpful in future purchases)			
Does vendor provide			
a. equipment			
b. installation (or is this contracted out, which may refer to experience level and support after the purchase)			
Software/hardware features (essential vs. nice to have)			
Does vendor offer the purchase of local servers/storage as well as web-based hosting?			
Student scheduling ability			
Automatic/manual operations of recording, data storage, and viewing permissions.			
Accessibility of viewing (at nursing institution vs. anywhere with Internet connections)			
Evaluative features for grading of performance			
Remote viewing (live or archived) for faculty			
Compatibility with other technology (patient simulators, computer platforms [PC vs. Mac], institutional ability to support streaming video)			
Data backup			
Data recovery			
Audiovisual solution functional elements			
Ease of use			
Flexibility of programming or case creation			
Security			
Virus protection			

(continued)

Exhibit 7.1	Audiovisual Solution Selection Comparisons Checklist *(continued)*		
	Vendor A	**Vendor B**	**Vendor C**
Cost of audiovisual solution			
Initial capital cost			
Licensing			
Add-on functions			
Annual maintenance agreements			
TOTAL COSTS			
Maintenance agreement(s):			
Equipment issues and/or failure			
Software issues and/or failure			

CAMERA, MICROPHONE, AND CONTROL-ROOM PLACEMENT

The following section of this chapter describes different considerations for the placement of recording equipment and the control room. Having early and continued conversations with simulation staff, faculty, and departmental administration as well as networking with other nursing simulation users will assist in the understanding of function and use of recording equipment and simulation control-room design. As audiovisual vendors may have participated in development of other sites, they can be a great resource to gain insight into simulation center designs specifically related to camera, microphones, and the control room, including types, location, and placement. These vendors may also offer services to assist with the general design and design and layout of rooms. Another great resource in gaining an understanding of room and equipment layouts is by getting out and visiting other simulation centers. A great deal can be learned by touring and speaking with other simulation professionals.

Camera and microphone placement will be affected by the size of the simulation suite as well as the number of cameras and microphones that will be placed. Single camera and microphone placements would typically be positioned to capture video and audio of the main focus of the nursing simulation suite, typically a patient's bed, nurses' station, and conference table. The camera can be placed at the foot of the bed (nurses' station or conference table) or from either side, far enough back to allow for viewing/recording of the entire bed and work space around the bed. The microphone would be placed directly over the bed or at the center of focus. Figure 7.1 shows a floor plan of this room configuration. Authors Dhingra and Kerns (2011) provide an in-depth description on health care simulation labs hardware and software design, which this author would encourage reading before deciding on a simulation lab design.

If the capital budget allows placement of a second camera and microphone, placement in an additional key focus area or from a corner of the room to allow a full room view would be optimal, as shown in Figure 7.2. An additional key focus area could be a counter work space, a sitting area, as well as a fuller view of the entire simulation suite. Key discussions with the audiovisual solution vendor, simulation consultant, and other design professionals will aid with the appropriate placement of cameras and microphones.

The ability to place a third camera and microphone or more would be dependent on the size of the simulation suite as well as the design of the room. One last consideration would be the placement of a bird's-eye view camera, which allows for viewing only from the control-room and does not allow audio or visual capture. This feature would allow for control-room staff to view student performance from over the focal area (patient's bed, nurses' station, or conference table) when the view from the one-way mirror into the simulation suite may be blocked by students or other simulation participants. The third camera and the bird's-eye view camera are shown in Figure 7.3.

Overall floor design should include strategic placement of the control room. A conceptual layout is shown in Figure 7.4. Control-room access and flow should allow for entering and exiting from both a main hallway as well as the nursing simulation suite. The use of these two access/exit points should be used to promote the "feel" of the simulation encounter. Typically, the hallway that

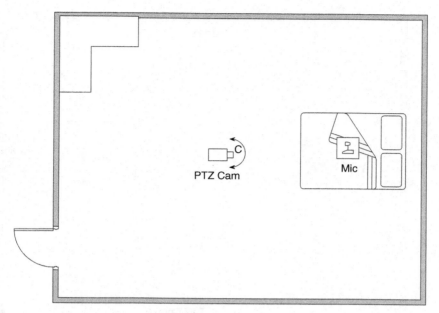

Figure 7.1   Camera and microphone placement—one each.
PTZ, pan, tilt, and zoom.

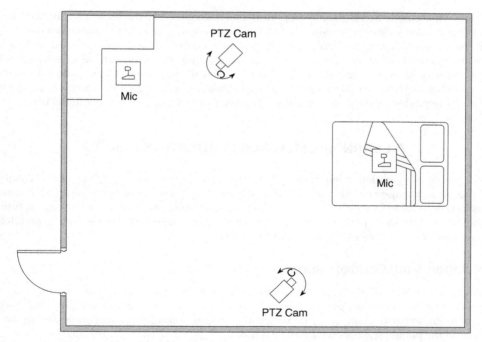

Figure 7.2   Camera and microphone placement—two each.
PTZ, pan, tilt, and zoom.

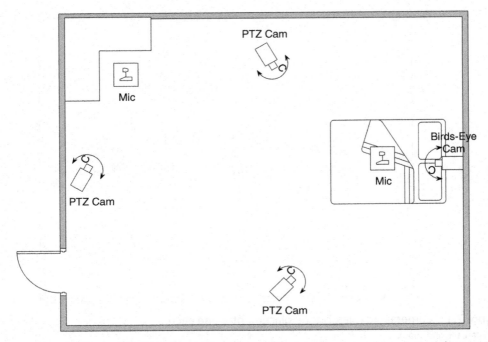

Figure 7.3   Camera and microphone placement—three cameras and two microphones and one bird's-eye view camera.

PTZ, pan, tilt, and zoom.

students would use to access the nursing simulation suite would be the same hallway that faculty would use to access the control room; should the student need to request assistance or a conference with the faculty member, this could take place just inside or outside of the same entrance of the simulation suite. The second access to the control room from the simulation suite is designed for quick and easy access by simulation staff and actors. Ideal space use would include a prep/prop room area between the control room and nursing simulation suite to gain easy access to equipment and props requested by the students, but which was not placed in the room for initial use.

A LEARNER-CENTERED SIMULATION CENTER

Development of a simulation lab environment brings about a variety of considerations regarding the use and management of the varied resources in an environment to support learning. Considerations include how to design and use a control room, how to use the video capture of health care simulation experiences, whether and how to implement simulation testing, and determining guidelines or polices for students and faculty.

Simulation Suite Control Room

Having a simulation suite control room as a part of the nursing laboratory environment is a relatively new phenomenon in nursing education. Ten years ago very few nursing programs used a control room, whereas today many nursing programs use a control room of some design, and if not, are in the planning stages for a control room.

Determining the type and style of control room(s) that are needed is based on a variety of factors, including student and faculty numbers, budget, mission, vision, and the plans for the use of the various simulation room(s). Control rooms can be used as a view-only

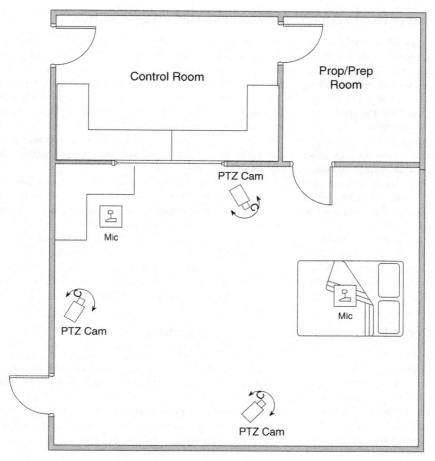

Figure 7.4 Control room and simulation suite conceptual layout.
PTZ, pan, tilt, and zoom.

style by way of a one-way mirror or an observe and record type of room, or an observe, record, and remote patient simulator operation center. Control rooms can be attached to a single simulation room or lab or they can be standalone stations monitoring events in a variety of rooms through cabling and audiovisual system controls (Seropian & Lavey, 2010). Having a design that allows for multiple uses provides for the greatest flexibility and varied options for use of space. When designing control rooms, it is important to include representatives from faculty, staff, and administration when consulting with architects and builders to ensure that all needs are considered. It is helpful to think futuristically because more possibilities will exist as the future becomes today's experience.

Control rooms in simulation laboratories provide a great number of assets for faculty and students. Faculty can be located away from the learning or testing environment, thus allowing for decreased student anxiety and less frequent faculty cueing and teaching during simulation scenarios. Other benefits include the ability to record events thereby allowing students to review and reflect on experiences and offering faculty the opportunity to view live or view and/or grade at another time. Faculty, other staff, or standardized patients can speak for a patient simulator or be the voice of other health care providers from the control room, lending to a sense of realism. Faculty new to the process can learn the methods for simulation scenario teaching or evaluation in the control room, unobserved by students.

To Record or Not to Record; Shakespeare Had an Easier Choice

Recording of all scenarios may not be necessary, so how do faculty determine when it is necessary? Decisions regarding the need to record are based on the goals of the simulation or laboratory experiences. It is necessary to determine whether experiences are formative or summative. If formative, debriefing following a simulation experience provides an opportunity for shared discovery rather than an evaluation process (Johnson-Russel & Bailey, 2010). Having a recording to return to can help the student to (a) review key events and reflect on actions/inactions for deeper learning, (b) reinforce appropriate behaviors, (c) gain insight from situations during or following debriefing, and (d) create an electronic portfolio for professional use. During debriefing, students and faculty review and discuss key highlights or critical situations that are particularly important to demonstrate clinical reasoning on the part of students.

During summative evaluation, the use of recording devices will allow students to be reviewed by one or more observers or raters thereby increasing interrater reliability. Students can be observed performing a variety of skills, including interpersonal communication, history taking, physical assessment, a variety of psychomotor skills, and clinical reasoning abilities, or any combination of these. These key concepts, if video recorded, provide an opportunity for giving detailed feedback, which can help students to learn and improve (Levett-Jones & Lapkin, 2014; Winters, Hauck, Riggs, Clawson, & Collins, 2003). Following testing situations, having the ability to return to a recorded scenario to reevaluate a situation can be very helpful in fairly and accurately assigning a grade to a student's performance, particularly if there is a grading discrepancy.

Video Recorded Simulation in the Classroom Setting

Traditional teaching methods are not adequate for today's students. Nurses need to be able to think on their feet, analyze patient situations quickly in order to respond effectively, and enhance patient outcomes. Neurobiology researchers are seeking ways to determine the role of the brain and its chemistry in how knowledge is acquired. Use of more action-oriented activities, such as simulation, help to enhance the brain's chemical energy, which helps when trying to make decisions, such as those needed in complex patient care scenarios. Use of simulation scenarios can help to support the associations made in the brain because it impacts a variety of student learning styles (Cardoza, 2011).

Studies have demonstrated that playing video games stimulates the release of dopamine (Koepp et al., 1998, as cited in Cardoza, 2011). Cardoza (2011) postulates that use of simulation in a scaffolding manner across a curriculum can possibly enhance learning and patterns of learning in the brain through the release of dopamine and adrenaline. There are research studies that support the use of recorded simulation to enhance learning.

Sharpnack, Goliat, Baker, Rogers, and Shockey (2013) used seven prerecorded simulation scenarios that incorporated quality and safety issues, such as incivility, delegation, prioritization, nursing management of care, as well as moral and ethical dilemmas in order to help students learn skills related to teamwork and collaboration. The combination of the video with structured questions and debriefing helped students to analyze and critically think through the clinical scenario and leadership situations. Results of the study demonstrated that use of the repeated videotaped simulation scenarios, along with debriefing and practice of skills, such as providing a situation, background, assessment, and recommendation (SBAR) report, were effective in improving critical thinking, communication, patient assessment, and safety-related competencies. Repeated use of the scenarios combined with practice of the required skills enhanced confidence as well and knowledge as demonstrated by posttest scores (Sharpnack et al., 2013).

Aiming to enhance leadership and safety practices of students, Cantrell, Mariani, and Meakim (2016) used two prerecorded videos, one demonstrating violations of safety principles and practices, the other depicting consistent safe practices along with an environmental safety check of a "patient's" physical setting. Students rotated through the video with the safety violations and completed the environmental review, identified safety violations in both, and then completed a group debriefing in which they discussed these violations as well as the nurse's role as a leader in achieving safety principles and practices. Discussion focused on communication (handoffs and transitions of care), use of the nursing process to minimize safety risks, promoting a blame-free environment, and appropriate delegation. Following the debriefing, students viewed the optimal video with the positive safety behaviors being demonstrated. Student feedback indicated that the activities were positive and contributed to their learning (Cantrell et al., 2016).

Video capabilities can help faculty with student visualization of simulation activities in the classroom while simultaneously being completed in the simulation lab. Burns, O'Donnell, and Artman (2010) described a program used for freshman nursing students to learn the nursing process whereby students as a class are presented 12 evolving patients' scenarios based on two relatively complex cases. The two cases were altered each time for six unique, yet similar experiences for students. The larger class group was in an auditorium and smaller groups were sent to the simulation lab to participate in the experiences while classmates watched via a link from the lab to the classroom. Each experience took approximately 5 minutes. Students were directed by graduate students in the simulation lab to guide and cue students through the process. Debriefing of the group was completed in the classroom and reflection focused on the nursing process steps used during the experience. This example provides a very creative use of audio or visual systems involving simulated experiences for larger groups of students.

Support of Skill Development

The literature also reveals a variety of helpful ways that educators have used situational recordings for student learning. Self-directed videotaping can be used to support student skill development for both formative learning and summative assessment. The following advantages may be possible: the process encourages student independent thinking; faculty makes more efficient use of their time as opposed to direct observation; review of practice videotapes allows the student to see their mistakes more clearly; students practice, which increases confidence, and students make mistakes and correct them before being evaluated. If working in pairs or teams, students can develop enhanced cooperative learning. There can be greater flexibility in time for faculty and students as opposed to a fixed testing schedule. (Winters et al., 2003).

Disadvantages for faculty and students can be: students have to coordinate efforts together, students' need to learn how to use the audiovisual equipment, difficulty visualizing procedures requiring detailed skills, the potential for technical difficulties, and a potential for weak students to work together. In addition, faculty may be unavailable to answer questions that may arise (Winters et al., 2003).

Other nursing authors have found additional benefits of video recording simulation experiences or portions of experiences. Chau, Chang, Lee, Lee, and Wooten (2001) used videotaped vignettes to promote critical thinking and to assist students in learning to manage important clinical situations. Guidelines were developed to assist faculty in discussion of the vignettes. Using a pre- or posttest design, they measured the effectiveness of the vignettes on student knowledge and critical thinking. Although the findings did not show a significant difference among the groups in critical thinking, the intervention groups' knowledge test scores were higher. There were positive outcomes attributed to helping students to relate better to clinical situations, and students were satisfied with the strategy. Faculty found that students were more capable of identifying their strengths and weaknesses by the end of the term.

Debriefing and Use of Video

Video has been used to improve student performance following high-fidelity simulations. Megel, Bailey, Schnell, Whiteaker, and Vogel (2013) assert that the use of video following simulation allows learners to actually visualize their performance as opposed to relying on memory of it, which makes their reflective abilities more accurate (Fanning & Gaba, 2007), helps to improve future behaviors (Anderson, Murphy, Boyle, Yaeger, & Halamek, 2006), and can create an awareness of the needs of other team members, thereby enhancing teamwork (Daniels, Lipman, Harney, Arafeh, & Druzin, 2008; Messmer, 2008).

Inconsistencies exist in the literature related to the effectiveness of video-facilitated debriefing and/or feedback (Levett-Jones & Lapkin, 2014); however, there seems to be evidence that it can support some behavior change. Cheng and colleagues (2014) carried out a systematic review and meta-analysis of the literature in order to characterize how debriefing is reported in the literature and to determine which features associated with debriefing lead to the best outcomes. They also wanted to determine the effectiveness of debriefing when combined with technology-enhanced simulation (TES). In the comparison of video-assisted debriefing versus non–video-assisted debriefing, the authors found that there was minimal difference in terms of benefits to participants between the two methods. The use of a shorter debriefing (less than 15 minutes) combined with a viewing of an expert modeling video of appropriate performance showed some benefit, although in this comparison, the results were not statistically significant.

Following previous studies that demonstrated positive outcomes for videotape reviews of performance, Scherer, Chang, Meredith, and Battistella (2003) conducted a study of medical practitioners managing trauma resuscitations over a 3-month period comparing verbal feedback alone versus videotape reviews of performance. The group who received verbal feedback alone did not have behavioral change over a 3-month period; however, those who received videotaped feedback had improved behavior after 1 month of feedback. The change in behavior was sustained over the remainder of the study. The authors suggest several possibilities for why videotape review enhances performance. Providing objective evidence of performance is the first step in bringing about a behavior change. It provides an opportunity to model appropriate behaviors and extinguish poor behaviors. Video also helps individuals to break down perceived self-efficacy, which is the discrepancy between the ways people think they are performing and the reality of the performance (Scherer et al., 2003).

Kaur-Dusaj (2014) completed a randomized controlled study with 74 associate-degree nursing students to determine the effects of video-assisted debriefing on student outcomes, including clinical judgment, self-confidence, and learner satisfaction with the simulation and facilitator. The author's findings demonstrated higher clinical judgment scores in the video-assisted debriefing group as opposed to the traditional debriefing group. Both groups had high scores in self-confidence, with no differences between the groups. There were also higher satisfaction scores with the simulation and the facilitator for the video-assisted debriefing group than those for the traditional debriefing group. Students in this study learned from the self-observation of both their successes and errors.

Grant, Moss, Epps, and Watts (2010) conducted a study to evaluate the effect of use of videotape-facilitated human patient simulation with practice sessions versus standard scenarios with practice and oral feedback to bring about the desired simulation behaviors. The desired simulation behaviors focused on communication, patient safety, general and problem-focused assessment, prioritizing care, carrying out appropriate interventions, and delegating to team members when caring for two patients in two 60-minute scenarios, which were evenly spaced throughout the semester. Undergraduate nursing students rotated roles throughout the practice sessions to provide ample opportunities to participate as the nurse in a variety of functional roles. In order to evaluate students, a third 60-minute scenario was completed by both groups at the end of the semester. Although there were no significant differences between the groups in the overall performance scores, the intervention group had higher mean scores on the majority of the desired simulation behaviors. Another significant finding and the supposition of the study was that assignment of student roles impacts on students' future performance. The authors suggest that students' roles should be rotated during simulation activities so that they have opportunities to perform the expected behaviors during simulation activities.

A crossover, comparative study was completed to evaluate students in an undergraduate critical care nursing program to compare verbal debriefing (V) with video-assisted verbal debriefing (VA + V). The intent of the video was to provide a visual reinforcement to the debriefing experience. Students participated in a cardiopulmonary arrest (CPA) simulation and faculty used a valid and reliable tool to evaluate student performance. Debriefing was guided with a standardized tool with key debriefing points for a 30-minute time period, with one group also reviewing the video of their performance. Students were evaluated for knowledge as well as skills. All students had higher skill scores on the second simulation, which was completed a week following the first simulation. However, the quality of skill performance and the time it took to respond was higher in the VA + V group. Knowledge scores were higher for the V-only group. Because the VA + V group only had 30 minutes to watch the video and complete a guided debriefing discussion, this may have impacted their knowledge score (Chronister & Brown, 2012).

Videotaping of clinical skills and vignettes can have a positive impact on student learning, can enhance simulation experiences, and provide an impetus for behavior change. Providing this opportunity for students seems a necessary option in today's learning environments.

Other Uses of Video Recording to Support Simulation and Learning

In addition to simulation recording for student learning, recording can provide other opportunities to support simulation efforts through recording of presimulation preparatory videos and to enhance classroom teaching. Alfes (2011) describes the use of a series of 5-minute videos to provide a patient handoff report and introduce simulated clinical experiences to students for scenarios completed in the simulation lab. Videos progress as the scenario evolves and fade as students meet their patient to provide care. Faculty, staff, and other people assume patient roles, scripts are prepared and props chosen to add to the realism of the video. The faculty, staff, and so on speak as the patient to set the stage for the simulated experience. Faculty believe that these videos heighten realism, interest, and immersion in the lab experiences, and find students less intimidated by simulation experiences following the video. Student feedback indicates that students enjoyed seeing the patient before engaging in the simulation.

Gantt (2013) conducted a study to examine how preparation can impact anxiety and therefore simulation performance. Over time, faculty realized that students needed more hands-on simulation practice, especially before an evaluative simulation. Deliberate practice and repeated performances by students were used initially. For this study, faculty used a series of simulation videos followed by extensive class discussion to prepare students for their evaluative scenarios. These included both formative and previously recorded summative scenarios. Following the intervention, analysis of the data revealed that there were no significant differences between the groups who were prepared using the videos and discussion and the other group. However, it did demonstrate that anxiety had an impact on student performance and score for the simulation experience, despite the preparation method used.

Recording for High-Stake Performance

Nursing education uses a variety of assessment modalities. With the growth of simulation there has been a great deal of discussion and controversy regarding the use of simulation for testing students' clinical skills and reasoning abilities. Although many simulation activities are used for formative learning, simulation testing experiences can also provide important feedback regarding a student's abilities and can also serve as a powerful learning experience as well.

Furman, Smee, and Wilson (2010) provided a summation of best practices from three organizations in order to ensure quality standards for simulation-based assessment. The authors determined that having a quality-control process in place helps to ensure valid and reliable assessments using simulation for formative or high-stakes assessment. This includes the use of standard protocols for case development and pilot testing of new cases as well as the use of a template for developing valid scoring instruments. Training of all participants, such as standardized patients, raters, and staff, are critical to variance reduction. Developing administrative standards to ensure timing systems accuracy, security of case materials and dealing with any examination irregularities, such as fire alarms, bathroom floods, or human error, all help to ensure a well-controlled and professional demeanor for the simulation environment.

Testing in and of itself can be helpful to enhance learning; Roediger and Karpicke (2006) conducted an assessment of research studies, which demonstrated that testing itself provides a powerful way of improving memory of material to be learned. The testing effect boosts retention of learned material. Although testing may be an indicator of what a student knows, the act of being tested also enhances an individual's ability to retain learned information.

Kromann, Jensen, and Ringsted (2009), conducted a study to determine whether using time for testing as a final activity in a resuscitation skills course for medical students increased the learning outcome of students when compared with providing them an equal amount of practice time. Both groups received an in-house resuscitation course. The intervention group had 3.5 hours of training followed by 30 minutes of testing. The control group received 4 hours of training, and during the last 30 minutes, they reviewed three or four scenarios (including one that would be used for the testing), followed by brief feedback. Both groups had outcomes assessed 2 weeks after the course was completed. Each participant had to demonstrate the skills in a scenario. The authors found that learning outcomes for the intervention group were significantly higher than the mean scores for the control group. The authors indicate that learning outcomes were enhanced with the use of testing in a skills-based course. It is their assertion that testing can have an effect on knowledge retention in skills learning.

When deciding to implement a simulation process for testing or grading, carrying out a trial process in advance of the actual event allows for anticipatory problem prevention. Recording of testing events may be needed to determine grades. Faculty can review recordings to ensure that grades match performance, particularly when an assigned grade can have a serious impact on a student's final grade for a course or there is disagreement regarding a performance appraisal.

Planning for Emergencies

Preparing for student simulation experiences requires days if not weeks to ensure a quality experience for users. Time spent configuring equipment and software for operations requires detailed attention to case development, student enrollment, development of surveys (both pre and post), and ensuring access to recorded videos, which will provide early identification of issues to lessen any impact of service to students and faculty. Development and implementation of a daily checklist of software and hardware health will aid in identification, reconfiguration, or repair of issues early on. Daily equipment checks should be conducted early enough (1 to 1.5 hours before live recording) to allow for contacting of the customer support team, determination of the issue(s), and reconfiguration of the equipment. Key software updates and equipment replacement should be scheduled for down periods, which will allow adequate time for installation and testing of simulation software and equipment. Spending time to create, develop, configure, implement, and test your simulation equipment may prevent academic emergencies or at least decrease the level of its impact.

Data Security

Electronic data security is an important aspect of managing learner simulation files for health care simulation professionals, but it is not generally understood. Knowledge of the Family Educational Rights and Privacy Act (FERPA, 2016) laws, including how electronic information is accessed, travels, and is stored, and requirements for workstation and device security, can be challenging.

FERPA was enacted to provide parents access to their child's educational records as well as to provide the right to privacy regarding grades, enrollment, billing information, and records. Electronic data, such as videos, electronic surveys, and tests, used within the simulation environment is considered part of the student's records and requires safeguards to protect privacy.

Electronic student records or data can be considered to be (a) data at rest, (b) data in use, or (c) data in motion (Raglione, 2015). *Data at rest* refers to information, such as student records, that can be stored on a hard drive and represents data in a state of relative security. Examples of hard drives are desktop computers, mainframe servers, and portable hard drives. Associated examples of electronic security for data at rest include antivirus software and firewalls. Caution should be used with the storage of FERPA-protected information on portable hard drives so as not to misplace, leave behind, or have information stolen, whereas servers and desktop computers are not easily lost or stolen. *Data in use* refers to accessing electronic data, via a computer or a handheld device, and being viewed, as in videos being observed or heard. Types of security that can protect data in use include user authentication such as signing on with a user identification (ID) and password. Information technology (IT) systems can monitor the number of attempted log-ons, which can be reviewed in case of a potential system attack. *Data in motion* is the phrase used for data that is moving or in the process of being transferred; specifically, leaving a network via the Internet by web, email, or via other Internet protocols. Data is very susceptible when it is in motion and protecting data will require specialized processes like encryption, use of a virtual private network (VPN), and other protective capabilities (Raglione, 2015). Understanding electronic data and its vulnerabilities will increase in importance with the growth and use of mobile devices. It is prudent to develop unit-specific policies and procedures to protect and safeguard the access, use, and movement of student records. Recurring safety audits of hardware and software should be conducted, documented, and inadequacies responded to in order to maintain a level of protection required by FERPA.

Data Backup

With the increased use of technology to record, store, and view student simulation experiences, simulation centers are dependent on the integrity of data storage in the hardware of computer systems. Electronic student records can be vulnerable in many ways, including hardware failure, natural disasters, lost or stolen equipment, human error, or malicious attacks. To offset any potential lost data, it is important to provide data backup to storage devices to allow for duplicate services in the event of lost data. Backup of videos and other data can be made to hard drives, portable devices, such as DVDs, CDs, USB drives, and remote servers (local and cloud based). Explore options with the IT department to determine which data backup process works best for your simulation center.

Selecting a Level-of-Service Agreement

Simulation technology hardware and software is an expensive endeavor. Technology is constantly changing and equipment wear and tear requires a level of service afforded by the amount of use and the budget of your simulation center. Costs of service agreements may be an initial consideration, but should not be the only one. Length of warranty coverage, replacement time period, and the ability to monitor performance and run diagnostics are some of the considerations needed when selecting the right level-of-service agreements. Additional considerations should include level of customer support team, service provided after installation, response time, education provided for operational staff, troubleshooting, and software configuration. Customer support considerations include accessibility of phone service for a standard number of operational hours; use of an email or ticket system, which allow for opening up and monitoring of issues; management of equipment breakage and other unusual occurrences. The ability to provide remote equipment monitoring, perform remote diagnostics, resolve issues, and conduct software updates is also key. Simulation vendors offer varied level-of-service agreements to meet the needs of your simulation center. It is important to query the sales team by asking direct questions regarding the cost of replacement parts or equipment, determining the average life of the equipment, and the availability for customer support in order to determine the level-of-service agreement that meets your simulation center's needs and budget.

GUIDELINES, POLICIES, AND PROCEDURES
TO EFFECTIVELY MANAGE A SIMULATION SUITE

The need for and type of policies and procedures that are necessary for a simulation suite will depend on various circumstances in your environment. Guidelines, policies, and procedures can assist in providing an optimal environment for working and learning, supporting the integration of simulation into the curriculum in a consistent manner, and ensuring the protection of equipment. An examination of how your mission, vision, philosophy, and curriculum impact your students, faculty, and staff and their interaction with the simulation environment will help to start the process.

Some important questions to be considered related to the operation of audiovisual recording equipment and patient simulators include the following:

1. What is important in your physical environment that must be addressed?
2. Who has access to recording and patient simulator equipment?
3. Who are super users as opposed to operators of equipment?
4. What rights and privileges need to be identified for users of recording and simulation equipment?
5. Who is responsible for equipment maintenance?
6. Who is/are the key contact person/people for the audiovisual recording and patient simulator companies?
7. How are problems reported and managed?

Development of procedures helps staff and faculty to become more comfortable with equipment management because they are able to follow a step-by-step process. Having access to easy-to-follow guides supports personnel as they learn to use equipment effectively.

Scheduling of Simulation Events and Setting Up the Environment

In addition to policies and procedures, consideration needs to be given to scheduling of simulations and resources via a calendar, database, or combination of resources. Ensuring sufficient space(s) and resources, including patient simulators, supporting equipment, standardized patients, and other resources, can be taxing, but are essential to the operation of a center. As a center's operations increase in complexity, including the increased number of faculty and participant users, a scheduling program becomes essential to daily operation and assurance of equitable availability of resources. Policies for faculty and participants regarding use of and scheduling for a variety of uses and resources within the simulation lab ensures clarity of purpose and protection of resources. A process and a tool can be developed for faculty requests for scheduling.

Simulation activities require realistic equipment in the environment and a detailed way for the environment to be set up for the encounter to seem plausible. The simulation lab manager or support personnel must take the lead in establishing a process for creating equipment resource list(s), or setup list(s). Lab equipment lists and photos with details of setup protocols are essential for helping lab staff set up simulation equipment as required by the educational activity.

Other policy considerations include equipment maintenance and repair, review and revision of job descriptions to coincide with job changes, equipment security, student dress, use of cell phones, borrowing of equipment and resources, inventory management, and training of faculty and staff. Training of faculty, standardized patients, and students is a key component of simulation management. Training includes information about cases, simulation, and audiovisual equipment, as well as debriefing standards. Defining the expectations for faculty in the environment is important, including their role(s) in managing the simulation, as well as other potential responsibilities, such as assisting with setup, cleanup, or supply management. In order for simulation to be effective, faculty need to learn to manage all facets of the environment and equipment.

Consent to Be Recorded

Another key policy related to students and standardized patients is to acquire consent to be video recorded. Video recording during simulation can be essential to the learning process. Development of a policy and form for the student to sign early in the program can ease the process as the student proceeds through the curriculum and simulation activities. It is essential to use legal resources to review the process and form help to ensure that both meet the standards for your program.

CONCLUSION

As the process of integrating audio or visual hardware and software is ever growing and technology advancements can be measured in months rather than years, it is the hope of the authors of this chapter that a logical and practical approach to the development of an audiovisual enhanced simulation program has been presented. This chapter outlines a process to investigate, select, and install state-of-the-art audiovisual equipment and software, including selection of a collaborative team, suggested methods for determining a program's needs and matching those needs to technologic resources, seeking and evaluating proposals from vendors as well as design considerations for placements of camera and microphones. Additional considerations related to the daily operation of the equipment and software as a learner-centered simulation center were explored. Topics discussed include center management, control-room functions, video recording or viewing policies and procedures, and considerations as to when to film or record. If you are recording or are exploring recording options for educational simulation experiences or high-stakes performance, it is our desire that this chapter provides valuable information to the reader to assist with your decision-making processes.

REFERENCES

Alfes, C. (2011). Short communication: Creating an introductory video library to set the simulation stage. *Clinical Simulation in Nursing, 8*, e1–e2. doi:10.1016/j.ecns.2011.03.001

Anderson, J. M., Murphy, A. A., Boyle, K. B., Yaeger, K. A., & Halamek, L. P. (2006). Simulating extracorporeal membrane oxygenation emergencies to improve human performance. Part II: Assessment of technical and behavioral skills. *Simulation in Healthcare, 1*(4), 228–232.

Burns, H. K., O'Donnell, J., & Artman, J. (2010). High-fidelity simulation in teaching problem solving to 1st-year nursing students: A novel use of the nursing process. *Clinical Simulation in Nursing, 6*, e87–e95. doi:10.1016/j.ecns.2009.07.005

Cantrell, M. A., Mariani, B., & Meakim, C. (2016). An innovative approach using clinical simulation to teach quality and safety principles to undergraduate nursing students. *Nursing Education Perspectives, 37*(4), 236–238. doi:10.3928/01484834-20150218-05

Cardoza, M. P. (2011). Neuroscience and simulation: An evolving theory of brain-based education. *Clinical Simulation in Nursing, 7*(6), e205–e208. doi:10.1016/j.ecns.2011.08.004

Chau, J., Chang, A., Lee, I., Lee, D., & Wotton, Y. (2001). Effects of using videotaped vignettes on enhancing students' critical thinking ability in a baccalaureate nursing programme. *Journal of Advanced Nursing, 36*(1), 112–119. doi:10.1046/j.1365-2648.2001.01948.x

Cheng, A., Eppich, W., Grant, V., Sherbino, J., Zendejas, B., & Cook, D. A. (2014). Debriefing for technology-enhanced simulation: A systematic review and meta-analysis. *Medical Education, 48*(7), 657–666.

Chronister, C., & Brown, D. (2012). Comparison of simulation debriefing methods. *Clinical Simulation in Nursing, 8*(7), e281–e288. doi:10.1016/j.ecns.2010.12.005

Daniels, K., Lipman, S., Harney, K., Arafeh, J., & Druzin, M. (2008). Use of simulation based team training for obstetric crises in resident education. *Simulation in Healthcare, 3*(3), 154–160.

Dhingra, S. S., & Kearns, L. (2011). Hardware and software. In L. Wilson & L. J. Rockstraw (Eds.), *Human simulation for nursing and health professions* (pp. 11–23). New York, NY: Springer Publishing.

Fanning, R. M., & Gaba, D. M. (2007). The role of debriefing in simulation-based learning. *Simulation in Healthcare, 2*(2), 115–125.

Family Educational Rights and Privacy Act. (2016). U.S. Department of Education. Retrieved from https://www2.ed.gov/policy/gen/guid/fpco/ferpa/index.html

Furman, G. E., Smee, S., & Wilson, C. (2010). Quality assurance best practices for simulation-based examinations. *Simulation in Healthcare, 5*(4), 226–231. doi:10.1097/SIH.0b013e3181da5c93

Gantt, L. T. (2013). The effect of preparation on anxiety and performance in summative simulations. *Clinical Simulation in Nursing, 9*(1), e25–e33. doi:10.1016/j.ecns.2011.07.004

Grant, J. S., Moss, J., Epps, C., & Watts, P. (2010). Using video-facilitated feedback to improve student performance following high-fidelity simulation. *Clinical Simulation in Nursing, 6*(5), e177–e184. doi:10.1016/j.ecns.2009.09.001

Jeffries, P. R. (2012). *Simulation in nursing education: From conceptualization to evaluation* (2nd ed.). New York, NY: National League for Nursing.

Johnson-Russel, J., & Bailey, C. (2010). Facilitated debriefing. In W. M. Nehring & F. R. Lashely (Eds.), *High-fidelity patient simulation in nursing education* (pp. 369–385). Sudbury, MA: Jones & Bartlett.

Kaur-Dusaj, T. (2014). *A randomized control study comparing outcomes in student nurses who utilize video during simulation debriefing as compared to those who utilize traditional debriefing* (Doctoral dissertation). Retrieved from http://search.proquest.com.ezp1.villanova.edu/docview/1560895429?pq origsite=summon

Koepp, M. J., Gunn, R. N., Lawrence, A. D., Cunningham, V. J., Dagher, A., Jones, T., ... Grasby, P. M. (1998). Evidence for striatal dopamine release during a video game. *Nature, 393*(6682), 266–268.

Kromann, C. B., Jensen, M. L., & Ringsted, C. (2009). The effect of testing on skills learning. *Medical Education, 43*(1), 21–27. doi:10.1111/j.1365-2923.2008.03245.x

Levett-Jones, T., & Lapkin, S. (2014). A systematic review of the effectiveness of simulation debriefing in health professional education. *Nurse Education Today, 34*(6), e58–e63.

Megel, M. E., Bailey, C., Schnell, A., Whiteaker, D., & Vogel, A. (2013). High-fidelity simulation: How are we using the videos? *Clinical Simulation in Nursing, 9*(8), e305–e310. doi:10.1016/j.ecns.2012.04.003

Messmer, P. R. (2008). Enhancing nurse-physician collaboration using pediatric simulation. *Journal of Continuing Education in Nursing, 39*(7), 319–327. doi:10.3928/00220124-20080701-07

Ness, A. (2006). *Preparing and evaluating a request for proposals: How to select a vendor.* Lexington, KY: National Association of Government Defined Contribution Administrators. Retrieved from www.nagdca.org/content.cfm/id/preparing_and_evaluating_a_request_for_proposals

NPower Network. (2011). Selecting the right technology vendor. Retrieved from https://www.adrc-tae.acl.gov/tiki-download_file.php?fileId=27666

Oakes, K. (2004). Do the due diligence! *T + D, 58*(4), 15–16. Retrieved from http://ezproxy.villanova.edu/login?url=http://search.proquest.com/docview/227005635?accountid=14853

Raglione, A. (2015). Best practices: Securing data at rest, in use, and in motion. Retrieved from https://www.datamotion.com/2015/12/best-practices-securing-data-at-rest-in-use-and-in-motion

Roediger, H. L., & Karpicke, J. D. (2006). The power of testing memory: Basic research and implications for educational practice. *Perspectives on Psychological Science, 1*(3), 181–210.

Scherer, L., Chang, M., Meredith, J. W., & Battistella, F. (2003). Videotape review leads to rapid and sustained learning. *American Journal of Surgery, 185*, 516–520. doi:10.1016/S0002-9610(03)00062-X

Seropian, M., & Lavey, R. (2010). Design considerations for healthcare simulation facilities. *Simulation in Healthcare, 5*(6), 338–345.

Sharpnack, P. A., Goliat, L., Baker, J. R., Rogers, K., & Shockey, P. (2013). Thinking like a nurse: Using video simulation to rehearse for professional practice. *Clinical Simulation in Nursing, 9*(12), e571–e577. doi:10.1016/j.ecns.2013.05.004

Winters, J., Hauck, B., Riggs, C. J., Clawson, J., & Collins, J. (2003). Use of videotaping to assess competencies and course outcomes. *Journal of Nursing Education, 42*(10), 472–476.

CHAPTER 8

Integration of Disability in Nursing Education With Standardized Patients

Suzanne C. Smeltzer, Bette Mariani, and Colleen H. Meakim

OVERVIEW AND BACKGROUND

It is estimated that almost 60 million people in the United States and more than 1 billion people worldwide live with a disability (World Health Organization [WHO], 2011). The number of people with disabilities in the United States makes this population the largest minority group in the country. *Disability*, a term that has many definitions, refers to limitations in one's ability to perform usual daily activities and social roles because of physical, cognitive, sensory, or emotional impairment, which is often due in part to environmental barriers (Iezzoni, 2006). Although disability may have a negative connotation in society and in health care, the word is neither positive nor negative and merely reflects one's ability to participate in activities and roles in a world made for those without disability. It does not imply dependence, reluctance, or unwillingness to participate.

Research indicates that individuals with disability often have difficulty obtaining health care and that the health care they receive is of lower quality than that provided to individuals without disability, despite the passage of the Americans with Disabilities Act in 1990 (Peacock, Iezzoni, & Harkin, 2015; WHO, 2011). Individuals with disability report poor communication, compromised care, negative attitudes on the part of health care professionals, lack of sensitivity, and fears related to quality of care—all issues of universal concern to the nursing and medical professions. In addition, people with disability report being stigmatized, stereotyped, ignored, and occasionally abused by health care professionals (Smeltzer, Avery, & Haynor, 2012; U.S. Department of Health and Human Services [USDHHS], 2002, 2005; WHO, 2011).

The lack of inclusion of disability-related content and the lack of exposure of health care professions students to individuals with disabilities during their education and training have been identified as major factors in disparities in health care that affect those with disabilities (Kirschner & Curry, 2009; USDHHS, 2005). Multiple calls have been issued in response to these health disparities to improve the knowledge, skills, and attitudes of health care professionals (Institute of Medicine, 2007; Smeltzer, Dolen, Robinson-Smith, & Zimmerman, 2005; USDHHS, 2005). Despite the multiple calls for action, progress in addressing these health care disparities has been slow.

One strategy consistently recommended to begin to address these health care disparities is to incorporate content and concepts related to disability in health professions' education and training programs (Kirschner & Curry, 2009; USDHHS, 2005). Strategies to integrate such content and concepts include (a) revision of course and program objectives with attention to competencies (i.e., knowledge, attitudes, behaviors, and skills) required to ensure quality health care for those with disabilities; (b) use of innovative teaching strategies and learning experiences that address the health-related needs of individuals with disabilities; and (c) provision of interactive experiences for all health professions students in which they have the opportunity to communicate with individuals with disabilities and to learn firsthand about the health disparities these individuals experience and the barriers they often encounter in their efforts to obtain health care. The inclusion of individuals with disabilities in these efforts is essential to ensure that future health care providers learn about disability-related issues from those most knowledgeable about their experiences and the barriers they encounter in their efforts to obtain health care. Further, the practice of including individuals with disabilities is consistent with a patient-centered approach and the expression, "nothing about me without me" (Iezzoni & Long-Bellil, 2012). This expression clearly conveys the importance of individuals with a disability having a role or voice in determining what is relevant when their health needs are being discussed and care and treatment are being determined. The inclusion of persons with disabilities as standardized patients (SPs) for teaching and testing purposes is essential to ensure that the responses of the "patient" are authentic and credible (Long-Bellil et al., 2011).

Villanova University College of Nursing faculty have had a long-standing interest in addressing the health disparities of people with disabilities and the use of strategies to improve their health and health care, including nursing care, in the nursing education program. A small group of faculty members, hereafter referred to as the Project Team, addressed the topic through the integration of SPs with actual disabilities in the curriculum and to an already functioning SP program with actors and students serving the role of patient. Important to the faculty was the need to accomplish this without disrupting the existing curriculum and without increasing faculty workload. Previous research findings have suggested that these two issues could potentially scuttle the project because nursing faculty generally have considerable content to teach to students and report having heavy teaching loads (Smeltzer, Blunt, Marozsan, & Wetzel-Effinger, 2015; Smeltzer, Mariani, et al., 2005).

WHY ARE PEOPLE WITH DISABILITY IMPORTANT TO BE INCLUDED AS SPs?

Inclusion of people with disability (PWD) as SPs is essential because these individuals have a unique perspective and expertise that other people who may act out a role do not have. They are most knowledgeable about living with the complexities of their disability and are most credible in discussing the consequences of their disability on their daily lives, health, and well-being. Inclusion of PWD as SPs also provides learners with the opportunity to learn from those who are the true "experts" and helps to dispel fears and preconceptions that learners may have about disability. An individual without disability who acts out the role of a patient with disability lacks the authenticity that is valued by students and may also harbor unrecognized personal misconceptions related to disability, which could be inadvertently conveyed to learners (Long-Bellil et al., 2011).

INTEGRATION OF SPs WITH DISABILITY ACROSS THE CURRICULUM

The goal of integrating a program of simulation that includes SPs with disability is to do so in a way that maximizes the value of this learning experience for students and for people with disabilities, with the least disruption to the academic program to allow for a smooth transition. Oftentimes, new curricular content is seen as difficult to implement, as most curricula are already so rich with content and concepts that faculty find it difficult to envision how they can fit "one more thing" into the program. The goal of this integration is to facilitate simulation experiences while assimilating these experiences into the curriculum in a meaningful way that fosters attainment of student learning objectives (Masters, 2014). A key factor to this integration is faculty support and investment in the significance of this curricular integration (Conrad, Guhde, Brown, Chronister, & Ross-Alaolmolki, 2011; Masters, 2014).

First, it is important to assemble a team of champions who are committed to adopting this important curricular intervention. Building a team with a shared vision, and supporting this team are key steps to success (Conrad et al., 2011). The team can develop a strategic plan outlining the goals and objectives of the program, key stakeholders, recruiting and training of SPs, financial considerations, and sustainability of the program. Part of the strategy is to keep the faculty well informed, to elicit their feedback and thoughts, to provide a clear picture of the plan, and provide for ongoing evaluation. Meeting with faculty gives a voice to their concerns, and helps them feel invested in the plan. It is important for faculty to understand why this is important not only to student learning, but also to the delivery of safe, quality care to people with a disability.

In a study by Brown, Graham, Richeson, Wu, and McDermott (2010), medical students demonstrated lower performance on objective structured clinical examinations (OSCEs) with SPs with disability than with those without disability. Brown and colleagues (2010) concluded that greater emphasis needs to be placed on teaching disability-related concepts and content throughout the curriculum. It is important to critically examine the existing curriculum to determine where it can be modified or adapted to include simulation-based learning experiences (SBLEs) with SPs with disability. There are two main goals of this curricular integration. The first goal is to have students learn about caring for patients with preexisting disability within the context of their current health problem to learn to provide quality care for people with disability. The second goal is to ensure a smooth transition along with curricular integration. These concepts about the care of people with disability are crucial to integrate into nursing's and other health care professions' curricula to assist students in learning to care for people with a disability.

PLAN FOR IMPLEMENTATION

Communication between the project team and the faculty is critical to the successful integration of the SBLEs with SPs with disability. The project team should develop a plan for transition, and discuss the plan with the course faculty, so they can understand how to best integrate the SBLE with SPs with disability and what the outcome will be for students and ultimately for patients. Next, a plan for the changes to existing curriculum and the SBLEs has to be designed. This could be as simple as adapting an existing communication learning strategy to include an SP with disability. In the original communication unit, the student may learn communication techniques through communicating with an SP without disability or with a student peer. In the SBLE that incorporates learning about PWD, the SBLE would include an SP with an actual disability. As the program progresses into sophomore, junior, and senior years, more opportunities can be identified to integrate SPs with disability into simulation experiences that already include SPs or human patient simulators.

A critical piece of the program of incorporating SBLEs with SPs with disability includes students receiving information to prepare them for the experience with an SP with disability. This includes readings that help to inform students about caring for PWD. Based on the International Nursing Association for Clinical Simulation and Learning Design Standard of Practice (Lioce et al., 2015), SBLEs include prebriefing, the scenario, and debriefing. The prebriefing addresses the objectives of the SBLE, as well as provides an overview of the scenario and the environment. The students participate in the scenario, followed by debriefing. In addition to the debriefing that is customary with an SBLE, if possible, the SP with disability can provide postscenario feedback to the students about their interaction with the SP with disability. Table 8.1 illustrates the changes made in one nursing curriculum to integrate SPs with disability into SBLEs.

An important part of the curricular integration is to provide continuous evaluation of the SBLE, the SPs with disability, the logistics of the program, and student feedback and to continually review the strategic plan.

Table 8.1	Sample SBLE Curricular Integration Plan	
Course Level and Name	**Original SBLE**	**Revised SBLE With SPWDs**
Freshman: Introduction to Nursing I	Communication content	Content along with videotaped communication SBLE, including a 25-year-old SPWD with a T-7 spinal cord injury and in-class activity
Freshman: Introduction to Nursing II Second semester	Summative capstone SBLE with vital signs, communication, and patient education	Summative capstone SBLE, including vital signs, communication, and patient education with SPWD
Sophomore: Assessment course	Musculoskeletal assessment SBLE	Musculoskeletal assessment SBLE with SPWD
Sophomore: Fundamentals of Nursing Course	Beginning shift-assessment SBLE	Summative capstone SBLE with SPWD
Junior: Maternal/Child Health Nursing Course		New SBLE with a postpartum SPWD: nurse completes discharge planning for mother and newborn
Senior: Home Health Nursing Course	Home care SBLE patient with heart failure who is noncompliant	Home care SBLE SPWD (who has an amputation) with heart failure who is noncompliant

SBLE, simulation-based learning experience; SPWD, standardized patient with disability.

RECRUITMENT OF SPs WITH DISABILITIES

Recruitment of individuals with disabilities can seem daunting when first planning an SP program that incorporates PWD. Initially, it may be difficult to identify where to find or recruit people with disability to fulfill the role of an SPWD. Networking through local organizations that support people with disability, such as the Post-Polio support group or the Amputee Coalition, is an excellent place to begin. Another strategy is to talk to other colleagues in health care and academic settings to determine whether they may know people who could fill these roles as SPs with disability. Initially, in the development of the program at Villanova University, one faculty member knew the nurse who coordinated a support group for people with post-polio syndrome. Most of these individuals have some degree of musculoskeletal and/or neurological impairment, but were mobile enough to get around, although some used walking aids (cane, crutches, wheelchair, or scooter). These interested individuals provided the first group of PWDS who served as SPs.

As the program expanded, other people with disabilities were through other faculty and staff who knew of individuals living every day with a disability and who were interested and willing to participate as an SPWD to help educate nursing students. They included a woman who had a stroke in her early 20s, a 30-year-old man with spina bifida, and a man in his mid-50s who had a traumatic leg amputation. As the program matured and life circumstances of individuals changed, there was a need for the project team to reach out to other disability-related groups. The project team identified the local Amputee Coalition through an Internet search, and contacted the organization to provide some information about the SPWD program and to determine possible interest in participation among its members. The group leader was eager to help, and shared the details of the program with the amputee support group. Interested members attended an informational meeting held by the director of simulation at the college of nursing, which ultimately led to additional people being hired as SPs with disability.

Other options could include advertising in newspapers, flyers, or church bulletins; attending meetings of groups at local churches or other types of communities; placing a call to community clubs or support groups and talking with other health care education program staff who run SP programs or with companies that make equipment for people with disabilities (Bosek, Li, & Hicks, 2007; Ferguson, McDonough, Stowe, & Sturpe, 2011; Wallace, 2007).

When recruiting SPWDs, it is helpful to hold an information session to explain the overall program, describe the role of the SP, and, if possible, to have a currently employed SPWD speak about his or her experience and feelings about the work in the program. As most recruits will not be experienced SPs or actors, use of pictures or video clips can assist in helping people gain a better understanding of what is expected of them in the SP role.

TRAINING OF SPs WITH DISABILITY AND PROVIDING FEEDBACK ON PERFORMANCE

Once hired, SPs with disability need training related to the overall program and policies, as well as the specific case(s) in which they will participate (Wallace, 2007). One caveat related to including an SPWD is that often a case has to be modified to align with the person's disability. If the goal for the SBLE is to assess musculoskeletal and neurologic systems, both a person with an amputation and one with spina bifida may be able to fulfill the role, but the specific disability may have an impact on some of the details of the SBLE and training of the SP.

Reviewing the case and providing details of the script are very important. When training SPs for a specific SBLE, it is important to consider the purpose (including formative vs. summative experiences) of the SBLE, the backstory of the scenario, the education level of the student, the objectives for the SBLE, and the script. When training is conducted with a group of SPs with disability, it is important to specify what the standardized portion of the case is, and what can be individualized based on the person's disability (Wallace, 2007). Pictures, demonstrations, or previous videos of the SBLEs, if available, are effective tools to help people who are new to the SP role to better understand what they are expected to do in the scenario. If an SBLE is to be used for testing purposes (summative), then case design and scripts are more prescribed; however, the SBLE objectives, health problem/situation, and case can still be built around the SP's specific disability.

New SPs with disability may need one or more opportunities to practice and receive feedback on their enactment of the role to develop confidence and skill. Once SPs with disability are trained and become more experienced, they can be extremely effective in helping to train other new SPs with disability for the role. The experienced SPWD can provide details about nuances, which occur during simulation activities and help prepare new SPs with disability for these situations.

Providing feedback to the SPs with disability is essential. Because these individuals are new to this type of role and take it very seriously, they desire feedback in order to improve their performance in their role(s) and in giving feedback to students (Smeltzer, Mariani et al., 2015). It is ideal if a simulation center has a resource person who can do this. If not, videos can be observed following an experience; faculty who are viewing scenarios can provide feedback directly or through the lab manager or SP trainer, or another more experienced SP can observe the new SP in action or in a recorded session with a checklist and provide feedback.

WRITING SBLEs FOR PEOPLE WITH DISABILITY

Writing SBLEs for PWD can be done in several ways. A generic type of SBLE can be written that could be relevant to many PWD, so that each individual's details can be applied to the case. For example, a case in which the patient is complaining of shoulder pain is relevant to many people who have a physical disability. Incorporating aspects of the person's disability into the SBLE helps the SPs with disability to be able to use their disability as a means to help learners appreciate what is important in the care of PWD. In some scenarios, the exact type of disability is not as important as the focus on using proper therapeutic communication (communicating directly with the person with disability, not his or her support person; using person-first language; sitting at eye level; asking questions about the impact of the disability on the person's/patient's ability to manage the problem/health issue/situation; and asking what help is needed before assisting) and assessing the disability and its impact on the problem/health issue/situation at hand.

Another approach to developing an SBLE is to develop it around the person's disability. An example is the development of a case of a woman whose status is poststroke at 20 years of age, who has left-sided lower extremity weakness and a flaccid left arm, and has just delivered her first baby. Using the person's actual disability and his or her true story makes for a very powerful scenario that can be easily enacted by the SPWD. In addition, an SBLE may be blended. For example, the scenario can be amended to accommodate the same situation (childbirth with a focus on healthy postpartum assessment, discharge planning, and home safety assessment) but using a scenario for a person with a different disability and different life story. The objectives for the scenario can remain the same. Writing or amending the scenario with input from the SPWD can be a key to making it work. Both parties (writer and SPWD) can collaborate on making the objectives for the SBLE meet the patient's story. Sometimes the SPWD's story may need some modification in order to meet objectives for the SBLE.

MANAGING SBLE ACTIVITIES WITH SPs WITH DISABILITY

It is important to consider the fatigue factor when running simulation days with SPs with disability. Individuals with a disability, and particularly those who are aging, can become fatigued more quickly than people who do not have a disability. Because of the disability, they require more energy to complete activities of daily living (University of Washington Rehabilitation Research and Training Center, n.d.). Consequently, they may need frequent breaks or to be scheduled in shifts to prevent fatigue that interferes with their ability to participate. When schedules are developed, it is important to include additional breaks and people, or have one SPWD in the morning and a different SPWD in the afternoon. It is also useful to have an extra SPWD available or to schedule another person as a backup in case the original person becomes ill. Another consideration is planning for handicap-accessible parking, building access and accommodation, and ensuring that there is access nearby to food, drink, and accessible bathroom facilities. In addition, inclement weather (e.g., snow) can be a factor in mobility, so having a backup plan for those types of situations is also important.

SPs WITH DISABILITY GIVING FEEDBACK TO LEARNERS

Inclusion of SPs provides a foundation for the development of professional communication skills (Weaver & Erby, 2012). Because intentional communication with a person with disability is one of the most important aspects of caring for a person with a disability, teaching SPs with disability to provide feedback to the students/learners about their communication is also essential. These key aspects should be included in the feedback to learners: Did the learner talk to me as a person directly and not only to the caregiver or support person? Did the learner treat me as an adult, demonstrate active listening and make eye contact with me, ask about my disability and its impact on my current situation, ask whether I need assistance with tasks rather than assume that I do or do not (Smeltzer, 2014)? Depending on the scenario objectives, other details could also be provided in the feedback if appropriate to the SBLE, such as did the student assess for risk of abuse, falls, depression, and/or secondary conditions and discuss the potential need for accommodations and modifications (Smeltzer, Mariani, & Meakim, 2017)? In addition to communication, SPs with disability can provide feedback about the style of questioning and learner's body language, both of which have an impact on the emotional connection during the interaction (Hill, Bronwyn, & Theordoros, 2010).

CONTRIBUTIONS OF SPs WITH DISABILITY

PWD are motivated to participate in health care educational programs because they have a desire to improve health care for future patients who have a disability. They find it to be a rewarding opportunity that offers them a new purpose in life and a chance to contribute to students' learning. It provides a personal sense of satisfaction and reward as they interact with students and see their growth as a result of their interactions with students, particularly related to the specific needs of PWDs (Smeltzer, Blunt et al., 2015).

CONCLUSION

The inclusion of SPWD in nursing education has the potential to improve the knowledge, attitudes and skills of students who will encounter individuals with disabilities in all health care environments, facilities, and home care settings throughout their professional careers. Simulations that incorporate SPWDs enable students to learn to communicate effectively, appropriately and sensitively with individuals with disabilities across the lifespan and with diverse types of disabilities. A well-planned strategy to integrate SPWDs in nursing education will enhance nursing students' learning experiences and faculty members' adoption of this innovative teaching approach with the goal of improving health care for persons with disabilities.

REFERENCES

Bosek, M. S., Li, S., & Hicks, F. D. (2007). Working with standardized patients: A primer. *International Journal of Nursing Education Scholarship, 4*(1), 1–12. doi:10.2202/1548-923X.1437

Brown, R., Graham, C., Richeson, N., Wu, J., & McDermott, S. (2010). Evaluation of medical student performance on objective structured clinical exams with standardized patients with and without disabilities. *Academic Medicine, 85,* 1766–1771. doi:10.1097/ACM.0b013e3181f849dc

Conrad, M. A., Guhde, J., Brown, D., Chronister, C., & Ross-Alaolmolki, K. (2011). Trans-formational leadership: Instituting a nursing simulation program. *Clinical Simulation in Nursing, 7,* e189–e195. doi:10.1016/j.ecns.2010.02.007

Ferguson, D., McDonough, S., Stowe, C., & Sturpe, D. (2011). Recruiting and training standardized patients—Tips and tools for success. Retrieved from http://www.aacp.org/meetingsandevents/pastmeetings/2011/Documents/Recruiting and training Standardized PatientsHandout .pdf

Hill, A. E., Bronwyn, J. D., & Theordoros, D. G. (2010). A review of standardized patients in clinical evaluation: Implications for speech-language pathology programs. *International Journal of Speech-Language Pathology, 12*(3), 259–270. doi:10.3109/17549500903082445

Iezzoni, L. I. (2006). Going beyond disease to address disability. *New England Journal of Medicine, 355*(10), 976–979. doi:10.1056/NEJMp068093

Iezzoni, L. I., & Long-Bellil, L. M. (2012). Training physicians about caring for persons with disabilities: "Nothing about us without us!" *Disability and Health Journal, 5*(3), 136–139.

Institute of Medicine. (2007). *The future of disability in America.* Washington, DC: National Academies Press.

Kirschner, K. L., & Curry, R. H. (2009). Educating health care professionals to care for patients with disabilities. *Journal of the American Medical Association, 302*(12), 1334–1335.

Lioce, L., Meakim, C. H., Fey, M. K., Chmil, J. V., Mariani, B., & Alinier, G. (2015). Standards of best practice: Simulation standard IX: Simulation design. *Clinical Simulation in Nursing, 11*, 309–315. doi: 10.1016/j.ecns.2015.03.005

Long-Bellil, L. M., Robey, K. L., Graham, C. L., Minihan, P. M., Smeltzer, S. C., & Kahn, P. (2011). Teaching medical students about disability: The use of standardized patients. *Academic Medicine, 86*(11), 1163–1170. doi:10.1097/ACM.0b013e318226b5dc

Masters, K. (2014). Journey toward integration of simulation in a baccalaureate nursing curriculum. *Journal of Nursing Education, 53*(2), 102–104.

Peacock, G., Iezzoni, L. I., & Harkin, T. R. (2015). Health care for Americans with disabilities—25 Years after the ADA. *New England Journal of Medicine, 373*(10), 892–893.

Smeltzer, S. C. (2014). Chronic illness and disability. In J. L. Hinkle & K. H. Cheever (Eds.), *Brunner & Suddarth's textbook of medical–surgical nursing* (13th ed., pp. 131–152). Philadelphia, PA: Wolters Kluwer/Lippincott Williams & Wilkins.

Smeltzer, S. C., Avery, C., & Haynor, P. (2012). Interactions of people with disabilities and nursing staff during hospitalization. *American Journal of Nursing, 112*(4), 30–37; quiz 38, 52.

Smeltzer, S. C., Blunt, E., Marozsan, H., & Wetzel-Effinger, L. (2015). Inclusion of disability-related content in nurse practitioner curricula. *Journal of the American Association of Nurse Practitioners, 27*(4), 213–221.

Smeltzer, S. C., Dolen, M. A., Robinson-Smith, G., & Zimmerman, V. (2005). Integration of disability-related content in nursing curricula. *Nursing Education Perspectives, 26*(4), 210–216. Retrieved from http://www.nln.org/newsroom/newsletters-and-journal/nursing-education-perspectives-journal

Smeltzer, S. C., Mariani, B., Ross, J. G., Petit de Mange, E., Meakim, C. H., Bruderle, E., & Nthenge, S. (2015). Persons with disability: Their experiences as standardized patients in an Undergraduate Nursing Program. *Nursing Education Perspectives, 36*(6), 398–400.

Smeltzer, S. C., Mariani, B., & Meakim, C. (2017). *Assessment of the patient with a disability checklist.* Washington, DC: National League for Nursing; Advancing Care Excellence for Persons with Disabilities (ACE.D) Program.

University of Washington Rehabilitation Research and Training Center. (n.d.). Aging well with a physical disability: Factsheet series. Retrieved from http://agerrtc.washington.edu/info/factsheets/fatigue

U.S. Department of Health and Human Services. (2002). *Report of the surgeon general's conference on health disparities and mental retardation. Closing the gap: A national blueprint to improve the health of persons with mental retardation.* Rockville, MD: U.S. Department of Health and Human Services. Retrieved from https://www.nichd.nih.gov/publications/pubs/closingthegap/Pages/index.aspx

U.S. Department of Health and Human Services. (2005). *The surgeon general's call to action to improve the health and wellness of persons with disabilities.* Rockville, MD: U.S. Department of Health and Human Services. Retrieved from http://www.ncbi.nlm.nih.gov/pubmed/20669510

Wallace, P. (2007). *Coaching standardized patients: For use in the assessment of clinical competence.* New York, NY: Springer Publishing.

Weaver, M., & Erby, L. (2012). Standardized patients: A promising tool for health education and health promotion. *Health Promotion Practice, 13*(2), 169–174. doi:10.1177/1524839911432006

World Health Organization and the World Bank. (2011). *World report on disability.* Geneva, Switzerland: Author.

CHAPTER 9

IV Simulation Curriculum Development

Shannon Krolikowski

INTRAVENOUS SIMULATION

Intensifying standards and increases in technology demand the transformation of education in colleges and universities worldwide. Nursing education is no exception. In the not-so-distant past, many of the skills and competencies necessary to substantiate a student nurses' capabilities transpired through practicing on a student nurse peer or other willing nursing program volunteer. These skills encompassed a vast spectrum of learning objectives, including such noninvasive nursing procedures as taking each other's blood pressures to more invasive procedures such as nasogastric tube and Foley catheter insertion.

Learning how to insert intravenous (IV) catheters is quite possibly the skill student nurses look most forward to acquiring during their nursing education. In the past, this skill was fairly easily taught and performed within nursing labs throughout the United States, with students using each other's veins for practice. In today's nursing labs, IV education has fallen on hard times as a result of financial and litigious concerns. IV catheters, which the students use for practice, continue to rise in cost, causing a substantial decrease in most lab coordinators already thinly stretched budgets, placing strict limitations on the number of IV starts allotted to each student. Another concern involves the possibility of a needle-stick injury occurring within the lab setting. Carefully developed policies and procedures must be in place if this predicament occurs, including the necessary follow-up bloodwork required by the involved students. Simulation solves these dilemmas by allowing students the opportunity to learn IV skills while taking away the potential risks to the nursing lab through the use of an IV simulator.

When students begin a simulation or skills lab, they enter into it with the somewhat mistaken expectation that they will perfect every nursing skill or task within this setting, and venture out into the nursing world with the ability to flawlessly perform any skill solicited of them. As much as nursing educators would like to imagine this as an accurate description of what transpires within simulation and skills labs, the realistic probability and actual syllabus objective descriptions state that the students walk away with the knowledge and understanding of how to safely and accurately perform these skills or tasks within the clinical setting. Perfection, or near to it, is what transpires within the actual nursing setting. No other skill needs to be more accurate than IV insertion.

Until approximately 5 years ago, from this author's experience, any skill learning performed by the nursing students occurred in the Fundamentals Laboratory (lab). This was the only lab available to the nursing students until the construction of the new Simulation Lab. Any instructional methods for implementing IV education transpired within the Fundamentals Lab during the student's second medical–surgical semester. The IV education was taught by whoever the designated lab instructor was and usually consisted of several different instructors who filled the many lab courses necessary to provide instruction to the entire second-level nursing student group.

The first step within the IV education protocol consisted of the students viewing a series of videos within the lab focusing on preparing a patient for an IV line, IV cannulation, care and maintenance of the IV site, and discontinuing an IV catheter. After viewing the videos, the lab instructor provided further instruction through lecturing. Subsequently, the students practiced IV cannulations on mannequin arms preloaded with simulated blood, with the instructor overseeing the attempts. Finally, following the mannequin arm practice, students were required to sign an IV Start Informed Consent form. On signature completion, the students commenced to practicing IV cannulation on each other as the lab instructor said a prayer for anyone who entered the lab that day, that he or she came in well hydrated. Those students who chose not to sign the informed consent observed the other students during their IV cannulation performances. The instructor was required to actively observe each student's IV cannulation attempt(s).

Several complications existed with the use of this IV program protocol. First, if the students did not sign the informed consent, they did not receive the opportunity to practice IV cannulation in a realistic fashion. Second, because the students were attempting IV cannulation on each other, a standardized method of assessment could not transpire because every student could not attempt IV cannulation on the same vein. Third, because each student's attempt had to be witnessed by the instructor, it resulted in a slow process with many students stating boredom. Not all of the students could gather around to observe the individual IV cannulation attempt, yet every student had to remain present until the opportunity presented itself for his or her turn under the instructor's surveillance. Finally, although the students who participated in the IV cannulation performances signed an informed consent releasing the university from any responsibility, the university was still at risk for potential liability from either the student who was performing the procedure or the student on the receiving end of the procedure.

Beside the noted complications with the preexisting IV program protocol and the decree from the university stating students no longer practice IV cannulations on each other, an addition to the simulation lab created the need to change the way IV education transpired. This addition was the purchase of Laerdal's Virtual IV simulator, that consists of the software, simulator, and the computer that houses the software and to which the simulator is attached. The Virtual IV simulator provides learners with the opportunity to learn and practice IV insertions noninvasively in a safe, controlled environment preparing them for real-world experiences within clinical settings. It would be irrational to purchase this equipment that cost in excess of $18,000 and not use it to its fullest potential.

This series of events created the need to develop and implement a new curriculum and protocol for the IV education within the school of nursing. Although essential to implement a new curriculum, past components of the old curriculum remain crucial. It is still necessary to teach students the proper technique of IV insertion and allow them to familiarize themselves with and learn how to manipulate IV equipment and supplies through the use of videos and mannequin arms. The addition of the simulator creates the need to orientate students on the operation of the Virtual IV simulator, develop the module sequence most appropriate for the students, and determine how competence is measured and achieved (Reyes, Stillsmoking, & Chadwick-Hopkins, 2008).

The Bachelor of Science in Nursing (BSN) students receiving training with the Virtual IV simulator successfully completed their fundamentals of nursing courses and clinical practicum, and mental health nursing courses and clinical practicum. These students are currently within their third semester of the program, which is comprised of level-one medical–surgical nursing courses, including a nutrition didactic course, medical–surgical nursing didactic course, clinical practicum, and simulation lab. Within their 2-hour weekly simulation lab, they experience not only a simulated medical–surgical nursing experience, but also learn a variety of nursing skills. Previous to this grouping of students, IV skills were not taught until the students' level-two medical–surgical nursing courses. Once the IV skills were taught, they were never revisited within any of the labs or classes remaining within the students' nursing education. The decision to change when this curriculum is delivered was based on the implementation of simulation within the BSN program education; the students' desire and eagerness to acquire IV skills; and the addition of the Virtual IV simulator, which allows further skill development throughout the remainder of the students' nursing education. Before learning how to insert an IV line, certain skills are acquired within this lab that is related to IV therapy. These skills include learning how to prime, hang, and administer primary and secondary IV tubing; learning how to calculate IV drip rates and IV push medications; learning how to perform a blood transfusion; understanding and using the various IV infusion pumps available within the hospitals in which clinical transpires; and learning how to dress, assess, and remove an IV site. Subsequently, the students learn how to insert an IV line through lecture, demonstration, and practice using a mannequin arm filled with simulated blood. Although the Virtual IV simulator allows the student repeated IV insertion practice opportunities, it remains important for the students to understand how to manipulate true IV catheters and equipment (Jung et al., 2012). This places the introduction and orientation of the Virtual IV simulator toward the end of the students' first semester of their sophomore year.

Virtual IV Experience Learning Objectives

- Students verbally state and demonstrate the correct operation of the Virtual IV simulator.
- Students demonstrate the ability to:
  - Properly select the correct equipment necessary to perform various intravenous cannulations using the Virtual IV simulator, obtaining a 90% or higher within the debriefing for each case scenario.
  - Follow the correct procedure when performing IV cannulation using the Virtual IV simulator, obtaining a 90% or higher within the debriefing for each case scenario.
  - Correctly secure and dress the IV catheter and properly dispose of used supplies when finished performing IV cannulation using the Virtual IV simulator, obtaining a 90% or higher within the debriefing for each case scenario.

A variety of practice case scenarios are available within the Virtual Products software and include varying ethnicities; six different levels of complexity; and trauma, medical, surgical, pediatric, obstetric, and geriatric cases (Laerdal, n.d.). The students' ranges of patient experiences to this point within their education include basic medical–surgical, geriatric, and mental health patient care. Therefore, the practice case scenarios involving medical or geriatric cases are used. The students are also limited to learning within the "S1" level within the Virtual Products software because this is the students' first introduction to IV insertion (Laerdal, n.d.). The practice case scenarios chosen within the Virtual Products software include the medical gastroenteritis case involving a Hispanic female and the upper respiratory infection case involving a geriatric female (Laerdal, n.d.). Subsequent to the students' introduction and orientation to the Virtual IV simulator, a sign-up sheet with slots representing 2-hour time blocks for use of the simulator is distributed, allowing the students to sign their name to the block of time that works best for them. Successful completion of a student's use of the Virtual IV simulator enables the student to begin the insertion of IV lines within the next semester's clinical setting under his or her instructor's observation. The student demonstrates successful completion of the Virtual IV simulator experience by achieving a 90% as determined by the Virtual IV software within both of the case scenarios the students are required to perform. The students have a 2-hour time block with unlimited attempts during this time frame to complete the simulation. In addition, feedback and debriefing are built into the IV simulation software and are provided at the end of each student's IV attempt, with video demonstrations of correct portions of the procedure offered. If a student is unable to accomplish a 90% within the 2-hour time block, additional time with the lab instructor to review IV insertion is scheduled followed by another time block with the Virtual IV simulator.

A complication that exists in learning how to use Laerdal's Virtual IV simulator is that one-on-one instruction is not provided by Laerdal. Whereas a majority of Laerdal's other simulation equipment comes with a 1- or 2-day training provided by a Laerdal educator following installation, the Virtual IV simulator does not. A small amount of instruction may accompany the installation of the Virtual IV simulator, but it is not enough to fully understand its use or potential within an educational setting. On installation, the educator is given an administrator user name and password that allows for the addition and management of students within the system.

The rational starting point to understanding Laerdal's Virtual IV simulator is found within the Virtual Products software in the form of the directions-for-use manual. The manual provides information on the installation or tear down of the Virtual IV simulator; Laerdal's explanation of the benefits, learning objectives and features of the simulator; a quick-start user guide, system overview, training, administration, and frequently asked questions (Laerdal, n.d.). Although the directions for use provide instructors with the basic information on the use of the simulator, it does not provide them with any guidance for curriculum implementation. It may also be perceived as slightly overwhelming to the novice user who has not yet attempted to use the simulator.

The next step to understanding the use of Laerdal's Virtual IV simulator is to observe the system tutorial found within the Virtual Products software. The system tutorial delivers a visual and verbal monologue on the use of the simulator, provides users with an explanation of the different areas that can be explored within the Virtual Products software, and explains the meaning of many of the symbols within the software (Laerdal, n.d.). A special section for the instructor can also be found within the Virtual Products software system tutorial that provides direction on how to add and manage students within the system (Laerdal, n.d.). Again, although the system tutorial provides directions for use, it does not provide any recommendations for curriculum implementation or provide step-by-step instructions for use, or any helpful hints. The tutorial moves fairly fast and is hard to remember when actually using the Virtual IV simulator.

On further exploration of the Virtual Products software, other features that may assist instructors or IV-skills novice users include the procedure video and the anatomical viewer (Laerdal, n.d.). The procedure video provides users with both verbal and visual education on initiating IV lines within a clinical setting, and displays health care providers starting IV lines on actual patients rather than a simulated arm. The anatomical viewer within the Virtual Products software provides views of a supinated or pronated arm and allows the learner to either add or delete skin, nerves, arteries, bones, veins, muscle, and connective tissue (Laerdal, n.d.). This offers the learners a supplemental approach to understanding where veins likely may be palpated, if not plainly visible.

After perusing the directions for use, system tutorial, procedure video, and anatomical viewer within the Virtual Products software, it is necessary for the instructor to practice using the newly acquired simulator. Within the Virtual Products software, two options, practice case scenarios and competency training, are available for use by the learners (Virtual IV In-Hospital Module, n.d.). Novice users should start with the practice case scenarios because as the name suggests, these scenarios provide opportunities for practice with the Virtual IV simulator. The competency training is more appropriate for advanced learners or assessment purposes because it provides learners with increasing complexity after each successful IV cannulation attempt. The competency training may be perfectly suited for students within their final, practicum semester before graduation to further increase their skill and confidence level.

Some instructors may encounter frustration when learning how to use the system because the only instruction received is that provided through the directions for use and system tutorial within the Virtual Products software (Laerdal, n.d.). Educators who do not have a thorough knowledge of the Virtual IV simulator experience difficulty when working with students that may increase the students' fear or anxiety related to their IV insertion skills (Walton, Chute, & Ball, 2011). The only feedback received is that given within the debriefing session after an IV cannulation attempt is made. It can be extremely difficult to pinpoint errors in technique when one has no experience with the simulator and does not have an expert on hand to assist in correcting errors. In addition, one error that is easy to make is not recognizing that a scroll bar exists on the side of the debriefing list. It is necessary to scroll to the very end of the document to completely view the debriefing of the attempt. It may take educators several hours before mastery of the simulator transpires. The author of this chapter has received a significant amount of training within simulation, including the Certificate in Simulation offered by Drexel University, and recommends a person experienced with simulation manage the implementation of the Virtual IV simulator to both the students and faculty using the simulator within the lab setting.

Until students receive the opportunity to initiate an IV line in a human patient, the mere thought of performing the task may instill a sense of terror within them. A large portion of the skill of starting an IV line is having an understanding of the supplies and steps involved. The Virtual IV simulator provides students with the opportunity to practice acquiring the proper supplies and following the correct procedure, providing feedback within the debriefing session that assists in increasing the confidence of the student when faced with performing the skill on a human patient (Johannesson, Olsson, Petersson, & Silén, 2010). The Virtual IV simulator provides an experience that standardizes the learning experience for the students, creating the opportunity for a streamlined process in which all the students learn the skill in the same way. In addition, the learning does not end with the newly acquired, basic medical and geriatric cases; it can be continued and built on within each subsequent semester. The addition of increasingly difficult and challenging IV attempts can be assigned with cases that are extremely relevant to the semester and clinical patients whom the student experiences.

CONCLUSION

It was determined that a 90% can be achieved (vs. 100%) without successfully completing the procedure and that this is acceptable. The rationale for this decision is that within the clinical setting, a nurse may not successfully feed the catheter into the vein every time, but it is still extremely crucial the proper technique for insertion is followed.

It is the responsibility of nursing educators who acquire new equipment to provide an enriching and rewarding learning experience the nursing students whom the equipment is intended to benefit. Implementation of IV simulation curriculum provides students with realistic experiences invoking critical thinking and increases the level of patient care and satisfaction provided by the students within the various health care environments in which they practice.

REFERENCES

Johannesson, E., Olsson, M., Petersson, G., & Silén, C. (2010). Learning features in computer simulation skills training. *Nurse Education in Practice, 10*(5), 268–273.

Jung, E. Y., Park, D. K., Lee, Y. H., Jo, H. S., Lim, Y. S., & Park, R. W. (2012). Evaluation of practical exercises using an intravenous simulator incorporating virtual reality and haptics device technologies. *Nurse Education Today, 32*(4), 458–463.

Reyes, S. D., Stillsmoking, K., & Chadwick-Hopkins, D. (2008). Implementation and evaluation of a virtual simulator system: Teaching intravenous skills. *Clinical Simulation in Nursing, 4*(1), e43–e49. doi:10.1016/j.ecns.2009.05.055

Laerdal [Computer Software]. (n.d.). Virtual IV in-hospital module. Retrieved from http://www.laerdal.com/us/item/280–04201

Walton, J., Chute, E., & Ball, L. (2011). Negotiating the role of the professional nurse: The pedagogy of simulation: A grounded theory study. *Journal of Professional Nursing, 27*(5), 299–310.

PART II

Innovative Nursing Scenarios in Diverse Settings for Diverse Students

CHAPTER 10

Tune Into Simulation Through Physical Examination Using Your Five Senses

Catherine Napoli Rice and Carolynn Spera Bruno

A. IMPLEMENTATION OF SIMULATION-BASED PEDAGOGY IN YOUR INDIVIDUALIZED TEACHING AREA

During the past several years, simulation pedagogy has taken off in leaps and bounds. The breadth of simulation design and implementation has become woven into the fabric of the majority of nursing education in the United States and beyond. As faculty members who teach in both graduate and undergraduate courses, we find that simulation can be challenging to both the novice and seasoned educator. Whether you are a novice or experienced educator remember that Rome was not built in a day and it is okay to move slowly through the simulation experience. Just as you can feel overwhelmed with changes in technology and have a hard time keeping abreast of all the latest and greatest "best practice" methodology, be aware that students also need time, patience, and practice to build their foundational skills. This particular chapter focuses on the use of simulation in the fundamental physical assessment course. We have found simulation to be quite useful in this setting as students can be quite hesitant to touch their student partners. We have had the opportunity to educate many students regarding how essential it is for them to learn, develop, and eventually master the skills of inspection, palpation, percussion, and auscultation. We try to instill in them a vivid awareness of the need to create an assessment environment that allows the nurse to maximize the accuracy of this assessment process while also instilling patient confidence in that process. As such, we emphasize the need to ensure that each student follows a structured, well-organized, and comprehensive preparation and execution process before and during each assessment activity. We explain to the students that this requirement is just as important when they use simulation technology as when dealing with real patients in order to establish a routine they will consistently use to ensure that each step of this process is consistently followed. The use of simulation technology is especially useful in creating the equivalent of "muscle memory" for the students because of the ability to do frequent and repetitive exercises using this technology. It is especially useful in assisting students to learn, develop, and mature their assessment skills.

B. EDUCATIONAL MATERIALS AVAILABLE IN YOUR TEACHING AREA AND RELATED TO YOUR SPECIALTY

The nursing department program offerings include a BS, RN to BS, and MS degree. The university nursing laboratories are each tailored for specific patient environments, which are equipped with high-fidelity simulators. Each simulation area is equipped with scenario-appropriate equipment and SMART Board technology. Items, such as hospital beds, stretchers, fluid infusion devices, fluid drainage systems, monitoring systems, crash carts, ventilators, medication dispensing system, and bedside tables, are available for creating a tailored scenario. Properties, such as clothing, eyeglasses, dentures, wigs, splints, wounds, compression boots, and miscellaneous other items, are readily available to allow the instructor to create a wide range of different patient dispositions. A video-recording device is available to capture student performance and is subsequently used to debrief students regarding their performance.

C. SPECIFIC OBJECTIVES FOR SIMULATION USAGE WITHIN A SPECIFIC COURSE AND THE OVERALL PROGRAM

The overall objective of this simulation scenario is to define parameters of physical assessment for faculty in the context of simulation technology and create an awareness of the need to develop and nurture these skills through the use of simulation technology. Traditionally, physical assessment has been taught in the classroom through a variety of techniques, including lectures, videos, faculty demonstrations, student partnering, and such, and generally it gets concluded with the students demonstrating accurate assessment skills on completion of each module. In an era of evolving technology, nursing graduates must be introduced to and equipped to manage the complexities of the technologic environment they encounter. During each physical assessment module, simulation technology can be a valuable educational tool for both faculty and students. Although we may rely on technology to provide health care personnel with useful patient information (such as heart rhythm using an EKG reading), it is important for students to recognize that although the EKG looks perfect in rhythm, rate, form, and amplitude, the patient could be dead. Students are taught that a diagnosis of "pulseless electrical activity," or PEA, means that the patient is clinically dead. It must be stressed to students that technology, although useful, is limited and is only one of many tools that should be accessed from their assessment tool kit. In fact, it is essential that students first develop and mature their personal assessment skills of inspection, palpation, percussion, and auscultation and then use technology to validate and refine the effectiveness of these skills.

To teach the art of assessment skills (*inspection, palpation, percussion,* and *auscultation*), faculty can direct students to think of themselves as "instruments" to be "tuned" into the process of assessment techniques. Early in the assessment process students are instructed to palpate a radial pulse and count the pulsations for 60 seconds. Depending on the amount of pressure the student uses he or she may report that he or she cannot feel anything. As musicians learn to tune their instruments, so, too, must student nurses learn to tune into physical assessment and quickly adjust their approach, or in this case depress more firmly on the artery.

A second objective of this simulation scenario is to provide a generic teaching template for each physical assessment module that can be tailored by the individual faculty member and includes structured, supportive, and evaluative elements. Learning modules are developed to be prescriptive in nature and are designed with the intent that the student master simple components of the assessment process in a step-by-step sequence before progressing to more complex assessment techniques. Students who successfully complete individual learning modules advance, whereas those who are unsuccessful are offered additional learning opportunities or experiences and remediation activities within an agreeable time frame. Before initiation of the module, students are provided with an evaluative/assessment rubric. On mastery of the module, the student may receive a "satisfactory" or "pass" as a part of a credentialing process. If the student is unsuccessful and unable to perform the assessment, the instructor advises the student in the following manner:

1. Have the student self-evaluate his or her performance using the corresponding skill performance checklist.
2. Instructor provides feedback on student evaluation to identify areas of strength and areas requiring improvement.

3. Instructor and student develop an individualized remedial plan, to include the following:
   a. A review of specific scenario requirements and expectations
   b. Student practicing specific skills in a nonrisk environment
   c. Student reperforms the required assessment skills for validation by the instructor

The timing of each module must be carefully planned and flow from the course content. In addition, the student who attends to the readings and corresponding available media (video demonstrations, etc.) tends to move quickly and efficiently through the learning process. Students should be counseled, however, as to the need to review and reflect on their performance regardless of how rapidly they appear to be progressing.

A formalized reflection process creates an opportunity for students to identify and articulate positive behaviors, areas for improvement, and methods to enhance or address these areas. Weekly reflections, however brief, serve to demonstrate to the student his or her unique development and provide positive reinforcement of the progress being made. Having students identify what they do that contributes to improving their own performance and then having these students share, anonymously, this information with their fellow students can foster a positive communal learning experience.

D. INTRODUCTION OF SCENARIO

Setting the Scene

The scene takes place in a long-term care nursing facility. The patient is an 84-year-old female with a past medical history of coronary artery disease, hypertension, and mild dementia. The patient's chief complaint is dizziness that began after waking this morning. The student nurse is assigned to conduct a general health assessment followed by a physical examination. On completion of the assessments, the student nurse prioritizes an individualized plan of care.

Technology Used

The patient is a high-fidelity human patient simulator (HPS). She is dressed in her nightgown, lying on her hospital bed, covered to her chest with a sheet, and in a semiprivate room with a female roommate of similar age in an accompanying bed. There is a wheelchair next to her bed, an overbed table, a telephone, a call bell, and a water pitcher with a plastic cup. The patient's head of bed is elevated 15°, only one side rail is raised, the bed is in the lowest position with locks secured, and the patient is sleeping on student arrival. The privacy curtain between the beds is open and the lights are dimmed. The person operating the simulator is allowed to answer questions and speak for the patient.

The student is provided with an opportunity to obtain all necessary equipment and forms before entering the patient's room. Equipment needed includes the following: simulator, video recording device, assessment tools such as alcohol hand sanitizer, clean gloves, blood pressure cuff, stethoscope, medical record, and so forth.

Objectives

1. Conduct a general survey of the patient
2. Obtain a health history and complete a physical examination

Description of Participants

Student nurse in long-term care rotation: The student should be prepared in patient assessment techniques, including *inspection, palpation, percussion,* and *auscultation*. The student should be knowledgeable about the equipment and forms necessary to accomplish this task.

The student should obtain the necessary tools and forms from the instructor before entering the patient's room.

An 84-year-old female patient in a long-term care setting: This role is played by a high-fidelity HPS. The HPS is lying down on her bed. The simulator operator responds with short, simple answers to questions posed by the student and indicates that she does not understand when questions are not presented in clear, simple terms. The "patient" should not volunteer any information and should indicate a degree of self-consciousness and hesitancy when "personal" questions are asked.

Instructor running the scenario: The person running the scenario is also operating the HPS (a high-fidelity simulator), unless another qualified operator is available. In that case, the instructor running the scenario observes and takes notes relative to scenario objectives.

E. RUNNING OF THE SCENARIO

The student is given guidance as to the specific objectives of the assignment. The student is told the time of day the assessment will be occurring and is provided with a basic health history of the patient based on forms the patient had completed when she first expressed concerns regarding a change in her health status. The student is expected to identify the tools and forms needed to conduct the assessment and is given the tools and forms requested. After making an introduction and explaining the purpose of the visit, the student should request permission of the patient to begin the interview assessment.

F. PRESENTATION OF COMPLETED TEMPLATE

Title

General Health Assessment and Physical Examination

Scenario Level

Novice

Focus Area

Basic assessment techniques include inspection, palpation, percussion, and auscultation.

Scenario Description

This chapter introduces concepts and techniques of physical assessment in the context of the nursing process. Simulation experiences provide opportunities to develop assessment skills in preparation for clinical courses in a minimal-risk environment. In addition, the simulation can be repeated as often as necessary for the student to gain confidence without exposing actual patients to the student's learning process.

On a note card: Provide the following information about the patient to the student: patient's name, demographics (gender, age, race, religion, occupation, height and weight), pertinent past medical history, presenting symptoms, illnesses, injuries and recent surgeries, current medications, allergies, significant other factors, social history, mental health history, and any other pertinent information. Identify your patient by name (first and last). Note the style of the following Patient Data Form.

Patient Data Form:

Name:

Demographics:

Pertinent Past Medical History:

Presenting Symptoms, Illnesses, Injuries, and Recent Surgeries:

Current Medications:

Allergies:

Significant Other Factors:

Social History:

Mental Health History:

Scenario Objectives

1. Use assessment techniques of inspection, palpation, percussion, and auscultation.
2. Collect data about an individual's health state.
3. Complete a health history and physical examination.

The American Association of Colleges of Nursing (AACN; 2008), *The Essentials of Baccalaureate Education for Professional Nursing* identifies practice-focused outcomes that integrate the knowledge, skills, and attitudes delineated in Essentials I–VIII. The time needed to accomplish each Essential varies, and each Essential does not require a separate course for achievement of the outcomes (AACN, 2008). The Essentials used in our evaluations are the following:

- Essential III: Scholarship for Evidence-Based Practice
- Essential IV: Information Management and Application of Patient Care Technology
- Essential IX: Baccalaureate Generalist Nursing Practice.

In addition, the National Council of State Boards of Nursing (NCLEX-RN®) test plan (2015), has correlated areas of congruency and are inclusive of the following: safe and effective care environment, health promotion and maintenance, and physiologic integrity.

Setting the Scene

Prescenario Setup Checklist

Equip your examination area with the following items (Jarvis, 2016):

Equipment needed

___Examination table
___Simulation device (man, woman, or child)
___Privacy screening
___Wall-mounted or gooseneck stand lamp
___Rolling stool
___Bedside stand or table
___Documentation (pen or pencil and forms)
___Platform scale with height attachment
___Skinfold calipers
___Sphygmomanometer
___Stethoscope with bell and diaphragm end pieces

___Thermometer
___Pulse oximeter
___Flashlight or penlight
___Otoscope/ophthalmoscope
___Tuning fork
___Nasal speculum
___Tongue depressor
___Pocket vision screener
___Skin-marking pen
___Flexible tape measure and ruler marked in centimeters
___Reflex hammer
___Sharp object (split tongue blade)
___Cotton balls
___Clean gloves
___Fecal occult blood test materials
___Gastric pH test strips

Scenario alternatives: If a high-fidelity HPS is unavailable, alternative simulation approaches would be to use a medium-fidelity simulator with student volunteers or other faculty to role-play.

Scenario Implementation

Evaluation Criteria
Required Student Assessment and Actions

___ **Hand hygiene:** Demonstrate performance of correct hand hygiene.

___ **Equipment:** Gather the appropriate equipment, and check that the equipment is functional before entering the examination area.

___ **Documentation:** Gather documentation and paperwork before entering the examination area, and validate that it is appropriate for this specific procedure.

___ **Request entry:** Knock on the patient's door to request entry to examination area.

___ **Personal introduction:** Introduce yourself (student identification [ID] badge must be visible, but do not rely on your name tag to serve as your introduction).

___ **Confirm patient identity:** Identify patient (ID band or whatever is deemed appropriate). If your patient does not have identification, then the student should not proceed until the patient's identity is verified and an appropriate ID band is placed on the patient.

___ **State purpose:** "I'd like your permission and cooperation to perform the following examination … "

___ **Query patient concerns:** Ask whether the patient has any questions, concerns, or other issues before start of the exam. It is important for students to recognize that in order to have a successful experience with the patient, the patient's immediate needs must be met before the initiation of an examination.

___ **Visually survey the patient:** During this introductory phase, it is important to visually survey the patient, as well as his or her environment.

___ Note whether the patient is awake, alert, and responsive or not.

___ Note patient's disposition (e.g., lying, sitting, standing, etc.).

___ Note the condition of the patient's physical environment (temperature of the room, cleanliness, equipment in use or on standby).

___ Note tubes, drains, intravenous (IV) lines, and so forth; identify what is present and, if there is a drainage amount, note its color, the presence of odor, and so forth. (For each scenario, the faculty can manipulate the simulation environment to create a realistic patient disposition and setting.)

___ **Set up examination field:** Have the student decide where to set up the examination field, assessing for cleanliness, clutter, garbage, and so forth. (The student may need to clean off the patient's overbed tray table, wipe down the surface to assure cleanliness, etc.)

___ Have the student practice/demonstrate physical examination assessment module, providing corrective feedback as appropriate.

Scenario-Concluding Steps

On completion of the documentation of the physical examination module, the student is expected to do the following:

1. Provide an opportunity for the patient to express concerns, questions, or seek clarification.
2. Thank the patient for his or her participation and cooperation.
3. Document according to the physical examination guidelines.
4. Place patient's bed height in the lowest position (if raised during the examination).
5. Lock wheels of bed, and reset safety alarms/devices as appropriate.
6. Ensure that the patient's personal dignity is maintained.
7. Ensure that the patient's call system is within easy access, and ask the patient to demonstrate how he or she would call for help/assistance if needed using the call system.
8. Position patient's assistive devices, bedside tray, and water pitcher, and so forth, within his or her reach.
9. Discuss with the patient what happens next (what should he or she expect, what is expected of him or her, who to turn to for assistance).
10. Determine who has the permission for status updates.

G. DEBRIEFING GUIDELINES

The instructor may debrief students individually or as a group.

1. Review learning objectives.
2. Students verbally recap the events as they remember them chronologically.
3. Students identify specific areas for improvement and end with their positive behaviors/critical thinking.
4. Students complete a written reflection exercise within 24 to 48 hours.
5. Faculty posts insightful student reflections anonymously for communal enrichment with the student's permission.
6. Instructor provides personalized feedback to the students.

H. SUGGESTIONS/KEY FEATURES TO REPLICATE OR IMPROVE

The advantages of using high-fidelity HPS are multifaceted and include the ability for frequent repetition of exercises, real-time responses, and realistic feedback, as well as an ability to avoid harm to the patients during the student nurse learning continuum. The use of high-fidelity HPS can be enhanced by creating a variety of scenarios across a wide spectrum of patient care settings.

The technology must be monitored regularly for optimum functioning. Suggestions for maintenance and updates are as follows:

1. Identify appropriate resource personnel responsible for the maintenance and updating of the simulation technology.
2. Identify service schedule for all simulation equipment and mechanism for reporting issues.
3. Identify users, and establish training program.

I. RECOMMENDATIONS FOR FURTHER USE

Tuning into physical assessment through the use of simulation technology is a wonderful teaching tool. Faculty should remember that "keeping it simple" is not always so simple or easily mastered by the student nurse. In order for the student to develop competency in basic assessment skills, patience, time, and practice are necessary. In addition, the use of positive feedback is critical for creating a successful learning experience.

J. HOW SIMULATION-BASED PEDAGOGY HAS CONTRIBUTED TO IMPROVED STUDENT OUTCOMES

Students use an end-of-semester course evaluation to provide faculty with feedback regarding the use of high-fidelity HPS technology in the laboratory setting. Although students report a very positive learning experience directly on completion of the course, the more compelling argument that this use of technology has merit is based on their actual encounters with patients in subsequent clinical visits. The competency level of students noted while they are engaged in the physical assessment of their patients offers overwhelming evidence that basic physical assessment skills developed through simulation are transferable to the patient setting.

K. EXPERT RECOMMENDATIONS AND WORDS OF WISDOM

Through the use of simulation, students have a unique opportunity to begin an exploration of the skill and techniques needed for physical assessment. Many students are under the impression that once they view a video/tutorial on a skill they will be able to perform it flawlessly. This certainly is a wake-up call to most students who need to be reminded that they did not learn to walk in 1 day or drive a car after one lesson. The frustration is not only felt by the students but by faculty alike. The old saying that practice makes perfect is certainly true in this setting.

L. EVALUATION OF BEST PRACTICE STANDARDS AND USE OF CREDENTIALED SIMULATION FACULTY

In 2014, The National League for Nursing along with Laerdal Medical and Wolters Kluwer Health developed and published "vSim® for Nursing Implementation Guide for Faculty.".

The guide provides strategies for use of vSim for Nursing in programs across all types of nursing education. It provides faculty with ideas to integrate vSim into existing curricula and offers ways to develop and/or enhance current teaching strategies. The guide is based on data collected from faculty who participated in pilot testing of vSim for Nursing during spring 2014 and who submitted feedback to the National League for Nursing. These faculty members provide instruction in a wide array of classroom, clinical, lab, and simulation settings (National League for Nursing, 2015).

Similar to this structured scenario, this guide provides faculty with a framework for deliberate practice, narrative pedagogy, and formative assessment. It is important to recognize and appreciate the deliberate and systematic approach this guide provides for faculty.

REFERENCES

American Association of Colleges of Nursing. (2008). The essentials of baccalaureate education for professional nursing practice. Retrieved from http://www.aacnnursing.org/Portals/42/Publications/BaccEssentials08.pdf

Jarvis, C. (2016). *Physical examination and health assessment* (7th ed.). St. Louis, MO: Saunders Elsevier.

National Council of State Boards of Nursing. (2015). NCLEX-RN examination: Test plan for the National Council Licensure Examination for Registered Nurses. Retrieved from http://ncsbn.org/RN_Test_Plan_2016_Final.pdf.

National League for Nursing. (2014). vSim for nursing. Retrieved from http://www.nln.org/centers-for-nursing-education/nln-center-for-innovation-in-simulation-and-technology/vsim-for-nursing-medical-surgical

FURTHER READING

Adamson, K. (2015). A systematic review of the literature related to the NLN/Jeffries simulation framework. *Nursing Education Perspectives, 36*(5), 281–291. doi:10.5480/15–1655

Hollenbach, P. M. (2016). Simulation and its effect on anxiety in baccalaureate nursing students. *Nursing Education Perspectives, 37*(1), 45–47. doi:10.5480/13–1279

Jumah, J. B., & Ruland, J. P. (2015). A critical review of simulation-based on nursing education research: 2004–2011. *International Journal of Nursing Education, 7*(3), 135–139. doi:10.5958/0974-9357.2015.00151.8

Rizzolo, M. A. (2015). The National League for Nursing Project to explore the use of simulation for high-stakes assessment: Process, outcomes, and recommendations. *Nursing Education Perspectives, 36*(5), 299–303. doi:10.5480/15-1639

Sittner, B. J. (2015). INACSL standards of best practice for simulation: Past, present, and future. *Nursing Education Perspectives, 36*(5), 294–298. doi:10.5480/15-1670

Stayt, L. C., Merriman, C., Ricketts, B., Morton, S., & Simpson, T. (2015). Recognizing and managing a deteriorating patient: A randomized controlled trial investigating the effectiveness of clinical simulation in improving clinical performance in undergraduate nursing students. *Journal of Advanced Nursing, 71*(11), 2563–2574. doi:10.1111/jan.12722

CHAPTER 11

Postoperative Care Following Appendectomy

Diana R. Mager and Jean W. Lange

A. IMPLEMENTATION OF SIMULATION-BASED PEDAGOGY IN YOUR INDIVIDUALIZED TEACHING AREA

This chapter incorporates students' knowledge of postsurgical patients, emphasizing operative assessment, problem recognition, interprofessional collaboration, and patient education for the prevention of postoperative complications.

In 2003, our School of Nursing received its first high-fidelity human patient simulator (HPS) as a gift from an adult learner who was graduating and wanted to leave something of import to the lab. At the time, Dr. Mager was the Learning Resource Center director, so when the manikin arrived, she began experimenting to test its capabilities. She thought that using HPSs to simulate patient care was an innovative way to teach, but realized that the machinery was quite complex to run. Dr. Mager also knew that it would be a leap for the faculty to begin using this complex technology.

We began with small steps. Drs. Lange and Mager decided to create a very simple scenario about a patient in pain and run it in Dr. Lange's medical–surgical course. Dr. Lange had attended workshops and demonstrations about how to conduct a simulated scenario and was willing to try out this new technology in her classroom. Together we designed a brief scenario about a patient who had an appendectomy and was in pain postoperatively. We created objectives and a check-list of desired student activities and set the date that the simulation would run live. We had no formal control room, cameras, or microphones at the time, so we ran the scenario in front of the classroom with four student volunteers while the other 60 students observed from their seats. Dr. Mager brought the manikin into the large auditorium on a stretcher and sat behind a rolling curtain running the controls. Dr. Lange introduced the simulation and facilitated the classroom discussion, while our faculty champion of simulation integration at the time, Dr. Suzanne Campbell, acted as the "on-call" health care provider. This allayed our anxiety about "going it alone" and broke the proverbial simulation ice. We have all come a very long way since that first scenario, but it was a starting point, and the scenario itself was rich and easy to run regardless of simulator fidelity level, amount of space available, or presence or lack of a control room.

B. EDUCATIONAL MATERIALS AVAILABLE IN YOUR TEACHING AREA AND RELATED TO YOUR SPECIALTY

Once the School of Nursing began to use simulation as a teaching–learning strategy, it was clear that an expanded laboratory with a formal control room was needed. A generous donation provided the funding to create The Fairfield University Robin Kanarek Learning Resource Center in 2006, including a control room flanked by two simulation rooms with one-way mirrors.

Ceiling-mounted cameras allowed simulations to be streamed live into two of the classrooms and recorded for debriefing. One room was designed so that it could be converted easily from an acute care patient room into an intensive care cubical by moving portable equipment in or out. Metal cabinets aligning one wall allowed for storage of various props and supplies used during simulations. Wall-mounted items included working oxygen/suction headwall unit, x-ray screen, hand sanitizer, sharps container/glove dispenser, and a flat-screen monitor to project images or lab values sent via the adjacent control room. Portable equipment housed in the room included high-fidelity simulator in a hospital bed, stretcher, intravenous (IV) pumps on poles, rolling vital signs station, linen cart, ventilator, EKG machine, wheelchair, and an overbed table.

One wall of the simulation room abutted the control room, where a handler controlled the HPS while watching the simulation through a double-sided mirror. Thus, although students could not see the control room, handlers could easily observe and record the simulation. Communication between the rooms was conducted via microphone, and the episode could be projected into nearby classrooms for viewing in real time, if desired. Once the control room was completed, Drs. Campbell, Lange, and Mager used streaming technology to demonstrate the use of simulation to faculty and staff during a business meeting. This, as well as the support of Drs. Mager and Campbell with planning scenarios and managing the control room, helped to accelerate faculty members' willingness to incorporate this new technology into their courses.

C. SPECIFIC OBJECTIVES FOR SIMULATION USAGE WITHIN A SPECIFIC COURSE AND THE OVERALL PROGRAM

Learning Objectives

We have added some complexity beyond the pain management and medication allergy to the following scenario so that it can be used with more experienced students, or simplified for the novice student. The primary objective of this scenario is to assess the prelicensure student's ability to conduct a thorough postoperative assessment, recognize abnormal findings, and cluster cues to diagnose actual and potential problems. Elements of patient education, interprofessional collaboration and communication, infection control, and judgment in medication administration are incorporated.

Student Learning Activities

To achieve the objectives of this more complex scenario, students need to have mastered the content on postoperative care, medication administration, and physical assessment, including identifying abnormal laboratory results.

Learning activities include:

1. Completion of reading related to postoperative care and appendectomy procedures
2. Review of basic laboratory interpretation, medication administration procedures, and dosage calculation
3. Review of procedures for postoperative bedside physical assessment and patient safety
4. Review of steps to perform dressing changes, wound assessment, and drain care

D. INTRODUCTION OF SCENARIO

Setting the Scene

The setting for the scenario is the hospital room of a 59-year-old man who presented to the emergency department the previous afternoon with abdominal pain. He was diagnosed with appendicitis, and is now 12 hours postoperation following a ruptured appendix and open appendectomy. The students arrive on the surgical unit at 7 a.m. for their clinical rotation and receive a verbal report from the night nurse.

Technology Used

The "patient" can be a low-, mid-, or high-fidelity simulator. In this case, a high-fidelity HPS was used. The patient was lying in bed with an IV running, a name band and red allergy bracelet in place, and a dressing applied to the right lower quadrant of his abdomen. Moulage to simulate an infected wound, pus-like yellow drainage on the dressing, and props, such as a wig, makeup, glasses, and an over-bed table with tissues, a cup of water, an incentive spirometer and an emesis basin, can be added for realism. For low-fidelity simulation, a standardized patient or another student could act as the patient.

Objectives

1. Use communication skills to identify themselves and their role, affirm the patient's identity
2. Perform a postoperative assessment on a patient in the acute care setting
3. Cluster cues to diagnose actual and potential patient problems (e.g., relate increased blood pressure [BP] and pulse to pain; recognize pain as a deterrent to coughing, deep breathing, and mobility; note increased temperature, pus-like drainage and elevated white cell count as indicators of infection)
4. Use clinical reasoning skills to decide on a course of action when discovering a potential medication error (allergy to a medication that is ordered)
5. Initiate interprofessional communication (with a physician or other health care provider) using appropriate communication skills
6. Provide patient education regarding prevention of potential postoperative complications

Description of Participants

Prelicensure student nurse in a medical–surgical course: Student preparation includes reading related materials: reviewing dosage calculations and basic laboratory value interpretation; practicing; medication administration, dressing changes, and drain care; and conducting a postoperative assessment. Students listen to the oral report and have electronic or written access to the medication record and laboratory results for electrolytes, blood urea nitrogen (BUN), glucose, and complete blood count (CBC). Faculty may wish to require that students wear uniforms and identification tags to mimic the clinical setting. It is expected that the students conduct a focused, postoperative assessment in a logical order, taking into account abnormal findings and/or patient-reported problems. Students must also assess the IV fluid rate, intake/output results, surgical site, recent and current vital signs, laboratory values, and the abdominal dressing. In addition, students are expected to incorporate appropriate postoperative patient education as they render care.

Adult patient in hospital room: A standardized patient with a script, or an HPS with preset vital signs and heart/lung/bowel sounds run by a handler may be used. The main script for this patient is to complain about terrible pain at the incision site ("9" out of 10) and to ask for pain medication.

On-call health care provider (physician, nurse practitioner): This role is designed to promote interprofessional communication, collaboration, and to encourage students to call a provider.

Faculty or staff running the scenario/handler: The handler may need to speak for the patient if using high- or mid-fidelity technology, and preset vital signs, lung and bowel sounds. If a standardized patient is being used instead, the faculty/staff member is there to observe and record whether and how the objectives are being met. In addition, notes may be kept that aid in debriefing later.

E. RUNNING OF THE SCENARIO

Before the scenario, an HPS is prepared by setting various pertinent findings for a patient who is in postoperative day 1, is in pain and showing signs of a wound infection. Initial vital signs (BP: 144/94 mmHg, pulse [P]: 98 beats/minute, respiratory rate [RR]: 20 breaths/minute; temperature [T]: 100.9°F; pulse oximetry: 94%), lung sounds (slightly diminished bilaterally), and bowel sounds (hypoactive) are preset. Based on standard care following perforation and an appendectomy, a 3-inch wound with a Penrose drain is present on the right lower quadrant (Mason, 2014), covered by a dressing containing a small amount of yellow pus-like drainage (vanilla pudding). The perimeter of the wound looks red. A wristband with the patient's name and a red bracelet indicating a morphine allergy are on the right wrist. An IV of 5% dextrose with normal saline (D5NS) is running into the left arm. Stethoscope, gloves, and a pulse oximeter are placed nearby. A medication record, intake/output flow sheet and laboratory results are available for students to review. When students approach the patient, he should be groaning and asking for pain medication. As students ask the patient questions and perform the assessment, the handler or standardized patient can answer. The scenario is designed to last approximately 15 minutes, not including the period of debriefing, which may take 30 to 40 minutes.

F. PRESENTATION OF COMPLETED TEMPLATE

Title

Postoperative care following appendectomy

Scenario Level

Prelicensure nursing students

Focus Area

Medical–surgical nursing course

Scenario Description

This scenario takes place at 7 a.m. in an acute care setting, in the room of a 59-year-old male who had an appendectomy following a perforated appendix the previous evening. Prelicensure students play the role of student nurses arriving at their clinical rotation, receiving morning report, and performing a postoperative patient assessment followed by any necessary interventions and patient education. Interprofessional communication is encouraged, and students are expected to use clinical reasoning skills to recognize problems and intervene appropriately. They are given the following information ahead of time:

Patient History

Patient: Mr. Joshua Rivera
Age: 59 years
Allergies: Morphine
Social history: Spanish is the preferred language for speaking, reading, and writing (speaks English).
Medical history: Hypertension, perforated appendix, 12 hours postop: appendectomy

Health Assessment Results

Students must examine the patient to obtain the following results:
    (Oriented to person, place, and time)

Vital signs: BP: 144/94 mmHg, P: 98 beats/minute, RR: 20 breaths/minute, T: 100.9°F; pulse oximetry: 94%
Pain: Patient moaning and rates pain as "9" out of 10
Skin: Pink, moist, no evidence of edema
Heart sounds: Normal but pulse slightly elevated (98); peripheral pulses present
Lung sounds: Slightly diminished bilaterally in lower lobes
Bowel sounds: Hypoactive, abdomen soft
Wound: Dressing in place to right lower quadrant, small amount of yellow pus-like drainage, Penrose
    drain inserted into 3-inch wound
IV site: D5NS running at 75 mL/hr; site intact in left arm, no redness or swelling present
Intake postoperatively: 1,180 (includes 120 mL of water and 60 mL Jello and 1,000 mL of IV fluid); out-
    put postoperatively: 650 mL urine via urinary catheter

Medication Record and Laboratory Results

Patient: Rivera, Joshua **DOB:** 2/21/1958	**Allergy:** Morphine
Medication List	**Time Due**
Metoprolol (Lopressor) 100 mg PO daily	08:00
Multivitamin 1 tab PO daily	08:00
Docusate sodium 100 mg PO daily	08:00
Cefoxitin 2 g IV every 6 hours[a]	12:00
Intravenous fluid: Dextrose 5% with normal saline at 75 mL/hr continuously	
PRN List	**Time Given**
Morphine sulfate IV 6 to 10 mg every 4 hours prn for severe pain	
Percocet 1 to 2 tabs PO every 4 hours prn for pain	
Tylenol 350 mg, 2 tabs PO prn for temp >101°F	
Phenergan 10 to 25 mg IM every 4 hours prn for nausea	
Laboratory Results (Use date scenario takes place)	**Reference Value**
Na: 141 mmol/L	135–145
K: 4.0 mmol/L	3.6–5.2
Cl: 101 mmol/L	100–108
HCO_3: 23 mmol/L	22–29
BUN: 12 mg/dL	6–21
Glucose: 101 mg/dL	70–140
Hgb: 12 g/dL	12–15.5
Hct: 42 **%**	34.9–44.5
WBC: 12.7 × 10(9)/L	3.5–10.5

BUN, blood urea nitrogen; Hct, hematocrit; Hgb, hemoglobin; IV, intravenous; IM, intramuscular; PO, per os; prn, pro re nata (as needed); WBC, white blood cells.

[a]*Source*: Solomkin et al. (2010).

On arrival on the unit, the night nurse gives the following report (read by a student):

> Mr. Joshua Rivera is a 54-year-old patient of Dr. Tracey's with a history of hypertension. He came into the emergency department (ED) yesterday with a temp of 103°F and severe abdominal pain, rule/out appendicitis. He had an appendectomy via laparotomy late yesterday. Mr. Rivera slept through the night, and his vital signs have been stable. He has a Penrose drain and his dressing is dry and intact. His Foley was removed at 6 a.m., but he has not voided yet. He has an IV running, has antibiotics ordered, and is on a soft diet. He has tolerated sips of water and Jello. His only other meds are a BP pill and he can have morphine for pain if needed but he has not requested any pain medication and has been sleeping, so I did not wake him up.

> Note: This report is designed to be a bit vague, as reports can sometimes be. In addition, the patient found on a bedside assessment may be quite different from the patient presented in report. When students perform their assessment, Mr. Rivera's dressing will no longer be dry, he will be in severe pain, and he has other medications ordered than what was mentioned in the report. He will have a drain in place, which will necessitate further investigation. Furthermore, he is allergic to morphine, a fact that has gone unnoticed by the providers thus far. The plan of care should also include monitoring Mr. Rivera's wound and his ability to void after catheter removal, tolerate food, regain bowel function, and ambulate. Patient teaching should include the importance of early mobility, deep-breathing exercises, and fluid intake to prevent complications.

Scenario Objectives

Key Elements from NCSBN-NCLEX-RN° Test Plan

The National Council Licensure Examination for a Registered Nurse (NCLEX-RN) test plan categories and subcategories (National Council of State Boards of Nursing, 2015) addressed in the simulation are as follows:

Safe and effective care environment: *Management of care* (advocacy, case management, client rights, collaboration with interdisciplinary team, continuity of care, establishing priorities, ethical practice, performance improvement [quality improvement], referrals), *Safety and infection control* (accident/error/injury prevention, handling infectious materials, reporting incident/event/irregular occurrence/variance, safe use of equipment, error prevention, handling hazardous and infectious materials, standard precautions/transmission based precautions/surgical asepsis); **Health promotion and maintenance:** Self-care, health promotion/disease prevention, principles of teaching/learning, techniques of physical assessment; **Psychosocial integrity:** Cultural awareness/cultural influences on health, therapeutic communication, therapeutic environment; **Physiological integrity:** *Basic care and comfort* (nutrition and oral hydration, elimination, personal hygiene, mobility/immobility), *Pharmacological and parenteral therapies* (adverse effects/contraindications/side effects/interactions, expected actions/outcomes, medication administration, parenteral/IV therapies, pharmacological pain management, dosage calculation), *Reduction of risk potential* (changes/abnormalities in vital signs, laboratory tests, potential for complications from surgical procedures and health alterations, system specific assessments, potential for alterations in body systems, therapeutic procedures), *Physiological adaptation* (alterations in body systems, fluid and electrolyte imbalances, pathophysiology, illness management).

AACN Essentials of BSN

The American Association of Colleges of Nursing (AACN, 2008) has created nine BSN Essentials that are used as a guide to building curriculum for baccalaureate nursing programs. The Essentials document

(2008) states that "Simulation experiences augment clinical learning and are complementary to direct care opportunities essential to assuming the role of the professional nurse" (2008, p. 4). The Essentials that are addressed in this simulation by objective are:

Essential II: Basic Organizational and Systems Leadership for Quality Care and Patient Safety
Essential III: Scholarship for Evidence-Based Practice
Essential IV: Information Management and Application of Patient Care Technology
Essential VI: Interprofessional Communication and Collaboration for Improving Patient Health Outcomes
Essential VII: Clinical Prevention and Population Health
Essential VIII: Professionalism and Professional Values
Essential IX: Baccalaureate Generalist Nursing Practice (AACN, 2008)

Setting the Scene

Equipment Needed

Video-recording device (optional); name and allergy bracelet with morphine listed; Penrose drain in wound with pus-like yellow drainage on dressing; incentive spirometer; gloves; D5NS infusing intravenously; BP cuff and stethoscope; intake and output, medication, and laboratory records.

Resources Needed

Student activity checklist; electronic resources available for students to look up information if needed.

Simulator Level

High- or mid- or low-fidelity HPS on gurney or bed, or person to role-play the patient

Participant Roles

Handler (to change settings in response to student actions and speak for the patient in response to student questions), student or faculty member (to read report as night nurse), faculty member (health care provider on call, recorder of student actions on the checklist), student nurses (up two to three students may share the care of Mr. Rivera, with a fourth as an observer).

Scenario Implementation

Initial Settings

___Apply wristband with allergy alert to morphine
___Medication record, laboratory results and intake/output sheets are available for students
___Simulate moaning on the manikin; facial grimacing if standardized patient
___Set manikin for hypoactive bowel sounds and slightly decreased breath sounds
___Place wound, Penrose drain covered with pus-like yellow drainage on dressing to right lower quadrant
___Set vital signs: BP: 144/94 mmHg; P: 98 beats/minute; RR: 20 breaths/minute; T: 100.9°F; pulse oximetry: 94%
___Make hand hygeine supplies available
___Place stethescopes, pulse oximeter, thermometer, and BP machine nearby

Expected/Required Student Assessments/Actions

Prelicensure nursing students are expected to listen to the night nurse's report, enter the patient's room, perform hand hygiene, introduce themselves and their student nurse role to the patient, and perform a postoperative assessment. Before starting the simulation, each participant should be assigned a particular role to play (e.g., one checks vital signs; one assesses heart, lung, and bowel sounds, and the wound; a third asks pertinent questions, another could review the medication record, lab report and intake/output record). Students should note the allergy to morphine and the morphine mistakenly ordered for pain.

Instructor Interventions

The instructor's role is to initiate the simulation, prepare the students by giving them patient background information, and provide resources as needed. If there are questions or concerns, they should be addressed before the start of the simulation. The instructor also acts as a facilitator and timekeeper, and runs the debriefing session. The evaluative criteria may be used by the instructor to assess student performance during the simulation.

Evaluation Criteria

Checklist of Interventions and Assessments

___Performs hand hygiene
___Introduces self and role in patient care
___Checks name band
___Notes allergy to morphine
___Assesses general condition/asks how patient is doing
___Assesses pain level (1–10 scale)
___Checks IV for proper fluid and rate
___Checks IV site
___Assesses vital signs
    ___BP (144/94 mmHg)
    ___P (98 beats/minute)
    ___RR (20 breaths/minute)
    ___T (100.9°F)
    ___Pulse oximetry (94%)
___Notes abnormal BP and elevated temperature
___Rechecks BP to confirm elevation
___Auscultates lungs
___Notes decreased breath sounds in bases
___Inquires about sputum production/amount and characteristics
___Evaluates the use of incentive spirometry
___Palpates pulses/checks capillary refill
___Dons gloves
___Observes dressing/wound
___Notes pus-like drainage (not mentioned in report)
___Auscultates bowel sounds
___Notes decreased bowel sounds
___Asks patient whether experiencing any nausea/vomiting
___Asks patient whether he has moved bowels or passed flatus postoperatively
___Asks whether patient is urinating
___Checks input and output (I&O) sheet
___Assesses ambulation status (has patient been out of bed?)

___Determines the need for a.m. medication (BP medication, vitamin, stool softener)
___Determines the need for pain medication (patient rates pain "9" out of 10)
___Notes allergy to medication ordered (morphine)
___Calls provider and pharmacy about morphine allergy
___Gives Percocet
___Rechecks (or states would recheck) BP 30 minutes after the medications are administered
___Evaluates response to pain medication (scale of 1–10)
___Reviews laboratory results
___Notes elevated WBC count
___Reports pus-like drainage and elevated WBC and temperature to provider
___Develops plan of care that includes:
   ___ Ambulation
   ___Pulmonary exercises
   ___Ability to void post catheter removal
   ___Food tolerance
   ___Bowel function
   ___Pain management
   ___Ongoing assessment of wound status
___Patient teaching and discharge plan
   ___Completes teaching regarding preventing postoperative complications:
   ___Cough, turn, deep breath
   ___Use of incentive spirometry
   ___Splinting
   ___Importance of early ambulation
   ___Importance of pain management

G. DEBRIEFING GUIDELINES

Issues to Consider

Students are sometimes anxious when participating in simulations, however, our experience has been that following the simulation experience, students invariably express how valuable it was to their learning. Simulation adds an action-oriented, problem-based learning approach to the classroom that allows better assimilation of content than listening to lectures or note-taking. It also adds interest and excitement to a course as students step up to participate in a situation in which they do not quite know what will happen, not unlike actual clinical settings. That being said, it is always possible that students miss a problem or issue that was strategically placed into the scenario, such as the medication error or signs of infection in the earlier scene. It is important that students do not feel judged or embarrassed for making a mistake, or for missing a cue. The safe environment of a simulation is used to prevent errors in real-life settings, and students may need reassurance surrounding this concept. It is also imperative to stress that students not "give away" the gist of the scenario to other students when leaving the simulation. They should go by the adage "Whatever happens in the sim room, stays in the sim room!" so that others may have the same learning potential that they experienced.

Student Questions

As in any learning setting, student questions pre- and postscenario should be encouraged. However, during this scenario, it is expected that they should proceed as if they are in a real setting, and seek answers to their questions as they would in the clinical environment. They can use resources, contact a provider, or ask the patient questions, but they should stay in character once the scenario begins rather than asking things like "Should I really document on the electronic record?" "Should I really pour the medication?" "Where do I get the IV bag?." By having students seek out answers in the manner that they would in the clinical arena, it may encourage critical thinking and autonomy.

Classroom/Observer Questions/Roles

Questions for Debriefing

1. What challenges did you face during this scenario?
2. What were some abnormal findings discovered on your assessment?
3. What problems/nursing diagnoses did you identify for this patient? (e.g., pain, risk for ineffective breathing pattern/infection, potential for altered elimination [gastrointestinal], infection, allergy?)
4. What nursing interventions would be appropriate for Mr. Rivera?
5. What additional information, if any, would you have liked to have had in report?
6. Are there any other lab results you would like to see? If so, what?
7. Is there anything you would change about your verbal communication with the patient or provider?
8. Is there anything you would change about your performance of the postoperative assessment?
9. If given more time, what else could you have explained or taught to the patient?
10. What did you think about the presence of a morphine order, when the patient was allergic to morphine?
11. Which other health team members might be appropriate in the management of this patient's condition (e.g. pharmacist, hospitalist, infection control nurse, wound care specialist)?

H. SUGGESTIONS/KEY FEATURES
TO REPLICATE OR IMPROVE

The first time we ran this scenario, it was the students' initial exposure to a simulation experience. Therefore, they were unfamiliar with the functioning of the HPS itself (e.g., where to listen to lung sounds, place the stethoscope to auscultate a BP, or to feel pulses). Since then we have learned that it is imperative to have time to orient students to the simulators. We have comprised a list of important "need to know" facts on a document named "Meet the Sims" that is distributed to students when they begin using simulation in courses. Students are oriented to the simulation room, the actual HPSs, and the expectations for participation (such as wearing a uniform, talking to the HPSs as though they are real people, etc.). We also recognize now that it is helpful to have materials, such as reports, patient information, and medication lists, available for observers as well as participants.

Our biggest lesson learned was regarding student preparation. Although we originally had objectives written for this activity, we did not share them with the students before running the simulation. At that time, simulation was quite new and we were experimenting with the process and with the HPSs. We initially thought it would be a great idea to "surprise the students" with this classroom activity and see what they had learned about the previously taught postoperative assessment content. We have learned through experience that has been validated by the International Nursing Association for Clinical Simulation and Learning (INACSL) best practices, that students need to have the objectives available before the simulation for richer potential learning (Lioce et al., 2013).

K. EXPERT RECOMMENDATIONS AND WORDS OF WISDOM

Start simple. Do not give up. Simulation is like anything else: Once you get familiar with it, there is nothing to be afraid of or to be intimidated by. Students love adventure, and using a different way to teach them in which they can participate in the teaching/learning dyad keeps the classroom interesting. Work smartly. You can take a simple simulation and, use it successfully to meet a few basic objectives and, rather than creating new scenarios, you can build on the same simulation to accomplish new objectives, as we did here. Simulations that develop over time and have added layers of information and complications are ways to level these experiences from more novice to more advanced courses.

This simulation could be presented as several scenarios, each increasing in complexity. For example, the first time it runs, perhaps the patient is admitted but has not yet gone to surgery, and the objectives may simply be to listen to report, wash hands, introduce self to patient, and perform a set of preoperative vital signs. The subsequent time it is presented the objective may be to conduct an entire postoperative assessment. By the third run, the patient may have been given the morphine that he is allergic to, resulting in an anaphylactic reaction. More complexity can be added as students become more familiar with medical–surgical content related to postoperative patients, by adding complications such as urinary retention, constipation, thrombosis, or paralytic ileus. Finally, the focus of the scenario could easily incorporate tenets of cultural awareness by having the postoperative patient fasting for a religious holiday.

By changing small components of any simulation, a vast variety of learning moments can be born. In any event, have fun with it. Sometimes things do not go perfectly; the simulator stops breathing and the students think it is a cardiac arrest scenario, when really the compressor blew. It's okay. It can all still be used as a learning moment.

L. EVALUATION OF BEST PRACTICE STANDARDS AND USE OF CREDENTIALED SIMULATION FACULTY

When we first developed this scenario in 2006, several faculty had attended conferences hosted by one of the leading HPS manufacturers. We also learned from more experienced conference attendees and the basic onsite training offered by the manufacturer. Eventually, we purchased some predesigned scenarios to use in our courses. Our faculty champion recognized the need for a wider range of scenarios and decided to coedit this text. These "ready-made" experiences can be adapted by faculty across schools for use in their programs. Many faculty in our school contributed chapters and, through the writing process, we learned about organizations such as the International Nursing Association for Clinical Simulation and Learning. In later iterations of our scenarios, the faculty had adopted its best practice standards to guide our debriefing practices and create uniform templates for scenario creation and evaluation (INACSL, 2013/2016).

Use of simulation has grown as a learning tool and, in many programs, counts for a portion of clinical hours. Universities need to support this growth financially. To that end, Fairfield University has hired a director of simulation, and has a number of faculty members persuing certification in Healthcare Simulation Education (CHSE). Also, with the new emphasis on interprofessional education, other disciplines are collaborating with nursing to create opportunities for students to learn with and about one another. Dr. Lange, now at Quinnipiac University, has successfully made the case to hire several dedicated personnel, including a director and a coordinator of operations that support the school's seven simulation labs and help faculty with scenario creation, delivery, and evaluation using a standardized template. A few years ago, Quinnipiac's Schools of Nursing, Medicine and Health Sciences formed an interprofessional simulation committee that works together to create cross-disciplinary student experiences, write grants, conduct studies regarding student outcomes, present results at conferences, and coauthor publications. We believe that we have only begun to explore the possibilities.

REFERENCES

American Association of Colleges of Nursing. (2008). *The essentials of baccalaureate education for professional nursing practice*. Washington, DC: Author. Retrieved from http://www.aacnnursing.org/Portals/42/Publications/BaccEssentials08.pdf

International Nursing Association for Clinical Simulation and Learning. (2013, updated 2016). INACSL standards of best practice: Simulation. Retrieved from http://www.inacsl.org/i4a/pages/index.cfm?pageID=3407

Lioce, L., Reed, C. C., Lemon, D., King, M. A., Martinez, P. A., Franklin, A. E., . . . Borum, J. C. (2013). Standards of best practice: Simulation standard III: Participant objectives. *Clinical Simulation in Nursing, 9*(6S), S15–S18. doi:10.1016/j.ecns.2013.04.005

Mason, P. (2014). Management of patients with gastric and duodenal disorders. In J. L. Hinkle & K. H. Cheever (Eds.), *Textbook of medical–surgical nursing* (13th ed., pp. 1261–1284). Philadelphia, PA: Wolters Kluwer/Lippincott Williams & Wilkins.

National Council of State Boards of Nursing. (2015). NCLEX-RN examination: Test plan for the National Council Licensure Examination for Registered Nurses. Retrieved from https://www.ncsbn.org/RN_Test_Plan_2016_Final.pdf

Solomkin, J., Mazuski, J., Bradley, J., Rodvoid, K., Goldstein, E., Baron, E., . . . Bartlett, J. G. (2010). Diagnosis and management of complicated intra-abdominal infection in adults and children: Guidelines by the Surgical Infection Society and the Infectious Diseases Society of America. *Clinical Infectious Diseases, 50*(2), 133–154. Retrieved from http://www.jstor.org/stable/27799535

CHAPTER 12

Medical–Surgical Skill-Based Scenarios

Karen M. Daley

A. IMPLEMENTATION OF SIMULATION-BASED PEDAGOGY IN YOUR INDIVIDUALIZED TEACHING AREA

At Western Connecticut State University, nursing students complete three levels of medical–surgical courses, each with an increasing breadth and complexity. The first course introduces common medical diagnoses found in chronic illness, long-term care, and restorative subacute care. In the middle medical–surgical course, students are introduced to common diagnoses requiring surgical intervention. In the third course, nursing care and interventions for complex patients, such as those in an intensive care unit (ICU), are studied within the context of the nursing process. Although the theory has been introduced in the foundation course, the second course is the first to include task and skill training related to acute care. Although medical–surgical experience has traditionally been performed on static task trainers, current nursing students have begun using a multipronged approach to task training. In the seminar portion of this middle surgical course, students are given the opportunity to read and review these skills in text and video. Instructors then demonstrate these skills in seminars and allow students to practice on static task trainers and manikins. In evaluations of the courses in the past, students did not seem to make the theory–seminar–clinical connections needed to transfer this knowledge as an integrated whole to their nursing practice. With a multipronged approach to read/study, view, and practice, however, we have found that the embedding of skills within a scenario or a case study that has been transformed into a scenario for use with a human patient simulator (HPS) was beneficial and increased their confidence in performing the skill on actual patients.

In addressing this need within a traditional nursing laboratory, an eight-bed nursing lab without computer or Internet access was renovated into a computer projection and instructor station with four student-use computers with Internet access and four beds with manikins. Videos of skills available online could then be projected and discussed by instructors and teachers, then reaccessed by students during open lab practice. In addition, these skill videos are available for students to view from home computers.

With the purchase of the department of nursing's first HPS, a section of the lab was designated as the simulation area and, over time, equipment was purchased to enhance the "realness" and usability of the area for simulation. A bed was taken out and replaced with a stretcher to make the HPS more mobile. Several small grants and summer curriculum funds provided both the equipment organization and time for constructing skill-based scenarios to match the existing skill-training modules. In addition, several more grants allowed updates and upgrades to the HPS as the technology became available. Although not used consistently by all faculty teaching the course, the availability of this high-fidelity learning tool gives each instructor the flexibility to teach at different levels of technology to meet student needs.

B. EDUCATIONAL MATERIALS AVAILABLE IN YOUR TEACHING AREA AND RELATED TO YOUR SPECIALTY AREA

As described previously, the simulation area used for these simulations is embedded in an existing nursing lab. It is an open area, with the HPS residing on a stretcher with an intravenous (IV) machine and pole nearby. In addition, this area even has a treatment cart that has become the simulation cart. In this cart are all the supplies needed for mock up of the scenarios and exclusively for use with the HPS. There are three hospital beds with static manikins and multiple partial task trainer manikins available, such as a pelvic model for urinary catheter insertion. Weekly objectives for the modules direct students and instructors to the equipment needed for each scheduled seminar. Each seminar coincides with a nursing concept being taught in the theory portion of the course. For example, when teaching about pain and comfort concepts in theory/class, students are asked in the seminar to review pain assessments, interventions to enhance a patient's comfort level, and evaluative criteria by which to judge the success of nursing interventions for the surgical patient. When taught as individual tasks, students learn how to administer shots and give IV pain medications. On the HPS within a scenario, students can interact with the HPS, assess the pain level of the "patient," decide which medication is appropriate, and measure the effectiveness of the medication. Unlike the static task training, the use of the HPS allows for practice with therapeutic communication and may involve contacting other health care professionals and possibly dealing with a patient with varying levels of pain relief. Safety techniques can be overlaid as well by asking the student to check the five rights of medication administration, put up side rails for the sedated patient, and concurrently assess the effects of the narcotic medications on the patient's respiratory system.

Five scenarios were created to supplement and complement learning within the seminar portion of the medical–surgical course (Nursing 255). This chapter presents these scenarios. Scenarios have similar objectives and expected outcomes based on the nursing process. Initially written as computerized scenarios with computer programming, each was rewritten with additional summer curriculum funds to better reflect the need of instructors and students for flexibility in implementing the scenarios. Currently, these scenarios are written as "on the fly," with the instructor running the scenario. Each scenario is simple and task oriented and is written to bring to life the common surgical nursing interventions.

At Western Connecticut State University, lab personnel may not be available, so each simulation must be run by an instructor who is trained in simulation. In some instances, this has resulted in the instructor enthusiastically jumping in with both feet to learn and use simulation. For others, lack of time and training opportunities are most often cited for nonuse of simulation. In addition, the classic task-training method is still a tried-and-true technique of effective teaching for most students, although students are requesting more simulation in this course each year.

C. SPECIFIC OBJECTIVES FOR SIMULATION USAGE WITHIN A SPECIFIC COURSE AND THE OVERALL PROGRAM

1. Student uses the nursing process to assess and intervene in a common surgical nursing problem.
2. Student develops a basic-level competency in performing a surgical nursing intervention.

D. INTRODUCTION OF SCENARIO

Setting the Scene

Each scenario includes a list of necessary equipment and supplies to mock up the HPS. These supplies are available in the simulation cart.

Technology Used

High-fidelity HPS

Objectives

1. Student uses the nursing process to identify a surgical nursing problem that needs intervention.
2. Student practices a selected skill within a scenario that integrates maintaining a standard of care, therapeutic communication, safety precautions, and psychosocial care.

In these simulations, The American Association of Colleges of Nursing (AACN) *Essentials of Baccalaureate Education for Professional Nursing Practice* (AACN, 2008) addresses Essential IX: Baccalaureate Generalist Nursing Practice. The National Council of State Boards of Nursing's (NCSBN) National Council Licensure Examination for Registered Nurses test plan categories and subcategories (NCSBN, 2016) are addressed in the simulation:

Safe and effective care environment: *Management of care* (establishing priorities, ethical practice, informed consent, legal rights and responsibilities), *Safety and infection control* (standard/transmission-based/other precautions/surgical asepsis, safe use of equipment); **Health promotion and maintenance:** Techniques of physical assessment; **Psychosocial integrity:** Coping mechanisms, therapeutic communications; **Physiological integrity:** *Basic care and comfort* (elimination, nonpharmacological comfort interventions, personal hygiene, rest and sleep), *Pharmacological and parenteral therapies* (dosage calculation, expected actions/outcomes, medication administration, parenteral/IV therapies, pharmacological pain management), *Reduction of risk potential* (diagnostic tests, laboratory values, potential for complications of diagnostic tests/treatments/procedures, system specific assessments, therapeutic procedures, vital signs), *Physiological adaptation* (hemodynamics, illness management).

Description of Participants

In these simple scenarios, the only participants are a small group of three to four nursing students and the HPS. Students seem to prefer this in contrast to be being "put on the spot" one by one. Students can portray a team of nurses using a group process to decide on care of the patients. Staff, or family members played by additional nursing students or faculty.

E. RUNNING OF THE SCENARIO

Each seminar topic area runs either 1 or 2 weeks for 3 hours each. The first hour usually involves discussion and application of the surgical concept being taught in class. The discussion involves taking that concept through the nursing process by integrating previously learned concepts with the new ones and reviewing common nursing interventions needed for the surgical patient in that topic area. During the second hour, the associated tasks are demonstrated, and the remaining time is given to the students for supervised practice. Students arrive ready to practice, having reviewed the skill content, viewed the associated videos, and, in the best case, having already tried to practice at home with their nursing kit.

During the designated practice time, two instructors are available to help with skills. When one is trained in the use of the HPS, that instructor works with the students who are ready to embed the skill into a scenario. The HPS is set up before the beginning of the scenario, and the scenario begins just as if the student were going to walk into a room to care for a patient. Students should identify and introduce themselves, check the identity of the patient, and begin a surgical assessment. During the assessment, a common surgical problem is found and interventions are needed to address the problem. A skill has to be performed to alleviate the problem and evaluation of the intervention follows.

F. PRESENTATION OF COMPLETED TEMPLATE

The following five medical–surgical skill-based scenarios have been included based on those written for this course. The scenario template is somewhat different from the templates used throughout the book in order to show the original "as written" format that is currently in use at the university.

Nursing 255—Scenario #1

Surgical Pain (Skill: Administration of Pain Medication)

A 63-year-old man was admitted yesterday for a left knee replacement. He is 1 day postop. During the student's morning assessment, he complains of pain.

Equipment Needed

____ IV setup
____ Syringe for pain meds
____ Stethoscope
____ Ace wrap for left knee

Objectives

1. Student will be able to identify source and level of pain.
2. Student will perform appropriate assessments in order to accurately assess pain level.
3. Student will correctly intervene to treat pain.

Settings for the Patient

Heart rate (HR): 108 beats/minute
Oxygen saturation (SpO$_2$): 93%
CO$_2$: 34%
Temperature (T): 37.2°C
Respiratory rate (RR): 20 breaths/minute
Blood pressure (BP): 96/64 mmHg
Vocals: "I've never had pain like this before!"

Interventions

____Identify self and patient
____Identify purpose of visit
____Perform surgical assessment
____Check incision
____Check vital signs
____Change BP to 110/80
____Vocals: "I don't feel well!"
____Assess pain on pain scale
____Check doctor's orders; select and administer IV pain meds
____Evaluate effectiveness
____Reposition patient with safety precautions for sedation

Settings

HR: 80 beats/minute
SpO_2: 98%
RR: 12 breaths/minute
BP: 120/80 mmHg
Vocals: "I feel better now." Repeat × 1

Evaluation

Patient states, "I feel better now." Level of pain is less than 5.

Nursing 255—Scenario #2

Hypovolemia

A 55-year-old woman, 2 days postop abdominal surgery with a large open wound. Wound is draining large amounts of serosanguinous fluid; patient is NPO (nothing by mouth) with a nasogastric tube (NG) tube.

Equipment Needed

___ IV setup
___ Stethoscope
___ Red-soaked abdominal wound dressing with drainage
___ NG tube

Objectives

1. Student will recognize need for overall assessment of patient and then recognize the signs and symptoms of hypovolemia.
2. Student will choose correct IV fluid and recognize need to hydrate patient.
3. Student will evaluate interventions appropriately.

Settings for the Patient

HR: 80 beats/minute
SpO_2: 98%
T: 37.2°C
BP: 100/80 mmHg

Interventions

___Identify self and patient
___Identify purpose of visit
___Perform surgical assessment
___Check IV
___O_2 in place
___Cardiac monitor on
___Check tubes/wound
___Increase HR to 92 beats/minute

___Change BP to 90/72 mmHg
___Vocals: "I feel dizzy"
___Reposition patient to low Fowler
___Check vital signs, assess wound, check labs, check input–output (I&O)
___Vocals: "I don't feel well"
___Redress wound, and assess IV fluid rate and solution. Choose appropriate solution and rate
___Check orders for antibiotic/anti-infective. Administer as ordered
___Change BP to 120/80 mmHg, RR to 12 breaths/minute, and HR to 80 beats/minute
___Document findings
___Vocals: "I feel better now"

Evaluation

Patient reports feeling better; BP returns to normal.

Nursing 255—Scenario #3

Wound Assessment (Skill: Surgical Wound Dressing Change)

A 57-year-old man, 1 day postop with open cholecystectomy. Patient has large abdominal dressing with Montgomery straps and a Hemovac drain.

Equipment Needed

___ Montgomery straps with dressing
___ Hemovac drain
___ Stethoscope

Objectives

1. Student will assess wound for signs and symptoms of healing or infection.
2. Student will perform appropriate interventions.
3. Student will evaluate wound and effectiveness of interventions.

Settings for Patient

HR: 80 beats/minute
SpO$_2$: 98%
T: 37.2°C
RR: 10 breaths/minute
BP: 120/80 mmHg

Interventions

___Identify self and patient
___Identify purpose of visit
___Perform surgical assessment
___Check that IV is running, oxygen and monitor are on
___Check tubes
___Check edema
___Check pulse
___Check dressing
___Assess wound

___Vocals: Moaning
___Redress wound, check labs, check I&O
___Administer anti-infective, document findings
___Vocals: "Thank you"

Evaluation

Student accurately assesses healing of surgical wound.
Student redresses wound with surgical asepsis.

Nursing 255—Scenario #4

Hypoxia (Skill: Administration of Supplemental Oxygen)

A 60-year-old woman, 1 day postop with right mastectomy. Patient has a large Ace wrap bandage around upper rib cage and a Jackson Pratt drain. Patient is receiving IV morphine for pain.

Equipment Needed

___Stethoscope
___Pulse oximeter
___O_2 setup
___Jackson Pratt drain
___IV setup

Objectives

1. Student will assess for and recognize signs and symptoms of hypoxia.
2. Student will intervene to treat hypoxia.
3. Student will evaluate interventions appropriately.

Settings for Patient

Bilateral wheezes at volume 9
SpO_2: 88%
RR: 22 breaths/minute
BP: 140/86 mmHg
Vocals: Cough, repeat × 1

Interventions

___Identify self and patient
___Identify purpose of visit
___Perform surgical assessment
___Focused respiratory assessment and auscultate lungs
___Vocals: "I don't feel well"
___Reposition patient with head-of-bed elevated
___Obtain pulse oximetry
___Administer oxygen: Select oxygen delivery device per standard of care
___Review the "cough and deep breathe" technique with patient. Have patient demonstrate and perform per protocol
___Review and have patient perform incentive spirometry per protocol

___Obtain pulse oximetry
___Reevaluate patient with focused respiratory assessment
___Change wheezes bilateral to volume 5, and increase SpO$_2$ to 99%
___Vocals: "I feel better now"

Evaluation

Student able to assess and treat hypoxia without it progressing.

Nursing 255—Scenario #5

Urinary Retention (Skill: Urinary Catheterization)

A 63-year-old man 1 day postop right knee replacement. Patient has a large Ace wrap bandage around right knee with a compression dressing in place. Patient was receiving IV morphine for pain on a patient-controlled analgesia (PCA) device that was discontinued this morning. He has now been on pain pills for 8 hours and has not been able to void since catheter was removed 6 hours ago.

Equipment Needed

___IV setup with PCA
___Urinary catheter kit
___Urinal
___Ultrasound probe to do a bladder scan

Objectives

1. Student will assess for and recognize signs and symptoms of urinary retention.
2. Student will intervene to perform bladder scan and urinary catheterization.
3. Student will evaluate interventions appropriately.

Settings for Patient

SpO$_2$: 98%
RR: 16 breaths/minute
BP: 140/86 mmHg
HR: 72 beats/minute

Interventions

___Identify self and patient
___Identify purpose of visit
___Perform surgical assessment
___Vocals: "I feel full, but I cannot seem to use the urinal"
___Assess bladder with bladder scan. Results: 650 mL urine in the bladder
___Explain reason for urinary catheterization and reposition patient
___Perform urinary catheterization
___Assess color and quantity of urine. Document
___Vocals: "I feel better now"

Evaluation

Student is able to assess and treat urinary retention.

G. DEBRIEFING GUIDELINES

Instructors may want to consider these reflection questions for use routinely after the implementation of the skill-based scenarios:

1. Was the correct nursing problem identified and addressed?
2. Was medical—and, if needed, surgical asepsis—maintained? How?
3. Did the nurse communicate effectively with the patients about the nursing problem and the interventions needed?
4. Were safety precautions taken at all times?
5. Did the implementation of the skill follow the standard of care described in the skill book?
6. In reflecting on the implementation of this scenario with real patients, what additional postsurgical problems would contribute to the assessment and implementation of your nursing intervention? In addition, what psychosocial issues may also need to be addressed in the postsurgical patient?
7. What was done well? What could be improved?

H. SUGGESTIONS/KEY FEATURES TO REPLICATE OR IMPROVE

As stated previously, these scenarios have not been fully implemented in this course because of time and training limitations. Each year, more instructors try some of the scenarios. In addition, an instructor who specializes in HPS technology offered to work with the students during open lab time as requested by students. The HPS has also been used after or as part of clinical time, which allows for a more focused interaction with students as a group. Use of these scenarios is a work in progress, as is true of many scenario implementations. Each year, more is added to improve the scenarios. The previous debriefing guideline questions were used for the first time as written this year.

I. RECOMMENDATIONS FOR FURTHER USE

Keeping the scenario as simple as possible is important at this point in the student's education. Skill competency is essential as these students move forward. At the end of the semester, the students must pass a skill practicum in order to pass the course. The HPS has been available for use as an option for skill testing in this skill practicum. Using the HPS on a more routine basis with these skills may provide the opportunity for students to learn skills in context by integrating patient interaction, therapeutic communication, safety precautions, and use of the nursing process within a scenario. In addition, frequent exposure to the HPS throughout the semester increases the students' comfort level in interacting with the simulator as a learning tool.

J. HOW SIMULATION-BASED PEDAGOGY HAS CONTRIBUTED TO IMPROVED STUDENT OUTCOMES

Students report that they enjoy interacting with the HPS and practicing "real" surgical patient situations before seeing these problems arise in clinical. Instructors in these seminars emphasize that these skill-based seminars are a safe place to learn and ask questions so that students enthusiastically try and retry to achieve the standard of care for each of the skills required. Within the context of a scenario, instructors are able to view student implementation of the nursing process step by step. In clinical, students often seek out instructors only after an assessment has been made that a surgical nursing problem needs to be addressed. From these perspectives, simulation-based skill/task training has improved student outcomes by increasing the students' confidence in their ability to perform selected nursing skills and increased the instructor confidence in the students' ability to accurately implement the nursing process in relation to selected surgical nursing skills. Embedding the skills in a scenario enables the student to enact the role of the nurse not only from a task-oriented view but also taking into consideration holistic patient care.

K. EXPERT RECOMMENDATIONS AND WORDS OF WISDOM

As time has passed since the introduction of this set of simulation-based skill/task training scenarios, similar scenarios have become more commonplace. Imbedding these skills within the context of a larger and more complex opportunity to use both learned skills and critical thinking is used frequently within programs where simulation-based pedagogy is embedded throughout. Skills trainers are now available for skill acquisition, both manually as well as virtually. I suggest a combination of the two until the student is comfortable with and ready for a skills test. Within the testing scenario, expanding the content to surround a demonstration of the skill is a more comprehensive assessment of a premedical surgical student's readiness for clinical competency by identifying a surgical nursing problem that needs intervention, and practicing a selected skill within a scenario that integrates maintaining a standard of care, therapeutic communication, safety precautions, and psychosocial care.

L. EVALUATION OF BEST PRACTICE STANDARDS AND USE OF CREDENTIALED SIMULATION FACULTY

Objectives that meet program standards, the NCLEX-RN® test plan (National Council of State Boards of Nursing, 2016), and AACN BSN Essentials have been outlined in the chapter. At the time of this scenario, there were no best practice simulation standards and no faculty training other than on-the-job through immersion in creating and implementing scenarios. In reviewing the International Nursing Association for Clinical Simulation and Learning (INACSL, 2013/2016) standards many years after the creation of these scenarios, many of the standards appear in a very early form. In addition, we were just at the point when simulation training was an idea and not the ideal. We have come a long way.

REFERENCES

American Association of Colleges of Nursing. (2008). *Essentials of baccalaureate education for professional nursing practice*. Washington, DC: Author. Retrieved from http://www.aacnnursing.org/Portals/42/Publications/BaccEssentials08.pdf

International Nursing Association for Clinical Simulation and Learning. (2013, updated 2016). INACSL standards of best practice: Simulation. Retrieved from http://www.inacsl.org/i4a/pages/index.cfm?pageid=3407

National Council of State Boards of Nursing. (2016). NCLEX-RN test plan. Retrieved from https://www.ncsbn.org/RN_Test_Plan_2016_Final.pdf

FURTHER READING

Doenges, M., & Moorehouse, P. (2014). *Nursing care plans: Guidelines for individualizing client care across the life span* (9th ed.). St. Louis, MO: F. A. Davis.

Fischbach, F., & Dunning, M. B. (2013). *A manual of laboratory and diagnostic tests* (9th ed.). Philadelphia, PA: Lippincott Williams and Wilkins.

Perry, P., Potter, P. A., & Ostendorf, W. (2013). *Clinical nursing skills and techniques* (8th ed.). St. Louis, MO: Mosby.

Potter, P., Perry, P. G., Stockert, P., & Hall, A. (2016). *Fundamentals of nursing* (9th ed.). St. Louis, MO: Mosby.

Smeltzer, S. C., & Bare, B. (2008). *Brunner and Suddarth's textbook of medical-surgical nursing* (12th ed.). New York, NY: Lippincott Williams & Wilkins.

Vallerand, A., & Sanoski, C. A. (2016*). Davis's drug guide for nurses* (15th ed.). Philadelphia, PA: F. A. Davis.

CHAPTER 13

Acute Management of Respiratory Distress in the Adult Patient

Monica P. Sousa and Linda H. Warren

A. IMPLEMENTATION OF SIMULATION-BASED PEDAGOGY AND AVAILABILITY OF EDUCATIONAL MATERIALS IN YOUR TEACHING AREA AND RELATED TO YOUR SPECIALTY

As new faculty we are looking at ways to improve our teaching techniques and optimize the resources available to us. High-fidelity simulators were not available when we graduated from our nursing programs. They are now a valuable resource and presently available to nursing educators. We are currently using high-fidelity patient simulators as medical–surgical/critical care instructors in the state university system. Dr. Linda Warren is a critical care nurse at a local medical teaching hospital and Dr. Monica Sousa is a clinical nurse specialist/cardiac educator in another medical teaching hospital. As educators we are not experts with patient simulation. However, we use simulation in seminar experiences to teach key concepts from lecture and reading assignments in order to encourage critical thinking among students in all phases of the nursing program. Some of our important focuses are evidence-based practice, standards of care, and patient safety. Simulation allows students to practice basic as well as complex skills in a nonthreatening environment. It also provides opportunities for standardized clinical experiences and addresses competencies in order to promote readiness for clinical practice. The acute care setting is a high-risk area with increasingly complex patients with multiple comorbidities. Students need to develop accurate assessment skills as well as the ability to think critically and react in emergency situations. Active listening skills during handoff communication are an important concept in this scenario. Nurses must use a holistic approach when assessing critically ill patients. They are also important members of the interprofessional health care team, who integrate problem-solving skills into their assessments in order to develop an effective plan of care for the patient.

B. EVOLUTION OF YOUR EXPERIENCES IN TEACHING AS YOU BEGAN TO USE SIMULATIONS

The intensive care unit (ICU) lab at Western Connecticut State University (WCSU) is equipped with SimMan® 3G by Laerdal. SimMan® 3G is easy to operate and allows programming of original scenarios or has preprogrammed scenarios available for use. Faculty has the ability to critique and give immediate feedback through debriefing to enhance student learning. SimMan® 3G also has various moulage elements to make scenarios more realistic. The computer technology allows instructors to follow a fixed program or manually change the scenario based on student reactions. In the spring of 2016, SimMan® 3G received the Laerdal Learning Application (LLEAP) upgrade to enhance the clinical simulation experience. The faculty received an 8-hour training from Laerdal on the new software.

The simulation lab can accommodate a group of six to eight students. Therefore, instructors can promote leadership, team-building, and critical thinking skills in the simulation process. The ICU lab is also equipped with an over-bed monitor for ease of visibility to the group. SMART Board technology is also located in the ICU lab to enhance student learning. A code cart is available for students to practice code management skills as well as preparation and administration of medications that may be required during an emergency situation.

Recently, a medication-dispensing system was purchased as well as a computer on wheels. We have used both to simulate the complete medication-administration process. Within the medication-dispensing system medications have been programmed and stocked, it is interesting to note that there are medications that have been stocked improperly. For example, look-alike/sound-alike medications are in the same drawer, and two of the same medications in different doses are in the same drawer. This was done to educate students to always look at the medication and perform the five rights of medication-administration during all phases of the medication-administration process.

In early 2016, the nursing department received funding to purchase the Harvey, the cardiopulmonary patient simulator. This simulator is a life-size mannequin that provides students with the opportunity to listen, feel, and see clinical cardiac and pulmonary findings. For example, for congestive heart failure students can listen to an S3 heart sound, feel the displaced point of maximum impulse (PMI), and visualize jugular venous distention (JVD). With the additional funding, the nursing department is building new simulation labs with the latest technology for simulation and debriefing. This will greatly expand our opportunities and use of simulation in all courses. We will be receiving a birthing simulator, newer SimMan human patient simulators (HPS), and actual control rooms. Currently, faculty stay in the same room to facilitate and control the simulation.

Simulation has enhanced our teaching experiences by providing students with hands-on learning. It encourages student engagement in the learning process by allowing the students to respond to various situations while providing a safe learning environment. It has also allowed us, as instructors, to be better able to assess student needs and learning styles that support and enhance learning using current digital technology (Fountain & Alfred, 2009; Leigh, 2008; Rogers, 2007). Simulation has also provided a way for us to link theory with clinical practice.

C. SPECIFIC OBJECTIVES FOR SIMULATION USAGE WITHIN A SPECIFIC COURSE AND THE OVERALL PROGRAM

Overall objectives of the scenario are for students to demonstrate critical thinking skills in the care of the complex patient. Students must be able to identify inconsistencies with hand-off communication, recognize symptoms, and establish treatment options for acute respiratory distress as a result of congestive heart failure or pulmonary edema. This scenario addresses Clinical Nurse Practice III of the bachelor of science in nursing (BSN) undergraduate program; the course objectives are:

1. Synthesize knowledge from the arts, sciences, and humanities with nursing theory as the basis for making nursing practice decisions for individuals experiencing complex illnesses.
2. Critically evaluate situations through the use of the nursing process to assess, diagnose, plan, implement, and evaluate the care provided to individuals experiencing complex illnesses.
3. Apply the nursing process to design, implement, and evaluate therapeutic nursing interventions to provide preventative, curative, supportive, and restorative care for individuals experiencing complex illnesses.
4. Selectively apply appropriate communication techniques, including written documentation, in the process of assessment, counseling, and therapeutic intervention with individuals experiencing complex illnesses.

5. Selectively apply appropriate teaching–learning strategies in the provision of health teaching for individuals experiencing complex illnesses.

6. Use the process of scientific inquiry and research findings to design and critically evaluate nursing interventions with individuals experiencing complex illnesses.

D. INTRODUCTION OF SCENARIO

Setting the Scene

A 72-year-old female patient named Mary Jane Brown was feeling her usual self up until a week ago. She began to feel increasingly more short of breath and unable to complete her normal activities of daily living before she needed to stop and catch her breath. She has been feeling palpations in her chest on and off during the past few days. She has also noticed that her ankles are swollen. Pertinent medical history includes coronary artery disease, diabetes, and hypertension. Current medications are Lopressor 25 mg twice a day, baby aspirin 81 mg daily, and Metformin 1 tab daily. Her daughter is with her today and mentioned that her mother has been going out to a local diner with some friends over the past few weeks and is worried she is getting overworked and not eating properly. The daughter called 911 when she found her mother breathing heavily and not looking good.

Emergency medical service (EMS) provided supplemental oxygen at 2 L by nasal cannula. Vital signs upon arrival to the emergency department (ED) are: heart rate (HR): 110 beats/minute, respiratory rate (RR): 28 breaths/minute, and blood pressure (BP): 138/88 mmHg. On hand-off report from the ED vital signs were: HR: 114 beats/minute, RR: 32 breaths/minute, BP: 146/88 mmHg, pulse oximetry: 92% on O_2 via nasal cannula at 2 L. The patient was reportedly very anxious and exhibiting signs of respiratory distress. Lungs on auscultation present with bibasilar crackles; +2 pedal and ankle edema is present; heart sounds are rapid and regular. Chest x-ray shows congestion of bilateral lung fields. Lasix 20-mg intravenous (IV) push was ordered and administered. IV fluids are ordered and infused to keep vein open (KVO). Cardiac monitor showed sinus tachycardia at a rate of 116 beats/minute. Patient weight is 101 kg and height is 62 inches (body mass index [BMI]: 40.7).

Patient is admitted to your unit in respiratory distress with indication of decreased cardiac output and cardiac compromise.

Technology Used

Patient simulator, video-recording device, medical equipment (e.g., patient monitor, oxygen flowmeter, pulse oximeter, BP cuff, and stethoscope), medical records, Foley catheter, x-ray, 12-lead EKG, and arterial blood gases (ABGs)

Objectives

1. Circulation, airway, breathing principle
2. Implement a focused cardiac and respiratory assessment
3. Demonstrate correct administration and evaluation of IV push medications and IV fluids
4. Identify the need to optimize cardiac output
5. Administer IV medication for cardiac stability
6. Identify discrepancies in hand off communication
7. Provide physical and emotional support to a patient in distress
8. Patient and family education

Description of Participants

Three to four junior/senior nursing students are needed to play the role of one primary nurse and three staff nurses on the unit. The scenario is videotaped to encourage peer participation and evaluation. The simulation is observed and supervised by the faculty. Other students are encouraged to take an active role in the simulation by reading the scenario, role-playing, or critiquing student performance.

E. RUNNING OF THE SCENARIO

Students will have completed at least two semesters of medical–surgical nursing courses to be adequately prepared. They will have completed lectures related to cardiac and respiratory emergencies. They will also have fundamental skills in assessment, taking vital signs, basic arrhythmia, and EKG interpretation. Before the simulation scenario, ground rules addressing trust and respect as well as expectations of the simulation exercise will be discussed. Students will be oriented to the simulation lab, including equipment, participant roles, specific objectives, method of evaluation, and time allocated for the scenario. One student will be given a copy of the demographics and the ED report to hand off to the other students, who will be managing the simulation scenario. They will have time to ask questions and participate in a postsimulation discussion.

This scenario takes approximately 20 minutes with an additional 15 minutes of debriefing time allowed for discussion and evaluation.

F. PRESENTATION OF COMPLETED TEMPLATE

Title

Acute Management of Respiratory Distress in the Adult Patient

Scenario Level

NUR 335: Clinical Nursing Practice III, Junior/Senior Critical Care Course

Focus Area

This chapter focuses on the management of a patient in pulmonary edema. The students must be able to look at the patient and assessment findings holistically.

Scenario Description

Students must be able to critically evaluate the information provided in the ED report presented earlier, identify the signs and symptoms of heart failure/pulmonary edema, and the rationale for the treatments provided. Simulation practice will consist of handoff communication, assessing respiratory and cardiac function, assessing signs and symptoms of pulmonary edema, demonstration of the administration of IV push medication, identifying medication actions and indications, demonstrating medication safety, and providing emotional support for a patient in distress.

Scenario Objectives

Overall, students are evaluated using the guidelines set forth by the American Association of Colleges of Nursing (AACN; 2008), *The Essentials of Baccalaureate Education for Professional Nursing Practice*. The BSN Essentials used in our evaluations are the following:

Essential II: Basic Organizational and System Leadership for Quality Care and Patient Safety
Essential III: Scholarship for Evidence-Based Practice

Essential IV: Information Management and Application of Patient Care Technology
Essential VI: Interprofessional Communication and Collaboration for Improving Patient Health Outcomes
Essential VIII: Professionalism and Professional Values
Essential IX: Baccalaureate Generalist Nursing Practice

In addition, we used the National Council of State Boards of Nursing NCLEX-RN® Test Plan as guidance for this simulation (National Council of State Boards of Nursing, 2016). The following are the areas we identified.

Safe and effective care environment: (collaboration with interprofessional team, continuity of care, establishing priorities, accident/error/injury prevention, reporting incident/event/irregular occurrence/variance, safe use of equipment, standard precautions/transmission-based precautions); **Health promotion and maintenance:** (health and wellness, health promotion and disease prevention, lifestyle choices, self-care, techniques of physical assessment); **Physiological integrity:** (assistive devices, elimination, nonpharmacological comfort interventions, nutrition and oral hydration, adverse effect/contraindications/side effects/interactions, expected actions/outcomes, medication administration, parenteral/IV therapies, dosage calculation, changes/abnormalities in vital signs, diagnostic tests, laboratory values, potential for complications regarding diagnostic tests/treatments/procedures, therapeutic procedure, system-specific assessment, medical emergency, fluid and electrolyte imbalances, pathophysiology, hemodynamics, unexpected response to therapies, illness management).

Setting the Scene

Equipment needed

Patient simulator, video-recording device, medical equipment (e.g., patient monitor, oxygen flowmeter, pulse oximeter, BP cuff, and stethoscope), medical records, Foley catheter, x-ray, 12-lead EKG, and ABGs.

Resources needed

Textbooks, computer access for database search (electronic medical record [EMR]), medication administration record (MAR) for barcoding purposes, and evidence-based practice personal digital assistant for point of care decision making.

Simulator level

Intermediate level because of the knowledge base of the nursing students.

Participant roles

Uses junior or senior nursing students in a baccalaureate nursing program. Each student is assigned a specific role for the scenario: ER nurse, unit nurse receiving report, or two additional nursing staff. ER nurse presents handoff report to receiving unit nurse.

Scenario Implementation

Guidelines for Running Scenario

- The ED report will be given by one of the students playing the role of the ED nurse.
- The other students will come to the patient simulator as the patient just arrived from the ED.
- Students should obtain a set of vital signs, connect patient to pulse oximeter, and cardiac monitor.
- A physical assessment with a focused assessment of cardiac and respiratory function should be performed.

Findings: Cardiovascular: HR: 120 beats/minute, sinus tachycardia; BP: 152/90 mmHg, peripheral pulses +1. Respiratory: RR: 36 breaths/minute, breathing labored-crackles 2/3 up bilateral, moist cough with frothy sputum. Gastrointestinal: hypoactive bowel sounds. Neurologic exam: alert and oriented, able to speak in two- or three-word sentences.

- Students should position patient in high Fowlers position and continue or increase oxygen therapy to maintain pulse oximeter greater than 92%.
- Students will interpret the results of their assessment. The values are slightly worse than what they were in the ED and patient appears to have worsening distress.
- Students should review signs and symptoms from their focused assessment, including the information provided in the ED report, to help identify and begin to formulate a plan of care.
- Students should recognize the signs and symptoms of pulmonary edema.
- Students should contact an advanced practice registered nurse (APRN) or medical doctor (MD) for orders specifically for Lasix IV push.
- Students should follow the seven rights of medication administration (right patient, right medication, right dose, right route, right frequency, right reason, and right documentation).
- Students may suggest a Foley catheter be inserted for accurate urine output.
- Students should reassess and evaluate the effects of the medication administered and consult with APRN/MD if additional medication is needed.
- Students should provide emotional support and reassurance to the patient as she is in distress.
- Students should educate patient and family regarding the medications that are given and the indications as to why the patient is receiving them. Education should also continue once stabilized regarding congestive heart failure.

Instructor Interventions

1. Instructors can help facilitate student's success by reinforcing the need to look at the patient holistically, and make the connection among the patient, presenting symptoms, and disease processes.
2. Encourage students to address and question possible issues or findings, including lab values and diagnostic procedures, as they pertain to the patient's treatment.
3. Assist students in the evaluation of medication interventions and patient response. Does the patient require more or different interventions?
4. If cardiac/respiratory arrest does occur what interventions will student's need to take?
5. Discuss available resources for this simulation, who can the students call upon (i.e., rapid response team, fast team, etc.)?
6. Other students can observe; if the students who are participating in the scenario are not progressing, others are encouraged to offer suggestions and ideas based on their knowledge and applications of theory and work in collaboration with their peers.
7. The scenario can be redesigned with different patient outcomes to challenge student's critical thinking skills.

Evaluation Criteria

Students should complete the following during the simulation:

___ Identify inconsistencies in the ED report—elderly female with cardiac history, in respiratory distress, crackles on auscultation, was administered Lasix IV push, but then had IV fluids infusing at KVO rate
___ Two patient identifiers before medication administration
___ Hand washing

___ Introduction of self to the patient and what one is going to do before task is done

___ Assess IV fluids hanging

___ Respiratory and cardiac assessment

___ Obtain vital signs

___ Identify signs and symptoms of pulmonary edema

___ Prepare and administer Lasix 80-mg IV push properly

___ Perform the seven rights of medication administration

___ Evaluate patient response to medication therapy

___ Explain the first line of treatment for a patient in pulmonary edema

___ Attach patient to cardiac monitor and pulse oximeter

___ Identify different methods of supplemental oxygen therapy

___ Identify and assess cardiac rhythm

___ Position patient properly to optimize respiratory efforts

___ Provide support and comfort to the patient

___ Educate patient and family regarding treatment and medications being administered

___ Explain rationale and demonstrate sterile technique in Foley insertion

___ Determine when to call a rapid response team or additional resources

G. DEBRIEFING GUIDELINES

1. What went well?

2. What could have been done differently?

3. Were treatments accomplished in the proper order for the patient?

4. What were the inconsistencies regarding the handoff report received from the ED?

5. What if the APRN/MD did not respond to give you orders for Lasix? Who might be the next in the chain of command?

6. What information do you need to make sure you have before contacting the APRN/MD? How do you relay the information (e.g., situation, background, assessment, recommendation [SBAR])?

7. How would you determine whether the patient needed to be transferred to a higher level of care?

8. What did the x-ray and blood work show?

9. How could this scenario be improved for the next time?

10. Discuss at what point a call should be made to the rapid response team or additional resource personnel. Who can you call for help? Encourage group discussion regarding the chain of command.

H. SUGGESTIONS/KEY FEATURES
TO REPLICATE OR IMPROVE

The important part of this scenario is to have the student understand that handoff communication is very important. Determine the key information needed to manage the patient. It is suggested that congestive heart failure and pulmonary edema be discussed in lecture prior to the scenario so that students have an understanding of the signs and symptoms. Instructors do not want to give too many hints to students, but encourage them to critically think about the situation at hand. Depending on the comfort level of both students and instructor, this scenario can easily progress to treating a patient in a code situation. The simulator can be programmed to continue to decompensate even after initial treatment. Students can then practice advanced cardiac life support (ACLS) skills.

I. RECOMMENDATIONS FOR FURTHER USE

High-fidelity simulation (HFS) can be adapted to any nursing discipline. The use of simulation requires faculty to develop a new set of skills (Jeffries, 2009). A recommendation for further use would be the development of a faculty research program in nursing education to promote faculty self-efficacy following the use of high-fidelity simulation. Faculty development and education related to new technology are an integral part of a successful pedagogical experience in nursing education. It's significant in that faculty must be able to administer and evaluate the effectiveness of HFS in relation to clinical situations experienced by nursing students. Through collaboration with colleagues, information and knowledge is then disseminated to other nursing educators through networking and partnerships.

J. HOW SIMULATION-BASED PEDAGOGY HAS CONTRIBUTED TO IMPROVED STUDENT OUTCOMES

HFS is a created experience to achieve pedagogical goals. Simulation is designed to help participants gain insight into complex relationships and develop critical thinking skills in a safe nonthreatening environment. HFS supports a pedagogical link between theory and practice. The use of simulation that imitates clinical situations enhanced with obstacles that confront students in acute care settings promote student learning and efficacy. Simulations afford students a safe, nonthreatening and protected environment in which they can learn and faculty can give immediate feedback through debriefing. Simulation also provides opportunities for students to learn, perform, experiment, problem solve, and develop critical thinking skills before entering the clinical area and providing care for patients. The ultimate goal of this new technology is to increase faculty efficacy that translates to enhanced student learning that will ultimately improve patient outcomes throughout the health care system (Bambini, Washburn, & Perkins, 2009; Jeffries, 2009; Leigh, 2008).

K. EXPERT RECOMMENDATIONS AND WORDS OF WISDOM

It is recommended that students have basic knowledge from lecture regarding congestive heart failure and pulmonary edema prior to the scenario. In addition, there should be a discussion regarding treatment of respiratory distress and medications most frequently used. Early recognition of signs and symptoms of respiratory distress is imperative to prevent patient deterioration necessitating an emergent rapid response or code situation. Furthermore, it is important that the students understand the importance of clear and concise communication during handoff report.

L. EVALUATION OF BEST-PRACTICE STANDARDS AND USE OF CREDENTIALED SIMULATION FACULTY

Recently we purchased the LLEAP upgrade to enhance the clinical simulation experience for our SimMan®3G. Along with this purchase, 10 faculty members were trained on the new software. We are currently undergoing construction of five new sim labs and we are utilizing the INASCL standards to design our simulation space and debriefing areas. We also have a position for a new lab coordinator and part of this person's responsibility will be to be a resource for faculty during simulation, setting up and breaking down simulation scenarios, working with students and making the labs accessible to all students at various times during the week. It is anticipated our use of simulation will increase significantly with the new position.

REFERENCES

American Association of Colleges of Nursing. (2008). *The essentials of baccalaureate education for professional nursing practice.* Washington, DC: Author. Retrieved from http://www.aacnnursing.org/Portals/42/Publications/BaccEssentials08.pdf

Bambini, D., Washburn, J., & Perkins, R. (2009). Outcomes of clinical simulation for novice nursing students: communication, confidence, clinical judgment. *Nursing Education Perspectives, 30*(2), 79–82.

Fountain, R. A., & Alfred, D. (2009). Student satisfaction with high-fidelity simulation: Does it correlate with learning styles? *Nursing Education Perspectives, 30*(2), 96–98.

Jeffries, P. R. (2009). Dreams for the future for clinical simulation. *Nursing Education Perspectives, 30*(2), 71.

Leigh, G. T. (2008). High-fidelity simulation and nursing students' self-efficacy: A review of the literature. *International Journal of Nursing Scholarship, 5*(1), 1–17. Retrieved from http://www.bepress.com/ijnes/vol5/iss1/art37

National Council of State Boards of Nursing. (2016). NCLEX-RN examination: Test plan for the National Council Licensure Examination for Registered Nurses. Retrieved from https://ncsbn.org/RN_Test_Plan_2016_Final.pdf

Rogers, D. L. (2007). High-fidelity patient simulation: A descriptive white paper report. *Healthcare Simulation Strategies,* 1–140. Retrieved from http://www.sim-strategies.com/downloads/Simulation%20white%20Paper2.pdf

FURTHER READING

Hinkle, J. L., & Cheever, K. H. (2016). *Brunner and Suddarth's textbook of medical-surgical nursing* (13th ed.). Philadelphia, PA: Lippincott Williams & Wilkins.

Sole, M., Klein D., & Moseley, M. (2013). *Introduction to critical care nursing* (6th ed.). St. Louis, MO: Elsevier.

CHAPTER 14

Trauma Resuscitation

Carolynn Spera Bruno and Catherine Napoli Rice

A. IMPLEMENTATION OF SIMULATION-BASED PEDAGOGY IN YOUR INDIVIDUALIZED TEACHING AREA

Simulation-based learning occurs in an innovative fashion for baccalaureate and nurse practitioner students. Integrated simulation learning, used within the curriculum, serves as an adjunct modality and, for undergraduate nursing students, it serves as partial fulfillment of the clinical requirement. The objective of simulation-based pedagogy is to provide opportunities for baccalaureate and nurse practitioner students to acquire critical thinking skills before encounters in the clinical setting. In addition, the development of role acquisition in the context of interprofessional learning is a key feature unique to simulation. The application of high-fidelity simulation lends itself to providing safe practice that can occur in a nonthreatening environment with support from faculty and peers. Repetition of high-risk clinical situations desensitizes the anxiety of students responding and participating in the delivery of high-acuity trauma resuscitation. Also, the students develop an "algorithm of response"—learned behaviors of rapid assessment and nursing intervention, formulated on evidence-based practice that may be employed during any precode, code, or resuscitation occurrence.

B. EDUCATIONAL MATERIALS AVAILABLE IN YOUR TEACHING AREA AND RELATED TO YOUR SPECIALTY

The Nursing Department at Western Connecticut State University (WCSU) offers bachelor of science (BS), RN to BS, and master of nursing (MSN) degree programs. Two of the three simulation facilities used at WCSU, which are designed to mirror critical care bays, are available for nursing students to practice skills and enhance contextual learning. An additional intensive care unit (ICU) laboratory will be completed in the next fiscal year, supported by federal assistance. The ICU simulation facility used for the critical care course houses a hospital bed, ventilator, emergency equipment, and the human patient simulator (HPS) with remote personal digital assistant (PDA) access. There are two adjoining laboratories, a classroom for instruction, and a smaller room designed as a library with textbooks. At the Yale School of Nursing (YSN), the simulation laboratory has an attached debriefing room equipped with a one-way viewing mirror and has full computer access that can be broadcast into larger classrooms. The simulation rooms are of generous proportion, and there is space to divide the class reasonably and to provide a quiet, private environment to run the simulation and debriefing.

C. SPECIFIC OBJECTIVES FOR SIMULATION USAGE WITHIN A SPECIFIC COURSE AND THE OVERALL PROGRAM

The overall objective of integrating simulation within the framework of the course curriculum is clear: to enhance student proficiency in performing critical care assessments and skills and to acquire new roles that provide collaboration, improved communication, and efficiency. Basic proficiency of appropriate nursing responses to precoded situations is imperative. Student nurses may have an opportunity to develop these skills with the assistance of simulation. This alleviates anxiety and provides an arsenal of responsive techniques to employ when delivering care to critically ill patients. Role-play and alternating these assignments facilitates teamwork and communication while providing safe care. An additional objective for student performance while working with high-fidelity simulation is to formulate pertinent differential diagnoses. Although some would argue that this is not a function of the role of nursing or consistent with the students' novice level, it is critical to assist students to anticipate nursing interventions based on the patient's medical presentation. Providing case scenarios whereby students can process and synthesize medical diagnoses builds confidence and proficiency while delivering excellent nursing care.

D. INTRODUCTION OF SCENARIO

Setting the Scene and Technology Used

Students are introduced to the HPS with as much reality as possible. The sights, sounds, and smells of the trauma bay are difficult to replicate. One way to address this may be to play an audiotape of background sounds customarily heard during trauma resuscitation. For the purpose of this simulation, the patient is arrayed as a trauma patient would be. Access to all the medical equipment in the ICU lab is available. The technology available for use includes oxygen and emergency resuscitation equipment, stethoscopes, ventilator, cardiac monitor, hemodynamic monitoring lines, intravenous (IV) lines and IV pump, code cart, nasogastric (NG) tube, suction equipment, Pleurovac drainage kit, and Foley catheter.

Objectives

The objectives of the participants are as follows:

1. Recognize precode indicators leading to acute deterioration of the trauma patient
2. Perform basic trauma assessment
3. Identify factors that place the patient at risk for physiologic deterioration
4. Increase proficiency in performing critical care skills
5. Assume roles to enhance proficiency in the clinical area
6. Communicate effectively within the team framework
7. Participate in debriefing exercise
   a. Identify stressors
   b. Identify areas for improvement (assessment, intervention, reevaluation, communication, and team proficiency)

Description of Participants

Student nurse in medical–surgical didactic course: The student should be prepared in patient assessment techniques, including *inspection, palpation, percussion,* and *auscultation.* The student should be knowledgeable about the equipment and forms necessary to accomplish this task.

The student should obtain the necessary tools and forms from the instructor before entering the patient's room.

A 21-year-old White female patient brought into an emergency department (ED) trauma resuscitation bay (Level 1 Trauma Center): This role is played by a high-fidelity HPS found lying on a stretcher. The simulator operator answers brief questions initially supplying the voice of the patient. The simulator operator responds with short, simple answers to questions posed by the student and indicates that she does not understand when questions are not presented in clear, simple terms. The HPS becomes short of breath. The patient becomes quickly disoriented to time and place. His conditions deteriorate, indicating a degree of altered level of consciousness.

Instructor/facilitator running the scenario: The person running the scenario is also operating the HPS (a high-fidelity simulator), unless another qualified operator is available. In that case, the instructor running the scenario observes and take notes relative to scenario objectives.

Family member: None present at this time.

E. RUNNING OF THE SCENARIO

Students are introduced to assigned ED roles. They are offered a clipboard and record data on a mock critical care flow sheet and medication record. Professional observers would be assigned to record elapsed time and interventions. Data from the trauma scenario is introduced as a "call in" from the paramedic as the trauma patient is transported to the ED. The "nursing staff" have only minutes to set up emergency equipment necessary for the first few minutes of initial resuscitation. Written resource materials are not readily available apart from IV drip calculation sheets. Access to learning resources is kept minimal, as this is similar to that experienced in a live resuscitation.

The trauma patient is unmasked, and the resuscitation is in play. Students are expected to proceed using available technology resources and personnel. Trauma resuscitation knowledge is based on previous lecture content. The instructor provides patient data sequentially outlined in the scenario template. Coaching and cues are offered as the scenario unfolds. Typically, assistance in recognizing differential medical diagnoses is provided. Additional prompts include timeliness of interventions, recognition of elapsed time, and communication. Proficiency in the basic resuscitation skills seems sound overall, although additional assistance is provided to novice nurses with directions offered for lifesaving activities. Positive reinforcement is consistently offered with the completion of appropriate assessments, recognition of differential diagnoses, successful nursing interventions, and effective communication.

F. PRESENTATION OF COMPLETED TEMPLATE

Twenty-four undergraduate students were divided into two groups and were introduced to the assignment. Groups of 12 students were considered large and, as a result, several students were assigned roles as extra observers. To offset the large class size during simulation, several trauma simulations were run, and roles were rotated. Groups of four to six students are considered to be ideal and have been used among the nurse practitioner cohorts at YSN. Additional exercises aimed at identification of cardiac dysrhythmias, hemodynamic waveforms, and instability were offered within the scenario.

Title: Trauma Resuscitation

Clinical Nursing Practice III, Nursing 335 (Critical Care Curriculum)

Focus Area

This is an emergency department trauma scenario for seniors and second-semester juniors and nurse practitioner students.

Scenario Description

This chapter introduces the concepts and techniques of physical assessment in the context of the nursing process. High-fidelity simulation provides opportunity for these undergraduate nursing students to apply advanced health assessment skills and delivery of care in the context of an acute, high-risk trauma resuscitation. Simulation may be paused during intensely stressful periods of time in order to provide reflective thought and corrective action or the scenario can continue to the end and reflection is provided afterwards in the debriefing.

Client profile: Sally is a 21-year-old White college student brought into the ED on Friday night after crashing her Jeep Cherokee Sport on I-84. Emergency medical technicians report that Sally, the restrained driver, sustained anterior chest injuries. The airbag was deployed, and vomit was detected on the dashboard. Sally smelled of alcohol. At the scene, Sally was found alert but disoriented to place and short of breath, with acute chest pain of 7/10 radiating to the thoracic area. Interventions at the scene include applying a cervical collar and backboard, O_2 at 4 L per minute, and a large bore peripheral IV of Lactose Ringer (LR) at 125 mL per hour. The initial Glasgow Coma Scale indicates a score of 14, blood pressure (BP) of 90/60 mmHg, pulse (P) 126 beats/minute and irregular, and respiratory rate (RR) of 30 breaths/minute; respirations are shallow and decreased to the right mid and lower lobe. Sally is taken by ambulance to the ED trauma bay of a nearby level I trauma center.

On arrival to the ED, paradoxical breathing and hemoptysis are present. Breath sounds are absent at the right midlobular region. It is determined that a chest tube should be placed to the right thorax. The chest tube immediately drains 200 mL of sanguinous fluid, and the Pleuravac is placed to 20 cm of suction. The patient is writhing on the hospital bed and moaning, "My chest hurts bad." Her level of consciousness deteriorates, and she begins to vomit. A blood gas is drawn and demonstrates a PaO_2 of 86%. The patient is given IV sedation by the certified registered nurse anesthetist (CRNA) and is nasally intubated. Bibasilar breath sounds are present. In order to monitor her, a Swan–Ganz catheter is placed to the left subclavian region with LR wide open. BP is 84/50 mmHg, P is 144 beats/minute, and RR is 12 breaths/minute and regular; O_2 saturation is 98% on FiO_2 of 40%, no positive end-expiratory pressurre (PEEP). The cardiac monitor shows sinus tachycardia with premature ventricular contractions. Jugular venous distention is present and is accompanied by muffled heart sounds. Faint peripheral pulses are palpable, and the skin is cool and moist. A suprapubic abrasion with a red, 5 × 8-cm line of demarcation is noted. An NG tube is inserted and placed at 60 cm continuous suction. A right radial arterial line is inserted by the CRNA. A 16 French indwelling Foley catheter is placed to straight drainage with a preset 200 mL of serosanguinous tinged urine output. Soft wrist restraints are placed on the patient to avoid self-discontinuation of treatment modalities. An arterial blood gas (ABG) is drawn, complete blood count (CBC) with differentials, chemistry panel, serum troponin, type and cross 4 units of packed red blood cells, and blood alcohol level are drawn from the arterial line. An EKG reveals ST elevation in anterior leads. A cervical-spine radiograph and chest x-ray (CXR) are taken. The Swan–Ganz catheter and nasal endotracheal tube are confirmed to be properly placed on CXR. A resolving hemothorax to the right midlobe is present on CXR. Focused abdominal sonography for trauma and an abdominal and pelvic ultrasound are ordered.

Verbally provide the following information about the patient to the students: Patient's name, demographics (gender, age, race, religion, occupation, height, and weight); past medical, surgical, family, social, and psychiatric history; immunization status; allergies; current medications; tobacco/alcohol/substances; presenting symptoms. Note style of the following patient data form.

Patient Data Form:

Name:

Demographics:

Past medical history *(reported by patient's parents via phone call):* Nothing significant; occasional urinary tract infections

Past surgical history: Status posttonsillectomy and adenoidectomy (S/PT&A) at age 15 years

Family history: Lives with parents and two younger siblings, aged 19 and 15 years; all are alive and well (A&W)

Social history: College student majoring in criminal justice at a local university; employed in a work study program in the university library; "A" student; well liked by peers and has many friends, including a boyfriend whom she has dated exclusively for 2 years

Psychiatric history: None

Immunizations: Up to date

Allergies: Morphine sulfate produces itching; penicillin (PCN) produces hives

Current medications: Multivitamin × 1 daily; oral contraceptive pill

Tobacco: None

Alcohol/drugs: Drinks socially on weekends; no other known substance usage

Presenting symptoms: Per scenario

Scenario Objectives

1. Maintains medical and surgical asepsis
2. Performs basic trauma assessment
3. Generates differential medical diagnoses pertinent to the initial assessment
4. Identifies primary nursing interventions
5. Recognizes factors that place the patient at risk of physiologic deterioration
6. Increases proficiency in critical care skills management
7. Assumes roles to enhance proficiency and communication in trauma resuscitation
8. Collaborates effectively with the interprofessional team regarding crisis intervention
9. Delegates nursing responsibilities to each team member
10. Enacts emergency response plan
11. Provides the need for interaction with family to maintain structural integrity
12. Uses safety devices appropriately
13. Participates in debriefing exercise
    a. Identify stressors
    b. Review areas for improvement (assessment, intervention, reevaluation, safety, communication, and team proficiency)

In *The Essentials of Baccalaureate Education for Professional Nursing*, the American Association of Colleges of Nursing (AACN, 2008) identifies practice-focused outcomes that integrate the knowledge, skills, and attitudes delineated in Essentials I to VIII. Although the predicted time needed to accomplish each Essential varies, each Essential does not require a separate course for achievement of the outcomes (AACN, 2008). The Essentials used in our evaluations are the following:

Essential II: Basic Organizational and Systems Leadership for Quality Care and Patient Safety, Objectives 1, 5

In addition, the National Council of State Boards of Nursing (NCSBN) NCLEX-RN® Test Plan for 2016 (NCSBN, 2016) addresses areas of congruency that correlate and are inclusive of the following: safe and effective care environment, safety and infection control, health promotion and maintenance, and physiologic integrity and adaptation outlined as follows:

Safe and effective care environment: *Management of care* (collaboration with interprofessional team, consultation, delegation, establishing priorities, informed consent, referrals), *Safety and infection control* (emergency response plan, injury prevention, standard/transmission-based/other precautions, safe use of equipment, use of restraints/safety devices); **Health promotion and maintenance:** (family systems, high-risk behaviors, immunizations, principles of teaching/learning, techniques of physical assessment); **Psychosocial integrity:** (chemical and other dependencies, crisis intervention, grief and loss, unexpected body-image changes); **Physiological integrity:** *Basic care and comfort* (elimination, mobility/immobility), *Pharmacological and parenteral therapies* (central venous access devices, parenteral/intravenous therapies), *Reduction of risk potential* (diagnostic tests, laboratory values, potential for alterations in body systems, potential for complication of diagnostic tests/treatments/procedures, potential for complications from surgical procedures and health alterations, system-specific assessments, therapeutic procedures, vital signs), *Physiological adaptation* (alterations in body systems, fluid and electrolyte imbalances, hemodynamics, illness management, medical emergencies).

Setting the Scene

Prescenario Setup Checklist

Equip your examination area with the following:

Stretcher
Simulation device (young woman)
Privacy screening
Rolling stool
Bedside stand or table
Documentation (pen or pencil and forms)

Equipment Needed

Airway equipment (emergency airway cart)-regulated O_2 equipment that includes mask, airway, adjuncts (oral/nasal airway), bag–valve–mask (BVM) ventilation device, endotracheal tubes, and laryngoscope with various blades
Crash cart—includes pharmacological agents according to the advanced cardiovascular life support (ACLS) protocol
Disposable trash can for garbage and contaminated equipment
Disposable needle box
EKG monitor
Oxygen source
Goose neck lamp/lighting
Immobilization devices
IV access cart—large-bore IV catheters, central lines, arterial lines
Otoscope/ophthalmoscope
Personal protective equipment—eyewear, footwear, gowns, gloves, and so forth
Pulse oximeter
Rapid volume infuser (prop)
Suction device with Yankauer suction catheter
Surgical procedure cart
Sphygmomanometer-noninvasive BP (NIBP)
Stethoscope with bell and diaphragm end pieces
Thermometer

The scene was set in designated simulation rooms in university settings. Federal assistance was provided at WSCU to expand the room capacity and technology. HPS on a hospital bed was used with a cardiac monitor in place. The following were provided to students: ventilator support; nasotracheal intubation (NTT); Ambu bag; oxygen; code cart equipped with a defibrillator; central-line catheters, IV machine with IV tubing, IV solution, and meds; Pleuravac; NG tube with suction canister; BP cuff; stethoscopes; automated BP cuff; and Foley catheters. Students recorded findings on trauma flow sheets and medication records. Interventions and time elapsed were recorded, the simulation level used high fidelity during the trauma scenario, remote personal digital access was available, and students had access to a substantial 17-inch screen to visualize the cardiac rhythm, hemodynamic profile, including central venous pressure and PA readings, and arterial waveforms.

Groups of 12 undergraduate students each participated in HPS case scenarios at WCSU. Each student nurse assumed assigned roles, including two trauma team responders, three ED nursing staff, one recorder, two runners, and four observers. On the other hand, the nurse practitioner cohort at YSN had four to six students assigned to participate in the scenarios including a responder, one nurse practitioner, one registered nurse, one recorder, and up to two observers. Written scripts were not observed but would be useful in future simulation exercises. Both cohorts (undergraduate and graduate) of students had nearby access to text resources, medication books, references, and laptops. The exercise, however, was to mimic a real-life trauma resuscitation scenario, so the use of resources during the resuscitation phase was minimal by design.

Three trauma scenarios were executed in approximately 45 minutes. Debriefing accounted for 15 minutes' additional time per scenario. Informal scripts were verbally provided for each player in the scene. Several students played the role of professional observer and were helpful in providing the response team with differential diagnoses, verbalizing appropriate nursing interventions, and keeping track of time elapsed.

Scenario Implementation

Initial Settings for the HPS

BP: 90/60 mmHg, P: 126 beats/minute and irregular, RR: 30 breaths/minute.

Required Student Action and Interventions

___Focused trauma assessment and alcohol evaluation
___Identify need to place chest tube and assist in chest tube insertion following protocol for insertion, assessment, and care
___Continue frequent respiratory assessment
___Focused cardiac assessment with recommendations for interventions
___NGT placement and assessment of proper placement
___IV access obtained
___Foley catheter insertion
___Identify blood tests
___Draw labs and send for the following tests (ABG, CBC with differential, chemistry panel, serum troponin, type and cross for 4 units of packed red blood cells, and blood alcohol level)

Instructor Interventions

Students have required some cues with basic communication skills. For example, asking, "Who is in charge?" helps them get started with communication and delegation skills. Asking the professional observer to provide a time check and summarizing the various assessments and interventions that have been performed helps keep students on track. Occasional attention to hemodynamic waveforms is requested. Clinical prompts to note respiratory pattern, muffled heart sounds, and safety measures in the form of soft wrist restraints may be necessary. The ventilator is an unfamiliar piece of equipment; prompts to interface with it are made.

This scenario was implemented without specific criteria to rate individual competency in performing skills during resuscitation. Students came to the scenario with competencies previously measured in another course. The simulation exercise involved group participation. It would be further enhanced in the future with specific criteria to measure individual competencies performed, in which case, additional instructor support will be necessary.

Evaluation Criteria

Students are evaluated on the basis of the degree to which they perform the skill in the appropriate sequence. Attention to the need for prompts is considered in Exhibit 14.1.

Exhibit 14.1	Evaluating Student Criteria in a Nursing Simulation Scenario		
Behavior	**Independent**	**Prompting**	**Appropriate Order**
Hand hygiene			
Documentation			
Personal introduction			
Confirm patient identity			
State purpose			
Query and respond to patient concerns			
Maintain medical and surgical asepsis			
Perform basic trauma assessment			
Generate differential medical diagnoses pertinent to initial assessment			
Identify primary nursing interventions			
Recognize factors that place patient at risk for physiologic deterioration, including arrhythmia identification			
Increase proficiency in critical care skills management			
Assume roles to enhance proficiency and communication in trauma resuscitation			
Collaborate effectively with interprofessional team regarding crisis intervention			
Delegate nursing or nurse practitioner responsibilities to each team member			
Enact emergency response plan			
Provide the need for interaction with family to maintain structural integrity			
Use safety devices appropriately			
Participate in debriefing exercises			
Identify stressors			
Review areas for improvement: assessment, intervention, reevaluation, safety, communication, and team proficiency			

Concluding Steps of the Scenario

On completion of the documentation of the physical examination module, the student is expected to do the following:

1. Provide an opportunity for patient and/or family to express concerns, ask questions, or seek clarification.
2. Thank patient for his or her participation and cooperation.
3. Document the exam according to physical examination guidelines.
4. Place patient's bed rails up × 4.
5. Lock wheels of bed, and reset safety alarms/devices as appropriate.
6. Ensure that patient's personal dignity is maintained.
7. Ensure that patient's call system is within easy access. If patient was conscious, ask patient/family to demonstrate how he or she would call for help/assistance if needed using the call system.
8. Position patient's bedside tray near bed.
9. Discuss with patient/family what happens subsequently (what should he or she expect, what is expected of him or her, whom to turn to for assistance).
10. Determine who has permission for status updates.

G. DEBRIEFING GUIDELINES

In concordance with International Nursing Association for Clinical Simulation and Learning (INACSL) Standard VI: The Debriefing Process (Decker et al., 2013), at the conclusion of the trauma scenario students engaged in planned debriefing that supported reflective learning. The simulation was discontinued and 15 minutes were allowed for debriefing and evaluation. The team's effort as it related to trauma care, communication, delegation, appropriateness and timeliness of interventions, and attentiveness to family needs was reviewed. Questions and points to review posed to the group were as follows:

1. What were the identified risk factors present in this case scenario?
2. Review the components of the primary assessment and secondary survey. Were the assessments complete? Did these assessments progress in a proper and timely sequence? If not, what were the factors that impeded the progression of the surveys?
3. What were the indicators of deterioration in the patient's condition, including arrhythmia identification?
4. List applicable differential diagnoses.
5. Based on the differential diagnosis list, which were the priority nursing interventions? Were these offered? If so, were these executed in a timely fashion?
6. Was written documentation maintained properly?
7. Was communication among team members clear?
8. Were roles clearly defined? Was there overlap? If so, was the overlap helpful or prohibitive?
9. Were proper referrals to the interprofessional team members made in a timely fashion?
10. Which referrals were made?
11. Was the patient's family/significant other cared for? Where were they placed during the resuscitation? Which members of the interprofessional team stayed with them to answer questions and offer support? When were they allowed to see the patient?
12. Did the scenario proceed in a timely and realistic fashion?
13. What overall improvements would you make when running this scenario again?
14. Which stressors have you identified?
15. Did you find the scenario was beneficial to your learning about trauma care? Explain.

H. SUGGESTIONS/KEY FEATURES TO REPLICATE OR IMPROVE

Suggestions to facilitate new learning would be to keep interventions simple. Allow students to formulate nursing interventions based on the top three medical differential diagnoses. In this trauma scenario, the priority nursing diagnoses were ineffective breathing pattern, risk for aspiration and decreased cardiac output related to cardiac tamponade, dysrhythmia, and/or shock secondary to organ trauma. Allow students to rerun the scenario after debriefing to integrate newly acquired knowledge and skills.

Additions to improve the simulation would include an audiotape of ED sounds to introduce the students to potential distractions during the exercise. The ability of the students to remain focused on the task and to delimit peripheral distraction would improve their delivery of care. The provision of a formalized checklist of skills performed would be helpful. In addition, limiting the group to a size of six students would be ideal in order to make individualized evaluations easier. The main aim of this scenario was to determine group process and teamwork. Having additional instructors present to record individual performance would add dimension to this exercise.

I. RECOMMENDATIONS FOR FURTHER USE

During the running of this simulation, I would recommend that the patient condition does not resolve completely after each successful intervention. Although this would prove extraordinary, it does not reflect the reality of resuscitation. It risks limiting the scope of critical thinking and group process that one hopes to achieve through the exercise. The inclusion of some student-generated deviations was also allowed during the scenario. This added great fun to the debriefing component of the exercise.

The trauma scenario would be recommended for use in critical care courses, competency review and evaluation for nurses new to critical care, mock code training, acute and primary care nurse practitioner education, and medical school education.

J. HOW SIMULATION-BASED PEDAGOGY HAS CONTRIBUTED TO IMPROVED STUDENT OUTCOMES

Simulation-based pedagogy is a unique and creative adjunct that adds dimension to nursing education. It provides opportunity for adaptive learning in a proactive, linear fashion. Acquired skills and competencies are fused in a safe, contextual manner during simulation exercises. A simulation scenario provides exposure to high-acuity skills the student might not otherwise master as a novice nurse. Application of advanced critical thinking skills occurs in real time with instantaneous measurable outcomes. The student has an opportunity to develop a set of algorithms for responsive behaviors in a supportive environment. These approaches are accomplished while alleviating student anxiety that normally accompanies a live patient encounter. The mastery of critical care skills is consolidated within the construct of the nursing process: assessment, nursing diagnosis, planning, intervention, and evaluation.

K. EXPERT RECOMMENDATION AND WORDS OF WISDOM

Simulation affords a safe environment for proactive learning that differs from traditional clinical encounters. Often, traditional learning occurs in a retrograde fashion. Students provide care for patients and then, after a period of reflection and integration, the nursing process is applied to the experience. In this manner, patient goals, interventions, and outcomes are measured and enhanced retrospectively. Adaptations to the clinical scenarios are improved through the use of point-of-care technology, such as iPads and SMART Boards for debriefing purposes. During simulation, however, instant recall of learned knowledge stored in the students' mental warehouse must be downloaded as the scenario rolls. The students evaluate the efficacy of their nursing interventions through immediate high-fidelity feedback. This feedback loop regulates self-correction with minimal instructor prompts. The instructor's role within the scenario is to coach. Simulation learning is intrinsically safe, adaptive, and fun. Student anxiety is lessened through repetitive practice of responsive actions and debriefing as a group process provides insight into the broad strokes of applied knowledge and team effort.

L. EVALUATION OF BEST PRACTICE STANDARDS AND USE OF CREDENTIALED FACULTY

The use of INACSL standards is observed by WCSU and Yale School of Nursing. In observance with the Standards of Best Practice: Simulation Standard V: Facilitator (Boese et al., 2013), instructors proficient in facilitating the complexity of simulation scenarios are key to student learning. The facilitators are clinician educators who extend student knowledge and learning by guiding the scenario, students' thought process, and their identification of evidence-based practice decisions along with clinical reasoning.

REFERENCES

American Association of Colleges of Nursing. (2008). *The essentials of baccalaureate education for professional nursing practice*. Washington, DC: Author. Retrieved from http://www.aacnnursing.org/Portals/42/Publications/BaccEssentials08.pdf

Boese, S., Cato, M., Gonzalez, L., Jones, A., Kennedy, K., Reese, C.,... Borum, J. C. (2013). Standards of best practice: Simulation standard V: Facilitator. *Clinical Simulation in Nursing, 9*(6S), S22–S25.

Decker, S., Fey, M., Sideras, S., Caballero, S., Rockstraw, L., Boese, T.,... Borum, J. C. (2013). Standards of best practice: Simulation standard VI: The debriefing process. *Clinical Simulation in Nursing, 9*(S6), S26–S29. doi:10.1016/j.ecns.2013.04.008

National Council of State Boards of Nursing. (2016). NCSBN simulation guidelines for prelicensure nursing education programs. Retrieved from https://www.ncsbn.org/16_Simulation_Guidelines.pdf

FURTHER READING

Bruno, C. (2014). Interpreting a 12-lead ECG. In J. Coviello (Ed.), *ECG interpretation made incredibly easy* (6th ed.). Philadelphia, PA: Lippincott Williams and Wilkins.

Bruno, C. (2014). Interpreting a rhythm strip. In J. Coviello (Ed.), *ECG interpretation made incredibly easy* (6th ed). Philadelphia, PA: Lippincott Williams and Wilkins.

Pellico, L. (2012). *Focus on adult health nursing*. Philadelphia, PA: Lippincott Williams and Wilkins.

Smeltzer, S., Bare, B., Hinkle, J., & Cheever, K. (2013). *Brunner and Suddarth's textbook of medical–surgical nursing* (13th ed.). Philadelphia, PA: Lippincott Williams and Wilkins.

Sole, M., Klein, D., & Moseley, M. (2012). *Introduction to critical care nursing* (6th ed.). St. Louis, MO: Elsevier.

CHAPTER 15

Advanced Cardiac Life Support

Sek-ying Chair and Ka-ming Chow

A. IMPLEMENTATION OF SIMULATION-BASED PEDAGOGY IN YOUR INDIVIDUALIZED TEACHING AREA

Changing trends in health care demand that nurses expand their roles to care for patients with increasingly complex health conditions. Such a challenge, along with a mandate to prepare students to become competent nurses working in the dynamic health care delivery system, leads nurse educators to look for effective training approaches and tools (Norman, 2012). Simulation-based learning, or virtual-reality learning, is an innovative teaching strategy used for nursing students to practice skills in a safe and controlled environment. It enables students to consolidate learning and develop competence through repeated and self-controlled practice, immediate debriefing from facilitators, and video recording (Cant & Cooper, 2010). It also can improve learners' knowledge and performance in clinical skills, consequently bridging the gap between theory and practice (Chakravarthy et al., 2011; Nestel, Groom, Eikeland-Husebø, & O'Donnell, 2011; Thomas, Johns, Marsh, & Anderson, 2014; Tsai et al., 2008). In simulation education, a clinical crisis can be planned as an essential tool used to facilitate students in making the transition to the real clinical setting as smoothly as possible and reducing their reality shock of entering clinical practice. Those skills not appropriate for learning and practicing in the real clinical setting because of ethical concerns about protecting the safety and best interest of patients are most suitable to be practiced under a simulated environment.

In the context of Hong Kong, apart from undergraduate nursing education in tertiary institutions, simulation-based pedagogy has been adopted for decades in health care professional training. With patient safety as the centerpiece of health care service, simulation-based pedagogy in invasive skills training is particularly valued for its capacity to provide students with exposure to realistic, context-rich scenarios, thereby facilitating a balance between the learning needs of students and the safety as well as care needs of patients. Multidisciplinary simulation and skills centers have been established in the local public health care sector to facilitate skills training and knowledge updates. A series of advanced team-based training and specialty emergency management courses have been launched, including an advanced surgical trauma course, obstetrics emergency workshop, airway management simulation training, and acute wound care workshop (Queen Elizabeth Hospital, Hong Kong, 2014). These simulation-based training activities aim to develop health care professionals' knowledge, skills, and attitudes while protecting patients from unnecessary risks, thus decreasing the possibility of litigation related to patient safety (Hicks, Coke, & Li, 2009; Hope, Garside, & Prescott, 2011; Lateef, 2010).

Cardiac arrest is an abrupt loss of cardiac functionality that accounts for more than 300,000 deaths worldwide annually (Kalus, 2012). For such a critical crisis, timely management with required knowledge and skills is essential as the survival rate declines 7% to 10% for every minute delayed in the initiation of resuscitation. The American Heart Association (AHA) advocated a "chain of survival" for patients with cardiac arrest, which emphasizes a series of

151

treatment and interventions that should be performed immediately to identify the patients' need for help and to activate the emergency response system. However, inexperienced nursing students and junior nurses may not have the opportunity to practice the skills or to get involved in managing a critical crisis in a real situation because of ethical considerations. Simulation-based learning is therefore adopted in our institution for advanced cardiac life support (ACLS) training to enable students to practice the skills and to obtain relevant experience.

B. EDUCATIONAL MATERIALS AVAILABLE IN YOUR TEACHING AREA RELATED TO YOUR SPECIALTY

The Nethersole School of Nursing at the Faculty of Medicine of The Chinese University of Hong Kong houses four simulation laboratories, each simulating a real clinical setting with sophisticated, high-tech specialized cardiopulmonary resuscitation (CPR) human patient simulators (HPSs; e.g., central and peripheral pulses, real cardiac and respiratory sounds, improved airway simulation) for student practice. Each simulation laboratory is equipped with two high-fidelity HPSs and one SimBaby®; hospital beds; a crash cart, including a defibrillator with a functioning electrocardiogram (ECG) and pacemaker; invasive and noninvasive airway supplies; fluid infusion devices; a fluid drainage system; an oxygen/suction headwall unit; a monitoring system; and an overhead table. A video-recording system with phones, video equipment, and microphones is available to record student performance, which can be used for debriefing and group discussion after the simulation scenario is completed. Outside the simulation laboratory there is a classroom-sized area where a projection screen has been set up.

The high-fidelity HPSs can respond to procedures and interventions in ACLS, and the simulation system also allows the educators to integrate the complexity of ACLS scenarios to meet the learning objectives. Therefore, great clinical variation in scenario designs can be captured and achieved without risking the safety of patients.

C. SPECIFIC OBJECTIVES FOR SIMULATION USAGE WITHIN A SPECIFIC COURSE AND THE OVERALL PROGRAM

In compliance with the extensive curriculum requirements stipulated by the Nursing Council of Hong Kong (The Nursing Council of Hong Kong, Hong Kong, 2016), a variety of scenarios have been designed through modification of the American Heart Association (AHA) guidelines according to the local health care situation and the learning needs of our students. The International Nursing Association for Clinical Simulation and Learning (INACSL) Standards of Best Practice: Simulation[SM] is also modified and used to guide the design and implementation of simulation scenarios to achieve the learning objectives within the local context and curriculum (INACSL, 2013/2016). The objective of integrating simulation-based training into the nursing curriculum is to enhance students' critical thinking skills in the care of patients with complex health care needs. Simulation-based training provides opportunities for students to get involved in managing crisis situations with less stress and to work as a team with classmates. Specifically, simulation-based ACLS training is incorporated into a theoretical course for year-4 students in the 5-year baccalaureate nursing program.

Learning Objectives

Through scenario-based ACLS simulation learning, students will be able to:

1. Describe client manifestations in cases of ventricular fibrillation (VF), pulseless ventricular tachycardia, and asystole.
2. Perform immediate resuscitation management, including airway management, application of various components in the emergency trolley, and defibrillation.

3. Increase proficiency in performing critical care skills for the management of VF, pulseless ventricular tachycardia, and asystole according to ACLS algorithms.
4. Understand the importance of a team approach in resuscitation.

Student Learning Activities

Before starting the simulation-based ACLS training, students are required to attend a 2-hour lecture for ACLS content regarding interventions according to different EKG algorithms, medication, defibrillation, cardioversion, and intubation. To facilitate effective learning, a big class of more than 200 students will be divided into 12 groups, with 16 to 17 students in each group. To have hands-on practice, each student will have to attend a 4-hour laboratory session that allows each student to be involved as a team member for teamwork practice at least once. During practice, each group will be divided into three teams and each team will have at least five members. Each member has a role to play in the team: one as team leader who is taking the lead to manage the situation and is also responsible for defibrillation, one is responsible for cardiopulmonary resuscitation (CPR), one is responsible for ventilation and intubation, one is responsible for medication and laboratory work, and one is responsible for documentation. Each team has 15 minutes for practice, that is, the whole group has 45 minutes in the simulation laboratory. The whole process will be video-recorded and the recording will be used for debriefing.

During skill practice, each team will have chances to practice ACLS, and the main focus is to develop students' ability to provide optimal artificial respiration and circulation. Students will also have numerous opportunities to provide chest compressions and artificial ventilation, prepare and administer medications, record the administration of medications, and give defibrillation.

D. INTRODUCTION OF SCENARIO

Setting the Scene

The scenario takes place in an Accident and Emergency Department (AED). The patient, a 73-year-old man, attends AED for decreased general condition and he complains of shortness of breath with poor oral intake in the past few days. Pertinent medical history includes an open-heart surgery undertaken 10 years ago but no history of dysrhythmia. The patient complains of chest pain at AED and a 12-lead EKG and cardiac markers have been performed. On admission, he is lethargic and not responding to verbal communication. During a reassessment, his condition suddenly changes and he becomes unresponsive.

Technology Used

A high-fidelity HPS, a crash cart equipped with a defibrillator and intubation devices, other medical equipment (e.g., pulse oximeter, blood pressure cuff, oxygen flow meter, intravenous infusion device, stethoscope, and medication tray), medical records, and a video recording system were used.

Objectives

1. Understand circulation, airway, and breathing principles.
2. Identify various dysrhythmias.
3. Perform immediate resuscitation management, including airway management, CPR, defibrillation, and administration of medications.
4. Assist in the intubation procedure.
5. Describe the principle and related care for defibrillation and automated external defibrillation.
6. Discuss how to manage VF, pulseless ventricular tachycardia, and asystole according to ACLS algorithms.
7. Document the assessment, intervention, and evaluation of findings.
8. Demonstrate a team approach to resuscitation.

Description of Participants

Each group, comprising approximately 16 to 17 students, will attend a 45-minute laboratory session. The students will be divided into three teams with at least five students per team, and each team will take turns practicing for 15 minutes in the planned scenario. Each team has:

- A team leader
- A member for ventilation and intubation
- A member for cardiac compression
- A member for medication administration
- A member for documentation

E. RUNNING OF THE SCENARIO

Students are introduced to their assigned roles. They are provided with the medical record of the patient with information about his past medical history, chief complaints, and current condition. The team leader approaches the patient to perform assessment and the patient suddenly becomes unresponsive. The student is required to respond to this critical condition and to identify the cardiac rhythms during focused assessment, then intervene appropriately according to the ACLS algorithm.

It will take approximately 15 minutes for each team to complete the scenario. After all three teams have completed the scenario, there will be a 20-minute debriefing for discussion and evaluation of the whole group.

F. PRESENTATION OF COMPLETED TEMPLATE

Title

Advanced Cardiac Life Support

Scenario Level

Undergraduate nursing students

Focus Area

Critical care nursing, senior year

Scenario Description

This scenario takes place at 10 a.m. in the waiting area of the AED. A patient (73-year-old man) attends AED for decreased general condition and shortness of breath with poor oral intake. On arrival to the AED, he also complains of chest pain. Students will play the role of RNs working at the AED. During reassessment at 11 a.m., the patient's condition suddenly changes and he becomes unresponsive. Students are expected to use critical thinking skills to identify what the problems are and intervene appropriately with reference to the following information provided to them beforehand:

Patient: Rene Tam (Mr.)
Age: 73 years
History: Open-heart surgery undertaken 10 years ago, with no history of dysrhythmia

Medication record: Lisinopril 20 mg PO QD (per os every day), Betaloc 50 mg PO BD (per os twice a day)
Health assessment results: EKG with normal sinus rhythm, heart rate (HR): 88 beats/minute, blood
  pressure (BP): 160/80 mmHg, SpO$_2$: 95% on room air, respiratory rate (RR): 22 breaths/minute,
  cardiac markers results pending, 12-lead EKG with ST elevation on II, III, and arteriovenous fistula
  (AVF) lead.

Scenario Objectives

The Nursing Council of Hong Kong has stipulated the curriculum requirements for preregistration
nursing programs in Hong Kong. Essential nursing techniques required for safe practice in clinical settings include basic life support for adults, children, and infants. ACLS is categorized under the cardiovascular and lymphatic system. The students should be able to identify various cardiac dysrhythmias and
intervene appropriately (The Nursing Council of Hong Kong, Hong Kong, 2016). Student actions include:

1. Identify various dysrhythmias.
2. Ensure safety and infection control.
3. Understand circulation, airway, and breathing principles.
4. Perform immediate resuscitation management, including airway management, CPR, defibrillation,
    and administration of medications.
5. Assist in the intubation procedure.
6. Describe the principle and related care for defibrillation and automated external defibrillation.
7. Reassess patient condition at appropriate intervals.
8. Document the assessment, intervention, and evaluation of findings.
9. Demonstrate a team approach in resuscitation.
10. Discuss how to manage VF, pulseless ventricular tachycardia, and asystole according to ACLS
    algorithms.

Setting the Scene

Equipment Needed

A high-fidelity HPS; a crash cart equipped with a defibrillator, intubation devices, including a laryngoscope with different blades, endotracheal tubes in different sizes, an endotracheal tube holder and a
carbon dioxide indicator, an Ambu-bag with a reservoir, a piece of oxygen tubing, oropharyngeal airways in different sizes, a suction catheter; and CPR records; other medical equipment (e.g., pulse oximeter, blood pressure cuff, oxygen flow meter, intravenous infusion device, intravenous fluid, stethoscope,
and medication tray); medical records; and a video-recording system.

Resources Needed

Resources needed include textbooks, AHA ACLS algorithms, computer access for database search and
evidence-based practice, and the student activity checklist. Students should practice CPR and review
ACLS algorithms before participating in the scenario.

Simulator Level

High- or medium-fidelity HPSs can be used, preferably with a computer monitor showing EKG rhythms
and vital signs.

Participant Roles

Five team members are needed. One student is the team leader, who takes the lead to manage the whole situation and is also responsible for defibrillation. Of the other four members, one is responsible for CPR, one for ventilation and intubation, one for medication administration and laboratory work, and one for documentation.

Scenario Implementation

All members of the team will be informed of their roles and provided with time to clarify their roles if needed. Other students in the group will be the observers. All students by rotation will have a chance to participate in the scenario, and each team has 15 minutes to practice.

Separate scenarios are developed for three types of dysrhythmias, including VF, pulseless ventricular tachycardia, and asystole. The scenario for VF is illustrated in Exhibit 15.1.

Exhibit 15.1 Resuscitation		
Student Actions	**Instructor Responses/Patient Condition Changes**	**Cardiac Rhythm**
→ Assess level of consciousness → Check carotid pulse (<10 sec) → Call for help → Start compressions (at least 100 per minute; at least 2″ depth; backboard or bed in CPR position; full chest recoil after compressions; repeat for five cycles) → Open airway (head tilt/chin lift if no evidence of head or neck injury) → Give breaths (good seal; two rescue breaths— each over 1 minute with visible chest rise; 100% oxygen) → CPR at 30:2 ratio	Mr. Tam is unresponsive, has no pulse, and is breathless	Unknown at this stage
→ Assess rhythm → Defibrillate with 150 joules (biphasic waveform) → Continue CPR until defibrillation is available → Team leader to check safety of defibrillation, including everyone is clear and oxygen source is away from immediate defibrillation area	EKG: VF Heart rate: 0 beats/minute Blood pressure: 0/0 SpO_2: 74% Respiratory rate: 0 CO_2: 20 mmHg	VF
→ Team leader to monitor effective CPR and instruct change of compressors every 2 minutes		
→ Resume CPR → Assist intubation → Administer epinephrine or vasopressin as per physician order → Check cardiac rhythm every 2 minutes → Defibrillate with 150 J	EKG: VF Heart rate: 0 beats/minute Blood pressure: 0/0 SpO_2: 74% Respiratory rate: 0 CO_2: 20 mmHg	VF

(continued)

Exhibit 15.1	Resuscitation (*continued*)	
Student Actions	**Instructor Responses/Patient Condition Changes**	**Cardiac Rhythm**
→ Resume CPR → Administer amiodarone or lidocaine as per physician order → Check cardiac rhythm every 2 minutes → Defibrillate with 150 J	EKG: VF Heart rate: 0 beats/minute Blood pressure: 0/0 SpO_2: 74% Respiratory rate: 0 CO_2: 20 mmHg	VF
→ Resume CPR for 2 minutes → Check cardiac rhythm → Repeat epinephrine or vasopressin as per physician order → Defibrillate with 150 J	EKG: VF Heart rate: 0 beats/minute Blood pressure: 0/0 SpO_2: 74% Respiratory rate: 0 CO_2: 20 mmHg	VF
	Patient converts to normal sinus rhythm	
→ Check pulse, respiration, and blood pressure	EKG: Sinus rhythm (SR) Heart rate: 61 beats/minute Blood pressure: 66/44 mmHg SpO_2: 91% Respiratory rate: 2 breaths/minute CO_2: 32 mmHg	SR
→ Maintain airway and breathing	EKG: Sinus rhythm Heart rate: 76 beats/minute Blood pressure: 88/72 mmHg SpO_2: 89% Respiratory rate: 2 breaths/minute CO_2: 42 mmHg	SR

CPR, cardiopulmonary resuscitation; EKG, electrocardiogram; VF, ventricular fibrillation.

Resuscitation Scenario

Students should complete the following during the simulation training:

___Identify condition changes and assess conscious level.
___Call for help.
___Implement infection control measures.
___Initiate immediate cardiac compressions.
___Perform airway management.
___Attach cardiac monitor and pulse oximeter to the patient.
___Perform cardiac rhythm assessment.
___Perform resuscitation management, including defibrillation and administration of medications according to ACLS algorithms.

___Reassess patient condition at appropriate intervals.

___Document the assessment, intervention, and evaluation findings.

___Properly position the patient to optimize respiratory efforts if cardiac activity resumes normally.

G. DEBRIEFING GUIDELINES

Issues to Consider

After the three teams of students have rotated to complete the scenario, there will be 20 minutes for debriefing, discussion, and evaluation of the whole group. Debriefing is a key element in simulation-based learning as this reflective learning experience allows participants to review their performance and the facilitator can provide additional feedback for improvements. In our institution, all simulation practices are video-recorded so that students can play back and reflect critically on their own performance (behaviors, communication patterns, emotional response, and intervention skills). The aim of debriefing is to reflect on one's actions so as to think critically about one's practice and clinical judgment, reinforce good practice, and learn from mistakes (Virginia Board of Nursing, 2013).

Questions for debriefing are as follows:

1. What are the learning objectives?

    Ensure the learning objectives are achieved.

2. What went well?

    Encourage students to identify the positive aspects of their performance.

    Ask for feedback from team members and observers.

3. What would you do differently if you could do it again?

    Encourage students to identify areas for improvement and to discuss alternatives to the intervention.

4. How would you facilitate better communication and collaboration with team members?

    Emphasize the importance of a team approach in resuscitation.

Student Questions

Students are encouraged to ask questions. They usually ask questions about the sequence of the actions and the skills of compression and ventilation. Students are also encouraged to provide feedback on the simulation activity and their perception of this teaching strategy.

Classroom/Observer Questions/Roles

Debriefing focuses on positive reinforcement without criticism. Errors in the simulation scenario are allowed, and no one will be punished or humiliated for mistakes. Students learn from mistakes, and observers, therefore, are encouraged to provide constructive feedback of the team's performance.

H. SUGGESTIONS/KEY FEATURES
TO REPLICATE OR IMPROVE

Team-based simulation has been considered an excellent tool to enhance effective teamwork and reduce miscommunication during the ACLS training (Dagnone, McGraw, Pulling, & Patteson, 2008). Scenarios are designed to assess how nursing students interact with a variety of team members, and how students respond verbally and nonverbally during the ACLS practice. Medical students can also be invited to join the simulation training, which will improve interprofessional collaboration and help nursing and medical students better understand their close partnership in their future careers.

If time is allowed, students may rerun the scenario after debriefing to integrate the newly acquired knowledge and skills into their practice.

I. RECOMMENDATIONS FOR FURTHER USE

Knowledge and skills for clinical practice should be better acquired through experience (Brewer, 2011; Buykx et al., 2011). In simulation scenarios, students are no longer recipients of didactic content, but are active learners. The dynamic and interactive nature of simulation-based pedagogy can enhance students' experiential learning and reflective practice, and facilitate students to identify gaps between knowledge and practice. The scenarios in the ACLS training require the integration and application of knowledge and skills rather than examining each as an individual function (Mundell, Kennedy, Szostek, & Cook, 2013; Yang et al., 2012). Students not only learn about how to manage such a crisis situation with less stress as mistakes are allowed, but also have a chance to work as a team with classmates.

Developing a checklist for evaluation is also recommended to facilitate effective discussion. Positive feedback is critical for creating a respectful atmosphere for debriefing.

J. HOW SIMULATION-BASED PEDAGOGY HAS CONTRIBUTED TO IMPROVED STUDENT OUTCOMES

Literature reveals that the majority of research regarding ACLS training using simulation has been conducted with medical students. High-fidelity simulation offers improved educational outcomes and better compliance with ACLS guidelines (Han et al., 2014; Ko, Scott, Mihai, & Grant, 2011; Langdorf et al., 2014). The majority of articles related to the use of simulation in ACLS training in the nursing field are about the descriptions of the application of ACLS simulation in a particular setting, although a growing body of literature has started to show the benefits of simulation-based ACLS training in various aspects of nursing education. Simulation, no doubt, is an innovative strategy, which can be used in ACLS teaching. The growing body of literature also supports the integration of simulation in ACLS training, facilitating the development of knowledge and skills in critical thinking, clinical judgment, decision making and problem solving, and promoting effective interprofessional collaboration.

In addition, team-based simulation has been considered an effective tool to enhance effective teamwork and reduce miscommunication during the ACLS training (Dagnone et al., 2008). Scenarios are designed to assess how nursing students interact with a variety of team members or how students respond verbally and nonverbally during the ACLS practice. Simulation-based pedagogy not only facilitates reflective learning but also helps students to enhance small-group behaviors and team-based competency. Ultimately, an effective medical team with a sense of group identity will be created (Dagnone et al., 2008). By allowing students to practice their team communication and interaction in a safe environment, they will be empowered to take on their new role and feel no risk of saying or doing something that would harm patients or embarrass themselves (Lewis, Strachan, & Smith, 2012; Zhang, Thompson, & Miller, 2011). Working in small groups, learners could also benefit from each other's successes and mistakes.

K. EXPERT RECOMMENDATIONS AND WORDS OF WISDOM

Xunzi, an ancient Chinese Confucian philosopher, once said: "I hear, I forget; I see, I remember; I do, I understand" (Etymology, 2016). The use of simulation as a teaching strategy in ACLS training is growing rapidly because of its potential to replicate clinical scenarios that allow students to integrate theory, practice, and critical thinking in a nonthreatening environment. The ultimate goal of the simulation is to enhance nursing competencies related to ACLS-related skills, thereby improving the efficiency of patient resuscitation.

L. EVALUATION OF BEST PRACTICE STANDARDS AND USE OF CREDENTIALED SIMULATION FACULTY

An AHA ACLS algorithm is used as an evaluation guideline to ensure best practice standards. A few teaching staff have been specially trained in the use of simulation-based pedagogy to design context-rich and culturally specific simulation scenarios and run simulation training sessions for students. All faculty members are capable of conducting debriefing with the video-recorded simulation practices to reflect critically about students' own performance and deconstruct events and mistakes that occurred during the simulation-based ACLS scenario for correction and future improvements (i.e., learning from mistakes; Henneman & Cunningham, 2005). Thus, the objectives of the ACLS training—development of knowledge and skills in critical and analytical thinking, clinical judgment, decision making, problem solving, and interprofessional collaboration—will be achieved.

REFERENCES

Brewer, E. P. (2011). Successful techniques for using human patient simulation in nursing education. *Journal of Nursing Scholarship, 43*(3), 311–317.

Buykx, P., Kinsman, L., Cooper, S., McConnell-Henry, T., Cant, R., Endacott, R., & Scholes, J. (2011). FIRST2ACT: Educating nurses to identify patient deterioration—A theory-based model for best practice simulation education. *Nurse Education Today, 31*(7), 687–693.

Cant, R. P., & Cooper, S. J. (2010). Simulation-based learning in nurse education: Systematic review. *Journal of Advanced Nursing, 66*(1), 3–15.

Chakravarthy, B., Ter Haar, E., Bhat, S. S., McCoy, C. E., Denmark, T. K., & Lotfipour, S. (2011). Simulation in medical school education: Review for emergency medicine. *Western Journal of Emergency Medicine, 12*(4), 461–466.

Dagnone, J. D., McGraw, R. C., Pulling, C. A., & Patteson, A. K. (2008). Interprofessional resuscitation rounds: A teamwork approach to ACLS education. *Medical Teacher, 30*(2), e49–e54.

Etymology. (2016). *Origin of "I hear, I forget; I see, I remember; I do, I understand."* Retrieved from http://english.stackexchange.com/questions/226886/origin-of-i-hear-and-i-forget-i-see-and-i-remember-i-do-and-i-understand

Han, J. E., Trammell, A. R., Finklea, J. D., Udoji, T. N., Dressler, D. D., Honig, E. G., . . . Schulman, D. A. (2014). Evaluating simulation-based ACLS education on patient outcomes: A randomized, controlled pilot study. *Journal of Graduate Medical Education, 6*(3), 501–506.

Henneman, E. A., & Cunningham, H. (2005). Using clinical simulation to teach patient safety in an acute/critical care nursing course. *Nurse Educator, 30*(4), 172–177.

Hicks, F. D., Coke, L., & Li, S. (2009). The effects of high-fidelity simulation on nursing students' knowledge and performance: A pilot study. *National Council of State Boards of Nursing Research Brief, 40*, 1–27.

Hope, A., Garside, J., & Prescott, S. (2011). Rethinking theory and practice: Pre-registration student nurses experiences of simulation teaching and learning in the acquisition of clinical skills in preparation for practice. *Nurse Education Today, 31*(7), 711–715.

International Nursing Association for Clinical Simulation and Learning. (2013, updated 2016). INACSL standards of best practice: Simulation. Retrieved from http://www.inacsl.org/i4a/pages/index.cfm?pageid=3407

Kalus, J. S. (2012). Introduction to advanced cardiac life support. In *Emergency cardiovascular pharmacotherapy: A point-of-care guide* (pp. 1–12). Bethesda, MD: American Society of Health-System Pharmacists.

Ko, P. Y., Scott, J. M., Mihai, A., & Grant, W. D. (2011). Comparison of a modified longitudinal simulation-based advanced cardiovascular life support to a traditional advanced cardiovascular life support curriculum in third-year medical students. *Teaching and Learning in Medicine, 23*(4), 324–330.

Langdorf, M. I., Strom, S. L., Yang, L., Canales, C., Anderson, C. L., Amin, A., & Lotfipour, S. (2014). High-fidelity simulation enhances ACLS training. *Teaching and Learning in Medicine, 26*(3), 266–273.

Lateef, F. (2010). Simulation-based learning: Just like the real thing. *Journal of Emergencies, Trauma, and Shock, 3*(4), 348–352.

Lewis, R., Strachan, A., & Smith, M. M. (2012). Is high fidelity simulation the most effective method for the development of non-technical skills in nursing? A review of the current evidence. *Open Nursing Journal, 6*, 82–89.

Mundell, W. C., Kennedy, C. C., Szostek, J. H., & Cook, D. A. (2013). Simulation technology for resuscitation training: A systematic review and meta-analysis. *Resuscitation, 84*(9), 1174–1183.

Nestel, D., Groom, J., Eikeland-Husebø, S., & O'Donnell, J. M. (2011). Simulation for learning and teaching procedural skills: the state of the science. *Simulation in Healthcare: Journal of the Society for Simulation in Healthcare, 6*(Suppl.), S10–S13.

Norman, J. (2012). Systematic review of the literature on simulation in nursing education. *Association of Black Nursing Faculty Journal, 23*(2), 24–28.

Queen Elizabeth Hospital, Hong Kong. (2014). Multi-disciplinary simulation and skills centre. Retrieved from http://www3.ha.org.hk/qeh/department/mdssc/en_index.html

The Nursing Council of Hong Kong, Hong Kong. (2016). A reference guide to the syllabus of subjects and requirements for the preparation of registered nurse (general) in the Hong Kong Special Administrative Region. Retrieved from http://www.nchk.org.hk/filemanager/en/pdf/sf04.pdf

Thomas, G. W., Johns, B. D., Marsh, J. L., & Anderson, D. D. (2014). A review of the role of simulation in developing and assessing orthopaedic surgical skills. *Iowa Orthopaedic Journal, 34*, 181–189.

Tsai, S. L., Chai, S. K., Hsieh, L. F., Lin, S., Taur, F. M., Sung, W. H., & Doong, J. L. (2008). The use of virtual reality computer simulation in learning Port-A cath injection. *Advances in Health Sciences Education: Theory and Practice, 13*(1), 71–87.

Virginia Board of Nursing. (2013). The use of simulation in nursing education. Retrieved from http://webcache.googleusercontent.com/search?q=cache:W2QBqTmpOecJ: https://www.dhp.virginia.gov/nursing/guidelines/90-24_Patient%2520Simulation.doc+&cd=5&hl=zh-TW&ct=clnk&gl=hk

Yang, C. W., Yen, Z. S., McGowan, J. E., Chen, H. C., Chiang, W. C., Mancini, M. E., . . . Ma, M. H. (2012). A systematic review of retention of adult advanced life support knowledge and skills in healthcare providers. *Resuscitation, 83*(9), 1055–1060.

Zhang, C., Thompson, S., & Miller, C. (2011). A review of simulation-based interprofessional education. *Clinical Simulation in Nursing, 7*(4), e117–e126.

CHAPTER 16

The Use of Simulation in the Recognition and Response of the Rapidly Deteriorating Patient

Sandra Goldsworthy

A. IMPLEMENTATION OF SIMULATION-BASED PEDAGOGY IN YOUR INDIVIDUALIZED TEACHING AREA

As simulation continues to gain traction in the preparation of undergraduate nursing students, specific strategies are being developed to enhance performance in the practice area. One such strategy includes a comprehensive high-fidelity simulation (HFS) intervention that is aimed at improving recognition and response to the rapidly deteriorating patient. The intervention includes pediatric- and adult-based acute care scenarios. Students are exposed to a hybrid approach to simulation through opportunities to complete both high-fidelity and virtual simulation cases. The simulation cases were developed and tested using best practices in simulation that included the International Nursing Association for Clinical Simulation and Learning (INACSL) Simulation Standard IX: Simulation design (Lioce et al., 2015), content expert panels, the use of peer-reviewed simulation case templates (Goldsworthy & Graham, 2013) and a "dry run" with subsequent refinement of all cases. Prebriefing of students was completed through required pre-readings, an overview of the learning objectives, and an orientation to the simulation learning space. In addition to the preparation of the students, the instructional team was also prebriefed by reviewing and running all of the cases, the evaluation tools, and participating in a dry run and setup of all learning stations.

B. EDUCATIONAL MATERIALS AVAILABLE IN YOUR TEACHING AREA AND RELATED TO YOUR SPECIALTY

The simulation intervention was completed in the simulation lab at the Faculty of Nursing, University of Calgary. The simulation lab has three simulation suites, three debriefing rooms, and a control room. High-fidelity human patient simulators (HFHPSs) were used for all six cases. The HFHPSs used in this initiative consisted of three adult HPSs, two pediatric HPSs, and one infant HPS. Every effort was made to closely mimic the actual practice environment and included such equipment as a baby warmer, blood bank, simulated urine, simulated blood, intravenous (IV) lines or saline locks, airway management equipment, defibrillators, crash cart, cardiac monitors, realistic dressings, and moulage as appropriate. In addition, each bedside had a patient chart, lab values, doctor's orders, and flow sheets for assessments and vital sign documentation. Examples of equipment to stage the scenario are described in an overview "recipe" card template (see example in Table 16.1).

Table 16.1	Simulation Overview Recipe Card
Learning objectives	**The student will:**
	1. Perform a focused cardiac assessment based on the patient's presentation.
	2. Recognize normal and abnormal assessment findings.
	3. Identify patient's worsening condition and notify with info to physician.
	4. Prioritize interventions based on findings and assessments.
	5. Document assessment findings.
	6. Administer medications accurately identifying indications, contraindications, and associated side effects.
	7. Accurately interpret any results and note abnormal lab values.
	8. Demonstrate advanced communication skills with a patient experiencing chest pain.
Equipment needed	Saline lock for right hand, nasal prongs, nitroglycerine, O_2 saturation machine, HFHPS, role name tags, clipboard for lab values, doctor's orders, vital sign flow sheet, IV pump, emergency equipment, resuscitation bag, oral airway, crash cart, identification band for patient, urinal, suction equipment and flow meter, scenario and script, pretest/posttest, debriefing questions, blood pressure cuff, thermometer.
Introduction	**Administer pretest**
	Mr. Dressup, a 54-year-old patient, is admitted to the medical floor with a diagnosis of R/O MI (rule out acute myocardial infarction). He has a history of hypertension and one previous MI.
Body of Scenario	Patient develops chest pain while initial assessment is taking place. His condition worsens after two sprays of nitro; he becomes unresponsive and goes into cardiac arrest.
Conclusion	Scenario ends while CPR is in progress and after code blue has been called.
Debriefing	Administer posttest
	see debriefing questions

CPR, cardiopulmonary resuscitation; HFHPS, high-fidelity human patient simulators; IV, intravenous; MI, myocardial infarction.

C. SPECIFIC OBJECTIVE FOR SIMULATION USAGE WITHIN A SPECIFIC COURSE AND THE OVERALL PROGRAM

Programmatic Level of Scenario: Prelicensure

The goal of the recognition and response to a deteriorating patient educational intervention was to strengthen our final year (term 7) baccalaureate nursing students' performance in reacting to and intervening appropriately in a timely manner to a change in patient condition.

D. INTRODUCTION OF SCENARIO

The setting for the scenarios in the deteriorating patient cases was an acute medical–surgical unit. A combination or hybrid approach of HFS and virtual simulation cases was used. Students completed 16 hours of HFS over 2 days. The high-fidelity cases were completed over 2 weeks (8 hours/day). In addition, all students were asked to complete one virtual pediatric case scenario and one virtual adult scenario during the HFS days. The technology used was the VSim° for Nursing: Medical–Surgical program (Wolters Kluwer/SLN/Laerdal, 2015).

E. RUNNING OF THE SCENARIO

Deteriorating Patient: High-Fidelity-Scenario Approach

Each high-fidelity scenario was run over 1 hour. Figure 16.1 shows the breakdown of the simulation case timing. The prebriefing period was 15 minutes in duration and included an orientation to the simulation space, HPS, role assignment, handover report, and pretest questions that were completed individually.

Each student was assigned a role and worked on the case in teams of four. Roles included primary nurse, secondary nurse, lab/diagnostician and a pharmacology role. The intent was that the primary and secondary nurse completed the initial assessment at the head of the bed and the lab/diagnostics and pharmacology students worked at the foot of the bed reviewing lab and diagnostic results and doctor's orders and communicated this information to the students completing the assessments. Each case was repeated on the second day of the HFS to allow for increased mastery of the acute care medical–surgical (adult and pediatric) competencies. High-fidelity cases included angina/cardiac arrest, chronic obstructive pulmonary disease (COPD)/respiratory failure, postoperative hemorrhage, pediatric sepsis, pediatric asthma, and neonatal seizures (Figure 16.2).

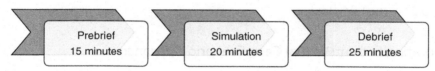

Prebrief	Simulation	Debrief
15 minutes	20 minutes	25 minutes

Figure 16.1   Timing of high-fidelity simulation delivery.

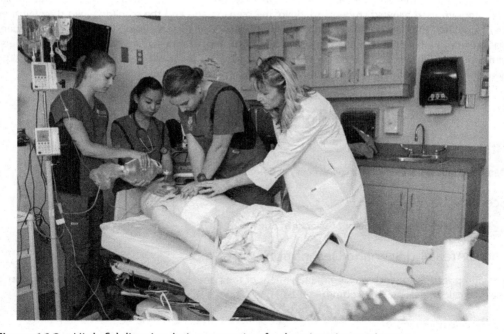

Figure 16.2   High-fidelity simulation scenario of a deteriorating patient.

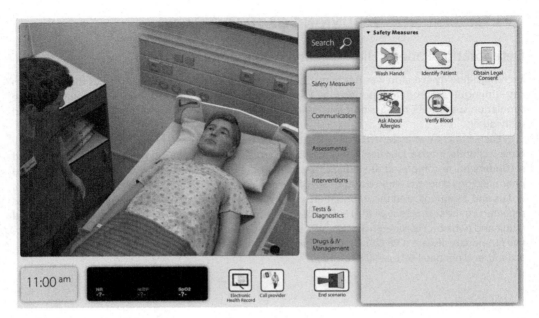

Figure 16.3   Virtual simulation.

Deteriorating Patient: Virtual Case-Scenario Approach

In the virtual cases, students can repeat the cases as many times as they want to achieve mastery with the case. The virtual cases included an electronic preparation guide to orientate students to the program and technology before beginning the case. Each case also had suggested readings and pretest questions and answers to further prepare the student before entering each of the virtual cases. The virtual simulation program used allowed students to "drive" the scenario and end the scenario when they felt they had completed the needed assessments and interventions. At the conclusion of the case, the student was provided with a pretest, guided reflection questions, and a debriefing log outlining a sample screen of the virtual simulation case and how the student performed in the case, as shown in Figure 16.3. The debriefing log also included comprehensive rationales for incorrect interventions and choices.

F. PRESENTATION OF COMPLETED TEMPLATE

Title

Deteriorating Patient Simulation (University of Calgary Case 2.0: Myocardial Infarction [MI])

Scenario Level

___Baccalaureate level (bachelor of science in nursing [BScN])

Focus Area and Scenario Description

Scenario purpose: To teach nursing management of the patient experiencing myocardial infarction in the medical/surgical practice setting.

Scenario number: 2.0
Scenario focus: MI/cardiac arrest

Admission type: Medical floor
Patient name: Ralph Dressup
Unique number: 1786601
Date of birth: January 8, XXXX
Scenario start day: Tuesday
Scenario start time: 1100
Admitting diagnosis: R/O MI
Secondary diagnosis: Hypertension
Recommended scenario run time: 20 minutes
Recommended debriefing time: 20 to 30 minutes
Learning resources: Barry, Goldsworthy, and Goodridge (2013)

Scenario Objectives

1. Perform a focused cardiac assessment based on the patient's presentation
2. Recognize normal and abnormal assessment findings
3. Identify patient's worsening condition and notify physician
4. Prioritize interventions based on findings and assessments
5. Document assessment findings
6. Administer medications accurately identifying indications, contraindications, and associated side effects
7. Accurately note abnormal lab values
8. Demonstrate competency in responding to an emergency situation

Setting the Scene

RN-to-RN Handoff Report

Mr. Dressup is a 54-year-old patient admitted to the medical floor with R/O MI. He has a history of hypertension and a previous MI 2 years ago. His vital signs are currently: blood pressure (BP): 92/52 mmHg, heart rate (HR): 52 beats/minute, respiratory rate (RR): 20 breaths/minute, O_2 saturation is 98% on room air, temperature: 37.1°C. He has a saline lock in his right hand. His extremities are warm and slightly diaphoretic. He is pale. Stat cardiac markers, complete blood count (CBC), and electrolytes have just been sent and results are pending. His blood work and doctor's orders are attached.

Scenario Implementation

Exhibits 16.1 and 16.2 present details of the full simulation.

> **Lab results:** Provided separately.
> **Doctor's orders/simulation hospital:** Provided separately.
> **Evaluation:** Students are then given a series of pre- and posttest questions, as listed in Exhibits 16.3 and 16.4, and evaluated using the competency checklist shown in Exhibit 16.5.

G. DEBRIEFING GUIDELINES

All instructors were provided with a debriefing guide and debriefing questions. Because instructor experience varied in simulation debriefing and delivery of simulation, a reactions phase and plus delta methodology for debriefing was chosen. Debriefing was completed directly at the bedside immediately

Exhibit 16.1	Simulation Scenario		

Simulation/Transition	Facilitator Action	Expected Student Behavioral Outcomes	Resources
Orientation	1. Describe the setting 2. Describe the simulation experience and review the learning objectives with the students. 3. Review simulator function if needed.		Simulator directions Manual
Pretest (optional)	4. Administer pretest (i.e., online, paper or i-clickers)		Presimulation quiz attached
Report (see instructor script)	5. Provide report using by one of the following options: (a) Audio (b) Video (c) Script (instructor read) (d) Script (student read)	1. The student is expected to take notes on worksheet during report.	–Review RN-to-RN handoff report –Smartphone download (and/or video) –Video
Start simulation	– Simulation may be preprogrammed but running it manually is recommended. – Select scenario 1.0.		–Simulator directions or manual if using preprogramming; otherwise have printed scenario script at hand.

Phase 1: Introduction

Physiologic state: HR: 52 beats/minute BP: 92/52 mmHg RR: 20 breaths/minute Temp.: 37.1°C SpO_2: 98% Saline lock: right hand Chest clear Appears pale and slightly diaphoretic	1. Patient situation progresses (see overview recipe card 1.0). 2. Hand (or phone from "lab") second set of ABG results. 3. If using preprogrammed scenario, select "Phase II—Body" of scenario from simulation software menu. *Recommended time to advance scenario = 8 minutes.*	1. Student performs focused cardiac assessment (patient c/o heaviness in chest). 2. Student demonstrates therapeutic communication skills and explains procedures. 3. Student initiates angina protocol, applies n/p: elevates head of bed, administers nitro at 5-minute intervals, and takes BP and VS. 4. Student safely and accurately administers required medications. 5. Student recognizes emergency situation, notifies physician. 6. Patient deteriorates and cardiac arrest occurs; student initiates high-quality CPR, calls for help, and activates a code blue.	

(continued)

Exhibit 16.1	Simulation Scenario *(continued)*		
Simulation/Transition	**Facilitator Action**	**Expected Student Behavioral Outcomes**	**Resources**
Phase 2: Body of scenario			
Physiologic state: No pulse Ventricular fibrillation	1. Patient situation progresses (see overview recipe card 1.0). 2. If a preprogrammed scenario, select "Phase III Conclusion" from the simulation software menu within 10 minutes. *Recommended time to advance scenario = 5 to 10 minutes.*	7. Patient deteriorates and cardiac arrest occurs; student initiates high-quality CPR, calls for help and activates a code blue. 8. Provides cardiac arrest team with an update (SBAR).	
Phase 3: Conclusion of scenario			
Asystole	*End scenario.* *Save debriefing log.*	9. Resuscitation is not successful; patient is not resuscitated.	

ABG, arterial blood gas; BP, blood pressure; c/o, complains of; CPR, cardiopulmonary resuscitation; HR, heart rate; RR, respiratory rate; SBAR, situation, background, assessment, recommendation; VS: vital sign.

Exhibit 16.2	Simulation Follow-Up		
Situation/ Transition	**Instructor Action**	**Expected Student Behavioral Outcomes**	**Resources**
Debriefing (20–30 minutes)	1. Allow students to discuss experience. 2. Discuss student performance. 3. Watch video of simulation (optional). 4. Administer postsimulation quiz (online, paper, response system). 5. Administer postsimulation survey (optional). 6. Instruct students to complete self-evaluation/reflection (optional). 7. Provide remediation as needed.	1. Student demonstrates ability to reflect on the scenario and discusses actions that were appropriate and reflects on interventions to modify for next time. 2. Student completes the posttest.	1. Debriefing/ reflection guide 2. Postsimulation quiz 3. i-clicker questions

Exhibit 16.3	Pretest Questions
Pretest Questions	**Expected Answer/Reference**
1. Describe the symptoms of someone experiencing an MI.	
2. Describe protocol for someone experiencing angina.	
3. Describe safety measures during defibrillation.	

Exhibit 16.4	Posttest Questions

Posttest Questions	Expected Answer/Reference
1. Describe appropriate airway management with a resuscitation bag.	
2. How long should one provider provide compressions for before switching compressors?	
3. If the patient would have been resuscitated, describe postarrest care.	

Exhibit 16.5	Competency Checklist (Case 2.0 MI)

Name: _____   Date:_____

Competency	Examples	Met	Unmet
Performs appropriate focused assessment.			
Demonstrates ability to immediately recognize abnormal vital signs.			
Elevates head of bed.			
Accurately administers nitroglycerine at 5-minute intervals assessing vital signs.			
Immediately recognizes lack of responsiveness and no pulse.			
Calls for help; activates code blue.			
Lowers bed; removes pillow.			
Provides compressions and ventilations at correct rate and frequency (30:2, at least 100/minute).			
Provides update to cardiac arrest team.			
Switches compressors every 2 minutes (5 cycles of 30:2).			
Appropriate management of airway with resuscitation bag (two providers, one-hand bagging vs. two).			
Accurate landmarking used for compressions.			
Documents on cardiac arrest record accurately.			

after each simulation and lasted approximately 40 minutes. In addition to debriefing, a posttest multiple-choice/short-answer quiz was delivered to assess knowledge after each simulation case.

H. SUGGESTIONS/KEY FEATURES TO REPLICATE OR IMPROVE

Suggestions for running the high-fidelity portion of the initiative include ensuring adequate time for set up, allowing for a "dry run," and having a backup instructor available if feasible. In relation to the virtual simulation cases, it is recommended that you provide the students with a thorough prebriefing on the technology and the associated help resources should they encounter any difficulty in running the case. Other important considerations for running this level of acute care simulation education is the level of preparation of faculty members. Competency for instructors in this area includes content expertise, simulation facilitation, and debriefing expertise. We have found that HFS delivery offers a tremendous mentoring opportunity for novice simulation educators and simulation experts to work side by side to build competency in simulation delivery.

I. RECOMMENDATIONS FOR FURTHER USE

There may be opportunity to expand the simulation initiative to other nursing specialties, to less experienced nursing students, and in a variety of geographical locations. There is also opportunity to conduct further research in understanding the role of simulation in improving competence and confidence in the recognition and response to rapidly deteriorating patients.

J. HOW SIMULATION-BASED PEDAGOGY HAS CONTRIBUTED TO IMPROVED STUDENT OUTCOMES

The current simulation intervention used to improve student performance in the recognition and response to the deteriorating patient was explored through a quasi-experimental study among our final-year undergraduate nursing students. In the study, the treatment group completed a 16-hour HFS intervention administered across 2 days (over 2 weeks). In addition, two virtual cases were completed by students between the 2 HFS days. The comparison group attended clinical practicum as usual with no addition simulation intervention. Measures included: a pre- and postclinical self-efficacy tool, general self-efficacy tool, a pre- and postknowledge test, and demographics. The study is completed and results will be available in a future publication.

K. EXPERT RECOMMENDATIONS AND WORDS OF WISDOM

Guidelines used in the deteriorating patient simulation initiative included:

- American Heart Association guidelines for emergency cardiac care (Neumar et al., 2015)
- INACSL standards for simulation (Lioce et al., 2015).

Practices that worked well with the deteriorating patient simulation initiative included:

- Repetition of all HFS cases to build confidence and competence
- Timing and flow of scenarios (six scenarios per day)
- Mixture of pediatric and adult acute care scenarios
- Well-defined roles (no observer role)
- Realistic settings (i.e., moulage, equipment)
- Mixture of cases run in simulation suites (adult cases) and pediatric cases run with instructor in room in a multibed (crib) room
- Mentorship of novice simulation faculty
- Enhances nursing student development through mentorship by simulation experts
- Dry run (pilot)
- Research conducted alongside education initiative
- Debriefing at the bedside created a "just in time" teaching/learning opportunity for key take home messages

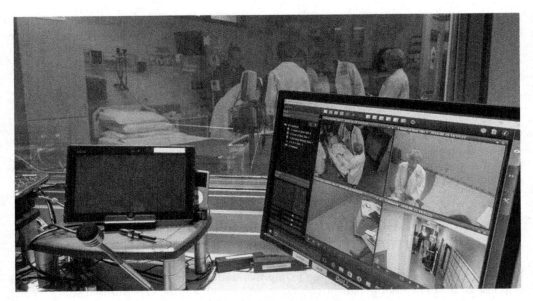

Figure 16.4   Control room for the deteriorating patient simulation.
Source: Photo by Adrian Shellard, courtesy of University of Calgary.

Adaptations could be made to adjust cases to a third-year baccalaureate student level; alternatively, the scenario complexity could be increased to prepare critical care or emergency novice nurses for transition into practice. Other adaptations and future plans include piloting this technique within the interprofessional context.

Additional technology used in the scenarios included student use of smartphones at the bedside for retrieval of pertinent reference material such as drug guides and lab or diagnostic references. In the control room, synchronized tablets were used for timing of the simulation, voice changers provided a realistic patient voice to match the gender/age of patient, and headsets were used to minimize noise distraction among instructors as shown in Figure 16.4. A direct telephone link was also available from the patient room to the control room for the student to call for help or provide an SBAR handover.

L. EVALUATION OF BEST PRACTICE STANDARDS AND USE OF CREDENTIALED SIMULATION FACULTY

At the University of Calgary, Faculty of Nursing, there is a dedicated simulation instructor team and a dedicated nursing simulation researcher and research team. The simulation team continually updates its knowledge through formal learning opportunities; all team members have master's degrees or doctorates. In addition, the simulation team frequently shares its experiences, innovations, and research findings at local, national, and international conferences and through peer-reviewed publications. The simulation lab at the University of Calgary follows international best practice guidelines in simulation.

REFERENCES

Barry, M., Goldsworthy, S., Goodridge, D. (Eds.). (2013). *Canadian medical–surgical nursing* (3rd ed., pp. 691–710). Toronto, Canada: Elsevier.

Goldsworthy, S., & Graham, L. (2013). *Simulation simplified: A practical handbook for nurse educators.* Philadelphia, PA: Wolters Kluwer.

Lioce, L., Meakim, C., Fey, M., Chmil, J., Mariani, B., & Alinier, G. (2015). Standards of best practice simulation standard IX: Simulation design. *Clinical Simulation in Nursing, 11*(6), 309–315. doi:10.1016/j.ecns.2015.03.005

Neumar, R. W., Shuster, M., Callaway, C. W., Gent, L. M., Atkins, D. L., Bhanji, F.,...Hazinski, M. F. (2015). 2015 American Heart Association guidelines update for cardiopulmonary resuscitation and emergency cardiovascular care. *Circulation, 132*(18), S315–S367. doi:10.1161/CIR.0000000000000252

Wolters Kluwer Health, National League for Nursing, & Laerdal. (2015). vSim for nursing: Medical–surgical. Retrieved from https://thepoint.lww.com/book/show/446600#/CoursePointContent/Show/c7c81e79-b0cd-4128-865b-375a0103c8c4?forceView=False&viewMode=Student&productAssetId=c7c81e79-b0cd-4128-865b-375a0103c8c4&behavior=Display&groupby=learningactivity&ts=1481871147507

CHAPTER 17

Medication Administration

Kellie Bryant and Beth Latimer

A. IMPLEMENTATION OF SIMULATION-BASED PEDAGOGY IN YOUR INDIVIDUALIZED TEACHING AREA

Medical and medication errors lead to more than 400,000 deaths per year (Makary & Daniel, 2016). Between 49% and 53% of new nurses (less than 1 year of experience) will make a medication error (Zimmerman & House, 2016). Causes for medication errors include miscommunication among health care providers, workload issues, lack of knowledge about the medication, failure to complete medication administration safety checks, look-alike/sound-alike medication names, rights, transcription errors, poor mathematical skills, distractions during medication administration, and dispensing errors from pharmacy (Leufer & Cleary-Holdforth, 2013). Nursing students report not feeling adequately prepared in the area of medication administration and safety due to lack of practice in the lab setting, limited opportunities to administer medication in the clinical setting, and lack of confidence in linking theoretical to practical learning (Vaismoradi, Jordan, Turunen, & Bondas, 2014). All of these factors attest to the importance of educating our students on safe medication practices to promote patient safety.

In an effort to provide students with additional practice of this essential nursing skill, the Clinical Simulation Learning Center (CSLC) required completion of one medication scenario for each student during their second, third, and fourth semester. These scenarios were developed in collaboration with the faculty teaching the course and the simulation staff. The scenarios are synchronized with lecture content and each semester the simulations increase in complexity. Students must successfully demonstrate selected critical criteria during the scenario in order to successfully pass the simulation. If students miss any of the critical criteria, they are required to attend a 1-hour remediation session.

The scenario presented in this chapter was based on a recommendation by the pharmacology professor to develop a scenario involving a patient having an allergic reaction to a prescribed medication.

B. EDUCATIONAL MATERIALS AVAILABLE IN YOUR TEACHING AREA AND RELATED TO YOUR SPECIALTY

New York University (NYU) Meyers College of Nursing's CSLC is designed to simulate the hospital and outpatient environment for both undergraduate and graduate students. The CSLC allows students to enhance their clinical skills and nursing knowledge in a safe learning environment. Our cutting-edge simulation center is larger than 10,000 square feet and consists of 21 simulation rooms to simulate medical–surgical rooms, outpatient examination rooms, and the home environment—all with video-recording capability. The CSLC is currently equipped with close to 30 human patient simulators (HPSs), including SimMan® 3G, Birthing Noelle, mid-fidelity manikins, and five pediatric manikins. In addition to the HPSs, the CSLC has a database of more than 20 diverse standardized patients (SPs) who are used for almost all graduate simulations and selected undergraduate simulation sessions. Each week more than 100 simulations sessions are conducted at the CSLC for more than 1,200 undergraduate BSN and graduate MSN students.

This scenario takes place in a simulation room with six beds, each of which has an over-the-bed table and bedside cabinet, with a diagnostic station above each bed. There are three workstations on wheels that contain patient mediations and a laptop computer for patient charting. In addition, there is a laptop and patient monitor at each bedside. Tablets are used for viewing of a video report on the patient and also used to evaluate each student.

C. SPECIFIC OBJECTIVES FOR SIMULATION WITHIN A SPECIFIC COURSE AND THE OVERALL PROGRAM

Specific course outcomes met with this scenario:

1. Prioritize increasingly complex evidence-based plans of care to achieve identified patient outcomes and set priorities
2. Reflect on client responses to nursing interventions in order to evaluate patient outcomes and care delivery
3. Advocate for high-quality safe and culturally competent patient-centered care for adults and older adults with common, increasingly complex, acute, and chronic health problems

Undergraduate program objectives:

1. Provide safe, high-quality nursing care using principles of leadership, quality improvement, and patient safety to improve patient outcomes
2. Integrate health-promotion and disease-prevention strategies across diverse settings and vulnerable populations to address health disparities and population health
3. Implement realistic patient-centered plans of care reflecting the variations and complexity of patients across the life span in all environments
4. Manage data and influence information technology to support the delivery of high-quality and safe patient care

Student Learning Activities

This postop orthopedic medication simulation was created for second semester upper division nursing students. During this orthopedic medication simulation the student is responsible for:

1. Reviewing the patient's chart using an electronic health record (EHR) system
2. Performing a focused physical assessment
3. Reviewing each medication using an appropriate drug resource guide
4. Performing appropriate nursing interventions based on the medication to be administered
5. Preparing the medication
6. Performing a three-way check
7. Charting the administration of the medication
8. Reassessing the patient after medication administration as needed

D. INTRODUCTION OF THE SCENARIO

Setting the Scene

The simulation takes place in the simulation center. The patient is currently on an orthopedic floor. The student receives the patient's report by viewing a videotaped report that is watched on a tablet and is expected to write down the report using a shift change report form provided in the room.

Technology Used

Each simulation is recorded using a simulation capture system. Tablets are used to complete an electronic evaluation tool that is later emailed to students after completion of the simulation. A simulated EHR system is used to create a chart for the patient. A workstation on wheels is used to store patient medication and includes a laptop to access the EHR system. A smart intravenous (IV) pump is used to administer antibiotics and IV fluids.

Objectives

The overall objective of the simulation is for students to safely administer medication by doing the following:

1. Perform focused assessment before medication administration
2. Demonstrate accurate medication administration skills using the six (rights) and three medication checks
3. Evaluate the patient response to treatment
4. Report any abnormal findings to the health care provider
5. Document administration of medication using the EHR system

Description of Participants

Implementation of our medication simulation involves two SPs and one faculty member to oversee the process. Mid- or high-fidelity manikins can be used in place of an SP. The SP will play the role of the patient, evaluator, and provide feedback to the student as part of the debriefing process. The faculty member's role is to orient the student to the simulation, ensure the SP is evaluating the student accurately, and provide final results (pass or fail) at the end of the session. The simulation staff prepare all necessary documentation for each scenario, create the patient's chart, and provide SP training for all medication simulations before the start of the semester.

E. RUNNING OF THE SCENARIO

Each medication simulation session is scheduled for 30 minutes: 10 minutes to listen to report, 15 minutes to complete the simulation, and 5 minutes for feedback. Students use an online booking system to schedule their session. The simulation staff post resources on the learning management system that students are expected to review before their medication administration session and include information on scheduling their session; description of the simulation experience, policy, and procedure on medication administration; sample evaluation tool; instructions on the use of the IV pump; and a video of a sample medication administration simulation session.

Thirty minutes before the start of the scenario, the SP arrives and is prepared for the simulation. Once the students arrive for their scheduled session, they are expected to review the video report for the patient via tablet. After 15 minutes, the faculty enter the room to escort the student to the simulation room, where they are oriented to the room.

The scenario begins with the student entering the room and accessing the patient's chart to review the orders. The student is expected to administer the prescribed antibiotic (cefazolin). Once the student administers the antibiotic, the patient begins to complain of "itching" throughout his or her entire body, including the throat. Students are expected to identify that the patient is having an allergic reaction, stop the infusion, and notify the health care provider.

During the simulation, the SP uses a tablet to complete the evaluation form. Once the 15 minutes are up or the student completes the simulation, the feedback process begins. The SP provides feedback first and the faculty provides the final results and identifies whether the student passed the simulation. If the student does not pass, the faculty inform the student of the need to attend a remediation session within the next 2 weeks. All students are emailed a copy of the evaluation form. Students who do not pass also receive a link to sign up for a remediation sessions.

F. PRESENTATION OF COMPLETED TEMPLATE

Title

Medication Administration Simulation: Orthopedics (Lawrence/Linda Bates; see Appendix A)

Scenario Level

Second semester undergraduate nursing student currently enrolled in a second medical–surgical clinical course

Focus Area

Medical–surgical nursing, pharmacology

Scenario Description

The patient is a 78-year-old female in room number 450 who is postop day 1 from internal fixation to the left ulnar and radius bones. The patient tripped over loose carpeting at home 2 days ago, which resulted in a compound fracture of her left ulnar and radial bones.

Patient history: The patient has a history of iron-deficiency anemia for the past 3 years, for which she takes iron sulfate 325 mg by mouth every day. She has had osteoporosis for the past 15 years. She was prescribed Boniva (ibandronic acid), however, she has not taken the medication in 3 years because of stomach pain and indigestion.

Health assessment results: *Latest vital signs:* heart rate (HR): 77 beats/minute, blood pressure (BP): 124/86 mmHg, respiratory rate (RR): 20 breaths/minute, SpO$_2$: 98% on room air, pain 3 out of 10. *IV access:* saline lock right forearm. *General appearance*: Withdrawn, appears stated age. *Neurological:* Alert and oriented to person, place and time, and situation. *Cardiovascular:* Regular heart rate and rhythm, no murmurs. *Respiratory:* Breath sounds clear bilaterally. *Gastrointestinal system*: Hypoactive bowel sounds in all four quadrants, has passed flatus today. Abdomen is non-tender and nondistended. *Genitourinary system*: Voided 200 mL clear yellow urine 1 hour ago. *Extremities:* Dressing to left forearm clean, dry, and intact. Pink fingers and full range of motion (ROM) of hands bilaterally, brachial pulses 2+ bilaterally. *Skin*: Warm, dry, and pale.

Medication record: Iron sulfate 325-mg tablet by mouth.

Cefazolin 1,000-mg intravenous piggyback tubing (IVPB) every 6 hours—due now.

Percocet (oxycodone 5 mg/Tylenol 325 mg) 2 tabs by mouth every 4 hours as needed (PRN) for pain—last dose 1 hour ago.

Scenario Objectives

Key elements from the National Council of State Boards of Nursing (NCSBN) National Council Licensure Examination for Registered Nurses (NCLEX-RN°) test plan (NCSBN, 2015) include:

Safe and effective care environment: *Management of care* (establishing priorities, collaboration with interdisciplinary team), *Safety and infection control* (accident/error/injury prevention, and safe use of equipment); **Psychosocial integrity:** (therapeutic communication); **Physiological integrity:** *Basic care and comfort, Pharmacological and parenteral therapies* (adverse effects/contraindications/side effects/interactions, dosage calculation, expected actions/outcome, medication administration), *Reduction of risk potential, Physiological adaptation* (unexpected response to therapies).

The simulation experience also allows students to practice the following key objectives of *The Essentials of Baccalaureate Nursing Education for Professional Nursing Practice* delineated by the American Association of Colleges of Nursing (2008):

Essential I: Liberal Education for Baccalaureate Generalist Nursing Practice, Objective 1
Essential II: Basic Organizational and Systems Leadership for Quality Care and Patient Safety, Objectives 7, 8
Essential IV: Information Management and Application of Patient Care Technology, Objectives 1, 3
Essential VI: Interprofessional Communication and Collaboration for Improving Patient Health Outcomes, Objective 2
Essential IX: Baccalaureate Generalist Nursing Practice, Objectives 3, 11, 13, 16

Setting the Scene

The scenario requires a room for students to receive the patient report. Students view a videotaped report using the tablet. Students are expected to write down report using a blank report sheet before starting the simulation.

Equipment Needed

___ Two tablets used for SPs to evaluate students
___ 1,000-mL bag of normal saline
___ IV pump
___ Ace bandage for left arm
___ Secondary IVPB tubing
___ Primary IV tubing
___ Simulated 50-mL secondary IV bags labeled "cefazolin 1,000 mg/50 mL"
___ Simulated Percocet 325 mg/5 mg tablets

Resources Needed

1. Simulated EHR chart or printed copy of patient's chart
2. Two SPs or HPSs
3. Script for SP
4. Scenario outline
5. Student evaluation form, which can be printed or programmed into Google forms as an online evaluation tool

Simulator Level

For this simulation we preferred to use two SPs. Another option for this scenario is to use mid- or high-fidelity manikin instead of SPs.

Participant Roles

In order to best utilize resources and decrease the cost of the simulation session, we use two SPs and one faculty member. The faculty member's role is to orient the students to the room and provide instruction to the students before they begin. The faculty member also coordinates the session ensuring the students log into the EHR system; input final grades into the tablet; and provides final feedback to students, including notifying students whether they require remediation.

The SPs are responsible for completing the evaluation tool using the tablet. At the end of the simulation, SPs will provide feedback to students regarding their performance and the care they received as a patient.

Scenario Implementation

Initial Settings

The SP is in the bed wearing a patient gown, left wrist wrapped with an Ace wrap, and a simulated IV site on the right forearm. Each SP has a tablet. Normal saline primary bag should be running from a smart IV pump at 75 mL/hour. The workstation on wheels is stocked with iron sulfate, cefazolin, and Percocet.

Expected/Required Student Assessments/Actions:

___ Washes hands on entering room
___ Introduces self to patient
___ Identifies patient and checks identification band
___ Speaks with patient in a therapeutic tone
___ Explains purpose of the interaction
___ Reassess pain
___ Assesses IV site
___ Reviews the EHR medication orders
___ Prepares to administer IV cefazolin using a three-way check
___ Explains purpose and side effects of medication before administration
___ Prepares secondary infusion
___ Begins IV cefazolin administration using smart pump
___ Recognizes patient's allergic reaction
___ Stops infusion
___ Notifies health care provider of patient's allergic reaction using situation, background, assessment, recommendation (SBAR) format

Instructor Interventions

The instructor's main role is to oversee the flow of the simulation and ensure that each session stays within the expected time frame. Instructor ensures that the SPs are prepared, all necessary equipment is readily available, the student is oriented to the room, and provides the final feedback to the students. At the end of the simulation, the faculty member must enter the grade into the learning management system and create a referral for remediation for each student who did not successfully pass the simulation.

Evaluation Criteria

Students must successfully meet all critical elements of the simulation, which are described on the evaluation tool (see Appendix B). If a student misses any of the critical elements, he or she must attend a remediation session. The remediation sessions are taught by our education specialist, who works with the student to review the criteria that were missed and provide an opportunity for additional practice. Once remediation is successfully completed, the education specialist will change the student's grade in the learning management system from "fail" to "pass." If the student has not successfully completed remediation, the education specialist will require the student to return for additional remediation.

G. DEBRIEFING GUIDELINES

Issues to Consider

Because of the limited time available for debriefing, students are provided with brief and focused feedback from the SP and the faculty. During this focused feedback the faculty and SPs not only review critical elements in the evaluation tool that were "not met" by the participant, but also provide positive feedback. If the student did not meet all the critical elements, students are required to sign up for a 60-minute intense remediation session. Remediation involves a review of the video of his or her simulation session, more detailed review of unmet criteria missed, and additional hands-on practice of medication administration skills. Students must be able to demonstrate proper technique and critical elements missed during their simulation in order to receive a passing grade.

Student Questions

1. How are you feeling right now?
2. What were some of the positive aspects of the care you provided?
3. What would you do differently if you were given another chance to complete this simulation?

Classroom/Observers Questions/Roles

The SP also provides feedback on how he or she felt, whether he or she was cared for from the patient's perspective, and also provide feedback on the student's performance.

H. SUGGESTIONS/ KEY FEATURES TO REPLICATE OR IMPROVE

Medication administration simulation should incorporate more than the psychomotor skill of giving a medication to a patient. Critical thinking can be enhanced using medication simulation through the inclusion of focused assessment, evaluation of laboratory values, and unexpected embedded challenges that require the use of clinical judgment such an allergic reaction. Another crucial key factor to replicate is a plan for remediating students who do not demonstrate safe medication practices. Before implementing a summative simulation, it is necessary to develop a remediation plan to address students who do not meet minimum requirements for safe medication administration to ensure students are equipped to administer medication in the hospital setting.

I. RECOMMENDATIONS FOR FURTHER USE

The template of this scenario can be replicated to create scenarios to meet the outcomes for other courses, such as pediatric and maternity courses. The medical conditions presented in the scenarios can be developed to meet specific course outcomes and increase in acuity as the student progresses through the curriculum. In the future, these scenario can be used for high-stakes testing once the scenarios have been tested for reliability and validity. If resources are available, the medication simulation can be repeated for students who did not successfully complete the simulation. The concept of medication administration simulations can be used to develop cases for nurse practitioner students and focus on prescribing the most appropriate medication based on the patient's clinical presentation.

J. HOW SIMULATION-BASED PEDAGOGY HAS CONTRIBUTED TO IMPROVED STUDENT OUTCOMES

Implementation of the medication administration simulation provides an opportunity for repetitive practice of an essential nursing skill. An anecdotal observation by faculty is that students continue to demonstrate safe medication practices during subsequent simulations sessions and during hospital-based clinical experiences. Students report a heightened awareness of the impact and potential for medication error and an increased confidence in their medication administration skills. Our expectation is that these desired behaviors will continue to be implemented during medication administration in the clinical setting.

L. EVALUATION OF BEST PRACTICE STANDARDS AND THE USE OF CREDENTIALED SIMULATION FACULTY

Many International Nursing Association for Clinical Simulation and Learning (INACSL) Standards of Best Practices guidelines were used during the creation and implementation of our medication administration scenario. The scenario was designed based on the elements outlined in Standard IX (Lioce et al., 2015). The scenario was developed based on a need for students to have additional practice with medication administration. The objectives developed for each scenario were measurable, congruent with the knowledge of the learner, based on evidence-based practice, and could be achieved within the 20-minute time frame. The format of the simulation was formative and based on a realistic case scenario. The facilitator role, level of debriefing, and evaluation were clearly defined. Standard IV was met by providing feedback after the simulation that acknowledged the learner's feelings and the instructor facilitated feedback from the SPs (Franklin et al., 2013). Students were adequately prepared for the simulation by multiple resources provided, such as sample evaluation templates, learning outcomes, and a video report of the patient. Pilot testing was conducted before implementation of the simulation to ensure the scenario was accurate, met objectives, and was effective.

REFERENCES

American Association of Colleges of Nursing. (2008). *The essentials of baccalaureate nursing education for professional nursing practice.* Washington, DC: Author. Retrieved from http://www.aacnnursing.org/Portals/42/Publications/BaccEssentials08.pdf

Franklin, A. E., Boese, T., Gloe, D., Lioce, L., Decker, S., Sando, C. R., & Borum, J. C. (2013). Standards of best practice: Simulation standard IV: Facilitation. *Clinical Simulation in Nursing, 9*(6), S19–S21.

Leufer, T., & Cleary-Holdforth, J. (2013). Let's do no harm: Medication errors in nursing: Part 1. *Nurse Education in Practice, 13*(3), 213–216.

Lioce, L., Meakim, C. H., Fey, M. K., Chmil, J. V., Mariani, B., & Alinier, G. (2015). Standards of best practice: Simulation standard IX: Simulation design. *Clinical Simulation in Nursing, 11*(6), 309–315.

Makary, M. A., & Daniel, M. (2016). Medical error—The third leading cause of death in the U.S. *British Medical Journal, 353*, i2139.

National Council of State Boards of Nursing. (2015). NCSBN–NCLEX-RN test plan. Retrieved from https://www.ncsbn.org/testplans.htm

Vaismoradi, M., Jordan, S., Turunen, H., & Bondas, T. (2014). Nursing students' perspectives of the cause of medication errors. *Nurse Education Today, 34*(3), 434–440.

Zimmerman, D. M., & House, P. (2016). Medication safety: Simulation education for new RNs promises an excellent return on investment. *Nursing Economic$, 34*(1), 49–51.

APPENDIX A

NYU Standardized Patient Script

Title of Case: Lawrence/Linda Bates Orthopedic Case

Scenario Summary	A 78-year-old was admitted yesterday for fracture of the left arm. You tripped on an area rug at home and fell 2 days ago. You had surgery yesterday to place plate and pins in your fractured left arm. During the scenario, you will take antibiotics and experience an allergic reaction. **YOU START COMPLAINING OF ITCHINESS THROUGHOUT ENTIRE BODY, INCLUDING THROAT, 3 MINUTES AFTER THE STUDENT HANGS YOUR ANTIBIOTIC.**
Setting	NYU SIM hospital, lying in bed on an orthopedic floor
Diagnosis	Compound fractures of left wrist
The Patient	
Name	Lawrence/Linda Bates
DOB	4/13/XX
Age	78
Behavior	Slightly annoyed with self that you are in the hospital because of a fall
Complaints	None at the moment. You just received Percocet and your pain level has reduced from 8/10 to 3/10 (you do not want any more pain medicine).
Physical Assessment Findings	Left wrist and lower arm will be wrapped with gauze and an Ace bandage
Past Medical History	Anemia, osteoporosis 15 years ago, stopped taking medication for osteoporosis 3 years ago (ibandronate/Boniva) because of stomach pains.
Medications	None
Allergies	None (see bold type in scenario summary)
Social History	
Family Life: marital status, kids	Spouse died several years ago, no children
Occupation	Retired
Smoking History	Denies

(continued)

(continued)

Alcohol History	Denies
Drug Use	Denies
Diet	Regular

Possible Student Questions	**Standardized Patient Response**
How did you fall?	I tripped on an area rug in my living room.
Is your pain better after the medication?	Yes
What is your pain score now based on a scale of 1 to 10?	8 before pain medication and now 3
Do you want any more pain meds?	No
Do you have any medical problems?	Anemia and osteoporosis
Are you on any medications?	I take iron pills every day. Was on Boniva but stopped 3 years ago due to stomach upset.
Do you have any allergies?	No
When was your dressing changed?	Earlier today
Can I examine your wrist?	"Yes, but it hurts when someone touches it."
(After antibiotic is given) Are you feeling ok?	"I feel very itchy all of a sudden. My whole body itches. My throat feels a little itchy, too."
Are you having a hard time breathing?	No, but my throat itches.

APPENDIX B

Medication Administration Competency Standardized Patient Checklist

	Met	Unmet
Introduction and Identification		
Washes hands before providing patient care (on entering the room).		
Introduces self to you by name and title.		
Provides patient privacy during patient care.		
Explains the purpose of the interaction.		
Asked you for your name and date of birth and checks ID band.		
Speaks to you in a therapeutic tone.		
Washes hands after providing patient care.		

CLINICAL SIMULATION CRITICAL ELEMENTS

	Met	Unmet
Pain Reassessment		
Asked about the location of your pain		
Asked about the severity of your pain (on a scale of 0–10)		
Cefazolin Medication Administration		
Med Check #1: Checks medication against MAR when removing from cart.		
States patient name (Lawrence/Linda Bates).		
States the name of the medication (cefazolin [Ancef]).		
States the dose of the medication (1,000 mg/50 mL).		
States route (IVPB).		
Medication given during correct time frame (every 6 hours).		
Med Check #2: Ensures correct medication against MAR while preparing.		
States Patient Name (Lawrence/Linda Bates).		

(continued)

(continued)

	Met	Unmet
States the name of the medication (cefazolin [Ancef]).		
States the dose of the medication (1,000 mg/50 mL).		
States route (IVPB).		
Medication given during correct time frame (every 6 hours).		
Med Check #3: Ensures correct medication and patient to EHR immediately before administering to patient at bedside.		
States patient name (Lawrence/Linda Bates).		
States the name of the medication (cefazolin [Ancef]).		
States the dose of the medication (1,000 mg/50 mL).		
States route (IVPB).		
Medication given during correct time frame (every 6 hours).		
Explained medication's purpose **before** giving you the medication.		
Explained medication side effects **before** giving you the medication.		
Secondary IV infusion		
Prepares secondary infusion correctly		
Checks the IV site before starting medication		
Wipes IV port above the pump with alcohol swab before connecting the IV antibiotic tubing,		
Sets pump rate to 100 mL/hr,		
Does not contaminate tip of IV tubing,		
Identifies an allergic reaction,		
Stops IV pump		
Notifies health care provider of patient's allergic reaction using SBAR report.		
Post Medication Administration		
Documents in the MAR		

EHR, electronic health record; IV, intravenous; IVPB, intravenous piggyback tubing; MAR, medication administration record; SBAR, situation, background, assessment, recommendation.
Shaded boxes represent critical elements required that must be MET in order to pass.

CHAPTER 18

Obstetric Emergency: Postpartum Hemorrhage[1]

Suzanne Hetzel Campbell and Wendy A. Hall

A. IMPLEMENTATION OF SIMULATION-BASED PEDAGOGY IN YOUR INDIVIDUALIZED TEACHING AREA

Experiences for the obstetric and pediatric clinical areas are becoming difficult to acquire for students, as increasing numbers of students compete for a small number of slots, and constraints on the numbers of students allowed in clinical settings continue to rise. In British Columbia, most of the family birthing units limit the number of students allowed to six and most health authorities require a 1:6 faculty/student ratio. In addition, students need to rotate through at least two areas—postpartum and intrapartum (labor and delivery)—which adds to the complexity of scheduling and student education. Students require preparation for assessments and skills required by these areas.

At present, simulation-based pedagogy has been implemented in this area with the use of an intermediate-fidelity pregnant human patient simulator (HPS) to demonstrate Leopold maneuvers; fundal height measurement; infant positioning in utero (e.g., for placement of external fetal monitors and to monitor the birth process); and, in some cases, to simulate the birth process (Cooper et al., 2012; Ferguson, Howell, & Parsons, 2014; Fox-Young et al., 2012; Gardner & Raemer, 2008). Other uses for this model could include the demonstration and practice of obstetric emergencies such as shoulder dystocia, prolapsed umbilical cord, placenta previa, and abruptio placentae. As postpartum hemorrhage (PPH) constitutes an obstetric emergency and remains a major cause of maternal morbidity and mortality in high- and low-resource countries (Chalouhi, Tarutis, Barros, Starke, & Mozurkewich, 2015), using a simulator offers an ideal opportunity for students to practice their skills in simulated PPH. The scenario presented in this chapter was modified and used at the University of British Columbia (UBC) School of Nursing (SoN) since January 2015. Student preparation requires readings, videos, and evidence-based practice protocols for PPH.

B. EDUCATIONAL MATERIALS AVAILABLE IN YOUR TEACHING AREA AND RELATED TO YOUR SPECIALTY

The UBC SoN has several rooms set up for simulation. The simulation lab was run over a 3-hour period with two faculty members and groups of six students exposed to the simulation at a time.

---

[1] This chapter appeared in the first and second editions of *Simulation Scenarios for Nursing Educators* (Campbell & Daley, 2009, 2013) and is based on the first author's experience using the simulation in a small, private, 4-year baccalaureate program. This third edition reflects the experience at a research-intensive institution in Canada with accelerated BSN students in their fourth term of a five-term education. Dr. Hall has added to the scenario for this student population and to reflect the international/Canadian perspective.

The PPH scenario takes place in the acute care area (a room set up like a patient room in hospital on a family birthing unit) using a medium-fidelity HPS (Laerdal's VitalSim Anne®). The faculty communicated with students directly and responded as the voice of the patient from behind curtained areas using the remote to effect vital sign (VS) changes. Students were requested to prepare for the simulation by completing a number of readings available on their learning management system. The readings included: Campbell and Daley (2013); Davidson, London, and Ladewig (2012a, 2012b); Hall (2014); and Leduc and colleagues (2009); see References and Further Reading.

C. SPECIFIC OBJECTIVES FOR SIMULATION USAGE WITHIN A SPECIFIC COURSE AND THE OVERALL PROGRAM

As PPH continues to be the leading cause of maternal death globally (Leduc et al., 2009; Rath, 2011), with one woman dying every 4 minutes (Rath, 2011), using simulation to educate health care professionals about teamwork in managing PPH should be a priority (Dolea, AbouZahr, & Stein, 2003; World Health Organization, 2010). This scenario aimed to assess nursing students' abilities to conduct thorough postpartum assessments, recognize abnormal findings, and act to determine a plan of action to enhance patient safety and emotional stability. The previous version of this scenario was designed as an in-class, advanced-level simulation for American third-year baccalaureate or first-year associate degree nursing students in their second semester. At UBC SoN, Canadian students exposed to the simulation were in an advanced course: Nursing Practice with Childbearing Families, offered in their fourth term of a five-term accelerated BSN program. The students in the UBC program had completed a medical–surgical course and an introductory course: Professional Nursing Practice with Childbearing Individuals and their Families. Students interested in pursuing a career in maternal-child nursing could select the advanced course from a number of specialty courses.

Student Learning Activities

- Review and practice normal postpartum assessment (text, videos, online materials)
- Review risk factors for postpartum complications (text, evidence-based-protocols, references)
- Review medications: pain, oxytocics, standard orders for postpartum medications (up-to-date pharmaceutical resources in your country)

D. INTRODUCTION OF SCENARIO

Setting the Scene

The setting is a hospital room on a postpartum unit of a tertiary-level institution. The students receive a report from the night nurse, an obstetric resident is available on call, and the infant is in the room being held by the father.

Technology Used

The medium-fidelity HPS is a female: genitalia are in place on this HPS, running manually, with initially normal vital signs (VS) (blood pressure [BP]: 100/70 mmHg, pulse [P]: 80 beats/minute, respiratory rate [RR]: 16 breaths/minute, temperature [T]: 36.9°C), but these are not visible on the monitor, and the pulse oximeter is not in place. The patient has a saline lock from IV antibiotics in labor for positive status for group B streptococcus (strep). She is wearing a pad with gauze panties that are soaked through with two grapefruit-sized clots (paste and food coloring). A boggy uterus displaced to the right is present in the medium-fidelity HPS using a fundal model. A wristband identifies the patient as "Mrs. Matilda Price." Stethoscopes, gloves, and a pulse oximeter are placed nearby for student use, as well as intravenous (IV) fluids (1,000 mL normal saline), a large-bore intravenous canula, IV tubing, blood transfusion set, suture materials, Foley catheter, packing materials, and blood products (Leduc et al., 2009; Perinatal Services BC [PSBC], 2011). Clean perineal pads, gauze panties, and a pericare bottle are nearby. Routine and as-needed (PRN) medications are also available (PSBC, 2011).

Objectives

1. Apply physiological knowledge to detect PPH.
2. Demonstrate critical and systematic thinking to manage PPH.
3. Incorporate all family members in the management of PPH to support emotional well-being.
4. Use empirical evidence to support approaches to managing PPH.
5. Work collaboratively with other members of the health care team to manage PPH.

Description of Participants

Mrs. Matilda Price, a 39-year-old First Nations woman of Coast Salish and Snohomish descent. Obstetric history: gravida 5, term 3, preterm 1, abortions 1, living 4. Augmentation of labor with Pitocin occurred and membranes were ruptured on Sunday morning. Had a vacuum-assisted delivery of 9 lbs. 8 ounces (4,309 g) male on Sunday at 4:30 a.m.; long labor—difficult delivery, pushed for longer than 1 hour. Midwife Robinson is on call for care of Mrs. Price, who is a clinic patient.

E. RUNNING OF THE SCENARIO

Before the simulation, students were requested to review readings available through the learning management system and provided with the patient history. Students were oriented to the simulation room and the HPS, shown the location of medications and supplies, and provided an opportunity to ask questions and clarify the situation. They were given report and told Mrs. Price is diaphoretic, with falling BP. Students were to identify the risk factors from the patient history and respond to the VS by performing a postpartum check, including information about the onset, duration, and amount of blood loss (PSBC, 2011). On assessing the fundal height and tone they found a boggy and displaced fundus, as well as lochia soaking the pad with two grapefruit-sized clots. Priority care involves calling for help, running IV fluids with 20 IU oxytocin, and performing bimanual fundal massage (PSBC, 2011). They should start oxygen by mask at 8 to 10 L/minute and monitor O_2 saturation. They would also insert a Foley catheter, to monitor urine output, recheck the fundal location, and continue bimanual uterine massage if still boggy, prepare a second line of uterotonic drugs, and anticipate laboratory studies (PSBC, 2011). They should recognize the potential for blood transfusions and surgery, dependent on the cause of the bleeding

F. PRESENTATION OF COMPLETED TEMPLATE

Title

Obstetric Emergency: PPH

Focus Area

Nursing 422: Nursing Care of the Childbearing Family, specialty clinical course in obstetrics for fourth-term nursing students in an accelerated baccalaureate program.

Scenario Description

The students arrive at 07:00 for clinical experience at a tertiary-level institution in a postpartum unit. They are assigned to care for Mrs. Matilda Price, a clinic patient being overseen by Ms. Robinson, midwife. The infant is under the care of Dr. Lavoy, a pediatrician, and at present is in the mother's room. The night nurse gives the following report:

Patient: Mrs. Matilda Price

Age: 39 years

DOB: As decided to configure the rest of the scenario

Allergies: No known drug allergies (NKDA)

History: Admission at 24 00 hours. Gravida 5, term 3, preterm 1, abortions 1, living 4 counting new 9-pound, 8-ounce (4,309 g) male born at 04:30. Breastfeeding: infant latched after delivery but is being held by the father because the mother is feeling very groggy and dizzy. Children at home are 6, 4, and 2 years old, two girls and a boy, respectively, being cared for by a grandparent.

Delivery history: Augmentation of labor with oxytocin and membranes ruptured artificially at 00:30. On admission had labored for 5 hours at home and per vaginal exam was 4-cm dilated and partially effaced. Vacuum-assisted delivery; after labor (9.5 hours)—difficult delivery, pushed more than 1 hour. At 2400, VS were as follows: BP: 100/70 mmHg, P: 80 beats/minute, RR: 16 breaths/minute, T: 36.9°C, hemoglobin (hgb): 12.0 g/L, and hematocrit (hct), 35%. The patient has a saline lock from IV antibiotics in labor for group B strep—positive status (received amoxicillin 1 amp ×3), 18-gauge needle is in place. Her fundus has been firm, midline, one fingerbreadth above umbilicus; lochia rubra, moderate amount; and the report indicated that episiotomy with 4th-degree laceration was intact when transferred to floor.

When students enter room, this is what they find:

- Monday morning at 07:00 VS: BP: 65/45 mmHg, P: 120 beats/minute, RR: 21 breaths/minute, T: 36.8°C
- Fundus: Boggy and displaced to right of umbilicus
- Lochia: Bright red, pad soaked with two grapefruit-sized clots
- Episiotomy with fourth-degree laceration: R-2, E-2, E-3, D-3, A-1 = 11; no signs of cervical lacerations, hematoma, or other problems
- Patient complains of dizziness, color is pale, and slight diaphoresis noticed on forehead
- Patient is not hungry and is very teary; lab values: group B strep positive, venereal disease research laboratory (VDRL) neg, HIV neg, white blood cell (WBC): 80,000, hgb: 9.7, hct: 30% (14% change from admission), blood type O+ (two units crossmatched and on hold)
- Father is present and holding the baby

PATIENT INFORMATION

Admission Date: TBD

Today's Date: Same as admission

Name: Matilda Price

Gender: F

Age/DOB: 39 years

Allergy Status: No known allergies

Previous Medical History (brief summary): No previous chronic illnesses or recent surgeries

Personal/Social History (brief summary if required): Married G5 T3 P1 A1, 4 children

History of Present Illness: Vaginal delivery of a 4,309-g male infant at 04:30 hours. Labor started at 19:00 previous evening. Labor was augmented with oxytocin and membranes were ruptured artificially at 24:00. First stage: 8 hours. Second stage: 90 minutes. Third stage: 30 minutes. A right-medio-lateral episiotomy was performed. Patient had active management of third stage with oxytocin 10 IU administered intramuscularly after delivery of the anterior shoulder. At final post-delivery check, her indicators were: BP: 100/70 mmHg, P: 80 beats/minute, RR: 16 breaths/minute, T: 37.2°C, hgb: 120 g/L, hct: 0.35 volume fraction. Her fundus was firm at 1 fingerbreadth above umbilicus. She voided 50 mL. Her episiotomy was intact and her lochia was moderate rubra.

Presenting Symptoms: Diaphoretic, increased capillary refilling time, cool and clammy extremities, anxiety, tachycardia (120 beats/minute), tachypnea (21 breaths/minute), oliguria, fundus boggy and displaced to right, lochia bright red with two grapefruit-sized clots, episiotomy intact, and no signs of hematoma (e.g., vaginal pressure and pain).

Diagnostics (relevant test results): Lab values not yet available.

Medication Record

Patient: Mrs. Matilda Price	**Allergy:** NKDA
Age/DOB: 39 years old	**Medical Provider:** Ms. Robinson, CNM

Notes: Nothing per rectum

Medication List:	**Time Given:**
Multivitamin one tab PO q a.m.[2]	08:00

PRN List:	**Time Given:**
Oxytocin (Pitocin, Syntocinon) 10 to 20 IU IM; one dose PRN heavy bleeding	
Methylergonovine maleate (Methergine) 0.2 mg IM every 2 to 4 hours PRN for heavy bleeding (hold with BP >140/90 mmHg or cardiac disease, five doses max)	
Ergonovine maleate (Ergotrate Maleate) 0.2 mg IM every 2 to 4 hours PRN for heavy bleeding (hold with BP >140/90 mmHg, five doses max);	
Ibuprofen (Motrin) 600 mg PO every 6 hours PRN for pain	

BP, blood pressure; IM, intramuscular; NKDA, no known drug allergy; PO, per os; PRN, pro re nata (as needed).

Scenario Objectives

1. Examine labor and delivery history to identify risk for hemorrhage, including augmentation or induction of labor (oxytocin use); dysfunctional or prolonged labor; medications used, such as anesthesia (halothane), magnesium sulfate, tocolytics (all cause uterine relaxation); interventions, such as use of vacuum or forceps, internal manipulation for retained placental fragments; inverted uterus. (*Debriefing:* This patient received Pitocin, had a prolonged labor with prolonged second stage [more than 1 hour], delivered a large infant by a vacuum extraction for delivery, and an episiotomy with fourth-degree laceration.)

2. Students introduce themselves to the patient, check wrist band, get information about present status, and explain the exam to be performed.

---

[2] Previous versions of this scenario included: Docusate sodium (Colace) 2 tabs twice a day as a standing order. This is still the case for many units in North America, but we decided to delete this from the case because the Canadian Agency for Drugs and Technologies in Health concluded "the available evidence suggests that docusate is no more effective than placebo in the prevention or management of constipation (Dioctyl sulfosuccinate or docusate [calcium or sodium] for the prevention or management of constipation; a review of the clinical effectiveness. Canadian Agency for Drugs and Technologies in Health concluded in a review of clinical studies that evidence suggests that docusate is no more effective than placebo in the prevention or management of constipation... the cited work allows for finding the research at the website https://www.ncbi.nlm.nih.gov/pubmedhealth/PMH0071211/#S8)

3. Obtain a history to determine whether there is a predisposition to hemorrhage. Risk factors include but are not limited to hypertensive disorders of pregnancy, previous hemorrhage, uterine overdistention (multiple gestation, polyhydramnios, or large infant—macrosomia), operative delivery, prolonged labor, and grandmultiparity (Leduc et al., 2009; Reichman & Samueloff, 2016). (*Debriefing:* This patient is indigenous, a grandmultiparity [fifth pregnancy].)

4. Perform an accurate postpartum assessment, including VS; fundal check for placement, firmness; lochia check (follow hospital protocol, but it may include describing blood loss by counting/weighing pads and Chux, recording the amount in specific time increments); bladder assessment; perineal check (describe any signs of lacerations, hematoma, etc.—use redness, edema, ecchymosis, discharge, and approximation [REEDA] scale) (Alvarenga et al., 2015).

5. Educate patient and partner regarding her status, provide accurate information, offer an opportunity to ask questions, and let her know when to contact the nurse (e.g., saturation of more than 1 pad in less than 1 hour). In addition, educate patient on normal findings and have her palpate her uterus and recognize firmness.

6. Determine patient's religious preference to establish whether blood transfusions is permitted (if they become necessary).

7. Given findings, evaluate more closely for hemorrhage, see student evaluation criteria.

The scenario also allows students to practice key elements from the National Council Licensure Examination for Registered Nurses (NCLEX-RN®) using the National Council of State Boards of Nursing (NCSBN; 2015) test plan categories and subcategories, including:

Safe and effective care environment: *Management of care* (Advocacy, Collaboration with interdisciplinary team, Establishing priorities), *Safety and infection control* (Accident/ Error/ Injury prevention, Emergency Response Plan, Safe Use of Equipment); **Health promotion and maintenance:** *Ante/intra/postpartum and newborn care, Developmental stages and Transitions, Techniques of physical assessment;* **Psychosocial integrity:** *Coping mechanisms, Crisis intervention, Cultural awareness/Cultural influences on health, Religious and spiritual influences on health, Support systems, Therapeutic communications;* **Physiological integrity:** *Basic care and comfort* (Elimination), *Pharmacological and parenteral therapies* (Medication Administration, Parenteral/intravenous therapies, Pharmacological agents/actions, Pharmacological pain management), *Reduction of risk potential* (Changes/Abnormalities in VS, Laboratory values, System Specific Assessments, Therapeutic Procedures), *Physiological adaptation* (Alterations in body systems, Fluid and electrolyte imbalances, Hemodynamics, Medical emergencies, Pathophysiology).

For this scenario, the American Association of Colleges of Nursing (AACN; 2008) *The Essentials of Baccalaureate Education for Professional Nursing Practice* items addressed include the following:

Essential V: Informatics and Healthcare Technologies, Objectives 2, 6
Essential VII: Interprofessional Collaboration for Improving Patient and Population Health Outcomes, Objective 2
Essential X: Master's-Level Nursing Practice, Objectives 3, 7, 8, 16

For this scenario, the College of Registered Nurses of British Columbia's (CRNBC; 2015) *Competencies in the Context of Entry-Level Registered Nurse Practice in British Columbia* addressed include the following:

1. Professional Responsibility and Accountability: Demonstrates professional conduct and that the primary duty is to the client to ensure safe, competent, compassionate, ethical care.

2. Specialized Body of Knowledge: Has knowledge from nursing and other sciences, humanities, research, ethics, spirituality, relational practice, and critical inquiry. Understands the requirements of self-regulation in the interest of public protection.

3. Competent Application of Knowledge: Demonstrates competence in the provision of nursing care: ongoing comprehensive assessment, health care planning, providing nursing care, and evaluation.

4. Demonstrates competence in professional judgment and practice decisions guided by the values and ethical responsibilities in codes of ethics for registered nurses.

5. Engages in critical inquiry to inform clinical decision-making, and establishes therapeutic, caring, and culturally safe relationships with clients and the health care team.

Setting the Scene and Scenario Implementation

Expected Activity Run Time: 30 minutes (see Appendix A)
Small-Group Discussion—refer to literature, self-evaluation: 30 minutes
Guided Reflection/Debriefing Time: 30 minutes

Initial Settings

____ Apply wristband
____ Have a printout of medications available to students on request
____ Simulate facial grimacing, diaphoresis on human HPS
____ Pad with large blood stain and two grapefruit-sized clots on HPS with gauze
____ Saline lock with IV setup available
____ VS set at BP: 100/70 mmHg, P: 80 beats/minute, RR: 16 breaths/minute, T: 37.2°C initially, with trend to change to BP: 65/45 mmHg, P: 120 beats/minute, RR: 21 breaths/minute, T: 36.8°C over the first 5 minutes of students entering the room

G. DEBRIEFING GUIDELINES

Debriefing/Guided-Reflection Questions for This Simulation

Knowledge considerations: risks factors for PPH, physiologic mechanisms associated with pregnancy and effects on assessments, interactions with infant including timely breastfeeding and skin-to-skin contact to release the birth parent's physiological oxytocin, indications of PPH, approaches to support family well-being, actions suitable within scope of nursing role, inter- and intraprofessional communication. Use an organized and systematic debriefing process such as reaction, analysis, summary.

Reaction Phase (Beginning)

Participants are encouraged to express their initial emotional reactions to the simulation and the instructor provides information or facilitates a conversation that clarifies the facts underlying the simulation. Questions are directed toward feelings, reactions, and observations.

- What went on/happened?
- How did you feel about that?
- Who else had the same experience? Who reacted differently?
- Were there any surprises/puzzlements?

Analysis Phase (Middle)

Allows participants to make sense of simulation events, their concerns, and to move toward accomplishing simulation objectives. Questions are directed toward making sense of the experience for the individual and the group and drawing on the principles or generalizations.

- How did you account for what happened?
- How might it have been different?
- What do you understand better about yourself/your group?
- What might we draw/pull from this experience?
- What did you learn/relearn?
- What does that suggest to you about (communication/conflict/etc.) in general?
- Does that remind you of anything? What does that explain?
- How does this relate to other experiences you have had?

Summary Phase (End)

This phase signals the end and reviews salient points. Translate lessons learned from the debriefing into principles that participants can take with them to improve their practice. The debriefer may summarize important points if the participants did not cover them or may recommend reading or activities participants can pursue to improve their responses. Questions are directed toward having participants summarize what they learned and how they apply this learning to practice.

- How could you apply/transfer that?
- Given similar circumstances, what might you do differently a subsequent time?
- How could you make it better?
- What modifications can you make work for you in your practice?

H. SUGGESTIONS/KEY FEATURES TO REPLICATE OR IMPROVE

This scenario was used with minimal preprogramming. Students requested a live demonstration of the event before becoming the nurses engaged in the simulation. Videotaping of the PPH scenario with faculty/student interaction for prebriefing of students before their exposure in the lab would be well received by students. Alterations in the case can occur easily to provide students with opportunities to demonstrate critical thinking and clinical decision making. Enhancing the realism of the scenario by using a microphone to answer students directly from the HPS could improve the experience. Having the simulation introduced at the end of the course following more student exposure to postpartum situations would be beneficial. Careful consideration of the medications on hand would be worthwhile, as would some prebriefing about types, dosages, and their usual administration.

I. RECOMMENDATIONS FOR FURTHER USE

This scenario is a high-risk case that could be used to educate new staff to family birthing units and obstetric floors, as well as undergraduate and graduate nursing students. Nurse practitioners and midwifery students would benefit from being part of this scenario. This scenario is also ideal for providing a foundation for interprofessional education of labor and delivery unit teams; an earlier version was transformed for use in a postgraduate medical education workshop for surgeons during an international conference (Campbell, 2013b). Late PPH (after 24 hours) can happen after discharge from the hospital and might be detected in outpatient clinics by other practitioners. In addition, this simulation could provide an opportunity for competency testing and accreditation checklists for hospitals that require a demonstration of staff members' abilities to manage obstetric emergencies. In the first and second edition of this text we had this scenario include a Caucasian woman with red hair, as there is no empirical evidence to support increasing risk of bleeding in red heads (Cunningham, Jones, Ansell, & Barry, 2010) and, given the evidence of increased risk for PPH for First Nations American women (Chalouhi et al., 2015), it is suggested that patient population might serve as a helpful reference group for PPH, as reflected in this version.

J. HOW SIMULATION-BASED PEDAGOGY HAS CONTRIBUTED TO IMPROVED STUDENT OUTCOMES

- This scenario was developed to test students' abilities to perform a complete postpartum assessment and to identify and take necessary actions in a timely fashion when abnormal results are found.
- Having collaboration between faculty and lab staff for the actual running of the scenario is key.
- Determining the best timing in the curriculum of the course and in the availability of the rooms and colleagues to assist is fundamental to effective simulation.
- During the debriefing, it is important to encourage the student who participated to provide some of his or her feedback before other feedback is offered by instructors, to decrease his or her feelings of evaluation by others.
- Focus on positive aspects of what students did.
- Gently introduce ideas about challenges or barriers to good care so that all students can participate in the brainstorming and critical thinking necessary to come up with new ideas.
- Have students journal for a few minutes afterward to reflect on the experience.
- Have clinical faculty observe student postpartum assessments after the scenario and note any significant changes. Have the students reflect on this in their final journaling for the course.

K. EXPERT RECOMMENDATIONS AND WORDS OF WISDOM

It was interesting to transition this scenario from a high-fidelity lab in the northeastern United States to a Canadian context with students at a higher level (fourth term) using medium-fidelity HPSs and very little technology. After running the PPH simulated scenario, the students requested a "live demonstration" of expected actions and interactions. The authors of this chapter then "played out" the scene, live in the classroom using a stretcher. They recruited a student to assist by playing a nurse; one faculty member enacted the patient role while the other enacted a nurse role and called for assistance from the second nurse as would be necessary in an actual PPH situation. The students commented that receiving the live-interaction demonstration first would have improved their performance during the scenario. They had not previously been exposed to maternity-based simulation scenarios so more "prebriefing" would be important for future classes. This experience provided good insight into the key components of simulation education, which include the ability to suspend disbelief, debrief in a manner that incorporates critical thinking and clinical decision making, and manage student fears with the realization that this previously healthy woman and mother of four could die so quickly from complications related to childbirth. Future use at British Columbia Women's Hospital with interprofessional groups and in other more rural and remote locations in the province would ensure updating present clinicians' preparation to manage PPH.

L. EVALUATION OF BEST PRACTICE STANDARDS AND USE OF CREDENTIALED SIMULATION FACULTY

International Nursing Association for Clinical Simulation and Learning (INACSL) *Standards of Best Practice: Simulation*[SM] (INACSL, 2013/2016) to provide prebriefing, facilitator roles, competency testing with specific objectives outlines, and careful planning for debriefing managing students sense of psychological safety and comfort with the learning environment.

REFERENCES

Alvarenga, M. B., Francisco, A. A., de Oliveira, S. M. J. V., da Silva, F. M. B., Shimoda, G. T., & Damiani, L. P. (2015). Episiotomy healing assessment: Redness, Oedema, Ecchymosis, Discharge, Approximation (REEDA) scale reliability. *Revista Latino-Americana de Enfermagem, 23*(1), 162–168. doi:10.1590/0104-1169.3633.2538

American Association of Colleges of Nursing. (2008). *Essentials of baccalaureate education for professional nursing practice*. Washington, DC: Author. Retrieved from http://www.aacnnursing.org/Portals/42/Publications/BaccEssentials08.pdf

Campbell, S. H. (2013a). Obstetric emergency: Postpartum hemorrhage. In S. H. Campbell & K. M. Daley (Eds.), *Simulation scenarios for nursing educators: Making it real* (2nd ed., pp. 137–148). New York, NY: Springer Publishing.

Campbell, S. H. (2013b, November). *Post-partum hemorrhage scenario*. Presented at the Royal College of Physicians & Surgeons, SimSummit Interprofessional Workshop, Vancouver, BC, Canada.

Campbell, S. H., & Daley, K. (2009). *Simulation scenarios for nurse educators: Making it real* (1st ed.). New York, NY: Springer Publishing.

Campbell, S. H., & Daley, K. (2013). *Simulation scenarios for nursing educators: Making it real* (2nd ed.). New York. NY: Springer Publishing.

Chalouhi, S. E., Tarutis, J., Barros, G., Starke, R. M., & Mozurkewich, E. L. (2015). Risk of postpartum hemorrhage among Native American women. *International Journal of Gynaecology and Obstetrics, 131*(3), 269–272.

College of Registered Nurses of British Columbia. (2015). *Competencies in the context of entry level registered nurse practice in British Columbia*. Vancouver, BC Canada: Author.

Cooper, S., Cant, R., Porter, J., Bogossian, F., McKenna, L., Brady, S., & Fox-Young, S. (2012). Simulation based learning in midwifery education: A systematic review. Women and birth: *Journal of the Australian College of Midwives, 25*, 64–78.

Cunningham, A. L., Jones, C. P., Ansell, J., & Barry, J. D. (2010). Red for danger: The effects of red hair in surgical practice. *British Medical Journal, 341*, c6931.

Dolea, C., AbouZahr, C., & Stein, C. (2003). Global burden of maternal haemorrhage in the year 2000. In *Evidence and information for policy*. Geneva, Switzerland: World Health Organization. Retrieved from http://www.who.int/healthinfo/statistics/bod_maternalhaemorrhage.pdf

Ferguson, T. D., Howell, T. L., & Parsons, L. C. (2014). The birth experience: Learning through clinical simulation. *International Journal of Childbirth Education, 29*(3), 66–72.

Fox-Young, S., Brady, S., Brealey, W., Cooper, S., McKenna, L., Hall, H., & Bogossian, F. (2012). The perspectives of Australian midwifery academics on barriers and enablers for simulation in midwifery education in Australia: A focus group study. *Midwifery, 28*(4), 495–501.

Gardner, R., & Raemer, D. B. (2008). Simulation in obstetrics and gynecology. *Obstetrics and Gynecology Clinics of North America, 35*(1), 97–127, ix.

International Nursing Association for Clinical Simulation and Learning. (2013, updated 2016). INACSL standards of best practice: Simulation. Retrieved from https://www.inacsl.org/i4a/pages/index .cfm?pageID=3407

Leduc, D., Senikas, V., Lalonde, A. B., Ballerman, C., Biringer, A., Delaney, M., . . . Wilson, K.; Clinical Practice Obstetrics Committee; Society of Obstetricians and Gynaecologists of Canada. (2009). Active management of the third stage of labour: Prevention and treatment of postpartum hemorrhage. *Journal of Obstetrics and Gynaecology Canada, 31*(10), 980–993.

National Council of State Boards of Nursing. (2015). NCLEX-RN examination: Test plan for the National Council Licensure Examination for Registered Nurses. Retrieved from https://www.ncsbn.org/ RN_Test_Plan_2016_Final.pdf

Paauw, D. S. (2015). Does Colace work? *Internal Medicine News.* Retrieved from http://www.mdedge .com/familypracticenews/article/104548/gastroenterology/myth-month-does-colace-work

Perinatal Services BC. (2011). *Registered nurse initiated activities: Decision Support Tool No.7: Postpartum hemorrhage.* Vancouver, BC Canada: Author.

Rath, W. H. (2011). Postpartum hemorrhage—Update on problems of definitions and diagnosis. *Acta Obstetricia et Gynecologica Scandinavica, 90*(5), 421–428.

Reichman, O., & Samueloff, A. (2016). The use of cervical sonography to differentiate true from false labor in term patients presenting for labor check. *American Journal of Obstetrics and Gynecology, 215*(6), 811–812.

World Health Organization. (2010). *Framework for action on interprofessional education and collaborative care.* Geneva, Switzerland: Author. Retrieved from http://www.who.int/hrh/resources/frame work_action/en

FURTHER READING

Davidson, M. R., London, M. L., & Ladewig, P. W. (2012a). *Olds' maternal–newborn nursing & women's health across the lifespan* (9th ed.). Upper Saddle River, NJ: Pearson Prentice Hall.

Davidson, M. R., London, M. L., & Ladewig, P. W. (2012b). *Clinical handbook for Olds' maternal–newborn nursing & women's health across the lifespan* (9th ed.). Upper Saddle River, NJ: Pearson Prentice Hall.

Hall, W. A. (2014). The high-risk postpartum woman. In R. J. Evans, M. K. Evans, Y. M. Brown, & S. A. Orshan (Eds.), *Canadian maternity, newborn, and women's health nursing* (2nd ed., pp. 741–773). Philadelphia, PA: Wolters/Kluwer, Lippincott Williams & Wilkins.

APPENDIX A

Clinical Course of the Simulated Scenario

Table 18.1 Clinical Course of the Simulated Scenario

HS Status Description	Parameters		Key Required Participant Activities	Time
	Mannequin	Instructor Responds/Cues	☐ **Reflect on Patient Risk Status for pph Given Past Obstetric History And Delivery History**	
08:00	**Physiological Parameters:** HR: 120 beats/minute BP: 65/40 mmHg RR: 21 breaths/minute **Cardiac:** Heart sounds normal (S1 S2) Thready pulse **Respiratory:** Breath sounds diminished to the bases with fine crackles. **GI:** Normal bowel sounds ×4	**Client Presentation:** Anxious, seems uncomfortable Diaphoretic **Cardiac Status:** Capillary refill >3 seconds Skin cool and clammy No edema noted. **Respiratory Status:** Abdominal breathing **Reproductive:** Boggy uterus at 2 cm above umbilicus peri pads soaked with blood and two large clots—est. 500-mL blood loss **Midwife's Orders When Called:** Start IV with crystalloid solution (normal saline and large-bore needle) with oxytocin 20 to 40 IU in 250 mL of IV fluid infused at an hourly rate of 500 to 1,000 mL. Undertake uterine massage. **Lab Will Be Called:** Hgb: 97 g/L; hct 0.26 volume fraction; blood type O+	☐ Wash hands. ☐ Introduce self. ☐ Check name band, two identifiers. ☐ Assess general condition—Ask about current status, pain levels; complete visual assessment. ☐ Assess vital signs (note difference from night report, recheck BP and pulse, temperature). ☐ Apply pulse oximetry. ☐ Check capillary refill. ☐ Don gloves for fundus, lochia, and perineal check. ☐ Palpate fundus (note boggy fundus). ☐ Assess pain level on 1 to 10 scale. ☐ Ask about voiding; including amount and time. ☐ Check for full bladder. ☐ Observe lochia (notes large clots and bright red lochia). ☐ Episiotomy with fourth-degree laceration 11/14 REEDA scale. ☐ Notice patient's complaints of diaphoresis. ☐ Fundus remains boggy, bleeding continues. ☐ Press call bell. ☐ Request second nurse to notify midwife for orders; obtain IV equipment and obtain catheterization equipment. ☐ Reassure patient and husband; maintain calm. ☐ Notice patient is sweating, cold, and clammy.	**15 minutes** **10 minutes**

(continued)

Table 18.1 Clinical Course of the Simulated Scenario *(continued)*

HS Status Description	Parameters	Key Required Participant Activities	Time
	Mannequin	Instructor Responds/Cues	☐ **Reflect on Patient Risk Status for pph Given Past Obstetric History And Delivery History**
			☐ Evaluate level of consciousness.
			☐ Massage uterus at fundus and express any blood clots.
			☐ Educate patient and family members regarding her status; provide accurate information; offer an opportunity to ask questions.
			☐ Determine need for oxytocic to contract uterus.
			☐ Determine need for pain medication.
			☐ Determine need for increased blood volume.
			☐ Administer NS.
			☐ Attempt to have client void on bedpan.
			☐ Provide emotional support to family and patient.
			☐ Encourage infant breastfeeding; support mother as needed.
			☐ Second nurse calls midwife, receives orders, and begins PPH protocol.
			☐ Prepare IV setup; check heparin lock site for any signs of infections.
			☐ Initiate oxytocin infusion (pre mixed). Administer oxytocin 20 IU/1,000 mL IV through second setup placed in the lowest port.
			☐ Apply oxygen as ordered.
			☐ Ensure voiding with Foley catheterization if necessary; monitor urine output.
			☐ Continue to monitor closely and provide support to client.
			☐ Reevaluate fundus—it is firm.

HS Status Description	Parameters	Instructor Responds/Cues	Key Required Participant Activities	Time
	Mannequin		☐ **Reflect on Patient Risk Status for pph Given Past Obstetric History And Delivery History**	
			Appropriate Interventions:	
			☐ Identify abnormal from normal findings.	
			☐ Recognize changing client status (deteriorating; urgent).	
			☐ Identify when to call the midwife or other HCP.	
			☐ Report to midwife using SBAR.	
			☐ Set up plan for monitoring of high-risk patient (including getting infant to breastfeed).	
			☐ Determine religious preference to establish whether blood transfusions are permitted if this becomes necessary in the future (modified from Campbell, 2013a).	
			Inappropriate Actions:	
			☐ Fails to recognize signs of hemorrhage.	
			☐ Does not begin immediate interventions to slow bleeding.	
			☐ Does not call for help.	
			☐ Does not call midwife.	

Setting/Environment

☒ ER
☒ Med–Surg
☒ Peds
☒ ICU
☒ OR/PACU

Equipment Attached to HPS:

☒ IV tubing with primary line fluids running at 100 mL/hr
☒ Secondary IV line running at 500–1,000 mL/hr
☒ IV pump
☒ Foley catheter <100 mL output
☒ PCA pump running

Equipment Available in Room:

☒ Bedpan/urinal
☒ Foley kit
☒ Straight catheter kit
☒ Incentive spirometer

(continued)

Table 18.1 Clinical Course of the Simulated Scenario *(continued)*

HS Status	Parameters	Key Required Participant Activities	Time
Description	Mannequin		

Description

☒ Women's center
☒ Behavioral health
☒ Home health
☒ Pre hospital
☒ Other: Postpartum unit

Simulator HPSs Needed: VitalSim

Props: Grapefruit-sized clots and red coloring on pad; newborn in room with father

Recommended Mode for Simulation (i.e., manual, programmed, etc.): Programmed

Instructor Responds/Cues

☒ IVPB with running at 125 mL/hr
☒ O$_2$
☒ Monitor attached
☒ ID band

Key Required Participant Activities

☐ Reflect on Patient Risk Status for pph Given Past Obstetric History And Delivery History

Time

☒ Fluids
☒ IV start kit
☒ IV tubing
☒ IVPB tubing
☒ IV pump
☒ Feeding pump
☒ Pressure bag
☒ O$_2$ delivery device (mask)
☒ Crash cart with airway devices and emergency medications
☒ Defibrillator/pacer
☒ Suction
☒ Other:

Medications and Fluids:
☒ IV fluids:
☒ Oral meds:
☒ IVPB:
☒ IV push:
☒ IM or SC:

Diagnostics available:
☒ Labs
☒ x-rays (images)
☒ 12-Lead EKG
☒ Other:

Documentation Forms:
☒ Physician/midwife orders
☒ Admit orders
☒ Flow sheet
☒ Medication administration record
☒ Kardex
☒ Graphic record
☒ Shift assessment
☒ Triage forms
☒ Code record
☒ Anesthesia/PACU record
☒ Standing (protocol) orders
☒ Transfer orders
☒ Other:

Roles/Guidelines for Roles:

☒ **Primary nurse**

☒ **Secondary nurse**

☒ **Clinical instructor**

☒ **Family member #1**

☒ **Family member #2**

☒ **Observer(s)**

☒ **Recorder**

☒ **Physician/advanced practice nurse**

☒ **Respiratory therapy**

☒ **Anesthesia**

☒ **Pharmacy**

☒ **Lab**

☒ **Imaging**

☒ **Social services**

☒ **Clergy**

☒ **Unlicensed assistive personnel**

☒ **Code team**

☒ **Other:**

Instructor Interventions:

■ Prebrief students involved in the scenario, act as patient, and help students recognize obstetric medical emergency, direct their care.

Important Information Related to Roles:

One family member will be a simulated baby. The primary nurse will discover the clots and saturated pads and call for help from a secondary nurse. The father will be delegated the care of the baby. The observer will be checking setting of priorities, assessment, management of family members, appropriate approach to getting help.

Student Information Needed Before Scenario:

☒ **Has been oriented to simulator.**

☒ **Understands guidelines/expectations for scenario.**

☒ **Has accomplished all presimulation requirements.**

☒ **All participants understand their assigned roles.**

☒ **Has been given time frame expectations.**

☒ **Other:**

Report Students Will Receive Before Simulation:

Time: 07:00 Vaginal delivery of a 4,309 g male infant at 04:30 hours. Infant latched following delivery but by 07:00 hours has not fed again. Father is in room holding infant. Other children are at home with family members. Other children are 6, 4, and 2 years of age. Due date was (calculate depending on time of scenario) for term birth. Labor started at 19:00. Labor was augmented with oxytocin and membranes were ruptured artificially at 24:00. First stage: 8 hours. Second stage: 90 minutes. Third stage: 30 minutes. A right- medio- lateral episiotomy was performed. Patient had active management of third stage with oxytocin 10 IU administered intramuscularly after delivery of the anterior shoulder. At final postdelivery check, her indicators were 06:00: BP: 100/70 mmHg, P: 80 beats/ minute, RR: 16 breaths/minute, T: 37.2°C, hgb: 120 g/L, hct: 0.35 volume fraction. Her fundus was firm at 1 fingerbreadth above umbilicus. She voided 50 mL. Her episiotomy was intact and her lochia was moderate rubra.

Nursing actions: Wash hands; introduce self; check wrist band; ask about current status; ask about pain levels; do visual assessment; take vital signs; don gloves; palpate fundus; ask about voiding, including amount and time; assess lochia; find clots and bright-red lochia. Reassure patient and family members. Press call bell, reassure patient, request help to recall midwife when second nurse enters the room, reassure husband, massage fundus, measure urine, monitor vital signs, prepare IV setup, provide emotional support for family and patient, administer O₂. Ask other nurse to assemble IV equipment. Do a Foley catheterization of patient if no voiding occurs.

(continued)

203

Table 18.1 Clinical Course of the Simulated Scenario *(continued)*

Significant Lab Values:

Lab will be called: Hgb: 97 g/L; hct: 0.26 volume fraction; blood type O+

Midwife Orders: Start IV with crystalloid solution (normal saline and large-bore needle) with oxytocin 20 to 40 IU in 250 mL of IV fluid infused at an hourly rate of 500 to 1,000 mL.

Undertake uterine massage.

BP, blood pressure; ER, emergency room; GI, gastrointestinal; HCP, health care personnel; hct, hematocrit; hgb, hemoglobin; HPS, human patient simulator; HR, heart rate; HS, human simulation; ICU, intensive care unit; IM, intramuscular; IU, international units; IV, intravenous; IVBP, intravenous piggyback; med–sur, medical–surgical; NS, normal saline; OR, operating room; P, pressure; PACU, postanesthesia care unit; PCA, patient-controlled anesthesia; peds, pediatrics; PPH, postpartum hemorrhage; RR, respiratory rate; SC, subcutaneous.

Source: Used with permission of Dr. Bernie Garrett, School of Nursing and Dr. Karim Qayumi, Faculty of Medicine, The University of British Columbia, Vancouver, BC Canada.

CHAPTER 19

Perinatal Grief: Threatened Spontaneous Abortion

Joan Esper Kuhnly and Meredith Dodge

A. IMPLEMENTATION OF SIMULATION-BASED PEDAGOGY IN YOUR INDIVIDUALIZED TEACHING AREA

The field of perinatal grief, or working with families that experience a pregnancy or neonatal loss, requires excellent communication and interpersonal skills. In an exploratory descriptive study, Modiba (2008) identified that midwives and physicians lacked appropriate knowledge of how to support mothers experiencing a pregnancy loss. Nurses, in practice, are the professionals who facilitate the bereavement process with parents. McCreight (2005), in an exploratory qualitative study, identified that nurses' own emotion and personal beliefs impact their own philosophy of caring for bereaved parents. Research by Chan and Arthur (2009) further identified that nurses need increased knowledge and training on how to cope with bereaved parents. They concluded that bereavement counseling education and preceptorship supervision should be included in nursing education to reduce the stressfulness of the experience, increase the confidence and expertise of novice nurses, and promote better care for bereaved parents. Another option to better prepare nurses and physicians for delivering bad news to parents in the clinical setting would be to use interprofessional simulations. Knight, Dailey, and Currie (2015) were prompted to include pastoral care and grief support in the debriefing process after nursing students were upset during a simulation of a fetal demise. Exposure to end-of-life situations in nursing student clinical experience is lacking and the simulation environment is ideal for this exposure. Knight's team determined that adding grief and pastoral support to the debriefing process provided emotional safety for students, modeled the supportive behaviors they could incorporate into their care, and strengthened the reflective learning process (Knight et al., 2015).

Since 2010, the Institute of Medicine (IOM) has identified the inclusion of interprofessional education as necessary and integral to learning for health care professionals (IOM, 2010). In clinical simulation, use of teamwork-focused and interprofessional simulation have been conducted using multidisciplinary obstetric simulated emergency scenarios (MOSES). Freeth and colleagues (2009) identified acquisition of new knowledge and insight and incorporation of new behaviors into practice when this team-based approach was used in learning. The research conducted by Shaw-Battista, Belew, Anderson, and van Schaik (2015) discusses how communication within a team can be improved by training with an interprofessional team. Interprofessional communication can greatly decrease medical errors and increase the quality of patient care. Similarly, Walker and colleagues (2014) support that a simulation-based scenario on a realistic obstetric and neonatal emergency not only improves communication and teamwork, but also reinforces evidence-based practice. The more realistic the scenario is, the better the opportunity for team collaboration and decision making to occur; the staff involved in the scenario needs to be able to immerse themselves in the scenario in order to gain the best experience. In a focus group study, Sørensen and colleagues (2015) report that there was no difference in learning between off-site clinical simulation and in situ simulation, and although it is important to aim for accurate fidelity, it was more important to maintain the psychological and sociological authenticity. This supports using the off-site clinical simulation center on campus for nursing student learning on such topics as perinatal grief, which all nursing students are less likely to experience in clinical settings. Sørensen's team did report more organizational impact with in situ simulation, but that would be more relevant for nursing students after graduation (2015).

The International Nursing Association for Clinical Simulation and Learning (INACSL), has nine standards that outline best practice guidelines for clinical simulation. Standard VIII, adopted in 2015, discusses simulation-enhanced interprofessional education (Sim-IPE); "Sim-IPE" is designed for the individuals involved to "learn about, from and with each other to enable effective collaboration and improved health outcomes" (Decker et al., 2015). In addition, "Sim-IPE empowers individuals to collaborate as a team in a controlled environment that replicates the health care setting. Participation in Sim-IPE has demonstrated improvement in the acquisition of knowledge, skills and attitudes, and behaviors of teamwork required to promote safe quality patient care" (Decker et al., 2015, p. 294). Using simulation with interprofessional teams gives them a safe learning environment to practice their communication skills and team collaboration for the best outcomes possible for the family involved in the bereavement process.

B. EDUCATIONAL MATERIALS AVAILABLE IN YOUR TEACHING AREA AND RELATED TO YOUR SPECIALTY

The University of Connecticut School of Nursing's Clinical Resource Laboratory has 10 state-of-the-art bed spaces, are all accessed by video from the control room. There is a health assessment lab with eight private rooms, a community room, and debriefing rooms. In addition, we have the ability to stream data live from the lab into the classroom and lecture hall and an electronic interprofessional health record system with bar code-scanning capability for medications. The health record and bar code system are used to enhance clinical realism in the simulation lab. We have one room designated as a labor, delivery, recovery, and postpartum (LDRP) room, with a high-fidelity human patient simulator (HPS), videotaping and microphone use, and a home care setting that we use as a low-fidelity outpatient clinic setting. A separate debriefing space is also available with video and audio display for the students to observe the scenario as it is happening. They can also use this space to discuss what they are observing during the simulation and to take notes to use as a discussion during the debrief.

This scenario was run on high-fidelity HPS in the LDRP space.

C. SPECIFIC OBJECTIVES FOR SIMULATION USAGE WITHIN A SPECIFIC COURSE AND THE OVERALL PROGRAM

As traditional undergraduate nursing students often have limited exposure to bereavement, especially of the perinatal kind, it is important to provide opportunities in their education to address perinatal grief. Historically, this scenario was run in the second semester of the senior year after exposure to the perinatal, medical–surgical, and pediatric environments, at which point, the students were more likely to have some end-of-life exposure. The students at this point have experienced simulation on obstetrical and postpartum assessment, intrapartum care and intervention, and obstetric (OB) and newborn emergencies in which they used low-, medium-, and high-fidelity HPSs. They are familiar with the LDRP room.

However, with the push to include more interprofessional education in the curriculum, we moved this simulation and made it part of a bigger unit "Unanticipated Outcomes in Perinatal Nursing." Other sections of this unit address fetal demise, and traumatic birth experiences. All sections require inclusion of grief counseling, psychosocial support of the mother and family, and a team-based approach to care. True, interprofessional education involves inclusion of other disciplines in learning as well. So, although currently this simulation included other professionals in the learning activity and guest debrief panel, the plan is to incorporate this simulation in a small-group activity with nursing, medical, social work, pharmacy, and chaplain students during the nursing students' final senior perinatal clinical semester. Through simulation, this experience helps students explore their own spiritual and personal beliefs regarding loss. Through exploring their own thoughts and experiences on grief, they are able to develop a grief framework that they can apply to their practice while working with patients and/or families experiencing a loss.

For scheduling purposes of panel participants, this scenario is videotaped and then shown to the class, after which the expert panel guides the debriefing session with the class. The debriefing process with a panel of experts is necessary to ensure student emotional safety and the availability of support for individual contact afterward, if needed. This has occurred when this scenario elicits a strong response because of a personal experience for the students or their family. Appreciating the impact of this experience and the students' reactions requires close faculty attention to the students' reactions and behaviors. Panel participants should include an obstetrician or midwife, a perinatal nurse, a perinatal or family-relevant social worker, and chaplain, in addition to the faculty. It is also ideal to include a mother or family who has experienced a loss, but this may or may not be available as it is a very difficult topic for some mothers to discuss. Guided reflection is necessary to provide some format, but, depending on the size of class, open discussion of responses, interventions, and feelings should be encouraged.

The faculty decided to focus on unanticipated fetal loss or loss of the "normal" pregnancy instead of using an example of a therapeutic abortion. As the debriefing panel would include a woman who had experienced an intrauterine fetal demise personally, it was not appropriate to discuss this scenario during the activity and debriefing period. However, another class included follow-up on the perinatal grief process and, at that point, the topic of therapeutic abortion was discussed. The faculty member's experience with fetal loss support groups helps parents in these two scenarios, although despite both experiencing a loss, they tend not to grieve in the same pattern.

D. INTRODUCTION OF SCENARIO

Setting the Scene

The setting was on a women's health/medical floor in a community hospital. The students received a report from the night nurse. The patient, 15 weeks pregnant, called her physician from home a couple of hours ago with complaints of abdominal cramping. He directed her to come into the hospital and said that he would see her first thing in the morning there. She has recently arrived to the floor.

Technology Used

This scenario was set up in any hospital bed with any type of high-fidelity human patient simulator (HFHPS) wearing an ID band. We set the HFHPS up with some moderate bleeding and clots on her underwear and sanitary pad. As it is a threatened spontaneous abortion, we did not use any fetus. The typical props available include a call bell, blood pressure (BP) cuff, stethoscope, gloves, sink or sanitizing station, sanitary pads, Chux, and wipes or linens.

Objectives

1. Assess perinatal bleeding and identify it as a threatened spontaneous abortion
2. Contact the physician to request a patient examination and perhaps an ultrasound
3. Use therapeutic communication to develop rapport and support with patient and family

Description of the Participants

Samantha Rodriguez is a 30-year-old White woman who is 15 weeks pregnant, admitted to the floor with cramping. Her spouse is with her and she has called her mother, who is coming in.

E. RUNNING OF THE SCENARIO

The night nurse gives a report on the patient, who has recently come on the floor from the emergency department (ED) with a pregnancy at 15 weeks gestation and complaints of cramping. There are no orders yet, but the worry is that she may experience another spontaneous abortion, in lay terms, a miscarriage. The students are called to the room shortly after report and the patient states she just felt a gush of blood on her pad and she is "afraid to look." The student should use universal precautions, introduce herself to the patient and family present in the room, and then assess the bleeding. We anticipate that the student would perform a baseline assessment, notify the physician of the updated status, request an examination by the physician, and perhaps an ultrasound. We also expect the student to access another available nurse to provide emotional support to the patient and family when she is calling the physician.

F. PRESENTATION OF COMPLETED TEMPLATE

Title

Perinatal Grief: Threatened Spontaneous Abortion

Scenario Level

Prelicensure

Focus Area

Senior Scenario

Scenario Description

Samantha Rodriguez is a 30-year-old White woman who is 15 weeks pregnant, admitted to the floor with cramping. She weighs 63 kg and is 5 feet, 3 inches tall. She is allergic to iodine and cephalosporin. Her history is significant for a therapeutic abortion (TAB) at 8 weeks at 18 years of age and a spontaneous abortion (SAB) at 12 weeks at 28 years of age. She denies smoking and alcohol or drug use during this pregnancy. Her surgical history includes an appendectomy as a child and she has no medical conditions. Her spouse is with her and her she has called her mother, who is coming in.

Scenario Objectives

The student assesses perinatal bleeding as a threatened spontaneous abortion, contacts the physician, and interacts appropriately with the patient and her family regarding potential perinatal loss.

The National Council of State Boards of Nursing (2010) National Council Licensure Examination for Registered Nurses (NCLEX-RN®) test plan categories and subcategories included in this scenario are as follows:

Psychosocial integrity: Grief and loss, Coping mechanisms, Family dynamics, Religious and spiritual influences on health, Therapeutic communication and support systems, Safety/infection control,

Standard precautions; **Health promotion and maintenance:** Developmental stages and transitions; **Physiological integrity:** Basic care and comfort and personal hygiene, Reduction of risk potential, Diagnostic tests, Potential for alteration in body systems, **Physiological integrity:** and Hemodynamics.

The American Association of Colleges of Nursing (2008) has created nine Essentials that are used as a guide to developing curriculum for baccalaureate nursing programs. The bachelor of science in nursing (BSN) Essentials addressed in this scenario are:

Essential II: Basic Organizational and Systems Leadership for Quality Care and Patient Safety—Knowledge and skills in leadership, quality improvement, and patient safety are necessary to provide high quality health care.

Essential III: Scholarship for Evidence-Based Practice—Professional nursing practice is grounded in the translation of current evidence into one's practice.

Essential VI: Interprofessional Communication and Collaboration for Improving Patient Health Outcomes—Communication and collaboration among health care professionals are critical to delivering high quality and safe patient care.

Setting the Scene

Equipment Needed

Typical props available should include a call bell, BP cuff, stethoscope, gloves, sink or sanitizing station, sanitary pads, Chux, and wipes or linens. This scenario is set up in any hospital bed with any type of HPS with an ID band. We set the HPS up with some moderate bleeding with some clots on her underwear and sanitary pad.

Resources Needed

As the patient is newly admitted and her doctor has not come in yet, the chart is minimally completed.

Simulator Level

High- or medium-fidelity HPS that has the ability for communication interaction.

Participant Roles

We assign two students to the role of Nurses 1 and 2 (the latter available as needed by Nurse 1). We use two other students in the roles of spouse and mother of the patient. If the HPS does not have voice ability, then the facilitator can be the HPS's voice from behind a curtain. Before starting the scenario, we hand out index cards to participants explaining their role. We also orient the students to the simulation and include an explanation that this is a nonthreatening environment and the best place for mistakes to happen. We also discuss the level of simulation at which this scenario is being run so that the students know whether they are able to take an actual BP, use the monitor, and so on (Meakim et al., 2013).

Scenario Implementation

The threatened spontaneous abortion scenario patient history and information, setup, and progression of the scenario are outlined in Exhibits 19.1 to 19.3. We use this format to promote consistency among

Exhibit 19.1	Patient Information

Admission Date: Today (Report at 7 a.m.)	Psychomotor Skills Required Before Simulation
Today's Date: ..../2017 **Brief Description of Client** 15 weeks pregnant admitted with cramping (threatened miscarriage)	– Interpersonal communication with patient and family – Vital sign (VS) – Use of sanitary pad/assessment of bleeding
Name: Samantha Rodriguez	**Cognitive Competencies**
Gender: F **Age:** 30 **Weight:** 63 kg **Height:** 5 ft. 3 in. **Race:** White	– Interpersonal communication with patient and family/perinatal grief – Stages of grief
Religion: Congregational	**Psychomotor Competencies**
Major Support: spouse	– Appropriate patient and family interaction regarding potential perinatal loss
Phone: 555-555-5555	
Allergies: ink, iodine, cephalosporin	
Immunizations: current	
Attending Physician/Team: Dr. Esper	
Past Medical History	
History of Present Illness – Intrauterine pregnancy with due date of: (25 weeks from now)	
Social History – Denies smoking, alcohol or drug use during pregnancy – Married, support person with her	
Primary Medical Diagnosis – Threatened spontaneous abortion	**Nursing Diagnoses** – Pain – Anxiety related to potential spontaneous abortion – Fear related to perinatal loss repeated
Surgeries/Procedures and Dates – 2004 TAB at 8 weeks – 2012 SAB at 12 weeks	

SAB, spontaneous abortion; TAB, therapeutic abortion; VS, vital sign.

faculty facilitating the simulation. It provides step-by-step instructions for setting up, planning, and running the scenario.

Evaluation Criteria

When we first started this scenario, we used a posttest on perinatal grief and an evaluation questionnaire that students completed, which was subjective, to "grade" the session. There was a lot of variability in the debriefing sessions depending on how the scenario went and the personal experiences of the students in each session. In an effort to create a consistent evidence-based method of evaluation for

Exhibit 19.2 | Scenario Preparation and Report

Setting/Environment	Medications and Fluids
Patient room, women's health/medical floor	None
Simulator HPS(s) needed	Diagnostics available
Noelle with elevator cushion in abdomen, in bed on Chux	Labs prenatal HCT 34

Props/Equipment Attached to HPS	Documentation/Forms
– ID band – Sanitary pad in underwear with spotting of "blood"	Copies of admission record for nurse to fill out

Equipment Available in Room	Recommended Mode for Simulation (i.e., Manual, Programmed, etc.)
– Handwashing station or sanitizer – Call button – Gloves – Maternal monitors for VS – Bed with HPS	Manual, load palette—"Threatened miscarriage" facilitator is voice for patient

Roles: Cards state	Report: Taking Place This Morning at 7 a.m.
– One to four observers: You are to observe and take notes on the scenario, provide positive and constructive suggestions for improvement. You cannot participate in the scenario or respond. – Nurse 1: Nurse on Women's Health Medical Floor – Nurse 2: Available for support to Nurse 1 – One spouse: You brought patient in from home. Act out your role as indicated. – One mother of patient: You met your daughter at the hospital when she called you this morning in a panic saying her spouse was bringing her to the hospital. Role play as indicated.	Samantha Rodriguez is a 30-year-old woman newly admitted this morning to room 12 of the women's health/medical floor. She came to the ED with c/o abdominal cramping starting at 5 a.m. this morning. She's 15 weeks pregnant. Her spouse and mother are with her. She just got to the floor at 6:45 a.m. and I put a call in to her OB. He said he will come in first thing this morning. The ED nurse told me Samantha's history is significant for a TAB at 8 weeks 13 years ago and a SAB at 12 weeks 5 years ago. Any questions? Oh, it looks like she just rang her call bell. Can you get it?
	Significant Lab Values
	Predelivery hct 34 g/dl, serology negative, O+ blood type
	Physician Orders
	None yet, doctor en route

c/o, complaints of; ED, emergency department; hct, hematocrit; HPS, human patient simulator; OB, obstetrician; SAB, spontaneous abortion; TAB, therapeutic abortion; VS, vital sign.

Exhibit 19.3	Scenario Progression Outline		
Timing (Approximate)	**HPS Actions**	**Expected Interventions**	**May Use the Following Cues**
First 10 Minutes	"Oh, I am glad you are here. I just felt a gush on m pad and I am afraid to look. Can you help me?"	**Process:** *Nurse 1:* – Washes hands, introduces self – Checks ID verification/band – Puts on gloves – Delegates second nurse to assess bleeding, or call doctor to ask for ultrasound	Based on student response, ad lib as indicated, but may use the following: "Do you think I have lost the baby?"
		Spouse: Could be anxious, sad, worried, angry . . . *Mother of patient:* Could be protective, worried, mad, angry, and so on.	"Oh, my God, not again! This cannot be happening!" "Can you do an ultrasound to check on the baby?" To spouse:" I am so sorry, Honey, I cannot keep our babies and we cannot afford another round of IVF."
		Nurse 2: Appropriate interaction with family and patient regarding potential loss	

HPS, human patient simulator; IVF, in vitro fertilization.

simulation, we switched to a checklist (Exhibit 19.4) that identified key points that would be accomplished in the scenario or identified through debriefing that students should have done. Training of the lab facilitators on open-ended debrief questions was important to avoid giving the answers as opposed to the group figuring out what it should have done to have provided a better experience for the family. Grading for the assessment checklist would be weighted based on the importance of information and the knowledge expected for the level of student. A total grade of 100% is earned if all components were completed for the simulation.

G. DEBRIEFING GUIDELINES

The most important part of this scenario is the debriefing. Therefore, continuing the evaluation checklist through the debriefing session is necessary because the technical response to the scenario is significant, but what is more salient is the interpersonal communication that is observed and the changes that could be suggested through debriefing. This is often when observers provide helpful insight of alternative options for communication that may be more appropriate. It is also when the students learn the most regarding this topic because of the discussion that follows. Often, students have had no experience with any type of perinatal loss, or death of any kind, and therefore, have no frame of reference from which to work for this scenario. If the scenario is run live, we use the checklist in Exhibit 19.4. If we are using the interprofessional expert panel debriefing, we use the following questions to guide the debriefing session. You, of course, may adapt these if you have curricular threads regarding loss and grief. In addition, if any faculty are certified by the End-of-Life Nursing Education Consortium (ELNEC), especially with perinatal content, your debrief may be guided by those criteria. "The ELNEC curriculum offers education

Exhibit 19.4	Evaluative Criteria

___Introduction of new nurse who is starting shift to the patient.

___Wash hands.

___ID check with patient.

___Appropriate interaction with anxious patient, spouse, and patient's mother (e.g., "I am sorry, I am sure this is distressing, we have got a call into the doctor and once he examines you, he will likely get an ultrasound so you can have more answers about what is happening.") (Not appropriate examples would be: "it will be okay, the important thing is that you will be okay, you are young, you can have another . . .")

___Appropriate assessment for bleeding, clots, volume, and cramping.

___Report of nurse to physician/provider includes introduction of self, patient situation and background, your assessment and request of what the nurse would like him or her to do: an evaluation, perhaps an ultrasound.

___Appropriate discussion on the phases of grief (denial/shock/disbelief, anger, bargaining, despair/depression, and acceptance).

___Appropriate discussion of the cultural issues that may affect this scenario. (How does this scenario compare to the students' knowledge of the Hispanic culture and grief? Does cultural knowledge avoid stereotyping or provide insight?)

___Appropriate identification of factors in this patient's history that could impact this situation. (The cost of infertility treatments, TAB at 18 years old—guilt? Secondary infertility after SAB 4 years ago—very wanted pregnancy, history of loss already.)

___Appropriate discussion of the impact of grief on the maternal and family relationships.

___Appropriate discussion of implications if there is incomplete excretion of products of conception when there is no heartbeat found on ultrasound (risk of infection, DIC, what VS/assessment/labs to look for).

___Identification of the subsequent physical and emotional needs this patient may require (methergine or hemabate, potential for a dilation and curettage surgical procedure, pain management, empathy, activation of support system, chaplain or social worker consults).

DIC, disseminated intravascular coagulation; SAB, spontaneous abortion; TAB, therapeutic abortion; VS, vital sign.

supported by research, as well as activities to develop skills and attitudes specific to enhancing palliative and end-of-life care" (O'Shea et al., 2015, p. 769).

Debriefing content to discuss:

1. This should include the scenario, RN response, and family involvement.
2. What can be said to women experiencing or potentially experiencing perinatal loss?
3. The stages of grief and how they apply to this scenario should be discussed.
4. What factors in this woman's history may impact her response?
5. Does her culture impact her response?
6. How could the financial burden factor into parents' response?
7. What do you think the effect of loss is on the mother–partner relationship and other family dynamics?
8. Content questions such as: Do you know of dead fetus syndrome and its implication? What subsequent steps, both physical and emotional, might you expect in this scenario?
9. Is there anything else you would like to discuss?

H. SUGGESTIONS/KEY FEATURES
TO REPLICATE OR IMPROVE

What is most necessary to remember is that this scenario may not be encountered by every nurse, but nursing students can apply the content learned through this simulation into end-of-life communication, emotional support of patients and families, and interprofessional collaboration.

I. RECOMMENDATIONS FOR FURTHER USE

Instead of embedded participants being nursing students for family reactions, the best option would be to have standardized patients, consistent actors, or volunteers serve in this capacity. We could also use staff or volunteers in this role.

J. HOW SIMULATION-BASED PEDAGOGY HAS
CONTRIBUTED TO IMPROVED STUDENT OUTCOMES

This scenario is unlikely to present itself to students in the clinical setting. Often, staff nurses do not want to burden a family undergoing this experience with a student nurse; therefore, experience in the simulation setting may be the only reference from which students develop a framework of care when patients experience a potential loss. This can be applied to more than the perinatal setting. Obviously, students' direct experience with potential loss in all settings is limited. McCreight (2005) stated that the more students have the opportunities to explore their feelings toward end of life in various settings, the more prepared they are to address it when they encounter it in clinical situations. Nursing education needs to include this content and simulations because they are the only way to consistently provide this opportunity for all students. All nurses appreciate that end-of-life issues regarding the psychosocial impact on the family are more difficult to provide than the physical postmortem care of the patient. With that knowledge, having this experience during their program of study prepares them best. Ensuring student emotional safety while learning in an interprofessional setting is the goal (Knight et al., 2015).

K. EXPERT RECOMMENDATIONS AND WORDS OF WISDOM

We recommend expanding application of the knowledge gained in this simulation to a small-group interprofessional education activity that includes medical, pharmalogical, social work, and chaplain students. By including these learners in the activity, it breeds interprofessional teamwork in practice after they graduate. This simulation is a rather low-tech scenario, but yet exposes students to communication patterns and end-of-life content that is applicable to other settings. It is also important to remember that learner's emotional support may be necessary, as this scenario may trigger personal memories or feelings. We were fortunate to have a nursing faculty member who specialized in psychology, who was also on our simulation team.

L. EVALUATION OF BEST PRACTICE STANDARDS
AND USE OF CREDENTIALED SIMULATION FACULTY

Our simulation program follows the standards of best practice for simulation as outlined in Chapter 1. We have a collaborative faculty model that uses some faculty's simulation expertise, content expertise, and networking alliances. Progression of this simulation, which was originally focused on nursing to the interprofessional realm, has added a richness to the learning experience.

REFERENCES

American Association of Colleges of Nursing. (2008). *Essentials of baccalaureate education for professional nursing practice*. Washington, DC: Author. Retrieved from http://www.aacnnursing.org/Portals/42/Publications/BaccEssentials08.pdf

Chan, M. F., & Arthur, D. G. (2009). Nurses' attitudes towards perinatal bereavement care. *Journal of Advanced Nursing, 65*(12), 2532–2541.

Decker, S., Anderson, M., Boese, T., Epps, C., McCarthy, J., Motola, I.,…Scolaro, K. (2015). Standards of best practice: Simulation standard VIII: Simulation-enhanced interprofessional education (Sim-IPE). *Clinical Simulation in Nursing, 11*(6), 293–297.

Freeth, D., Ayida, G., Berridge, E. J., Mackintosh, N., Norris, B., Sadler, C., & Strachan, A. (2009). Multidisciplinary obstetric simulated emergency scenarios (MOSES): Promoting patient safety in obstetrics with teamwork-focused interprofessional simulations. *Journal of Continuing Education in the Health Professions, 29*(2), 98–104.

Institute of Medicine. (2010). *The future of nursing: Leading change, advancing health: Report recommendations*. Washington, DC: National Academies Press. Retrieved from https://iom.nationalacademies.org/~/media/Files/Report%20Files/2010/The-Future-of-Nursing/Future%20of%20Nursing%202010%20Recommendations.pdf

Knight, C. C., Dailey, K. D., & Currie, E. R. (2015). An introduction to unexpected grief for pre-licensure nursing students: A simulation and interprofessional expert panel regarding fetal demise. *Nursing Education Perspectives, 36*(6), 414–416.

McCreight, B. S. (2005). Perinatal grief and emotional labour: A study of nurses' experiences in gynae wards. *International Journal of Nursing Studies, 42*(4), 439–448.

Meakim, C., Boese, T., Decker, S., Franklin, A. E., Gloe, D., Lioce, L.,…Borum, J. C. (2013). Standards of best practice: Simulation standard I: Terminology. *Clinical Simulation in Nursing, 9*(6S), S3–S11.

Modiba, L. M. (2008). Experiences and perceptions of midwives and doctors when caring for mothers with pregnancy loss in a Gauteng hospital. *Health SA Gesondheid, 13*(4), 29–40.

National Council of State Boards of Nursing. (2010). NCLEX-RN examination: Test plan for the National Council Licensure Examination for Registered Nurses. Retrieved from https://www.ncsbn.org/2010_NCLEX_RN_TestPlan.pdf

O'Shea, E. R., Campbell, S. H., Engler, A. J., Beauregard, R., Chamberlin, E. C., & Currie, L. M. (2015). Effectiveness of a perinatal and pediatric End-of-Life Nursing Education Consortium (ELNEC) curricula integration. *Nurse Education Today, 35*(6), 765–770.

Shaw-Battista, J., Belew, C., Anderson, D., & van Schaik, S. (2015). Successes and challenges of interprofessional physiologic birth and obstetric emergency simulations in a nurse-midwifery education program. *Journal of Midwifery & Women's Health, 60*(6), 735–743.

Sørensen, J. L., Navne, L. E., Martin, H. M., Ottesen, B., Albrechtsen, C. K., Pedersen, B. W.,…van der Vleuten, C. (2015). Clarifying the learning experiences of healthcare professionals with in situ and off-site simulation-based medical education: A qualitative study. *BMJ Open, 5*(10), e008345. doi:10.1136/bmjopen-2015–008345

Walker, D., Cohen, S., Fritz, J., Olvera, M., Lamadrid-Figueroa, H., Cowan, J. G.,…Fahey, J. O. (2014). Team training in obstetric and neonatal emergencies using highly realistic simulation in Mexico: Impact on process indicators. *BMC Pregnancy and Childbirth, 14*, 367.

FURTHER READING

Lindsay Miller, J., Avery, M. D., Larson, K., Woll, A., VonAchen, A., & Mortenson, A. (2015). Emergency birth hybrid simulation with standardized patients in midwifery education: Implementation and evaluation. *Journal of Midwifery & Women's Health, 60*(3), 298–303.

CHAPTER 20

High-Risk Infant of a Diabetic Mother: Hypoglycemia

Suzanne Hetzel Campbell, Natalia Del Angelo Aredes,
Luciana Mara Monti Fonseca, and Julie de Salaberry

A. IMPLEMENTATION OF SIMULATION-BASED PEDAGOGY IN YOUR INDIVIDUALIZED TEACHING AREA

University of São Paulo, Brazil, School of Nursing of Ribeirão Preto

The School of Nursing has been interested in active methods of learning, including simulation as a core strategy, which was first implemented in child health in 2010. One of the major challenges of implementing simulation pedagogy into the curriculum was the ratio of students to professors, which was solved by including trained graduate students in the process to assist faculty. These students were enrolled in masters, or doctoral-level courses; registered nurses matriculated in an internship for pedagogy in nursing and researching in teaching, simulation, or child health areas. Thus, we started to have volunteer actors assume diverse roles in the scenarios and more partners to prepare new cases, participate in running the scenarios in lab, and collaboratively conduct debriefing.

We use simulation to develop scenarios that are consistent with the emerging issues in public health; thereby better preparing students to deal with challenges in the context of the Brazilian public health system. Students report that simulated practice has helped them solve similar problems in the clinical setting after training and discussing with peers and facilitators. Therefore, we have found simulation to be an excellent strategy to improve skills in cognitive, procedural, and attitudinal learning—stimulating helps the students to apply the knowledge built into clinical situations and respond appropriately. Subsequent steps include to fully integrate simulation throughout the curriculum, to expand multiprofessional simulation, and to stimulate collaborative communication and practice among physicians, nurses, physiotherapists, nutritionists, and others.

University of British Columbia School of Nursing, Vancouver, BC, Canada

Given the constraints on practice sites for specialty areas, including pediatric and neonatal intensive care, the University of British Columbia (UBC) School of Nursing in Vancouver, BC, Canada, has developed flexible learning options, including clinical practice and learning with the use of simulation, that cover potential high-risk situations that all students need to be aware of and have some practical knowledge to provide safe care. In the present curriculum, some students take an advanced maternity course that covers the topic of high-risk newborn care. As they do not have an opportunity to practice in the neonatal intensive care unit (NICU) during the clinical rotation for this course, a scenario like this can provide students with the foundational knowledge and skill set needed to manage similar circumstances in the clinical area.

British Columbia's Women's Hospital and Health Centre, Vancouver, BC, Canada

British Columbia's Women's Hospital (BCWH) is the provincial referral and academic center for high-risk maternal–fetal medicine and advanced neonatal intensive care. In collaboration with UBC Faculty of Medicine and BC Children's Hospital, BCWH provides interdisciplinary and discipline-specific teams a variety of simulation learning experiences in our Simulation Center. Simulations are planned both with and without the use of the human patient simulators (HPS) to prepare the teams for a variety of complex care scenarios, for example, those that may require obstetrical, surgical, neonatal, and pediatric specialists at delivery.

BCWH recognizes that patients' optimal experience of health care services is one in which team communication is consistent, accurate, effective, and supports best outcomes. Communication errors are the most common cause of adverse patient events and have been linked to the differences in which health care providers learn to communicate, the embedded hierarchical power imbalances in the clinical setting, and a culture and approach to mistakes that may not support a "safe" learning environment (M. Leonard, Graham, & Bonacum, 2004; B. Leonard, Shuhaibar, & Chen, 2010). Focusing team learning on interdisciplinary communication and promoting a culture of safety may improve teamwork in both critical and routine care (Haller et al., 2008), and thus positively influence patient care outcomes. Simulation supports our interdisciplinary teams to gain situational awareness, determine critical language, and learn from and with each other through facilitated debriefing with the goal of preventing harm and promoting optimal care standards.

BCWH uses simulation to support standardized learning programs, such as the Neonatal Resuscitation Program (NRP; 2016) and the Advanced Care of the at-Risk Newborn (AcORN; 2016), to test and evaluate new clinical services, and to validate postpartum and neonatal nursing education such as managed postpartum hemorrhage, maternal escalation of care, and neonatal hypoglycemia scenarios. The growing complexity of perinatal health care requires attention to both technical skills and nontechnical skills; team interactions can benefit from intentional rehearsal and reflection (Freeth, Ayida, Berridge, Sadler, & Strachan, 2006). Simulation-based learning requires an organizational commitment that supports a clinician's time, equipment and space, team training, as well as support for the education of team members who facilitate the simulation debriefs. It has been shown to be an effective learning strategy in obstetrical emergency knowledge translation for midwives and obstetricians (Crofts et al., 2007) and in nursing education (Cant & Cooper, 2010). There is a limited understanding of the full impact of interdisciplinary education (Malt, 2015) on practice outcomes in simulation-based nursing education (Cant & Cooper, 2010) because of the heterogeneity of the various programs and outcome measures.

BCWH draws on a crisis resource management approach (Murray & Foster, 2000) in which trained facilitators are believed to be a key component to effective simulation learning. Facilitator development focuses on the development of knowledge and skills in order to provide interdisciplinary teams with feedback and an opportunity to reflect in a safe and supportive learning environment (Murray & Foster, 2000). A scripted debrief supports the facilitator in managing the complexity the debriefing by ensuring a standardized and practical approach (Eppich & Cheng, 2015), which has been shown to improve facilitator performance (Cheng et al., 2013).

B. EDUCATIONAL MATERIALS AVAILABLE IN YOUR TEACHING AREA AND RELATED TO YOUR SPECIALTY

The UBC School of Nursing

As described in Chapter 18, the UBC SON has several rooms set up for simulation. This simulation scenario was initially developed at Fairfield University School of Nursing and used from 2008 to 2012 with third- and fourth-year baccalaureate students during their obstetrical/maternal–child rotation. A room set up as a neonatal intensive care unit (NICU) with a high-fidelity infant–patient simulator (HFIPS—Laerdal's SimBaby®) under a warmer, with oxygen/suction wall mounts, and vital signs displayed on the monitor. Four students participated in the scenario while their classmates viewed live-streaming video in the classroom next door. The faculty communicated with students from the control room as needed. Students prepared for the simulation by completing a number of readings and videos available on their learning management system.

British Columbia Women's Hospital and Health Center

The Simulation Center at BCWH and Health Centre (BCWHHC) includes innovative educational space with more than 20 rooms for running team-based simulation scenarios, clinical skills rooms, and classrooms. The fully equipped simulation environments are designed to closely resemble the current clinical care environment in an effort to assist staff to "suspend" disbelief in order to promote the most "true-to-life" learning experiences. There are nine high-fidelity HPSs, including premature and term infants and pregnant mothers. In addition to clinical practice, our Perinatal Research Imaging Center provides researchers, clinicians, and educators access to a computerized ultrasound pregnant-woman simulator that is programmed to reveal fetal anomalies and normal findings in pregnancy. In addition to high-fidelity, facilitated simulation scenarios, BCWHHC engages learners in a variety of related learning activities that include workshops, in situ simulations, or "mock codes."

University of Sao Paulo

The Simulation Center of Nursing Practice includes five rooms prepared for running hospital scenarios and a simulated house for running home visits in the context of primary care. One of the simulation rooms is prepared for high-fidelity scenarios and includes videoconference capabilities and a control room. There are three adult high-fidelity and several medium-fidelity simulators, including adults, a high-fidelity obstetric simulator, and infants (including preterm babies) or children. Simulation has been used as an effective strategy for teaching and learning in a variety of disciplines within nursing at this university. This method of teaching has created spaces to focus on cognitive, attitudinal, and procedural skills and to discuss clinical reasoning in health care situations. In addition to their focus on nursing practice, the labs have been used to implement multiprofessional simulation and team training as well.

C. SPECIFIC OBJECTIVES OF SIMULATION USAGE WITHIN A SPECIFIC COURSE AND THE OVERALL PROGRAM

Learning Objectives

This scenario prepares students for newborn assessment, especially related to high-risk situations like the development of hypoglycemia. It is expected that students identify the condition early so as to avoid invasive interventions and respiratory distress, using nonpharmacological methods to solve the clinical problem, if possible.

Research shows a 60% increased risk of excessive fetal weight gain (large-for-gestational age [LGA]) and a fourfold increased risk of neonatal hypoglycemia among the infants of diabetic women, including women with gestational diabetes mellitus (GDM; Maayan-Metzger, Lubin, & Kuint, 2009). This increase in number of large newborns in this population is explained by maternal hyperglycemia leading to fetal hyperinsulinemia, increased glucose usage, and adipocyte accumulation in the fetus (Amaral, Silva, Ferreira, Silva, & Bertini, 2015). The reasons that infants of diabetic mothers (IDMs) are admitted to the NICU include neonatal hypoglycemia, macrosomia, respiratory distress syndrome, electrolyte imbalance, and trauma (Amaral et al., 2015). In addition, hypoglycemia can cause and aggravate tachypnea, leading to respiratory distress (Hermansen & Mahajan, 2015).

Learning objectives for this simulation include maintenance of postnatal glucose homeostasis in IDMs (Adamkin, 2011), with prioritization of minimizing mother–infant separation and promoting successful breastfeeding. Adopting a standardized approach that identifies infants at risk of low blood sugar, coupled with early and structured breastfeeding approaches, has been shown to be an effective strategy to manage hypoglycemia and reduce admissions to the NICU (Csont, Groth, Hopkins, & Guillet, 2014). However, the exact blood glucose (BG) levels in infants that lead to central nervous system (CNS) damage and long-term outcomes (Straussman & Levitsky, 2010) remains unknown. Therefore, it is necessary to educate students to properly assess, monitor, and respond to both asymptomatic and symptomatic infants based on up-to-date evidence-based practices (Adamkin, 2011; Thornton et al., 2015).

Research indicates that mothers cite percieved inadequate milk supply as one of the main reasons for stopping breastfeeding (Hill & Aldag, 2007; Li, Fein, Chen, & Grummer-Strawn, 2008). What message do we send to students working with mothers if breastfeeding is not the first intervention in the asymptomatic at-risk infant, especially when we recognize that health information related to breastfeeding when delivered by physicians and nurses increases the intiation of breastfeeding (Dyson, McCormick, & Renfrew, 2005). The use of simulation to support breastfeeding for mothers and their newborns at risk of hypoglycemia could support long-term breastfeeding outcomes and the education of the next generation of health professionals on the importance of breastfeeding for mother and infant, as a possible alternative to pharmacological and invasive health procedures in asymptomatic IDMs.

For this reason, there is an option with this scenario to take more than one approach—as an unfolding case or two separate scenarios. In the first version, there is an asymptomatic IDM, who is at risk of developing hypoglycemia. The student can act with early feeds (especially within the first hour of life), monitor the infant's vital signs, and encourage frequent feeding, informing the mother and educating her as care is provided. This monitoring would occur for the first hour and also encourage skin-to-skin contact and rooming in, according to Baby-Friendly Initiative (BFI) guidelines (Breast Feeding Committee for Canada, 2012). As the case unfolds or as a second scenario, the student arrives on the scene with a symptomatic infant who is cold, which would require feeding the infant (use donor breast milk if unable to breastfeed), warming the infant, and finally, if these actions do not relieve the symptoms, interventions, such as dextrose infusion and oxygen support, would be provided. In both endpoints, the students have the opportunity to learn more about newborn assessment, clinical reasoning in hypoglycemia, therapeutic communication and education to the mother, and critical thinking regarding association between gestational history and symptoms to assess, given the infant's clinical status. A "stop and freeze" approach could be used, especially if the participants are team practitioners in situ in the clinical setting. If actions are significantly different from the suggested care pathway, the facilitator could use questions to guide the team back.

This scenario provides an opportunity to reinforce the importance of the mother–infant dyad, breastfeeding, and skin-to-skin contact; to support the health outcomes of mother and infant; and to illustrate the relevance of early identification of signs and symptoms reinforcing critical thinking and clinical reasoning/decision making in everyday practice.

Student Learning Activities

- Perform an accurate newborn assessment.
- Identify the risk factors for the infant of a diabetic mother.
- Assess patient's physiologic changes for risks of hypoglycemia and respond to findings.
- Perform BG monitoring and prepare to treat the patient's condition.
- Communicate with mother regarding the newborn's status and with other team members to develop a plan of care, using an integrated approach with the parents.

D. INTRODUCTION OF SCENARIO

Setting the Scene

Identification and Initial Response

The mother and infant are in the immediate postdelivery area, either a delivery suite or single room maternity care. The mother is a 35-year-old White woman with insulin-dependent gestational diabetes who had a vacuum-assisted delivery 1 hour ago after a long, difficult labor. Shift handover has occurred. The nurse enters the room and the mother is supported to breastfeed the asymptomatic infant and given information about frequent feeding and need for BG monitoring in the first 12 hours of life. She is told that some IDMs will need an intravenous (IV) line in addition to feeding in the first 12 hours (Adamkin, 2011; Aziz et al., 2004, reaffirmed 2015).

Decompensation

The infant's blood sugar is low at 2 hours and the infant is now exhibiting symptoms that require the newborn to be admitted into the tertiary-level NICU.

Technology Used

Laerdal SimBaby® is in the room with mother initially and may transition to a pale infant under a radiant warmer. Mother's role is acted by faculty, another student, or standardized patient.

Objectives

1. Describe the assessment of the newborn who is at risk for postdelivery complications related to maternal history gestational diabetes.
2. Incorporate preventive measures in the care of the newborn delivered to a gestational diabetic mother, specifically at risk for hypoglycemia.
3. Obtain a maternal and delivery history to determine factors that may have put the newborn at risk for hypoglycemia and other complications.
4. Perform an accurate newborn assessment.
5. Examine the newborn for signs of hypoglycemia and other complications.
6. Perform interventions according to newborn health status using critical thinking and clinical reasoning.
7. Educate parents regarding the newborn's status and plan of care.

Description of Participants

Participants' roles: One night-shift nurse reporting to the day-shift nurse; 1 day-shift nurse, getting a report and examining the patient, 1 nurse assisting the examining nurse as a licensed practical nurse (LPN) or health care aide (HCA)—all of whom work with the registered nurse to complete tasks; one family member (mother of the patient), the mother, should ask a lot of questions and demonstrate interest and genuine emotional concern for the welfare of the baby during the simulation; and one observer documents the communication, body language, and interventions.

Infant: A 2-hour-old baby boy named James Jones, White; weighs 9 pounds, 8 ounces (4.309 kg); length is 21 inches (53 cm). Initially acts hungry, but, if not fed and given skin-to-skin contact with the mother during the running of this scenario, the infant then becomes jittery and lethargic, with circumoral cyanosis, chest retractions, nasal flaring, and expiratory grunt.

Mother of the infant: If the student nurse introduces themselves—you say, "Hi." If not, mother says, "Who are you? What are you doing?" Throughout the experience, if the student nurse does not engage you, tell you what they are doing, or ask permission before doing things, you continue to inquire, act frightened, and concerned. Say: "This is all my fault, is it not? I tried not to eat sweets and to keep my sugar in control, but I cheated once in a while. Did I make my baby sick?" If the student does not suggest breastfeeding and skin-to-skin contact to the mother in order to correct asymptomatic hypoglycemia, the case continues with clinical complications introducing symptoms. To stimulate the student to continue the clinical evaluation, the mother can touch the baby and ask the nurse: "Is it normal to be jittery like this? I think my baby is pale, too."

General Considerations

The following are instructions for the mother of the infant:

1. Mother is currently sitting in a wheelchair (or chair) alongside the radiant warmer in the NICU.
2. Mother introduces herself when asked by the RN, LPN, or HCA.
3. Mother is very concerned about the baby's appearance and condition and is asking a lot of questions about the assessment and care given to the baby like: "Is my baby okay?" "Is there anything wrong with my baby?" "Why is my baby shaking and so pale?" "What are you doing to my baby?" "Why did you take blood from my baby?" "Does that hurt my baby?"

Student nurse: Introduce self and explain to mother what is going on. Describe the pathophysiology of IDM transition to newborn life, and what you are going to do before you act. Incorporate mother into the plan of care.

Second student nurse: Assist with measuring vital signs and support primary nurse as asked.

Observer: If there are four students in the simulation, one can act as observer/evaluator and be given the checklist for the skills required for this scenario.

E. RUNNING OF THE SCENARIO

It is expected that students recognize the risks involved in care for this infant considering a history of GDM, foreseeing the possibility of injuries related to birth trauma, and quickly identifying signs of hypo-glycemia or respiratory distress. The scenario can have two endpoints—after rapid identification of signs of hypoglycemia the expected care is to encourage breastfeeding and skin-to-skin contact, stabilizing the baby clinically in a noninvasive approach. As the case unfolds, either the student is delayed in iden-tifying signs or notices that the infant becomes tachycardic, jittery, and demonstrates difficulty breath-ing (grunting, chest retractions, and nasal flaring) and requires interventions such as venous access for dextrose infusion and oxygen support.

Depending on the faculty's intention, whether the scenario is started with an asymptomatic or symptomatic infant, American Academy of Pediatrics (AAP) guidelines and steps as described in the lit-erature are followed (Adamkin, 2011). With both endpoints, the running of the scenario varies according to the time of response presented by the students in the simulation, so the facilitator must be alert to begin new symptoms in the SimBaby˚ to represent additional complications and signs of respiratory distress if the student takes too long to identify the hypoglycemic episode, or if the interventions (breastfeeding and skin-to-skin contact) are not successful.

Otherwise, if starting with an asymptomatic infant, when the student is able to identify hypoglycemia considering gestational diabetes history and symptoms in accordance with the clinical case, and encourages early feeding and monitoring with the mother, the scenario does not evolve to the second endpoint, because the problem is resolved by implementing breastfeeding and skin-to-skin contact with the mother.

The scenario also involves the opportunity for the student to educate the mother about the situation, risks, and health interventions, explaining to the family the symptoms they are seeing in the newborn, how they are connected to the baby being an IDM, and what possible interventions will work. Power sharing is expected by showing the mother how to identify signs of hypoglycemia in her baby and educating her on what can be done if it happens again.

F. PRESENTATION OF COMPLETED TEMPLATE

Title

High-Risk Newborn—Hypoglycemia

Scenario Level, Focus Area, Scenario Description

Provided in Exhibit 20.1.

Scenario Objectives

The scenario also allows students to practice key elements from the National Council Licensure Examination for Registered Nurses (NCLEX-RN˚) using the National Council State Boards of Nursing test plan (NCSBN; 2015) categories and subcategories, including:

Safe and effective care environment: *Management of care* (advocacy, collaboration with interdisciplinary team, establishing priorities), *Safety and infection control* (accident/error/injury prevention, emergency response plan, safe use of equipment); **Health promotion and maintenance:** *Ante/intra/ postpartum and newborn care, Developmental stages and transitions, Techniques of physical assessment*; **Psychosocial integrity:** *Coping mechanisms, Crisis intervention, Cultural awareness/Cultural influences on health, Religious and spiritual influences on health, Support systems, Therapeutic communications*; **Physiological integrity:** *Basic care and comfort* (nutrition and oral hydration), *Pharmacological and parenteral therapies* (medication administration, parenteral/ intravenous therapies, pharmacological agents/action), *Reduction of risk potential* (changes/ abnormalities in vital signs, laboratory values, system specific assessments, therapeutic procedures), *Physiological adaptation* (alterations in body systems, fluid and electrolyte imbalances, hemodynamics, medical emergencies, pathophysiology, unexpected response to therapies).

For this scenario, the American Association of Colleges of Nursing's (AACN; 2008) *The Essentials of Baccalaureate Education for Professional Nursing Practice* items addressed include the following:

Essential V: Informatics and Healthcare Technologies, Objectives 3, 6
Essential VI: Interprofessional Collaboration for Improving Patient Health Outcomes, Objectives 1, 2, 4, 5, 6
Essential VIII: Professionalism and Professional Values, Objectives 1 to 4, 6 to 12
Essential IX: Baccalaureate Generalist Nursing Practice, Objectives 1 to 19, 21

For this scenario, the College of Registered Nurses of British Columbia (CRNBC; 2015) *Competencies in the Context of Entry-Level Registered Nurse Practice in British Columbia* include:

1. Professional Responsibility and Accountability: Demonstrates professional conduct and that the primary duty is to the client to ensure safe, competent, compassionate, ethical care (includes accountability and responsibility, recognition of individual competence and roles and responsibilities of registered nurses, demonstrates critical inquiry in relation to new knowledge and technology, exercises professional judgment).
2. Specialized Body of Knowledge: Has knowledge from nursing and other sciences, humanities, research, ethics, spirituality, relational practice, and critical inquiry.
3. Competent Application of Knowledge: Demonstrates competence in the provision of nursing care: ongoing comprehensive assessment, health care planning, providing nursing care, and evaluation.
4. Demonstrates competence in professional judgment and practice decisions guided by the values and ethical responsibilities in codes of ethics for registered nurses. Engages in critical inquiry to inform clinical decision making, and establishes therapeutic, caring, and culturally safe relationships with clients and the health care team.

Scenario Implementation

This scenario can accommodate two different expected endpoints or unfold from one case into the next, as desired by the faculty. Everything in the scene related to structure, equipment, and simulation level remains the same, while the infant outcomes change and require different care:

Endpoint 1: Asymptomatic infant skin-to-skin with mother and breastfeeding; hypoglycemia is successfully resolved.

Endpoint 2: Symptomatic infant cannot feed, is jittery, has increasing pallor and an increased respiratory rate and increased work of breathing (retractions, low oxygen saturation levels), and presents other symptoms related to hypoglycemia (Reuter, Moser, & Baack, 2014). Provide expressed human milk (EHM) +IV glucose, and increased monitoring in a NICU.

Evaluation Criteria

Specific participant expected actions are embedded in the exhibit.

The scenario should promote feeding, ideally breastfeeding (in the absence of respiratory distress) as the first step and part of the ongoing approach even if IV fluids are required. If the baby is unable to feed, then care would be escalated. Evaluation criteria in this scenario relates to students' actions and there is a possibility of altering the endpoints, changing the expected actions. Criteria were grouped according to cognitive, procedural, and attitudinal learning levels, as follows:

1. Understanding of natural methods of glycemic level recovery through breastfeeding and prevention of respiratory complications by promoting optimal newborn transition and stabilization through skin-to-skin contact (cognitive and procedural skills)
2. Clinical knowledge to identify the need for a different intervention if the first attempt failed, as intended with the second endpoint in which other symptoms can be added, such as respiratory complication and hypotonic tonus (cognitive and procedural skills)
3. Student demonstrates an ability for therapeutic communication in an integrated approach creating an opportunity to partner with the infant's mother, explaining to her the possibilities of intervention and effectively educating her about the baby's clinical condition, as well as offering her support and options of breastfeeding and skin-to-skin contact (cognitive and attitudinal skills)
4. Effective communication with other health care professionals (attitudinal skill)

Setting the Scene and Scenario Implementation

Expected activity run time: 20 minutes
Small-group discussion: refer to literature, self-evaluation: 10 minutes
Guided reflection/debriefing time: 30 minutes

Exhibit 20.1	Clinical Course of the Simulated Scenario		
Parameters	**Cues**	**Key Required Participant Activities**	**Time**
Human Patient Simulation (HPS)	**Instructor Responds/Cues**		
Physiological Parameters: HR: 110 beats/minute BP: 64/42 mmHg T: 97.6°F/36.4°C **Cardiac** P: 164 beats/minute **Respiratory** Rate: 68 breaths/minute O_2 saturation: 85% **Blood Glucose** 38 mg/dL	**Client Presentation:** Endpoint 2: Decompensation: Infant is pale and jittery. **Respiratory Status:** Transition from rapid (68/minute breathing to labored, with O_2 saturation dropping to 93 [85]%), if feeding does not work, then chest retractions, nasal flaring, expiratory grunt all occur.	☐ Wash hands ☐ Introduce self to mother ☐ Check name band of baby ☐ Ask mother how the baby is doing ☐ Obtain a maternal history to determine factors that may have put the newborn at risk for hypoglycemia and other complications ☐ Examine the labor-and-delivery history to identify risk factors that may have put the newborn at risk for hypoglycemia and other complications ☐ Identify the infant as LGA ☐ Places infant on monitor ☐ Assess vital signs __ BP __ P __ RR __ T ☐ Find normal data ☐ Don gloves ☐ Perform an accurate newborn assessment and respiratory status ☐ Examine the newborn for signs of hypoglycemia and other complications ☐ Performs D-stick via heel stick (38 mg/dL) ☐ Report to neonatal nurse practitioner (by phone) what is going on ☐ Draw labs	10 min 5 min 5 min
		Endpoint 1 ☐ Ask baby's mother whether it is possible to breastfeed at that moment, explaining motive and advantages of this procedure ☐ Helps mother to establish good position to breastfeed and setup skin-to-skin contact ☐ Evaluate whether suck if adequate, considering newborn's hypotonic status	**Endpoint 2** ☐ Recheck VS ☐ Find abnormal P/BP/T ☐ Newborn is pale and jittery, now with a poor suck, hypotonic with developing signs of nasal flaring and retractions ☐ Prepare to start IV for D10W under neonatal nurse practitioner direction/order ☐ Install nasal cannula and oxygen

(continued)

Exhibit 20.1	Clinical Course of the Simulated Scenario *(continued)*		
Parameters	**Cues**	**Key Required Participant Activities**	**Time**
		☐ Maintain observation at the monitor ☐ Rechecks VS ☐ Don gloves ☐ Perform repeat heel-stick ☐ Monitor infant's condition ☐ Maintain infant's body temperature ☐ Incorporate preventive measures in the care of the newborn delivered to a gestational diabetic mother specifically at risk for hypoglycemia ☐ Educate mother regarding the newborn's status and plan of care ☐ Explain procedures ☐ Support mother	☐ Incorporate preventive measures in the care of the newborn delivered to a gestational diabetic mother specifically at risk for hypoglycemia ☐ Give IV of D10W according to hospital's protocol after NP or MD's prescription ☐ Perform repeat heel-stick 1, 4, and 6 hours after infusion ☐ Monitor infant's condition ☐ Maintain infant's body temperature ☐ Educate mother regarding the newborn's status and plan of care ☐ Explain procedures ☐ Support mother	

Fidelity (Choose All That Apply to This Simulation)

Setting/Environment:

☒ Delivery suite/LDR room or Newborn Nursery/NICU

Patient Simulator(S) Needed:

☒ SimBaby*

Infant is in the room with mother initially—may transition to a pale infant under a radiant warmer

Recommended Mode for Simulation (i.e., manual, programmed, etc.):

Some preprogrammed with on-the-fly capability

* Comment I: Point-of-care results often read higher than lab values and thus BG can be

Patient Simulator:

Second episode—symptomatic infant

☒ Pale and jittery (baby powder on face)

☒ Poor suck

☒ Hypotonic

☒ Nasal flaring

☒ BP cuff on

☒ Pulse oximeter on

☒ ID band (James Jones)

Patient Description:

Name: Baby Boy James Jones

Mother: Mrs. Althea Jones (A.J.)

Age: 2 + hours

Race: Caucasian

Equipment on Table:

☒ Bottle labeled "Pumped Milk—James Jones"

☒ Bottle labeled "Similac w/ Iron 24 Cal"

☒ Thermometer

☒ Heel-stick equipment

☒ Accu-chek paper strips

☒ Alcohol wipes

☒ Glucosemeter* (with result 38 mg/dL) with strips

☒ IV start kit

☒ SpO$_2$ monitor and probe

☒ Infant nasal cannula

☒ Lab reports

☒ EKG monitor/defibrillator/pacer

☒ Oxygen source/delivery

(continued)

Exhibit 20.1	Clinical Course of the Simulated Scenario *(continued)*

Fidelity (Choose All That Apply to This Simulation)

overestimated (Adamkin, 2011; Straussman & Levitsky, 2010), the authors do not recommend waiting for the lab.

Gender: Male
Weight: 9 pounds, 8 ounces
Height: 21 inches

Equipment Near Isolette/ Overhead:
☒ Stethoscope
☒ PPE (goggles, gloves, etc.)
☒ Reference material/pen/paper
☒ BP cuff
☒ Crash cart
☒ Radiant warmer
☒ Suction

Medications and Fluids:
☐ IV fluids: D10W
☐ Ointment: Erythromycin
☐ IM administration of vitamin K
Medications: Vitamin K IM to left thigh and erythromycin ointment to both eyes upon admission

Diagnostics Available:
☐ Labs

Documentation Forms:
☐ Apgar score
☐ Silverman–Anderson Index

Roles/Guidelines for Roles
☐ **Neonatal nurse practitioner (by phone)**
☐ **Mother:** If the student did not suggest breastfeeding and skin-to-skin contact in order to correct asymptomatic hypoglycemia, the mother will state, "When can I feed my baby?" The baby continues to decompensate. The scenario continues as more clinical symptoms are introduced. To stimulate the student to continue clinical evaluation, the actress representing the mother can touch the baby and says to the nurse: "Is it normal to be jittery like this? I think my baby is pale, too."
☐ **Instructor:** The instructor can intervene as if he or she was the nurse practitioner or medical doctor prescribing the IV dextrose and eventually supports the data collection about abnormal findings. It is important for the instructor not to conduct the resolution of the simulation case, but to be alert and give hints when necessary acting as he or she would in a real situation assuming the role of NP or MD.

Significant Lab Values:
MD/NP would order blood gases

Student Information Needed Before Scenario:
☐ Has been oriented to simulator
☐ Understands guidelines /expectations for scenario
☐ Has accomplished all presimulation requirements
☐ All participants understand their assigned roles
☐ Has been given time frame expectations

Report Students Receive Before Simulation:
Time: Gravida 5, term 3, preterm 1, abortions 1, living 3 and now new 9-pound, 8-ounce, full-term male on Sunday at 3:07 a.m. Breastfed for about 45 minutes after delivery with an intermittent latch and is now being observed in the NICU. Children at home are 6, 4, and 2 years old, two girls and a boy, respectively. Husband was present for birth but headed home to care for other children. Mother was diagnosed at 24 weeks with insulin-dependent gestational diabetes; however, she has poorly managed and controlled her blood glucose levels throughout the rest of the pregnancy.

(continued)

Exhibit 20.1	Clinical Course of the Simulated Scenario *(continued)*

Fidelity (Choose All That Apply to This Simulation)

Augmentation of labor with oxytocin early Saturday morning; vacuum-assisted delivery; long labor with a difficult delivery, pushed >1 hour. Membranes ruptured Friday evening.

The newborn is being admitted to the tertiary-level NICU. The mother is a 35-year-old White with insulin-dependent gestational diabetes who had a vacuum-assisted delivery 1 hour ago after a long difficult labor.

Nursing Actions:

Vitamin K IM to left thigh and erythromycin ointment to both eyes on admission.

BG, blood glucose; BP, blood pressure; D10W, dextrose 10% in water; HR, heart rate; IM, intramuscular; IV, intravenous; LGA, large for gestational age; NICU, neonatal intensive care unit; NP, nurse practitioner; P, pulse; PPE, personal protective equipment; T, temperature; VS, vital signs.

Used with permission of Dr. Bernie Garrett, School of Nursing, and Dr. Karim Qayumi, Faculty of Medicine, The University of British Columbia, Vancouver, BC Canada.

G. DEBRIEFING GUIDELINES

Important Issues to Discuss

It is necessary for students to understand the pathophysiology of IDMs, significant risk factors such as newborn danger signals—metabolic alterations: hypoglycemia; BG less than 30 mg/dL in first 72 hours or less than 40 mg/dL after 72 hours; temperature instability: axillary less than 36.5°C (97.7°F) or more than 37.5°C (99.5°F); Respiratory signs: apnea for more than 20 seconds, tachypnea more than 60 breaths/minute, nasal flaring, chest retractions, asynchronous breathing movements (see–saw respirations), and expiratory grunting. Specifics related to homeostatic control of newborns have been identified earlier in the chapter and many good references and recommended readings are suggested throughout.

Student Questions

Questions for Students Who Were Part of the Scenario

Initial reaction: go for you—were there things that concerned you?

1. What went well—what did you feel good about?
2. Are there points at which you would have liked to have done something differently?
3. What surprised you most in this scenario? How did you feel about the outcomes?

General Questions for Debriefing Related to the Case Itself

1. What physiological transition was being portrayed in this scenario?
2. What key assessment factors, vital-sign parameters, and lab tests were necessary?
3. How did you ensure you were following the known standards of care for this situation?
4. What were the crucial nursing interventions and evaluation points necessary?
5. Identify one key takeaway for use in your next clinical experience.

Questions for Students Observing in the Classroom

1. What did you initially notice about the patient? What problems did you identify?
2. What would you have included in the problem-focused assessment that was not included?
3. What additional data would you have wanted that was not collected?
4. What priority problem did you identify for this patient? What are the potential problems for this patient?
5. What further education and support would you give to the parents of this patient?

Orientations According to International Nursing Association for Clinical Simulation and Learning (INACSL) Guidelines

Students are oriented to the room and the participant roles are described to each individually. They have had a class detailing the high-risk newborn and the infant of a diabetic mother with explanation of assessments, the pathophysiology, and the neonatal energy triangle (Aylott, 2006).

They Are Given a Brief Patient History

- Newborn infant, male, 2 hours since birth
- Birth weight 9 pounds, 8 ounces (4,307 kg)
- Mother has history of insulin-dependent gestational diabetes since 24 weeks gestation
- Prolonged labor with vacuum-assisted delivery

Instructions to the Students

1. Be prepared to introduce yourself to the mother, check all equipment being used. Obtain a more complete maternal medical, obstetrical, and delivery history. Obtain information on postdelivery infant care and breastfeeding.
2. Prepare to discuss and conduct a problem-focused newborn assessment based on the nurse's report and your observations. Use all equipment available. Acquire subjective and objective data in order to properly assess, provide support and care, educate parent, and maintain patient safety.
3. After recognizing the patient's problem, be prepared to take further action to address the identified problem and to care for the patient.
4. Implement any further data collection, including subjective and objective data, in order to identify and investigate any other potential problems or complications.
5. Be prepared to include all necessary education and support and work collaboratively with the available health care team.

H. SUGGESTIONS/KEY FEATURES TO REPLICATE OR IMPROVE

This scenario was initially created for students in an obstetric undergraduate course. The intent was for them to quickly assess, manage the mother's anxiety, and call for backup while identifying hypoglycemia with necessary interventions. With the advent of mother–baby care according to Baby Friendly Hospital Initiative (Baby-Friendly USA, 2016) and NeoBFHI (2015) guidelines, we decided to provide two endpoints for this scenario. One in which the first intervention is skin-to-skin care and offer of breast milk to calm the infant and increase their blood sugar while decreasing the risk of respiratory depression. If this does not change the outcome, then the student would place the infant under a warmer and provide IV therapy to bring the blood sugar back to normal. Evidence-based guidelines suggest: early feeding (within 1 hour) in the asymptomatic at-risk infant with monitoring at 1 hour; check glucose 1 hour after first feed (at 2 hours of life) and, if BG more than 40, continue to feed and monitor for the first 12 hours. At-risk infants include late preterm, term small for gestational age (SGA), term LGA, IDM, and IDM/LGA (Adamkin, 2011; Csont et al., 2014).

I. RECOMMENDATIONS FOR FURTHER USE

Throughout this chapter suggestions for alternative uses have been described. Although initially developed for teaching BSN nursing students in their third or fourth year, this scenario is adaptable for graduate students (including neonatal nurse practitioners) and can be used in situ in the clinical setting to educate/orient new staff to this specialty area and to help practitioners keep their skill set and team skills well honed. The inclusion of invasive and noninvasive alternatives makes it replicable in poorly resourced areas without high-fidelity simulation capability, and either endpoint can be practiced. The potential life-threatening aspect of this condition makes it important for all health care practitioners to be skilled in recognizing the symptoms early and treating them quickly.

J. HOW SIMULATION-BASED PEDAGOGY HAS CONTRIBUTED TO IMPROVED STUDENT OUTCOMES

Students remark that whether they are actually participants in the live simulation or observing from the classroom, they feel that they enhance their confidence and recognition of a similar situation in clinical practice. By considering the debriefing questions and discussing with their classmates the experience, what might be done differently, and what was surprising, they gain confidence and skill in making sound clinical decisions and acting quickly when they see signs and symptoms that an infant is in trouble. As this is rolled out in Brazil and at BCWHHC, end-of-simulation evaluation to provide faculty/administrators with feedback regarding the use of high-fidelity HPS technology in the laboratory setting or in situ is collected to continue to improve the quality of the scenario and better meet student and practitioners needs.

K. EXPERT RECOMMENDATIONS AND WORDS OF WISDOM

This scenario has changed from a strictly high-risk situation for end-of-term baccalaureate nursing students to an option to reinforce patient-centered care, noninterventive solutions that protect the breastfeeding dyad and maternal confidence, and an unfolding case that allows multiple situations to evolve. We are exploring use of this simulation with students in Brazil and in situ with interdisciplinary teams in a tertiary-level institution with a level-three NICU. Being aware of updated guidelines and policies and protocols within one's own country, region, and health authority/ institution, and incorporating those guidelines appropriately enhances the learning for students and seasoned practitioners. Reviewing the pathophysiology of IDM, neonatal respiratory distress and hypoglycemia, as well as benefits of zero separation for the mother–infant dyad and encouraging breastfeeding are key learning outcomes.

L. EVALUATION OF BEST PRACTICE STANDARDS AND USE OF CREDENTIALED SIMULATION FACULTY

The earlier sections describe how the scenario was initially developed to follow the INACSL Best Standards: Simulation[SM] (2013/2016). The creation of the scenario and its use and tweaking since 2008, addressed the development of objectives that met program standards of the NCLEX-RN

Blueprint as well as AACN BSN Essentials and CRNBC RN competencies. Faculty who developed the scenario have had more than 10 years of working with simulation and are prepared to facilitate and debrief using the identified guidelines. Testing the scenario in Brazil and in situ in a practice site with multiple team members is the subsequent goal.

REFERENCES

American Association of Colleges of Nursing. (2008). *The essentials of baccalaureate education for professional nursing practice.* Washington, DC: Author. Retrieved from http://www.aacnnursing.org/Portals/42/Publications/BaccEssentials08.pdf

Advanced Care of the at Risk Newborn. (2016). Acute care of at-risk newborns. Retrieved from http://www.cps.ca/en/acorn

Adamkin, D. H. (2011). Postnatal glucose homeostasis in late-preterm and term infants. *Pediatrics, 127*(3), 575–579. doi:10.1542/peds.2010–3851

Amaral, A. R., Silva, J. C., Ferreira, B. D. S., Silva, M. R., & Bertini, A. M. (2015). Impact of gestational diabetes on neonatal outcomes: A retrospective cohort study. *Scientia Medica, 25*(1), 1–6. doi:10.15448/1980-6108.2015.1.19272

Aziz, K., Dancey, P.; Canadian Paediatric Society, Fetus and Newborn Committee. (2004). Screening guidelines for newborns at risk for low blood glucose. *Paediatric Child Health, 9*(10), 723–729. Reaffirmed February 1, 2016. Retrieved from http://www.cps.ca/en/documents/position/newborns-low-blood-glucose

Baby-Friendly USA. (2016). Baby Friendly Hospital Initiative. Retrieved from https://www.babyfriendlyusa.org/about-us/baby-friendly-hospital-initiative

Breast Feeding Committee for Canada. (2012). The Baby-Friendly Initiative (BFI) in Canada. Retrieved from http://breastfeedingcanada.ca/documents/BFI_Status_report_2012_FINAL.pdf

Cant, R. P., & Cooper, S. J. (2010). Simulation-based learning in nurse education: Systematic review. *Journal of Advanced Nursing, 66*(1), 3–15.

Cheng, A., Hunt, E. A., Donoghue, A., Nelson-McMillan, K., Nishisaki, A., Leflore, J.,...Nadkarni, V. M.; EXPRESS Investigators. (2013). Examining pediatric resuscitation education using simulation and scripted debriefing: A multicenter randomized trial. *JAMA Pediatrics, 167*(6), 528–536.

College of Registered Nurses British Columbia (CRNBC) (2015). Competencies in the Context of Entry-Level Registered Nurse Practice in British Columbia, Pub. No. 375. Retrieved from https://www.crnbc.ca/Registration/Lists/RegistrationResources/375CompetenciesEntrylevelRN.pdf

Crofts, J. F., Ellis, D., Draycott, T. J., Winter, C., Hunt, L. P., & Akande, V. A. (2007). Change in knowledge of midwives and obstetricians following obstetric emergency training: A randomised controlled trial of local hospital, simulation centre and teamwork training. *BJOG: An International Journal of Obstetrics and Gynaecology, 114*(12), 1534–1541.

Csont, G. L., Groth, S., Hopkins, P., & Guillet, R. (2014). An evidence-based approach to breastfeeding neonates at risk for hypoglycemia. *Journal of Obstetric, Gynecologic, and Neonatal Nursing, 43*(1), 71–81.

Dyson, L., McCormick, F. M., & Renfrew, M. J. (2005). Interventions for promoting the initiation of breastfeeding. *Cochrane Database of Systematic Reviews, 2005*(2). doi:10.1002/14651858.CD001688.pub2

Eppich, W., & Cheng, A. (2015). Promoting excellence and reflective learning in simulation (PEARLS): Development and rationale for a blended approach to health care simulation debriefing. *Simulation in Healthcare, 10*(2), 106–115.

Freeth, D., Ayida, G., Berridge, E. J., Sadler, C., & Strachan, A. (2006). MOSES: Multidisciplinary obstetric simulated emergency scenarios. *Journal of Interprofessional Care, 20*(5), 552–554.

Haller, G., Garnerin, P., Morales, M. A., Pfister, R., Berner, M., Irion, O.,...Kern, C. (2008). Effect of crew resource management training in a multidisciplinary obstetrical setting. *International Journal for Quality in Health Care, 20*(4), 254–263.

Hermansen, C. L., & Mahajan, A. (2015). Newborn respiratory distress. *American Family Physician, 92*(11), 994–1002.

Hill, P. D., & Aldag, J. C. (2007). Predictors of term infant feeding at week 12 postpartum. *Journal of Perinatal & Neonatal Nursing, 21*(3), 250–255.

International Nursing Association for Clinical Simulation and Learning. (2013, updated 2016). INACSL standards of best practice: Simulation. Retrieved from https://www.inacsl.org/i4a/pages/index.cfm?pageID=3407

Leonard, B., Shuhaibar, E. L., & Chen, R. (2010). Nursing student perceptions of intraprofessional team education using high-fidelity simulation. *Journal of Nursing Education, 49*(11), 628–631.

Leonard, M., Graham, S., & Bonacum, D. (2004). The human factor: The critical importance of effective teamwork and communication in providing safe care. *Quality & Safety in Health Care, 13*(Suppl. 1), i85–i90. doi:10.1136/qshc.2004.010033

Li, R., Fein, S. B., Chen, J., & Grummer-Strawn, L. M. (2008). Why mothers stop breastfeeding: Mothers' self-reported reasons for stopping during the first year. *Pediatrics, 122*(Suppl. 2), S69–S76.

Maayan-Metzger, A., Lubin, D., & Kuint, J. (2009). Hypoglycemia rates in the first days of life among term infants born to diabetic mothers. *Neonatology, 96*(2), 80–85.

Malt, G. (2015). Cochrane review brief: Interprofessional education: Effects on professional practice and healthcare outcomes. *Online Journal of Issues in Nursing, 20*(2), 12.

Murray, W. B., & Foster, P. A. (2000). Crisis resource management among strangers: Principles of organizing a multidisciplinary group for crisis resource management. *Journal of Clinical Anesthesia, 12*(8), 633–638.

National Council State Boards of Nursing. (2015). NCLEX-RN examination: Test plan for the National Council Licensure Examination for Registered Nurses. Retrieved from https://www.ncsbn.org/RN_Test_Plan_2016_Final.pdf

NeoBFHI. (2015). The NeoBFHI: The Baby-Friendly Hospital Initiative for neonatal wards. Retrieved from http://www.ilca.org/main/learning/resources/neo-bfhi

Neonatal Resuscitation Program. (2016). Neonatal resuscitation program. Retrieved from http://www.cps.ca/nrp-prn

Reuter, S., Moser, C., & Baack, M. (2014). Respiratory distress in the newborn. *Pediatrics in Review, 35*(10), 417–428; quiz 429.

Straussman, S., & Levitsky, L. L. (2010). Neonatal hypoglycemia. *Current Opinion in Endocrinology, Diabetes, and Obesity, 17*(1), 20–24.

Thornton, P. S., Stanley, C. A., De Leon, D. D., Harris, D., Haymond, M. W., Hussain, K.,...Wolfsdorf, J. I.; Pediatric Endocrine Society. (2015). Recommendations from the pediatric endocrine society for evaluation and management of persistent hypoglycemia in neonates, infants, and children. *Journal of Pediatrics, 167*(2), 238–245.

FURTHER READING

Aylott, M. (2006). The neonatal energy triangle. Part 2: Thermoregulatory and respiratory adaptation. *Pediatric Nursing, 18*(7), 38–42.

Davidson, M. R., London, M. L., & Ladewig, P. W. (2008). *Olds' maternal–newborn nursing & women's health across the lifespan* (8th ed., pp. 743–745, 1159–1165). Upper Saddle River, NJ: Pearson Prentice-Hall.

Stanford Hospital Guidelines. Hypoglycemia of the newborn. Retrieved from http://www.stanford-childrens.org/en/topic/default?id=hypoglycemia-in-the-newborn-90-P01961

Suprenant S., & Coghlan M. A. (2016). Distress in the newborn: An approach for the emergency care provider. *Clinical Pediatric Emergency Medicine.* doi:10.1016/j.cpem.2016.03.004

CHAPTER 21

Pediatric Nursing Care Clinical Simulation Scenarios for Prelicensure Students

Mary Ann Cantrell, Colleen H. Meakim, and Kathryn M. Reynolds

A. IMPLEMENTATION OF SIMULATION-BASED PEDAGOGY IN YOUR INDIVIDUALIZED TEACHING AREA

As experienced in other areas of clinical practice, pediatric clinical sites are becoming sparse in health care systems that are dedicated exclusively to the care of children and their families. Likewise, available and meaningful clinical learning experience in suburban and rural-based settings are limited. In addition, the strong emphasis of safety practices within pediatric-based institutions limits the scope of practice of prelicensure nursing students.

The following four pediatric-based clinical scenarios were created by two pediatric faculty members and a simulation-based expert at Villanova University, College of Nursing, who holds a certification as a Certified Healthcare Simulation Educator (CHSE). At Villanova University, College of Nursing pediatric clinical learning experiences for undergraduate learners are augmented with these four formative simulation scenarios offered during the 7-week pediatric clinical experience, along with a summative clinical scenario conducted after the 7-week clinical practicum. The pediatric clinical practicum is offered in the first semester of the fourth year for traditional undergraduate baccalaureate students. These learners were previously enrolled in a 12-week adult medical–surgical clinical, an adult complex (critical care) clinical experience, and a mental health and women–infant clinical practicum.

This chapter describes these four formative scenarios, which involve the care needs of a young child with asthma; a preschool-age child who is postoperative, recovering from a laparoscopic surgery for a ruptured appendix; an adolescent with sickle cell disease (SCD) who is experiencing vasoocclusive crisis; and a 9-month-old infant who is undergoing a well-child checkup. These formative scenarios are offered between the third and sixth week of the 7-week practicum course. Students in groups of seven to eight participate in the scenarios. The four scenarios are all done within a 6-hour day. Two students actively participate in each scenario and the remaining five to six students are observers. All students are prebriefed, which includes an orientation to the patient care setting, specifically the equipment being used in the scenario. There is a debriefing session following each scenario, which is described later in this chapter. The facilitator observes from a control room and can be the voice of any person the student needs to collaborate with, such as a health care provider, a pharmacist, or a respiratory therapist.

The companion pediatric nursing theory course provides the theory content, including nursing interventions for each of these disease processes as well as content addressing the psychosocial needs of the children and their families. It is intended that the theory content of these disease processes is taught before students participating in these formative scenarios. The preparation materials, which include information about the scenarios, are posted on the Blackboard learning management system (LMS) and are available to students at the start of the pediatric nursing theory course. These materials can be downloaded and students can complete the necessary preparation-for-learning activities before the simulation-based learning experiences (SBLEs). Faculty materials related to the scenario and debriefing methods are made available privately to faculty on the LMS.

B. EDUCATIONAL MATERIALS AVAILABLE IN YOUR TEACHING AREA AND RELATED TO YOUR SPECIALTY

The simulation lab in which the scenarios are implemented is a state-of-the-art facility that includes one floor of laboratory spaces in which students can experience skills preparation and simulated clinical experiences. This 12,000-square foot Simulation and Learning Resource Center (SLRC) includes six clinical simulation labs with six to 10 beds or examination tables in each room, five standardized patient rooms, and three simulation rooms (one of which is a simulated operating room). There are computers in between beds or individually in smaller rooms to permit access to electronic health records and resource information; audiovisual equipment for visualization and/or recording of simulation scenarios is available in all rooms. Students also have access to eight adult human patient simulators (HPSs), nine pediatric HPS, and one birthing HPS, as well as seven medication-dispensing machines and many other types of task trainers, equipment, and supplies to create a realistic simulated learning environment. Two to three staff and the director of the SLRC are available to assist the faculty and students during these simulation teaching–learning experiences.

C. SPECIFIC OBJECTIVES FOR SIMULATION USAGE WITHIN A SPECIFIC COURSE AND THE OVERALL PROGRAM

The simulation teaching–learning experiences are intended to support the learning objectives for the entire practicum course, which are:

1. Use reliable sources of information to implement evidence-based care of children, adolescents, and families.
2. Apply health assessment findings and clinical reasoning to family-centered care of children and adolescents.
3. Demonstrate selected patient care skills.
4. Integrate the concepts of genetics, culture, ethnicity, spirituality, and development into the care of children, adolescents, and families.
5. Use information management and technology in the care of children, adolescents, and families.
6. Demonstrate effective therapeutic and professional communication in providing care to children, adolescents, and families.
7. Incorporate patient safety, dignity, and quality family-centered care with children and adolescents.
8. Integrate professional values, health care policy, and ethical principles in the care of children, adolescents, and families.
9. Relate the scope of practice and responsibilities to the role of the professional nurse in the care of children, adolescents, and families.
10. Translate the principles of teaching and learning into the care of children, adolescents, and families.

SCENARIO 1

D. INTRODUCTION OF SCENARIO

Setting the Scene

Scenario 1. Adolescent with SCD admitted for vasoocclusive crisis

Technology Used

- Patient actor and parent actor
- Video clips of previously filmed scenario in stages could be used if the simulation is conducted as part of a classroom teaching–learning experience
- An HPS can be used, but it is more difficult to simulate the degree of pain and respiratory distress with an HPS versus a standardized patient or person

Equipment needed: See Exhibit 21.1.
Resources needed: Access to an online drug formulary or a pediatric drug text such as the Lexicomp Online | Clinical Drug Information (www.wolterskluwercdi.com/lexicomp-online)

Exhibit 21.1	Equipment Needed
Video-recording device, medical equipment (e.g., patient monitor, oxygen hookup, IV pump/pole, pulse oximeter, blood pressure cuff, and stethoscope), medical record (electronic or paper)	
Vital sign display: If no monitor is available, vital signs can be placed on a card for students to view when students assess the patient's vital signs; also the scenario can include a pulse oximetry machine with a sticker that identifies an initial reading of 86%, and later on in the scenario a second sticker can be placed to signify the pulse oximetry reading increased to 90%—(after treatment). Other alternatives are use of a computer and monitor from another manikin or a PowerPoint display showing vital signs for various scenes. The parent can change the display as needed during the scenario.	
Vital sign settings at the beginning of the scenario: (HR: 112 beats/minute, BP: 104/70 mmHg, RR: 32 breaths/minute, temperature: 39.5°C [103.1°F]; SpO$_2$:86%)	
Patient-controlled analgesia pump or simulated pump hanging on a pole with a device to look as if patient is controlling PCA pump for morphine administration	
Ventriloscope (a simulation stethoscope that uses a wireless transmitter to play sounds stored as MP3 files on a sound card, allowing students to hear abnormal sounds in a simulated patient care setting; Ventriloscope will be "playing" crackles). An alternative is using a Laerdal sounds trainer with a device that simulate crackles.	
IV solution 5% dextrose, 0.45% NSS on IV pump noting the rate of 175 mL/hr; with a secondary port for IV antibiotic administration.	
IV medication infusion pump for administration of morphine	
MSO$_4$ in a multidose vial that reads: "15 mg/1 mL for rescue dose of morphine."	
Vial of hydromorphone (Dilaudid) 1.5 mg/mL (used as a distracter)	
Three of each syringe sized: 1 mL, 3 mL, 5 mL (students need to select the appropriate-sized syringe)	
Liquid Tylenol dose—650 mg (325 mg/5 mL)	

(continued)

Exhibit 21.1	Equipment Needed *(continued)*

Tylenol tabs 325 mg/tab

Plastic medicine cups

Oxygen setup with flowmeter and humidification bottle, with O_2 mask set at 1–2 L FiO_2 via face mask, which is off patient when the nurse enters room.

Directions for actor

Patient gown

Name band for patient—Jack/Jackie Sullivan—that includes patient's full name with MRN and DOB.

Incentive spirometer

Identification bracelet with full name, MRN and DOB

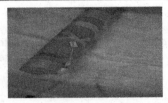

A swimming pool "noodle" with IV catheter and extension set inserted and a bag hanging beneath it to simulate patient's arm; set on bed next to patient, so IV can actually be administered (see photograph)

BP, blood pressure; DOB, date of birth; HR, heart rate; IV, intravenous; MRN, medical record number; NSS, normal saline solution; PCA, patient-controlled anesthesia; RR, respiratory rate.

Objectives

1. Complete patient assessment of an inpatient with sickle cell anemia.
2. Obtain a pertinent history related to the patient's current health status.
3. Provide priority nursing interventions related to patient's current situation.
4. Communicate effectively with patient and family member during scenario.
5. Communicate as needed with other medical personnel during scenario.
6. Safely administer medications related to the adolescent's care needs as described in the scenario.

Description of Participants

Two student nurses assume the role of direct patient care providers. The patient is Jackie, a 13-year-old female in the hospital with a known diagnosis of sickle cell anemia who was admitted for a painful vasoocclusive crisis. A family member is at the patient's bedside and is appropriately concerned.

E. RUNNING OF THE SCENARIO

A 13-year-old adolescent with a confirmed diagnosis of sickle cell anemia has been admitted to the pediatric inpatient setting and is experiencing a vaso-occlusive crisis. The patient is complaining of pain in legs, belly, and arms and states that her vision is blurry, she is dizzy, and is having difficulty breathing.

Two direct care providers are at the patient's bedside to address the patient's physical, and psychosocial care needs based on maintaining physiological safety, followed by psychosocial care needs.

F. PRESENTATION OF COMPLETED TEMPLATE

Title

Nursing Care of the Adolescent With Sickle Cell Anemia

Scenario Level and Focus Area

Senior-level course—Health Care of Children and Adolescents

Scenario Description

This scenario introduces concepts of pain management for a child experiencing acute pain, as well as potential signs and symptoms of respiratory and neurological functioning that can affect her physiological safety. The scenario allows learning opportunities for students to prioritize care needs according to the National Council Licensure Examination for Registered Nurses (NCLEX-RN®) standards of care.

Setting the Scene and Scenario Implementation

The setting is a hospital room in an acute care pediatric-based medical health care system. The patient was admitted at 12 noon and it is now 4:00 p.m. (1600). The report is received from another nurse. Exhibit 21.2 provides chart information for this patient.

> **Prebriefing:** 10 minutes
> **Expected activity run time:** 20 minutes
> **Debriefing:** 30 minutes

Clinical Course of the Simulated Scenario

Students are expected to come prepared, having completed the written preparation questions (see text that follows). Prebriefing includes an orientation to the environment, reviewing expectations, determining roles, and getting a patient report. Following prebriefing, the facilitator, who is usually a faculty member, observes from the control room.

Student Preparation to Be Completed Before the Scenario Participation

Students should know the following information before the simulation:

1. For a patient with SCD, what are the important questions to ask regarding past medical history and why?
2. When completing a pain assessment for a patient with SCD, what assessments are important to perform and why?
3. When completing a neurological assessment for a patient with SCD, what assessments are important to perform and why?
4. What are the important components of a respiratory assessment for a patient with SCD and why?
5. Why do some clients with SCD experience cerebral vascular attacks (CVAs) and/or transient ischemic attacks (TIAs)? If this is in the patient's history, what are the significant clinical care actions to take?
6. What are the critical nursing interventions for a patient with SCD? Prioritize these interventions.
7. Why is morphine sulfate administered to a patient with SCD?
8. Why is Tylenol administered?
9. What is the importance of intravenous (IV) fluid therapy for a patient with SCD?

Exhibit 21.2	Chart Information

Weight 50 kg

Urinalysis with urine-specific gravity = 1.030 (Normal [N] = 1.010–1.025)

Chemistry panel with the following abnormal results: BUN = 21 mg/dL (N = 10–20 mg/dL); sodium = 132 mEq/L (N = 135–145 mEq/L); potassium is on the low side, 3.5 mEq/L (N = 3.5–5 mEq/L)

CBC with the following abnormal results: WBC = 20,000 mm^3 (N = 5,000–10,000 mm^3); hgb 6 (N = M: 14–18 g/dL; F: 12–16 g/dL); hct 17 (N = M: 42–53%; F: 37–47%)

Reticulocyte = 4.5 (N = 0.5–1.5)

Intake and output sheet

Physician order sheet (see subsequently)

BUN, blood urea nitrogen; CBC, complete blood count; F, female; hct, hematocrit; hgb, hemoglobin; M, male; WBC, white blood cell.

Physician Orders

1. Admit to the inpatient hematology unit
2. Patient-controlled analgesia (PCA) pump: morphine sulfate in D5W 1:1 concentration; basal rate of 2 mL/hr; bolus: 1.0 mg; lockout time 15 minutes
3. Morphine sulfate 7.5 mg IV every 4 hours (therapeutic range is 0.1–0.2 mg/kg every 4 hours) for breakthrough pain
4. 650 mg Tylenol (acetaminophen) elixir orally every 4 hours, as needed (prn) for a temperature greater than 38.5°C
5. Intravenous fluid therapy (IVF) D5.45 normal saline solution (NSS) with 20 mEeq of KCl at 175 mL/hr (2 × maintenance)
6. Cardiorespiratory monitor with continuous pulse oximetry
7. Humidified O$_2$ at 1 to 2 L to maintain saturation at or above 90%
8. Chest physiotherapy (PT) and incentive spirometry every 2 to 4 hours
9. Strict intake and output monitoring
10. Initial settings for monitor:
    Temperature: 39.5 (C°) 103.2 (F°)
    Pulse: 112 beats/minute
    Respiratory rate: 32 breaths/minute
    Blood pressure: 104/70 mmHg
    Pulse oximetry: 88%

Monitor display changes as students interact with the patient:
- If oxygen mask is put back on patient: SpO$_2$ increases to 90%; Respirations decrease to 26 (trend over 30 sec). Lung sounds: coarse crackles in all lungs filed bilaterally
  o If the student initiates chest PT or incentive spirometry, then pulse oximetry increases to 93%
  o If Tylenol is given temperature decreases to 101.7°F (38.7°C)
  o If rescue dose of morphine is given: heart rate reduces to 87; respiratory rate (RR) reduces to 24 (trend over 45 sec)

Participant Roles

Patient/Actor Instructions

You are Jackie, a 13-year-old adolescent in the hospital. Your diagnosis is sickle cell anemia with vasoocclusive crisis and splenic sequestration. Exhibit 21.3 provides a script for patient responses to nurse's questions.

In persons with SCD, the red blood cells become crescent or sickle-shaped and become inflexible. The abnormal cells stick inside the capillaries, blocking blood flow to vital organs. Persons with sickle cell anemia can have symptoms such as yellow-appearing eyes and skin, pale skin, delayed growth, bone and joint pain, increased risk for infections, development of leg ulcers, eye damage, anemia, and damage to the organs affected by the obstruction.

Vasoocclusive crisis—a type of sickle cell crisis in which there is severe pain caused by infarctions (areas of the body that are not receiving blood supply) that may be in the bones, joints, lungs, liver, spleen, kidney, eye, or central nervous system). Splenic sequestration crisis occurs when the spleen enlarges and traps the blood cells. Aplastic crisis results when an infection causes the bone marrow to stop producing red blood cells.

An IV solution is being administered to you via peripheral intravenous catheter (PIV); you are in significant body pain, specifically, in your legs, belly, and arms. You have on an oxygen mask to help you breathe better. You are having difficulty breathing, sometimes you make a "grunting sound". When the nurse assesses your breathing, she will use the When the nurse assesses your breathing, she may use a device (such as a Ventriloscope® or other device) to allow the students to hear abnormal breath sounds. It will show that you have noisy lungs with mucus in them. You have a fever. When you respond, act as if you are uncomfortable. Move your arms and legs continually to stress that you are in pain. Moan when you speak and keep your focus on how much you hurt. You can only focus on yourself and your pain. When asked the following questions, respond with the statements in Exhibit 21.3.

Parent/Actor Instructions

You are the parent of Jackie, a 13-year-old female in the hospital with a diagnosis of sickle cell anemia who is experiencing a vasoocclusive crisis and splenic sequestration (see preceding text for explanation). You are very worried about your child, and hate to see her in so much pain. You hover and appear concerned. The students will need to do an assessment of Jackie before giving her pain medication. They will have some trouble because Jackie has a hard time focusing on them because of the pain. The nurse should give Jackie pain medication (morphine) and Tylenol for fever, but Jackie cannot swallow pills, so medication has to be in liquid form. Prompt the course of the clinical encounter along, if needed, by saying things like:

- **Pain**: "I've never seen her in so much pain. It's really scaring me."
- **Morphine**: "I've never given that medication before. What will it do to her?"
- **Fever**: "She feels so hot."

Exhibit 21.3	Script for Nurse and Patient
Tell me how your symptoms began or what happened to bring you to the hospital?	**State:** My symptoms started about 2 days ago.
Have you ever been hospitalized before?	**State:** Yes, I have had four prior hospitalizations.
Have you ever had a stroke?	**State:** Not that I know of.
On a scale of 1 to 10, can you describe your pain?	**State:** It is a 10 out of 10 all over, but especially in my legs, belly, and arms. I also have a terrible headache.
Are you dizzy, do you have blurred vision?	**State:** Yes.
Are you having trouble breathing?	**State:** I cannot take a deep breath, it hurts too much.
When was the last time you went to the bathroom?	**State:** I guess it was before I came to the hospital yesterday.

- **Headache, especially if the headache continues and is not being addressed by the nurse:** "Should the doctor know about the headache? I am worried about this because I heard that people can have strokes if they have a severe headache with sickle cell."
- If Jack/Jackie needs help with coughing, help him or her up to cough and breathe deeply.

Formative Evaluative Criteria

See Appendix A for the critical actions that are expected to be demonstrated by the two students who actively participated in the scenario.

SCENARIO 2

D. INTRODUCTION OF SCENARIO

Setting the Scene

Scenario 2. A young child with an asthma exacerbation

Technology Used

Simulator: Pediatric high-fidelity HPS—young child (toddler)

Equipment needed: This scenario includes simulator, video-recording device, medical equipment (e.g., patient monitor, oxygen setup, bandages, pulse oximetry meter, blood pressure cuff, and stethoscope), medical record (electronic or paper) as well as items listed in Exhibit 21.4.

Resources needed: Drug Guide for Nurses or access to an online drug formulary, such as the Lexicomp Online | Clinical Drug Information (www.wolterskluwercdi.com/lexicomp-online)

Exhibit 21.4	Equipment Needed

Toddler-sized HPS in crib with VS monitor with intravenous access in arm
Lubricant for nose to create nasal mucus
O_2 at 1 L/min with a pediatric nasal cannula
Nasal bulb syringe
Percussor
Suction canister hooked to wall suction, with catheters available
Bottle of sterile water
At bedside, a spacer with a mask (aero chamber); student will add medication from medication cart
Medication cart with medicines as identified in orders
Report in ISBAR format and orientation to surroundings (Thomas, Bertram, & Johnson, 2009)
Physician order sheet
IV pump for fluids and medication to be used when student calls physician and receives order for IV fluids and methylprednisolone

ISBAR, identify, situation, background, assessment, recommendation; IV, intravenous; VS, vital signs.

Objectives

1. Perform an assessment of a child in the hospital in an acute asthmatic situation
2. Perform nursing interventions in a prioritized manner related to patient's asthma to ensure physical safety
3. Effectively communicate with family members during scenario to reduce their fears and concerns and increase their understanding of their child's health status
4. Safely administer medications related to the care of the patient described in the scenario
5. Communicate with other health care providers as needed

Description of Participants

Two students collaborate to provide care. An actor plays the role of the child's mother who is at her child's bedside (could be another student or standardized patient; a script is provided as follows). Other students involved in this simulated learning experience will be in the role of observers. The faculty member (facilitator) plays the role of physician or a health care provider who is called during the scenario.

E. RUNNING OF THE SCENARIO

A toddler who is in respiratory distress has been admitted to the pediatric inpatient setting with the admitting diagnosis of asthma exacerbation. The two direct care providers are at the patient's bedside to address physical and psychosocial care needs based on meeting physiological safety needs, followed by psychosocial care needs of the mom, in an effort to practice family-centered care.

F. PRESENTATION OF COMPLETED TEMPLATE

Title

A Toddler With an Asthma Exacerbation

Senario Level and Focus Area

Senior-level course: Health Care of Children and Adolescents

Scenario Description

Jake is a 13-month-old child hospitalized with the diagnosis of asthma exacerbation. He has been receiving continuous nebulizer treatments and has now transitioned to nebulizer treatments every 2 hours. The 8 a.m. assessment revealed a 95% pulse oximetry reading in room air, respiratory rate (RR) of 36 breaths per minute, and overall, Jack appeared comfortable. As Jake's nurse, you enter the room at 10 a.m. to administer the 10 a.m. nebulizer treatment and perform a focused assessment.

Setting the Scene and Scenario Implementation

The setting is a hospital room in an acute care pediatric-based medical health care system. The toddler who is experiencing an asthma exacerbation and has recently transitioned from continuous nebulizer treatments to nebulizer treatments every 2 hours. As the patient's direct health care provider, the student nurses enters the room to provide care. Exhibit 21.6 provides the settings for the human patient simulator at the start of the scenario.

Prebriefing: 10 minutes
Expected activity run time: 20 minutes
Debriefing: 30 minutes

Clinical Course of the Simulated Scenario

Students are expected to come prepared, having completed the written preparation questions (see text that follows). Prebriefing includes an orientation to the environment, reviewing expectations, determining roles, and getting a patient report. Following prebriefing, the facilitator, who is usually a faculty member, is in the control room.

Students should know the following information before the simulation:

1. For a child with asthma, what are the important questions to ask regarding the past history and why?
2. What are the important details of a respiratory assessment for a child with asthma and why?
3. What are the critical nursing interventions for a child with asthma?
4. Why is epinephrine administered and why is it administered subcutaneously?
5. What is important about continuous Ventolin nebulizer treatment for a patient with asthma?
6. Discuss oxygen therapy for the asthmatic child.
7. What is important about fluid therapy for a patient with asthma?
8. What is methylprednisolone (SoluMedrol)? Why is it often administered to a child experiencing an acute exacerbation of asthma?

Students receive the following SBAR (situation, background, assessment, recommendation; Exhibit 21.5) report before starting the scenario:

Exhibit 21.5	SBAR Communication
Situation	Jake Miller is a 13-month-old admitted with asthma exacerbation.
Background	Pt. has no known allergies. Full code. History of present illness: pt. was admitted via ED last evening in acute respiratory distress. Pt. was diagnosed with asthma 8 months ago and had a cold last week. On presentation to the ED—pt. was SOB, respiratory rate was 50, SpO_2 was 85%. Use of accessory muscles and cyanosis were noted. Pt. responded well to respiratory treatments.
Assessment	Pt. was just transferred to our unit 1.5 hours ago.
	Neuro: Pt. is resting comfortably and is sleeping intermittently. A parent is at bedside. Temperature is 98.0°F (36.7°C)
	Cardiovascular (CV): Heart rate is 96 beats/minute, blood pressure 90/52 mmHg. Good capillary refill. Extremity pulses present and +2.
	Respiratory: breath sounds are clear. RR = 32 breaths/minute. Pulse oximetry is 95% on 1 L of FiO_2 via nasal prongs. No mucus drainage noted from nose.
	GI: No BM. Pt. has not eaten.
	GU: Last diaper change was 2200 in ED. Patient's current diaper is dry.
	Skin: IV saline lock in right forearm is patent. No rashes noted.
	Weight is 12 kg.
Recommendation	Perform a beginning shift assessment.
	Continue to monitor respiratory status.
	Follow MD orders.
	Patient's parents have been at bedside all night and are quite anxious— provide education as appropriate.

BM, bowel movement; ED, emergency department; GI, gastrointestinal; GU, genitourinary; IV, intravenous; Pt., patient; RR, respiratory rate; SOB, short of breath.

Exhibit 21.6	Initial Settings for Human Patient Simulator

- Simulation baby in crib: Setup of manikin/Display vital signs on monitor.
- Pulse oximetry—88%
- Heart rate: 160 beats/minute
- Respiratory rate—42 breaths/minute (with grunting)
- Inspiratory and expiratory wheezes and set to have intercostal retractions
- Lips cyanotic
- Information on cards: Nasal flaring
- Lubricant for nose to create nasal mucus
- O_2 on at 1–2 L FiO_2 via a mask

Physician Orders

Physician orders/chart information (initial):

1. Admit to pulmonary unit
2. Diet—regular as tolerated
3. Vital signs (VS) every 2 hours
4. Strict intake and output
5. Maintain peripheral IV in right arm
6. Cardiorespiratory monitor with continuous pulse oximetry
7. Administer oxygen 1 to 3 L FiO_2 to maintain SpO_2 >93%
8. Albuterol metered-dose inhaler (MDI: 90 mg/puff) 6 puffs every 2 hours
9. Arrange for parents to attend asthma class before discharge
10. Flu vaccine before discharge

Physician orders to be given when student has contacted the doctor about Jake's (patient) present respiratory status:

1. Begin IV fluids of D5 ¼ normal saline (NS) + 20 mEq KCl/L IV and PO (per os) to equal 45 mL/hr
2. Administer methylprednisolone (SoluMedrol) 24 mg IV STAT
3. Methylprednisolone 12 mg IV every 12 hours (12 hours after the initial loading dose)

The monitor displays changes as students interact with the patient:

- Increase oxygen to 2 L/min FiO_2, SpO_2 increases to 87%
- Increase oxygen to 3 L/min FiO_2, SpO_2 increases from 88% to 89%
- Provide Albuterol inhaler, SpO_2 increases to 90%; respirations increase to 65 breaths/minute
- Administer methylprednisolone (SoluMedrol); SpO_2 increases to 95%; pulse decreases to 130 beats/minute; respirations 40; baby coos.

Required student assessments and action:

1. Obtain baseline RR and repeat RR after treatment, if treatment is given, RR will decrease to 32 after treatment.
2. Assess and describe breath sounds; determine baseline before and after treatment, if treatment is given (wheezing will continue).
3. Student will use bulb or wall suction to clear Jake's nasal passages.
4. Student will not leave Jake's bedside.

5. Note Jake's nasal flaring, work of breathing (WOB), grunting, and retractions (this will be done in students description of assessment findings).
6. Assess level of consciousness (LOC), baseline at which the child is irritable before and after treatment; he is lethargic.
7. Administer Albuterol MDI as ordered.
8. Increase FiO_2 from 1 to 3 L (pulse oximetry only increases to 90% after O_2 increase and respiratory treatment).
9. Call respiratory therapist or doctor from phone in room.
10. Work with parent to address the child's crying related to hunger and thirst.

Facilitator Interventions

You can provide cues when phone call is made to the physician (or pediatric NP [nurse practitioner] or CNS [clinical nurse specialist]) or respiratory therapist.

> **Standardized patient (SP):** While serving as the mom or dad, please discuss your fears about the child's difficulty breathing with the nurse(s).
>
> **Parent instructions:** You are the parent of Jake, who is a toddler in the hospital with diagnosis of an acute exacerbation of asthma. Has had asthma in the past, diagnosed at 5 months of age—it is usually controlled with breathing treatments. It is 8:00 in the morning and you came to the emergency department (ED) around 10:00 last night.

On admission, Jake was receiving continuous nebulizer treatments and has now transitioned to a dose every 2 hours.

The 8 a.m. assessment revealed normal VS and the child appeared comfortable. The baby HPS will be used as Jake (your baby). He will be on an oxygen mask or nasal cannula.

The nurse enters the room to administer the 10 a.m. inhaler spacer treatment and perform the 10 a.m. assessment (Jake's VS will have changed from the previous nurse visit).

Jake will be wheezing, grunting, and have nasal congestion. His nostrils will be flaring (he is trying to get more air in), and his lips will be blue. He also will have retractions in his lung area (all of these symptoms mean that he is in respiratory distress). You will appear anxious and upset because your baby seems to be getting worse again. The nurse will need to give the baby a breathing treatment to help him.

When asked **"How is Jake doing?"** (or a similarly phrased question):

- **Say:** Jake is acting restless and irritable. It looks like he is working hard to breathe.
- **Say:** His lips are blue...oh my...what does that mean?

The nurse will take VS. **If he or she does not respond in a timely manner in performing a VS assessment:**

- **Say:** Nurse, I am worried, he isn't looking well...you have to help him.
- **Say:** "I don't know what is going on and I am afraid!"
- **Say:** "The monitor is beeping, what does that mean?"

If/when given medication:

- **Ask:** How does the medicine work? Why will that medicine help my child?

Jake was hospitalized yesterday evening and has been very lethargic. He has not been eating or drinking since his arrival to the hospital. He loves his bottle, and has not been able to drink it since he got to the hospital. Now he is crying and you think he is hungry. You want to feed him and are upset because he is crying. His diaper will be dry, indicating that he is dehydrated. You will ask the nurse about wanting to get him a bottle, and feel upset because of his dry diaper and crying (seeming to be hungry).

- **Say:** "Nurse, He seems to be hungry. He's crying and I think I need to give him his bottle of milk. He hasn't wet his diaper in a while, so I know he needs to eat."

Formative Evaluative Criteria

See Appendix B for the critical actions that are expected to be demonstrated by the two students who actively participated in the scenario.

J. INTRODUCTION OF SCENARIO: SCENARIO 3

Setting the Scene

Scenario 3. An infant receiving a well-child checkup

Technology Used

Medium to high-fidelity simulator with VS capability and fontanel, if available. Exhibit 21.7 outlines the other equipment needs and used for this scenario.

Objectives

1. Perform a well-child focused developmental assessment (using *Maxishare Milestones: A Growth and Development Guide* [Children's Hospital of Wisconsin, 2004]).
2. Perform a growth assessment, including height, weight, head circumference, and nutrition. Exhibit 21.8 provides specifics on the patient as recorded in their chart.
3. Obtain child's health history, including (a) general health; (b) eating; (c) sleeping; (d) play; (e) temperament; (f) immunizations; (g) vitamin supplements including fluoride; (h) elimination.
4. Discuss upcoming developmental milestones for child.
5. Teach the parent about immunization and the current American Academy of Pediatrics immunization schedule.

Description of Participants

Participants are student nurses providing direct care for the child and parent; parent (mother or father) present (only one parent is present, not both); patient (a well, older infant); student observers.

Exhibit 21.7	Equipment Needed

Current CDC or WHO growth charts for children 0 to 36 months

Current CDC vaccination schedules

A published or online drug guide for nurses or access to an online drug formulary such as the Lexicomp Online | Clinical Drug Information and the *Maxishare Milestones: A Growth and Development Guide* (Children's Hospital of Wisconsin, 2004) or another growth and developmental guide

Stethoscope

Oral thermometer

A mock immunization record that reports that the child has had appropriate immunizations for months 2 and 4, **but not** month 6

K. RUNNING OF THE SCENARIO

A 9-month-old infant is receiving a well-child checkup. The child is not up to date with immunizations and parent has concerns regarding immunizations. Parent is also feeding child whole milk instead of formula. The infant, Joseph DiGiacamo, is the youngest of three children, with a 3-year-old brother (Tyler) and a 5-year-old sister (Aurora), who live at home with their mom, dad, and their pug, Princess. Both parents work. Mom has an established day-care center in her home and is so busy with the children in her day care that she sometimes gets a little overwhelmed with all of the children. Dad is a businessman who travels a significant amount of the time. Because of traveling, Dad knows some information, but sometimes is unclear with the details.

L. PRESENTATION OF COMPLETED TEMPLATE

Title

Nursing Care and Assessment of 9-Month-Old Receiving a Well-Child Checkup

Senario Level and Focus Area

Senior-level course: Health Care of Children and Adolescents

Scenario Description

This scenario introduces the concepts of growth and development; growth assessment, including height, weight, head circumference, and nutrition assessment; immunization status as well as overall well-child care needs to the students learning the care of well children. The nursing students' goal is to take a complete and accurate health history of the child as reported by the primary caregiver.

Setting the Scene and Scenario Implementation

Prebriefing: 10 minutes
Expected activity run time: 20 minutes
Debriefing: 20 to 30 minutes

Clincial Course of the Simulated Scenario

Students are expected to come prepared having completed the written preparation questions (see text that follows). Prebriefing includes an orientation to the environment, reviewing expectations, determining roles, and getting a patient report. Following prebriefing, the facilitator, who is usually a faculty member, is in the control room.

Student preparation to be completed before the simulation:

1. What are the developmental milestones you should inquire about and/or physically see in a healthy 9-month-old?
2. What are the next set of developmental milestones you are likely to see for a 9-month-old child?
3. When would you be concerned, or what would concern you, about milestones missed in a 9-month-old's development? If a 9-month-old has not met all of the developmental milestones, when would you consider a referral to a specialist and to whom would you refer?
4. What immunizations are necessary for a 9-month-old? What side effects are the most common? How would you educate the caregivers about the management of side effects of immunizations? How would you deal with a situation in which the parent expresses concern about the possible link

between immunizations and autism? How would you handle a caregiver who refuses immunizations? How would you explain the importance of immunizations?

5. What are the nutritional needs of a child this age? Are there any changes in needs from a 9-month-old to a 12-month-old?

6. What are the possible nutritional causes of anemia in an infant?

Additional Student Preparation Requirements

1. Review of *Maxishare Milestones: A Growth and Development Guide* (Children's Hospital of Wisconsin, 2004) or another child developmental guide for developmental milestones for a 9-month-old child (students are expected to bring the *Maxishare Milestones: A Growth and Development Guide* to the simulation). Exhibit 21.9 provides Milestones expected for a 9-Month-Old.

2. Read a pediatric theory text on the growth and development of a 9-month-old infant.

3. An infant HPS will be used in this scenario. The infant will be sleeping during assessment; apical heart rate (AHR) will be 100; and RR will be 24. Height, weight, and head circumference will be plotted on a growth chart. Growth chart will already have these measurements from birth, and at the 2-month and 4-month visits (6-month checkup data are missing). The baby will also have a pacifier around its neck on a string (a safety hazard). Mom/dad will answer questions. They will make light of the fact that 6-month immunizations were missed. The child's level of development will be normal except for 6-month missed immunizations.

Physician Orders

1. Complete a physical examination, including VS, height, weight, head circumference, and nutrition.

2. Obtain child's health history, including (a) general health, (b) eating, (c) sleeping, (d) play, (e) temperament, (f) immunizations, (g) use of vitamins/fluoride, (h) elimination patterns, (i) home safety assessment. Exhibit 21.8 provides specifics on the patient as recorded in their chart.

Required Student Assessments and Actions

Safety assessment: (a) ensure patient is in the parent's lap or on examination table with the parent's hand on the child, (b) assess for strangulation risk (pacifier string around neck), and (c) assess risk for medical equipment out of child's reach.

   Developmental assessment: using the *Maxishare Milestones: A Growth and Development Guide* (Children's Hospital of Wisconsin, 2004) or from the Centers for Disease and Control and Prevention (CDC; www.cdc.gov/ncbddd/actearly/milestones)

   Other assessments: Obtain and properly document height, weight, and head circumference on the correct growth chart that includes (a) obtain apical rate, RR, temperature; (b) evaluate apical rate, RR for age; (c) discuss 6-month immunizations after checking for allergies and obtaining consent; (d) teach the parent the importance of scheduled well visits and the immunization schedule (provide up-to-date information on the CDC's recommended immunization schedule; (e) provide resources available to the parent through the community, and provide well-child teaching and anticipatory guidance related to nutrition, sleep, development, safety, dental care, and use of fluoride.

Exhibit 21.8	Chart Information
Patient:	Joseph DiGiacomo (Patient is 9 months old at this visit)
DOB:	**4/25/XX**

Facilitator instructions: None
Parent/actor instructions:

You are the parent of Joseph. When asked, please respond as noted:

- *General health:* **Say:** He seems fine. He has not been sick.
- *Eating:* **Say:** He eats sometimes, but he is kind of picky. Not eating much of the toddler food. He takes a bottle pretty easily though.
    a. He feeds himself the bottle. (If asked, **say:** "Starting to drink from a cup, but easier to use bottle.")
    b. How many bottles per day: four bottles of "milk." If asked about what type of milk, you are feeding him whole milk. You are not giving him juice regularly—just now and then (if asked).
    c. (N.B. This will be a problem as the child is really too young for whole milk; he should still be getting formula. He should be eating toddler food: baby cereal with fruit in morning, food that is "mushy" with little bits of banana or soft vegetables in it for lunch and dinner. Maybe dry Cheerios for snacks).
- *Sleeping:* **Say:** He sleeps OK, only fussy when teething.
- *Play:* **Say:** We have a lot of toys from the other two kids and the day care. He likes to play with toys and big blocks.
- *Temperament:* **Say:** He is an easy baby; he does not cry much.
- *Immunizations:* You are behind on immunizations—as you missed the 6-month well-child visit. **Say:** Oh, did we miss his last visit? Oh, I didn't realize that…too much going on. I saw on the news about babies developing autism, and they think it is associated with the immunizations. I am kind of worried about that…maybe we shouldn't be giving him any more of the immunizations.
- *Take vitamins/meds?* Yes, takes liquid vitamins prescribed but no other meds.
- *Fluoride drops?* No. *Fluoride in water?* You do not know.
- *Voiding (urine)—How many diapers a day are changed for being wet?* Five to six diapers per day
- *Bowels (feces)? Does he have bowel movements each day?* Yes, once per day … it is usually formed (stool) and brownish in color.

Exhibit 21.9	Milestones for a 9-Month-Old

Your baby now can pull himself up to a standing position from sitting.

He can stand while holding onto someone or something.

Baby uses the "pincer grasp" holding tiny objects between his thumb and forefinger.

He can walk while holding onto furniture.

Baby drinks from a cup.

He can stand alone for a few seconds or perhaps longer.

Baby says "Mama" or "Dada."

He understands the meaning of "no."

Baby responds to simple commands (such as "Give Mommy the toy").

Actively participate in games such as "pat-a-cake" and "peekaboo," "so big," sing "One, Two, Buckle My Shoe"

Toys: Stacking, sorting and building toys; toys to enhance physical development such as standing and cruising; toys with dials and buttons; language development toys

The nurses will teach you about immunizations and may tell you what to expect from Joseph developmentally during the time between now and his next examination.

Formative Evaluative Criteria

See Appendix C for the critical actions that are expected to be demonstrated by two students who actively patriated in the scenario.

M. INTRODUCTION OF SCENARIO: SCENARIO 4

Setting the Scene

Scenario 4. A preschool-age child who is in the immediate postoperative recovery period

Technology Used

Medium-fidelity pediatric HPS. Exhibit 21.10 provides the list of equipment needed.
Resources needed: Drug guide for nurses or access to an online drug formulary, such as the Lexicomp Online | Clinical Drug Information

Exhibit 21.10	Equipment Needed

- Moulage placed on manikin's back to simulate a rash

- Identification bracelet with "Jose Chavez" and date of birth

- Steri-strips at site of laparoscopy (appendectomy)

- Noodle IV arm (right arm, see photo on p. 236) with IV pump with medication setup. Lactated Ringer's solution administered at 60 mL/hr

- Oxygen with mask attached to an oxygen setup, but not on the patient

- Wall computer with bedside chart information and ability to look up medications as needed

- Items in medication cart or medication drawer:

  ○ Tylenol suppository (325 mg is dose)

  ○ Liquid children's Tylenol (270 mg is dose)

  ○ Syringes of vancomycin 300 mg/60 mL

  ○ Vials—labeled morphine sulfate 2 mg/mL

  ○ Vials—labeled epinephrine 1:1,000

  ○ Vials—labeled epinephrine 1:10,000

  ○ Syringes—labeled diphenhydramine 25 mg/mL

- Postop orders

- Faces Pain Assessment Scale

IV, intravenous.

Objectives

1. Perform essential focused assessments on a 5-year-old child to ensure physical safety.
2. Interact and communicate with the child using age- and developmentally appropriate strategies.
3. Develop a plan of care for pediatric patient with complications following surgery.
4. Administer rectal, IV, and intramuscular medications to a preschool-aged child.
5. Evaluate changes in patient status and intervene appropriately.

Description of Participants

Participants are two student nurses who provide direct care for the patient, child HPS with someone acting as the voice of the child, parent at bedside, health care provider who is called regarding rash on child's back, student observers.

N. RUNNING THE SCENARIO

Jose Chavez is a 5-year old boy who has just been transferred from the postanesthesia care unit (PACU) to the pediatric medical–surgical unit following a laparoscopic appendectomy. Jose was brought into the ED by his parent; Jose was experiencing right lower abdomen pain suggestive of symptoms of appendicitis. While in the ED his appendix ruptured and he was immediately taken to surgery for a laparoscopic appendectomy.

O. PRESENTATION OF COMPLETED TEMPLATE

Title

A Preschool-Age Child in the Immediate Postoperative Period

Scenario Level/Focus Area

Senior level: Health Care of Children and Adolescents

Scenario Description

This scenario introduces concepts and nursing care interventions to safely and effectively care for a child who is recovering from abdominal surgery who subsequently experiences a reaction to an antibiotic prescribed related to a ruptured appendix.

Setting the Scene and Scenario Implementation

> **Prebriefing:** 10 minutes
> **Expected activity run time:** 20 minutes
> **Debriefing:** 20 to 30 minutes

Clinical Course of the Simulated Scenario

Students are expected to come prepared having completed the written preparation questions (see text that follows). Prebriefing includes an orientation to the environment, reviewing expectations, determining roles, and getting a patient report. Following prebriefing, the facilitator, who is usually a faculty member, is in the control room.

Students should know the following information before the scenario:

1. What is the pathophysiology of appendicitis?
2. Discuss normal postoperative care for a child who has undergone abdominal surgery.
3. What complications are associated with abdominal surgery in children?
4. What complications are associated with a ruptured appendix?
5. What are the potential complications of antibiotic medications?
6. Discuss interventions for treating an allergic reaction related to antibiotic therapy.
7. How is pain assessed in a preschooler?
8. Discuss the expected Erikson developmental stage for a preschool child.

Chart Information

Students will receive a report before the start of the scenario including a verbal report (see Exhibit 21.11 for the SBAR Communication), Laboratory Values, and Providers Orders (See Exhibit 21.12).

Laboratory Values

- Chemistry panel with the following results: Sodium: 140 (N = 138–145 mEq/L), potassium: 4.0 (N = 3.5–5 mEq/L), creatinine: 0.3 mg/dL (N = 0.3–0.7 mg/dL), glucose: 80 mg/dL (N = 60–100 mg/dL)
- Complete blood count (CBC) with the following results: white blood cell (WBC): 16,000 mm^3 (N = 5.5–15.5 [×10^3/μL]), hemoglobin: 13.5 (N = 11.5–15.5 g/dL), hematocrit: 40 (N = 35–45 %), neutrophil count: 79% (N = 54–62%), platelets: 200 (N = 150–400)
- WBC result: 16,000 (N = 5.5–15.5); patient's weight is on chart: 20 kg.

Exhibit 21.11	SBAR Communication
Situation	Jose Chavez is a 5-year-old male who was just transferred from the PACU to our floor (pediatric surgical unit) and had a laparoscopic appendectomy 3 hours ago.
Background	Patient is a full code. Allergic to penicillin. Diagnosed with acute appendicitis and had a laparoscopic appendectomy 3 hours ago. Procedure went well. Recovery in PACU was normal.
Assessment	Patient assessment upon transfer to our unit.
	Neuro: Patient just beginning to wake up. He is very groggy but can state his name. Last temp was 98.8°F (37.1°C) complaining of slight pain—rating it a 2 out of 10.
	CV: HR is 90 beats/minute, BP: 96/66 mmHg. Good cap refill, less than 3 seconds. Good extremity pulses (+2).
	R: Breath sounds are clear. RR = 18 breaths/minute. No adventitious sounds.
	GI: Pt. has steri-strips at surgical site, which is clear, dry, and intact. No bowel sounds yet. Pt. is withheld from fluids/solids by mouth (NPO).
	GU: Pt. has not urinated since transfer to our floor.
	Skin: IV in R forearm is patent. IV fluids infusing at 60 mL/hr.
Recommendation	Follow standard postop care (as per institution's standards of care).
	MD orders are at the bedside.
	Educate parents to post-op care and the role they can play.

BP, blood pressure; CV, cardiovascular; GI, gastrointestinal; GU, genitourinary; HR, heart rate; IV, intravenous; NPO, nothing per os; Pt., patient; PACU, postanesthesia care unit; R, respiratory; RR, respiratory rate.

Exhibit 21.12	Provider Orders

1. Admit to pediatric surgical unit

2. Vital signs every 4 hours

3. Cardiorespiratory monitor with continuous pulse oximetry

4. IV: Lactated Ringer's at 60 mL/hr

5. Vancomycin 300-mg IV every 6 hours; begin upon transfer to unit

6. Morphine 1-mg IV every 2 hours as needed for pain

7. Acetaminophen 270-mg oral every 4 hours as needed for temperature greater than 38.3°C (100.94°F)

8. Acetaminophen 350 mg rectally every 4 hours as needed for temperature greater than 38.3°C (100.94°F)

9. Diet: NPO

10. Activity: Ambulate three times per day

IV, intravenous; NPO, nothing per os.

Initial Settings for Human Patient Simulator

A 5-year-old-sized HPS will be used and will present with the following VS at the start of the scenario: Temp: 38.5°C (101.3°F), heart rate: 82 beats/minute, RR: 18 breaths/minute, and blood pressure: 94/66 mmHg.

Verbal orders to be given when student calls provider regarding patient's reaction to the vancomycin are listed in Exhibit 21.13.

Exhibit 21.13	Verbal Orders

1. Discontinue vancomycin.

2. Administer epinephrine 1:1,000 solution 0.2 mL subcutaneously stat (0.01 mL/kg/dose).

3. Administer diphenhydramine 20 mg IV stat and q 6 hours as needed for complaints of itching.

4. Take VS every 15 minutes until stable.

IV, intravenous; q, every; VS, vital signs.

HPS settings change as students work through the scenario:

- If the student administers Tylenol (acetaminophen), temperature changes after 1 minute to: 37.9°C.
- After patient receives vancomycin, SPO$_2$ decreases to 87%; patient is wheezing and complains of itching.
- If action is taken, and epinephrine is administered, oxygen saturation increases to 93%, and the breath sounds are now clear.

Required student assessments and action:

1. Complete bedside safety assessment: two-patient identifier, IV fluids (correct solution and rate), IV catheter site assessment, bedside equipment (function of monitors and correct setting limits; position of bed height and side rails; functioning oxygen equipment and bag/mask).

2. Perform physical assessment reflective of typical assessment parameters for a 4-year-old child.
3. Evaluate VS and interpret findings.
4. Assess pain using appropriate pain evaluation scale for age.
5. Assess surgical site.
6. Assess infusion site.
7. Communicate effectively and educate patient and family using developmentally appropriate terminology.

Identify symptoms of allergic response and perform the following:

1. Stay with the patient, stop infusion of vancomycin.
2. Notify health care provider of changes in patient status using ISBAR communication technique (identify, situation, background, assessment, recommendation; Thomas, Bertram, & Johnson, 2009).
3. Mantain ongoing evaluation of respiratory status.
4. Apply allergy band on patient.
5. Document vancomycin allergy and notify pharmacy.

Initiate appropriate interventions:

1. Administer acetaminophen per rectum (PR) using the six rights (a) right dose, (b) right indication, (c) right route, (d) right mediation, (e) right patient, (f) right time of medication administration.
2. Administer morphine sulfate (IV/intramuscular [IM]/intravenous piggyback [IVPB]) using the six rights of medication administration and two-RN checks.
3. Administer vancomycin (IV) using the six rights of medication administration.
4. Administer epinephrine (IM) using the six rights of medication and two-RN checks.
5. Draw up medication and label it with the patient's name and name of drug before administering it to the patient.
6. Encourage coughing/deep breathing and ambulation.
7. Explain reason for nothing per os (NPO) status.
8. Reevaluate response to antipyretic, pain medication, and epinephrine.

Patient Actor Instructions

Facilitator interventions: Assume the role of health care provider or any other person with whom the students need to collaborate.

Patient instructions: Almost immediately you demonstrate signs of a postop blood infection with an oral temperature of 38.5 C° (101.3°F). You **say:** "I feel hot, Mommy, can I have something to drink?" The nurse will need to give the patient (you) Tylenol for this fever. Tylenol should be given rectally (a suppository). If the students attempt to administer it orally—you **say:** "Oh, good, I can have something to drink now." When the nurse attempts to administer the suppository, you **say:** "NO! Mommy, I'm afraid that's going to hurt."

You are ordered an antibiotic postop, which the nurse should prepare to administer. Once administered, you experience an allergic reaction and **say:** "My back is itchy and I can't breathe." The nurse will give you medication (epinephrine), which will clear these symptoms—they may also put oxygen on you. For your pain, they will ask you to point to a scale with happy or sad faces to demonstrate your level of pain. Your pain level is high, so a "sadder face" will be selected on the Faces Pain Scale. You can indicate a face on the scale that corresponds to a numerical rating of "8."

Parent Actor Instructions

When Jose is asked how he is doing, let Jose speak first then you can also **say:** (a) I am relieved that Jose did well in surgery, (b) I am concerned about Jose's pain but expected him to have some, (c) he feels WARM to me. (You touch his forehead.)

Past History

You know your son is allergic to penicillin. (If asked, please **say:** "He got a terrible rash after taking penicillin once for an ear infection when he was 2.")

There is no other remarkable medical history. This is the first time Jose has ever been in the hospital. All pediatric appointments are normal. Only if asked indicate that the patient is adopted so there is no family medical history.

As the nurse enters the room she will observe and do the following:

Child appears very warm and has a recorded temperature of 38.5 C (101.3 F) and will touch the HPS and say that the patient feels warm:

- VS: Temperature of 38.5°C (101.3°F).
- You should touch the HPS and say that patient feels warm to you.
- You (the parent) will appear relieved that surgery went well, you can be "mildly concerned" about temp and your son's complaints of pain.

Nurse will most likely ask the patient about the pain. Anticipate the nurse to:

- Show the HPS a FACES pain chart. (The patient will indicate that he feels like the sad face and/or has a pain score of "8.")
- You should indicate that he pointed to the "8."
- Nurse may ask more questions to help describe and quantify the pain.
- Nurse should also allay your concerns—as postop pain and postop temperature are not uncommon. Nurse should also mention that patient has a temperature.
- Nurse should go to get ordered medicines for your son that include drugs for pain, fever, and antibiotics.

Medication Administration

1. Administer Tylenol rectally for fever.

   Regarding rectal Tylenol: Your child will respond by acting scared or in disbelief that he needs to have medicine in his "bottom." You can reassure him and help roll him over.

   If the nurse attempts to administer Tylenol oral elixir—you can **say:** " I didn't think he could drink anything yet. Is it okay if I give him some juice, too?"

2. Morphine IV for pain

   Regarding morphine: "What will it do to him? I hope it helps."

3. Antibiotics

   Regarding antibiotic that will be hung on the IV line:

   If nurse does not tell you why she is administering the antibiotic—you can **say:** "What's that medicine for?"

Allergic Reaction

Once the antibiotics begin to infuse, your son will have an allergic reaction. This will include behaviors or complaints from him that include "itchiness on the back" and some difficulty breathing. On the nurse's assessment may also note that his pulse-oximetry level has dropped and that he is wheezing—both suggest a severe reaction. The nurse should stop the infusion immediately and place the oxygen mask on your child and call the doctor immediately.

You should appear to be fearful and scared. **Say:** "Is everything okay?

If asked about any known allergies:

Say: "I know he is allergic to penicillin, but my son is adopted and we do not have family history." You have no further information about other known allergies.

The nurse will administer a subcutaneous injection to your son to stop the allergic reaction—this medication improves Jose's breathing and lessens his itching.

Additional information:

Nurses should interact with the child in an age-appropriate manner. The nurse may use distraction techniques in an attempt to lessen Jose's perception of pain. You may **say:** "Let's watch your favorite TV show on the computer." You can also try to divert by telling him he did really well. Suggest that when he is feeling better you will take him to his favorite place for pizza.

Formative Evaluative Criteria

See Appendix D for the critical actions that are expected to be demonstrated by the two students who actively patriated in the scenario.

P. DEBRIEFING GUIDELINES

For each of these pediatric SBLEs, the structured debriefing method, debriefing for meaningful learning (DML), is used (Dreifuerst, 2011, 2015) in accordance with International Association for Clinical Simulation and Learning (INACSL) Standard VI: Debriefing (Decker et al., 2013). This method informs the debriefing discussion to include prior experiences, educational preparation, reflection, and the current clinical situation in order to guide students' development of the knowledge, skills, and attitudes necessary to be an effective and safe nurse. According to Dreifuerst (2011), this debriefing method supports development of metacognition, leads to a stronger conceptual understanding and application of the nursing process within the context of patient care, and potentiates meaningful learning through a change in clinical reasoning and clinical judgment. To implement the DML method, Dreifuerst developed a series of worksheets that students complete both alone and together with the simulation facilitator (faculty member). The first worksheet, immediately completed following each scenario, asks the following questions: *a. What is the first thing that comes to mind about this simulation experience? b. What went right and why? c. What would you do differently and why?* In addition, this worksheet asks the students to frame the client's story. The next phase of the DML focuses on students' reflection on their thinking-in-action, thinking-on action, and later thinking-beyond-action, which includes specific reflective questions for each category. During this phase, the faculty facilitator and students complete a concept map, which helps them focus on these key problems. The next worksheet focuses on each major nursing diagnosis or problem identified in the scenario and students are asked to complete information about nursing interventions, expected client responses, and an evaluation and summary of client progress toward desired outcome(s). During all phases, students are questioned using the Socratic and other methods to assist them to create new, different, or enhanced frames of mind.

Q. SUGGESTIONS/KEY FEATURES
TO REPLICATE OR IMPROVE

Key features to replicate and improve these scenarios would be the consistent adherence to the "INACSL Standards of Best Practice: Simulation^{SM}" (INACSL, 2013/2016; Lioce et al., 2015). Continued updating of these scenarios is warranted as these standards are updated. A specific feature to improve on is further development of scripts for SPs and facilitators to improve the fidelity of the scenarios across student groups.

R. RECOMMENDATIONS FOR FURTHER USE

One recommendation we offer is engaging students in the observer role so as to create an active learning experience for them. In the observer role, students critically examine observed behaviors for evidence that these critical behaviors are demonstrated and use the checklist customized for each scenario to guide their observations. The observer tool (checklist) for each scenario is provided in the appendices. It must be emphasized to these students that they are expected to actively participate in the debriefing using their observations to enhance the discussion of the patient and/or situation(s) and their focused observations of the enactments of scenario are critical to the group's learning.

S. HOW SIMULATION-BASED PEDAGOGY HAS CONTRIBUTED TO IMPROVED STUDENT OUTCOMES

With the inception of these scenarios and for several years following, the scenarios were evaluated each semester among all learners (students) who participated in them. Ten questions were asked, four were on a 5-point Likert-type scale and five were open ended and included those in Exhibit 21.14.

Findings to these questions provided a robust, positive assessment of students' appraisal of the scenarios. Based on students' evaluations and faculty feedback, changes have been made to enhance the scenarios to make them accurate and reflective of current practice standards of care. Specifically, they have been updated according to practice changes with a greater emphasis on medication administration, increased fidelity to actual patient situation, SP role—educating them and providing instructions related to how to give feedback. The scenarios have been enhanced by including a parent(s) role and voices to HPS responses.

Exhibit 21.14	Survey of the Simulation Experience

1. The prep materials for this simulation experience helped me to prepare for my roles in the scenarios.

2. The scenarios seemed realistic to me while I was participating.

3. The scenarios provided me an opportunity to practice critical thinking skills.

4. I think I will be better able to perform in a related clinical situation after participating in these scenarios.

5. I understood my role in the scenario. My role was: [student provide response]

6. The debriefing sessions helped me to understand the clinical situations and the most appropriate actions to take.

7. Overall, I think this was a valuable experience.

8. What was most helpful/beneficial about this scenario? [open-ended response]

9. What did you like LEAST about this scenario? [open-ended response]

10. In what ways could this scenario be improved? [open-ended response]

T. EXPERT RECOMMENDATIONS AND WORDS OF WISDOM

As standards of best practices evolve, these scenarios should be revised and updated to reflect the state of the science in simulation pedagogy. The scheduling of these scenarios to reflect what has been taught in the companion theory course and allowing a sufficient amount of practice experience in the actual practice settings are always considerations for optimal student learning in these SBLEs. The preparation and the prebriefing, especially having students view "the scene" before the implementation of the scenarios, enhances learning and decreases students' anxiety.

U. EVALUATION OF BEST PRACTICE STANDARDS AND USE OF CREDENTIALED SIMULATION FACULTY

These scenarios were developed, revised, and are implemented under the guidance of a simulation-based expert who holds a Certified Healthcare Simulation Educator certificate. Having this expert involved in these scenarios is essential to their quality and rigor. The objectives of each scenario reflect and support the objectives of the clinical practicum course in which these scenarios are implemented. Of the American Association of Colleges of Nursing (AACN; 2008) nine BSN Essentials, these scenarios met the following:

Essential II: Basic Organizational and Systems Leadership for Quality Care and Patient Safety
Essential VI: Interprofessional Communication and Collaboration for Improving Patient Health Outcomes
Essential IX: Baccalaureate Generalist Nursing Practice.

REFERENCES

American Association of Colleges of Nursing. (2008). *The essentials of baccalaureate education for professional nursing practice*. Washington, DC: Author. Retrieved from http://www.aacnnursing.org/Portals/42/Publications/BaccEssentials08.pdf

Children's Hospital of Wisconsin. (2004). *Maxishare milestones: A growth and development guide* (6th ed.). Milwaukee, WI: Maxishare, Seeger Health Resources.

Decker, S., Fey, M., Sideras, S., Caballero, S., Rockstraw, L., Boese, T., . . . Borum, J. C. (2013). Standards of best practice: Simulation standard VI: The debriefing process. *Clinical Simulation in Nursing, 9*(Suppl. 6), S26–S29. doi:10.1016/j.ecns.2013.04.008

Dreifuerst, K. T. (2011). Debriefing for meaningful learning: A reflective strategy to foster clinical reasoning. *Clinical Simulation in Nursing, 7*(6), e250. doi:10.1016/j.ecns.2011.09.023

Dreifuerst, K. T. (2015). Getting started with debriefing for meaningful learning. *Clinical Simulation in Nursing, 11*(5), 268–275. doi:10.1016/j.ecns.2015.01.005

International Nursing Association for Clinical Simulation and Learning. (2013, updated 2016). INACSL standards of best practice: Simulation. Retrieved from https://www.inacsl.org/i4a/pages/index.cfm?pageID=3407

Lioce, L., Meakim, C. H., Fey, M. K., Chmil, J. V., Mariani, B., & Alinier, G. (2015). Standards of best practice: Simulation standard IX: Simulation design. *Clinical Simulation in Nursing, 11*(6), 309–315.

Thomas, C. M., Bertram, E., & Johnson, D. (2009). The SBAR communication technique. *Nurse Educator, 34*(4), 176–180. doi:10.1097/NNE.0b013e3181aaba54

APPENDIX A

Scenario 1. Nursing Care of the Adolescent With Sickle Cell Anemia

Student Observer Tool

Criteria	Done/Time	Comments

Identifies self and patient

Uses hand hygiene

Completes assessment of safety checks (rescue equipment available [Ambu bag, oxygen supplies]), bed in locked position, parameters of monitors, intravenous solutions (correct solution and rate); allergy alert bracelet (if applicable); side rails properly up; fall risk bracelet (if applicable).

Asks appropriate history questions to include:

- Two patient identifiers (medical record number and name)
- Onset of symptoms
- Pain history
- Treatment of pain at home
- Previous number of hospitalizations
- History of CVA
- Temperature history

Assesses patient for:

- Pain; location, duration, level, temperature
- Abdomen for tenderness (not too deeply)
- LOC, headache, dizziness, speech, use of arms and legs, pupillary response to light
- Respiratory: pulse ox, RR, WOB, grunting, nasal flaring, chest retraction
- Fluid balance: weight, mucous membranes, tenting, check IV site and IV fluids, check urine specific gravity, check I &O sheet

Interventions:

- Administers morphine sulfate as ordered
- Teach patient about PCA pump
- Drew up medication and labelled it before going to give to patient (with patient's name and name of drug)
- Checks for compatibility of medication with IV solution

(continued)

(continued)

Criteria	Done/Time	Comments
• Administers Tylenol as ordered		
• Provides other comfort measures: back massage, heating pad, guided imagery		
• Provides or asks to give chest PT and incentive spirometry treatment		

CVA, cerebral vascular attack; I&O, intake and output; IV, intravenous; LOC, level of consciousness; PCA, patient-controlled analgesia; PT, physical therapy; RR, respiratory rate; WOB, work of breathing.

APPENDIX B

Scenario 2. Young Child With an Acute Asthma Exacerbation

Student Observer Tool

Criteria	Done/Time	Comments
Obtains baseline RR and repeat a RR assessment after treatment.		
Assesses and describes breath sounds, determining baseline and assessing after treatment, if treatment is given.		
Student uses bulb suction to clear Jake's nasal passages.		
Student does not leave Jake.		
Student notes Jake's nasal flaring, WOB, grunting, and retractions (this will be seen in students description of assessment findings).		
Calls respiratory therapist from phone in room.		
Calls physician as needed.		
Assess LOC—at baseline (initial) assessment reveals the child is irritable and after treatment he is lethargic.		
Administers Ventolin as ordered.		
Increases FiO_2 to 50%.		
Discusses dry diaper and mother's concerns of child not drinking.		
Provides support to mother as needed.		

LOC, level of consciousness; RR, respiratory rate; WOB, work of breathing.

APPENDIX C

Scenario 3. An Infant Receiving a Well-Child Checkup

Student Observer Tool

Criteria	Done/Time	Comments
Performs developmental assessment using *Maxishare Milestones: A Growth and Development Guide* (Children's Hospital of Wisconsin, 2004) or another child developmental guide		
Assesses the following:		
• Gross motor skills		
• Fine motor skills		
• Cognitive skills		
• Play		
• Social development		
Obtains health history, including:		
• Eating		
• Sleeping		
• Toys		
• Discipline		
• General health		
• Immunizations		
• Obtains and properly documents height, weight, head circumference.		
• Obtains apical rate and RR.		
• Evaluates apical rate, RR for age.		
Discusses 6-month immunizations after checking for allergies and obtaining consent.		
Teaches parent importance of scheduled well visits and immunization schedule.		
Teaches parents about specific immunizations using the vaccine information sheets.		
Provides resources available to mother through the community.		
Provides well-child teaching, proper nutrition, sleep, development, safety, and so on.		

RR, respiratory rate.

APPENDIX D

Scenario 4. A Preschool-Aged Child Who Is in the Immediate Postoperative Recovery Period
Student Observer Tool

Criteria	Done/Time	Comments
Completes bed side safety assessment (using two patient identifiers): intravenous fluids (correct solution and rate), intravenous catheter site assessment, bedside equipment (function of monitors and correct limit settings, position of bed height and side rails).		
Performs physical assessment on 5-year-old.		
Evaluates vital signs and interprets findings.		
Assesses pain using appropriate tool.		
Assesses surgical site.		
Assesses infusion site.		
Communicates effectively with patient and family using developmentally appropriate terminology.		
Identifies patient's and family's potential emotional distress and describes supportive measures.		
Identifies symptoms of allergic response.		
Stays with patient; turns off vancomycin.		
Notifies health care provider of changes in patient status using ISBAR.		
Performs ongoing evaluation of respiratory status.		
Outs allergy band on patient.		
Documents vancomycin allergy and notifies pharmacy.		

Interventions:

- Administers acetaminophen PRN using the six rights of medication administration.
- Administers morphine sulfate using the six rights of medication administration and a two-RN check.
- Administers vancomycin using the six rights of medication administration.
- Administers epinephrine using the six rights of medication administration and a two-RN check.

(continued)

(continued)

Criteria	Done/Time	Comments
Drew up medication and labelled it before administering it to the patient (with patient's name and name of drug).		
Encourages coughing/deep breathing/ambulation.		
Explains reason for NPO status.		
• **Reevaluates** response to anti-pyretic, pain medicine, and epinephrine.		
Communicates effectively with patient and family regarding changes in patient status and treatment modalities.		

ISBAR, identify, situation, background, assessment, recommendation, NPO, nothing per os; PRN, as needed.

CHAPTER 22

Preparing Prelicensure Nursing Students for Clinical Practice in Pediatric Acute Care Settings and Interprofessional In Situ Simulation

Maureen M. Ryan and Melissa Holland

A. IMPLEMENTATION OF SIMULATION-BASED PEDAGOGY IN YOUR INDIVIDUALIZED TEACHING AREA

Within the collaborative curriculum at the University of Victoria (UVic), pediatric theory is taught in the classroom and psychomotor skills laboratory and applied in a variety of community and inpatient settings in the first 2 years of the program. However, more than two thirds of the student population do not have the opportunity to practice "hands-on" nursing care in acute care pediatric units before entering clinical practice in their senior year. As nursing education continues to evolve, there is the ongoing question as to whose responsibility it is to support preparation for nursing within specialty areas—academia or practice (Campbell & Lloyd, 2005; Chua, Mackey, Ng, & Liaw, 2013; Rosser, 2015)?

A partnership was developed between the faculty at the School of Nursing, UVic, and the nurse leaders at the Island Health Authority (IH), Vancouver Island, British Columbia, to address a mutual concern—how to prepare senior nursing students for acute pediatric nursing care? In our setting, twice a year, our generalist pediatric unit at Victoria General receives prelicensure nursing students who have transitioned into semiindependent practice practicums; students work under direct supervision of a staff nurse, following the nurse's shift pattern, and are assessed by a clinical instructor from the university who meets with them after each set of shifts to evaluate their progress.

Simulation pedagogy has been integrated into our pediatric clinical placements with low-fidelity simulation as a key tool for transitioning to this specialty area. High-fidelity simulation is then used as part of the evaluation process as the semester progresses, which sets the students up for successful participation in interprofessional simulation experiences that take place in situ within the pediatric and pediatric intensive care unit (PICU) settings at Victoria General Hospital (and described in Chapter 48). UVic School of Nursing created my (Maureen Ryan) faculty position clinical simulation coordinator responsible for instilling simulation pedagogy in the BSN curriculum. I (Maureen) am a certified trainer providing simulation training, support, and evaluation to a team of clinical instructors including Melissa Holland (coauthor) in the prelicensure program. In addition, simulation learning events in clinical practice are situated within the Canadian Association of Schools of Nursing (CASN; 2015) guidelines for simulation and clinical practice and meet the International Nursing Association for Clinical Simulation and Learning (INACSL) Standards of Best Practice: Simulation^SM from recommended design standards through to participant evaluation and professional integrity (INACSL, 2013/2016).

C. SPECIFIC OBJECTIVES, INTRODUCTION OF SCENARIO, AND RUNNING OF THE SCENARIO

Low-Fidelity Simulation—Orientation

Before entering practice on the pediatric in-patient units, there is an expectation of students' self-directed review of introduced pediatric theory and skills in years 1 and 2 before participating in a low-fidelity simulation learning event for a "hands-on" review of pediatric nursing practice. We use a multipurpose clinical teaching space with a crib rolled in to facilitate a clinical setup. As much as possible, hospital pajamas, linens, and basic supplies are used to support familiarity with products used within the clinical setting, depending on the age and stage of different pediatric patients. Our orientation events focus on concepts that will require critical thinking to transfer knowledge from previous adult settings to the unique pediatric setting.

Learning Objectives

1. To review senior nursing students' psychomotor skills and family-centered care practices
2. To orientate and ensure senior nursing students' readiness for pediatric practices in a semi-independent role at IH

Each session commences with a review of the room setting, equipment, learning objectives, and participant expectations. We use formative assessment and corrective learning as emphasized during debrief.

Scenario

"You have been working with a 6-year-old patient with significant stomatitis, which has made it difficult for her to maintain adequate oral intake. She has no underlying comorbidities, and has been ordered an intravenous (IV) line to be started for maintenance fluids and antibiotics."

The student describes the steps for preparation and communicates with the low-fidelity human patient simulator (LFHPS). The instructor gives a developmentally appropriate response, which usually would include a refusal by the patient, because of the unknowns or anticipated pain. The student needs to work through how to proceed (e.g., hands-on site assessment, limb positioning, therapeutic hold, and communication with a child) alongside consideration of what supports (resources or personnel) he or she may need to enable the best outcome for this patient, including having family members present at the bedside. As part of the debriefing, the instructor offers additional learning to enable best practices in pediatric nursing and policies shaping pediatric nursing at IH.

High-Fidelity Simulation—Midsemester Evaluation

Within the 6 weeks of their clinical practice, we evaluate prelicensure nursing via a series of six high-fidelity simulation experiences. Students are expected to review the scenario descriptions before attending the learning event, including recommended prebrief reading.

Learning Objectives

1. To evaluate student's ability to successfully demonstrate progress in meeting the leveled entry-to-practice competencies as outlined by the College of Registered Nurses British Columbia (CRNBC; 2015) and provide feedback on how to successfully meet those leveled competencies by the end of term

2. To assess student readiness for interprofessional team practice following the National Interprofessional Competency Framework (Canadian Interprofessional Health Collaborative [CIHC], 2010) evidenced by demonstrated scope of practice and role identity alongside team communication in an urgent situation

Setting the Scene

These simulations are either run within our clinical simulation lab facilities or use mobile high-fidelity simulation equipment available within the pediatric clinical area. In the next section, we provide an example of one of six required simulation learning events. Exhibit 22.1 lists the required resources needed to run the scenario.

F. PRESENTATION OF COMPLETED TEMPLATE

Ideally, a technician or second instructor is available to assist in simulation progression by playing the role of the patient and operating the high-fidelity human patient simulator (HFHPS) via a progression chart outlined in Exhibit 22.2. The instructor is free to attend to the simulation progression and complete the Exhibit 22.3 assessment checklist. One student will play the role of the parent and is given the Exhibit 22.4 cue sheet. Before launching the learning event, the instructor reviews the equipment, setup, and learning objectives (INACSL, 2013/2016).

A reflective practice narrative on the scenario may be added as needed. The reflective practice narrative asks the student to reflect on the learning event from an experiential standpoint, and then locate the experience in the larger context of evidence-based practice with a view to shaping entry to practice competencies.

I. EXPERT RECOMMENDATIONS AND WORDS OF WISDOM

Moving from simple simulation to strategically introducing more complex situations, the student ultimately joins the interprofessional in situ simulation described in Chapter 48. This allows prelicensure students to apply their learning in a way that naturally engages them with their clinical environment. Several adaptations to our approach include the use of a pre- and posttest administered to assess student knowledge before simulation and following simulation to assess knowledge base and gain. We are currently implementing that strategy using the National Council Licensure Examination (NCLEX; newly introduced in Canada) and mapping student readiness for licensure examinations. Mentioned in our introduction is the challenge we have in accessing a pediatric acute care placement for all of our nursing students before

Exhibit 22.1	Equipment and Resources for Managing the Simulated Experience

Sim child

Oral/IV medications: Phenobarbital/Ativan

Medication resources available online: pedmed.org, IH drug monograph, IH syringe reconstitution table

IV pumps, syringes, secondary med tubing

O_2 supplies

ID bracelet, allergy bracelet

Hand sanitizer

Patient chart (clipboard with orders, vital signs, medication record, fluid balance sheet)

Parent cue sheet

IH, Island Health Authority; IV, intravenous.

Exhibit 22.2	Scenario Progression
Information reviewed in prebrief	**Learning objectives:** • Communicate effectively during patient handover. • Identify the appropriate phenobarbitol dose for this pediatric patient. • Identify the potential complications related to prolonged seizures. • Recognize the signs and symptoms of typical and atypical seizures. • Prioritize treatments and interventions for seizures. • Collaborate with the interdisciplinary health care team using situation, background, assessment, recommendations (SBAR) communication. • Take the leadership role in a patient adverse event articulating the role of the nurse with respect to patient-centered care and the interprofessional health care team.
Information given on initiation of scenario	Jill is a 5-year-old girl with a known seizure disorder who has been recovering from a viral infection and experienced multiple seizures yesterday evening at home. She was brought to the hospital in the ambulance and assessed in the ER. Phenobarbitol levels were checked and came back below therapeutic levels. She came to the floor overnight and, as you are reviewing your charts for your day shift, the call bell rings. Mom states, "She is having another seizure!" Diagnosis: Seizure disorder and mild developmental delay Current medications: Ranitidine 75 mg twice a day; phenobarbitol 90 mg twice a day Allergies: Penicillin, latex, and sensitive to dairy Weight: 32 kg **Admission orders:** Diet as tolerated Activity as tolerated Take neurological VS q 4 h peripheral intravenous to keep vein open or saline lock Ativan 2 mg IV for seizure activity >5 min Phenobarb 95 mg PO twice daily Repeat phenobarbitol levels tomorrow morning
Information as participant proceeds with assessment	**Initial assessment with seizure vital signs:** Blood pressure (BP): 100/66 mmHg HR: 120 beats/minute RR: 22 breaths/minute SpO_2: 94% Temperature: 37.5°C **Head-to-toe assessment:** Neurological: Evident seizure activity with rapid eye movement, shaky/jerky movements to extremities Cardiac: Mild tachycardia, normal, no noted rhythm abnormalities Respiratory: Clear chest, irregular respiratory rate Integument: Faint mottling to peripheries Musculoskeletal: Rigidity to limbs with dyskinetic movements to extremities Gastrointestinal: Flat, nontender abdomen Genitourinary: Incontinent of urine

(continued)

Exhibit 22.2	Scenario Progression *(continued)*	
Alternative pathways depending on participant interventions	If the student does not start timing seizure or assessing the level of consciousness using the AVPU Scale Chameides, Ralston, American Academy of Pediatrics, & American Heart Association, 2011) or Pediatric Glasgow Coma Scale (Teasdale, 2014), assess vitals after 2–3 minutes: BP: 100/58 mmHg HR:132 beats/minute RR: 18 breaths/minute SpO_2: 89%	If student does start timing seizure and assessing level of consciousness, assess vitals after 1 minute: BP: 100/58 mmHg HR:132 beats/minute RR: 18 breaths/minute SpO_2: 89%
	If student applies O_2 appropriately, after 1–2 minutes: O_2 saturation: 94% RR: 14 breaths/minute	If student applies O_2 appropriately, right away: O_2 saturation: 94% RR: 14 breaths/minute
	Pt. is still seizing at 5 min. If student does not administer Ativan: BP: 96/50 mmHg HR: 165 beats/minute RR: 12 breaths/minute SpO_2: 94% Potential complication: respiratory arrest	Pt. is still seizing at 5 min. If student does administer Ativan: Reassess following medication: BP: 99/65 mmHg HR: 122 beats/minute RR: 20 breaths/minute SpO_2: 96% Patient stops seizing and returns to baseline
Debrief	Participant: 1. What do you think was happening in this scenario? 2. What so you think went well? 3. What did you have difficulty with? 4. Is there anything you would have changed/done differently? 5. What (if anything) will you carry forward in your nursing practice as a result of this learning event?	Learning objectives: As you listened to the report on the patient, did you have any further questions to ask before prioritizing care for Jill and her family? What are the priorities forming in your mind even in approaching Jill having heard Mom's comment? What manifestations of seizures would cause you concern? What other options do you have for Ativan administration? What did you note to be important in terms of communicating with patient and/or parent? What was the priority reporting (SBAR) required and to which member of the interprofessional team was the report given?

BP, blood pressure; ER, emergency room; HR, heart rate; IV, intravenous; PO, per os; Pt., patient; q, every; RR, respiratory rate; VS, vital sign.

Exhibit 22.3	Critical Action Checklist—Seizure	
Critical Actions	**Criteria**	**Score**
1 Sanitizes hands.	Does NOT wash hands.	0
	Washes hands.	1
2 Introduces self and care intent.	Does NOT introduce self/care intent.	0
	Introduces self/care intent.	1
Vital Signs/Physical Assessment		
3 Obtains vital signs.	Does NOT obtain vital signs.	0
	Obtains vital signs partially or inaccurately.	1
	Obtains vital signs completely and accurately.	2
4 Assesses neurological vitals.	Does NOT assess neurological vitals.	0
	Assesses neurological vitals.	1
5 Assesses pain.	Does NOT assess pain.	0
	Assesses pain.	2
Medication Administration		
6 Checks Ativan dose.	Does NOT identify correct dose.	0
	Identifies correct dose.	2
7 Prepares Ativan dose.	Does NOT appropriately prepare Ativan.	0
	Appropriately prepares Ativan.	2
8 Reassesses and recognizes changes.	Does NOT recognize changes.	0
	Recognizes changes when patient/family speaks.	1
	Recognizes changes in physiologic condition.	2
Communication		
9 Receives patient report/asks pertinent questions.	Fails to recognize missing information in the patient handover and does not ask questions.	0
	Recognizes missing information in the patient handover and asks questions.	2
10 Uses closed-loop communication among health care team.	Does NOT use closed-loop communication.	0
	Uses closed-loop communication some of the time.	1
	Uses closed-loop communication all the time.	2
11 Contacts provider.	Does NOT contact provider.	0
	Contacts provider.	2
12 Uses SBAR.	Does NOT use SBAR or give structured report to provider.	0
	Partially uses SBAR to communicate to provider.	1–3
	Fully uses SBAR to communicate to provider.	4

(continued)

| Exhibit 22.3 | Critical Action Checklist—Seizure   (*continued*) | |

Critical Actions	Criteria	Score
13 Discusses interventions with patient and family.	Does NOT discuss intervention with patient and family.	0
	Partially discusses interventions with patient and family.	1
	Discusses interventions with patient and family.	2
14 Provides psychological support to family.	Does NOT provide psychological support.	0
	Does provide psychological support.	1
Interventions		
15 Administers O_2.	Does NOT administer O_2.	0
	Does NOT administer O_2 correctly.	0
	Administers O_2 correctly.	2
16 Repositions patient or objects in patient's bed space to support safety.	Does NOT reposition patient or objects.	0
	Does reposition patient and/or objects in bed space.	2
17 Reassesses patient and vital signs throughout simulation.	Does NOT reassess patient and vital signs.	0
	Reassesses patient some of the time.	1
	Reassesses patient and vital signs consistently.	2

SBAR, situation, background, assessment, recommendations.

| Exhibit 22.4 | Parent Cues |

If asked on assessment, parent can indicate that Jill's seizures are often flicking or rolling eye movement, followed by shaky or jerky limb movement that can be slight or very evident.

If asked when Jill's last seizure was, parent can indicate that she has had no seizures since coming to hospital.

As seizure continues to progress, parent can become increasingly agitated and upset and **say:** "Why is she still seizing? What is going on? This is not like her!"

licensure examinations. We plan to pilot a simulation laboratory experience offering the six scenarios to students who will not "practice" in the clinical area but may participate in the interprofessional simulations and have an opportunity for "hands-on" application of knowledge of pediatric nursing.

We have recently implemented a written assignment, the reflective practice narrative, an assignment consistently used in our curriculum to encourage a deeper reflection on the simulation learning events. Students are expected to review the clinical case presented in the scenario and the practice requirements within the evidence-based literature and write a narrative complete with critical consideration of evidence to date that contrasts with their personal experiences and projections of practice requirements on entry to practice. They outline further learning goals and identify ways in which they will take up resources to support their learning.

We continue to hear from students that very shortly after their simulation experience, they had "the exact thing happen in clinical." They are excited because they are able to relate how they were able to recognize the deteriorating patient, or they were able to be actively involved in addressing the issue because they understood what was happening and could make suggestions using their own clinical judgment. Students who acknowledged being a little fearful to be put into a primary role during inter-professional simulation are given the opportunity to thoughtfully work through communication with team members to successfully address complex situations.

REFERENCES

Campbell, S., & Lloyd, H. (2005). Shared interests. *Nursing Management, 12*(7), 28–30.

Canadian Association of Schools of Nursing. (2015). *Practice domain for baccalaureate nursing education: Guidelines for clinical placements and simulation.* Vancouver, BC, Canada: College of Health Disciplines, University of British Columbia. Retrieved from http://www.casn.ca/2015/11/practice-domain-for-baccalaureate-nursing-education-guidelines-for-clinical-placements-and-simulation

Canadian Interprofessional Health Collaborative. (2010). A national interprofessional competency framework. Retrieved from http://www.cihc.ca/files/CIHC_IPCompetencies_Feb1210.pdf

Chameides, L., Ralston, M., American Academy of Pediatrics, & American Heart Association. (2011). *Pediatric advanced life support.* Dallas, TX: American Heart Association.

Chua, W. L., Mackey, S., Ng, E. K., & Liaw, S. Y. (2013). Front line nurses' experiences with deteriorating ward patients: A qualitative study. *International Nursing Review, 60*(4), 501–509.

College of Registered Nurses of British Columbia. (2015). Competencies in the context of entry level registered nursing practice in British Columbia. Retrieved from https://www.crnbc.ca/Registration/Lists/RegistrationResources/375CompetenciesEntrylevelRN.pdf

International Nursing Association for Clinical Simulation and Learning. (2013, updated 2016). INACSL standards of best practice: Simulation. Retrieved from http://www.inacsl.org/i4a/pages/index.cfm?pageid=3407

Rosser, E. (2015). Generalist or specialist in nurse education? *British Journal of Nursing, 24*(2), 120.

Teasdale, G. (2014). The Glasgow structured approach to assessment of the Glasgow Coma Scale. Retrieved from http://www.glasgowcomascale.org/faq

Developmental Assessment and Communication With Pediatric Patients and Their Families

Lee-Anne Stephen and Anne Kent

A. IMPLEMENTATION OF SIMULATION-BASED PEDAGOGY IN YOUR INDIVIDUALIZED TEACHING AREA

Pediatric clinical experiences can cause considerable anxiety for the undergraduate nursing student, primarily because of fear of making a mistake that could harm a child (Oermann & Lukomski, 2001). The lack of confidence in developing relationships with families is common, especially in situations in which families observe student assessments and interactions with their children. Students have concerns about including parents in the assessment process and doubt their ability to answer parent questions. Earlier experience with children does little to minimize the insecurity surrounding the examination of and communication with a sick child as their response is often unpredictable.

Simulation can help to decrease students' anxiety and provide them with the opportunity to gain the clinical knowledge and skill required to confidently enter the clinical setting (Megel et al., 2012). In order to support our students learning, we developed three pediatric clinical scenarios using children of different stages of growth and development and used this simulated experience to replace a 7.5-hour clinical day.

B. EDUCATIONAL MATERIALS AVAILABLE IN YOUR TEACHING AREA AND RELATED TO YOUR SPECIALTY

The School of Health Studies at the University of the Fraser Valley (UFV) houses four dedicated medium- and high-fidelity simulation rooms, three single suites, and one two-bed suite. An advanced software program provides live viewing of the simulated learning event to the debriefing room. This software is equipped with annotated playback capabilities to highlight key learning opportunities during the simulated event. The human patient simulators (HPSs) include one high-fidelity adult, two medium-fidelity adults, one medium-fidelity child, and one medium-fidelity baby.

C. SPECIFIC OBJECTIVES FOR SIMULATION USAGE WITHIN A SPECIFIC COURSE AND THE OVERALL PROGRAM

Learning Objectives

The objectives of this learning activity are to incorporate developmentally appropriate care into the assessment of children; to understand the unique communication needs of each age group; and to engage with family members to provide safe, atraumatic care to children.

The simulation day was designed for students in the second year of the BSN program as an orientation to the clinical experience. Many of these students have very little experience with children and no experience in caring for the hospitalized child.

Student Learning Activities

1. Review assessment and communication strategies for:
   an infant presenting with poor feeding
   a preschooler admitted with dehydration
   an adolescent with type 1 diabetes
2. Review communication strategies with different family forms in the acute care setting

D. INTRODUCTION OF SCENARIO

Setting the Scene

All three scenarios occur in the acute pediatric care setting of a regional hospital. Each child requires hospitalization but none are acutely ill; each has family members at the bedside.

Technology Used

Medium-fidelity human patient simulators are used for all three scenarios. The simulators include an infant simulator (for the infant scenario), a child (for the preschool child), and an adult (for the adolescent patient). Live-feed equipment for video-recording is helpful but not necessary.

The focus of the three scenarios is communication, so standardized patients could be used for both the patient and the family member.

Objectives

1. Discuss the role of the family when caring for an infant, preschool child, and adolescent.
2. Discuss developmentally appropriate strategies when communicating with an infant, preschool child, and adolescent in a health care setting.
3. Demonstrate communication with the family during infant, preschool child, and adolescent assessment using relational nursing practice.
4. Demonstrate a head-to-toe assessment of an infant, preschool child, and adolescent using atraumatic care and developmentally appropriate communication and assessment strategies.

E. RUNNING OF THE SCENARIO

Students have reviewed the learning activities before arrival. The briefing session includes a review of the objectives, the student confidentiality agreement, the expectation of professionalism, and the use of constructive feedback. It should last about 30 minutes. The challenges of realism in the simulated environment, as opposed to a real-life, active, verbal child, should be discussed. Time should also be provided for an orientation to the simulation suite, patient-care planning, questions, and a description of participant roles (Exhibits 23.1 and 23.2).

Exhibit 23.1	Description of Participants
Infant	Emily Sarah Smith is 2 months old. She was brought to the hospital because her mother felt that she was not her usual self; she had been lethargic and was not feeding well. Emily's mother is in a common-law relationship with Emily's father. Both have very busy careers and rely on Emily's grandmother to provide care.
Preschool child	Noah Eric Jones is age 5 years. He was admitted because of moderate dehydration following a tonsillectomy 5 days earlier. Before the procedure, he had recurrent tonsillitis, but according to his aunt was otherwise healthy. Noah has lived with his aunt since he was 2 years old, as neither parent could care for him. There are five other children in the household and the aunt is single.
Adolescent	Melissa Jane Steward, age 14 years, was admitted 2 days ago because of hyperglycemia and ketonuria. She was first diagnosed with type 1 diabetes when she was 6 years old and her condition has been managed well until 6 months ago. This is her second admission in 6 months for the same condition. Melissa's blood sugars are now stable and she is preparing for discharge. Her parents, who separated recently, are both present.

Exhibit 23.2	Outline of Scenarios
Infant scenario	The infant is lying quietly in her crib when the students enter the room. The students should communicate with the mother and grandmother and complete an across-the-room assessment of the child. Emily's grandmother verbalizes that there is nothing wrong with the infant. Emily's mother should look visibly upset, tired, and annoyed with the grandmother. The students will do a physiological assessment of the child and will find nothing abnormal.
	The students should try to get to the heart of the family conflict. If they do, they will discover that Emily's mother feels guilty about not spending enough time with her child because of the necessity of full-time work and her inability to breastfeed. Emily's mother is also concerned about her own mother's health and ability to care for Emily. Emily's grandmother thinks her daughter should resign from her job to care for her child. If the students cannot facilitate a family conversation they should ask about the grandma's comfort level and find a seat for her in a different room. This will demonstrate their ability to prioritize whose concerns take precedence and give them an opportunity to listen to Emily's mother's story without interruption.
Preschool child scenario	The preschool child is sitting in a hospital bed. His aunt is sitting in a chair at his bedside checking messages on her phone. Noah should have a teddy bear and a coloring book. The students should comment on the teddy bear after they have introduced themselves. The students should assess his pain choosing a developmentally appropriate scale, administer an analgesic, encourage fluid intake, and link poor oral intake and subsequent dehydration to painful tonsil beds. The aunt, who is very distracted by her phone, should be drawn into the conversation. Unknown to the students, the aunt is trying to arrange day care for her other children. She asks the students, several times, whether she can leave, and wants to know how long it will be before Noah is discharged.
Adolescent scenario	The students should introduce themselves to the patient and then the family. They should start to establish a therapeutic relationship with the family and discuss the possibility of involving social work because of the frequency of hospitalizations in the past 6 months. When doing the assessment, they should ask the adolescent whether she would like the family to remain in the room. The students will need to consider the developmental needs of the adolescent and determine how to support her in her illness journey. The focus of this simulation is on listening and challenging stereotypes.

The students start with the adolescent scenario, followed by the preschool child scenario, and close the day with the infant scenario. If there is time, students can repeat the scenario of their choice.

F. PRESENTATION OF COMPLETED TEMPLATE

All scenarios should be used with second-year BSN students and all are focused on pediatrics and family care (Exhibit 23.3).

Exhibit 23.3	Scenario Template for All Three Pediatric Scenarios	
Infant scenario	**Preschool-Age Scenario**	**Adolescent Scenario**
Shift report:	*Shift report:*	*Shift report:*
Patient woke every 4 to 5 hours for feeds. Tylenol was given at 6 a.m. for a temperature of 39.0°C. Mom and Grandma are at the bedside. Emily last fed at 6 a.m.	Patient did not sleep well. Around-the-clock Tylenol was given for pain. The last dose was given at 4 a.m. Noah's aunt is at the bedside. Encourage fluids today.	Patient slept well. Mom spent the night. Patient ready to be discharged. Discuss social work referral with the patient and her family.
Patient: Emily Sarah Smith Age: 2 months Allergies: No known allergies Weight: 5 kg Last vitals: BP: 75/45 mmHg, HR: 100 beats/minute, RR: 35 breaths/minute, Temp: 39.0°C, O_2 saturation: 98% on room air	Patient: Noah Eric Jones Age: 5 years Allergies: No known allergies Weight: 15 kg Last vitals: BP: 90/55 mmHg, HR: 75 beats/minute, RR: 26 breaths/minute, Temp: 37.1°C, O_2 saturation: 99% on room air, pain 5/10	Patient: Melissa Jane Steward Age: 14 years Allergies: Penicillin and cats Weight: 45 kg Last vitals: BP: 105/60 mmHg, HR: 60 beats/minute, RR: 16 breaths/minute, Temp: 37.0°C, O_2 saturation: 100% on room air
Medical history:	*Medical history:*	*Medical history:*
Previously healthy. Admitted because mother felt her infant was lethargic, had a decreased appetite, and was warm to touch.	Dehydration following tonsillectomy. Before the removal of tonsils, Noah experienced frequent colds and would snore loudly at night. He appears to be small for his age.	Diagnosed with type 1 diabetes at 6 years of age; has been admitted twice in the past 6 months for hyperglycemia and ketonuria. Before these admissions, she managed her chronic illness very well. She attends the diabetic outpatient clinic.
Family/social history:	*Family/social history:*	*Family/social history:*
Emily's parents are in a common-law relationship. Both work shifts; her father is a paramedic and her mother is a police officer. Emily is their first child and was born just after her mother graduated from the police academy. Emily's mother did not qualify for maternity leave, so the couple relies heavily on Emily's grandmother for child care.	Noah has lived with his aunt since he was 2 years old. His aunt is a single parent who has five of her own children. His mother is homeless and addicted to drugs and is only allowed to have supervised visits with him. The identity of his father is unknown. Noah loves to watch TV, has started kindergarten, and gets along very well with his cousins. He is enrolled in soccer this year.	Melissa's parents have recently separated and do not get along. Her father has a new girlfriend and Melissa and her mother are struggling with this. She has two sisters, aged 10 and 12 years. She was an "A" student and a member of the school band, but since the separation of her parents her grades have started to slip and she has become moody. She is not managing her diabetes well.

BP, blood pressure; HR, heart rate; RR, respiratory rate.

The American Association of Colleges of Nursing (AACN; 2008) *The Essentials of Baccalaureate Education for Professional Nursing Practice* objectives that these scenarios address are as follows:

Essential VIII: Professionalism and Professional Values—Objectives 6 and 9
Essential IX: Baccalaureate Generalist Nursing Practice—Objectives 1, 4, 5, 8, 21.

Scenario Objectives

The students in each scenario are expected to develop therapeutic relationships with the families and children they care for. They should come prepared to interact with children of different developmental stages and complete assessments in an atraumatic manner. Relational practice skills should be used to gain an understanding of the families in each of the scenarios.

The scenario allows students to practice key elements from the Test Plan for the National Council Licensure Examination for Registered Nurses (NCLEX-RN®) of the National Council of State Boards of Nursing (NCSBN; 2015) test plan, including: **Health promotion and maintenance** (Developmental stages and transitions, Techniques of physical assessment); **Psychosocial integrity** (Family dynamics, Therapeutic communication, therapeutic environment); and **Physiological integrity:** physiological adaptation (Illness management).

For this scenario, the College of Registered Nurses of British Columbia's (CRNBC; 2015) *Competencies in the Context of Entry-Level Registered Nurse Practice in British Columbia* (2015) addressed include the following:

1. Professional responsibility and accountability: Self-regulation competencies 1, 4, 7, 14
2. Knowledge-based practice: Specialized Body of Knowledge competencies 27, 28, 32; Ongoing Comprehensive Assessment competencies 37, 38, 39, 41, 42; Health Care Planning competencies 47, 52; Providing Nursing Care competencies 57, 59, 61, 67, 69, 71, 72
3. Ethical practice: Ethical Practice competencies 89, 90, 91, 92, 93, 94, 95, 97

Setting the Scene

Equipment Needed

The equipment needed for all scenarios includes an appropriately sized stethoscope, O_2 saturation monitor with age-appropriate reading apparatus, thermometer, and a medication administration record (MAR). Exhibit 23.4 provides additional resources for each scenario.

Exhibit 23.4	Equipment by Scenario
Infant	*Equipment:* Diapers, wipes, rattle, musical mobile, teddy bear, chair for grandma, bedside table, crib, IV, D5W *Physicians orders:* TFI—120 mL/kg/d Labs already done—blood and urine culture done, but waiting for results Feed ad-lib—formula IV D5W running at TKVO Daily weight VS q 4 hours Ampicillin 125 mg IV q 6 hours Gentamicin 12.5 mg IV q 8 hours Tylenol 50 mg PO q 4–6 hours PRN

(*continued*)

Exhibit 23.4	Equipment by Scenario (continued)

Preschool child	*Equipment:* Teddy bear, coloring, books, pain assessment tools, stickers, juice, small drinking cups or syringes to encourage fluid intake *Physicians orders:* VS q 4 hours Oral rehydration protocol Soft diet Tylenol 225 mg PO q 4–6 hours prn Ibuprofen 150 mg PO q 6–8 hours PRN
Adolescent	*Equipment:* Magazines, iPad or laptop computer, resources for teens with diabetes and for peer groups, diabetic teaching material, BP cuff, phone *Physicians orders:* BS QID and at hs VS q 6 hours Referral for social work/counseling Insulin as per doctor's discharge orders. Reassess insulin requirement in outpatient clinic in 1 week.

BP, blood pressure; BS, blood sugar; D5W, 5% dextrose in water; hs, before bed; IV, intravenous; PO, per os; PRN, as needed; q, every; QID, four times a day; TFI, total fluid intake; TKVO, to keep vein open; VS, vital signs.

Participant Roles

Two primary nurses (Nurse 1 and Nurse 2) will provide care to the child and family. They should spend time before the simulation discussing how they will work as a team. For example, one nurse might do the assessment while the other distracts the child or speaks with the family.

Students assigned the role of the observer do not watch this scenario live. Instead, the observer students work in the debriefing room on a pen-and-paper care plan for the patient. They need to describe what strategies they would use when communicating with the child and family. Their answers are written on flip chart paper, so they can be reviewed during debriefing (Exhibits 23.5 and 23.6).

Exhibit 23.5	Participant Role Descriptions for Scenarios

Roles for infant scenario	***Mother***—You feel guilty because Emily is formula fed, but you could not breastfeed because of your work schedule. You are anxious about Emily because she is your first child, so you ask the student nurses what they are doing and why they are doing it every time they perform an intervention. You also wonder whether your lack of experience has led you to be overly cautious, but you feel intuitively that something is wrong with your baby. You are frustrated with Emily's grandmother because she keeps telling you that you are doing things wrong and you also feel guilty because Emily's grandmother needs to provide child care. ***Grandmother***—You feel that Emily's mother is overreacting by bringing Emily to the hospital. You have a sore hip, so cannot stand for long periods of time. If you do not have a chair, make sure you ask for one. During the time the student nurses are in the room keep acting as though you think Emily is fine. You should frequently interrupt.

(continued)

Exhibit 23.5	Participant Roles and Scripts for Scenarios (continued)

the conversation when the students try to get information from Emily's mother. If Emily's mother tries to do anything with Emily, suggest a different approach. You feel Emily's mother should resign from her job so that she can care for Emily.

Infant—The infant should cry if the students do not follow assessment from least invasive to most invasive and if they do not include the family. The infant should coo when appropriate distraction methods are used or when the family is involved.

Roles for preschool child scenario	**Noah**—You had a bad experience when your tonsils were removed, so the student nurses make you very nervous. If the student nurses talk to you about your teddy bear you will answer their questions more completely; otherwise, only answer with one word and very quietly.
	If the student nurses use language that is not developmentally appropriate—that is, *pain* instead of *hurt*, *abdomen* instead of *stomach*, you should ask your aunt what the nurse means. If the student nurses do not start with a focused pain and intake assessment, start to tell them that your throat hurts and feels scratchy.
	Aunt—You are very distracted because you are planning child care for your other children, so you are on the phone. Keep asking the student nurses whether you can leave and when they think Noah will be discharged. Do not be very concerned or appear very involved in what is happening with Noah. Keep quiet or use only one-word answers unless you are asked open-ended questions. The student nurses should discover that you want to leave because your other children are staying with a friend who is not always very reliable.
Roles for adolescent scenario	**Mother**—You are stressed and worried about your daughter's health, but you have an accusatory stance toward her for not following the diabetic regimen. You do not know how to get your daughter to follow the protocol. You feel she is bad tempered and hard to get along with. Your relationship is filled with tension, as is your relationship with your ex-spouse.
	Dad—If the mother says anything you should disagree with her. You do not feel she knows anything about your daughter's personality or health care habits. You favor your daughter and feel that she is doing her best and that her mom needs to do more for her.
	Melissa—When your parents are in the room your attitude is hostile and sulky. You do not want to be here so you are not listening. You provide limited responses to any questions from the nurses. You are more antagonistic to your mother than to your father. If the student nurse asks you whether you want your parents in the room during an assessment, tell them no. If they do not ask, tell them that you would like your parents to leave. Once your parents have left you start to share your story with the student nurses. You tell them that your mother is always nagging you. Sometimes you forget to give yourself insulin at school because you are too busy and it is boring to always have to check your sugars. Your parents are always telling you what to do and get mad if your sugars are high or low so it is better not to bother and the results do not really matter because you knew how much insulin you need and can "guesstimate." A friend has told you about a diet blog for losing weight and that your stomach gets nice and flat when you skip your insulin.

Scenario Implementation

Exhibit 23.6	Initial Settings for the HPS/equipment
Infant scenario	Hospital room with an infant in a crib: Grandmother and mother are standing by the crib. The HPS should be wearing a sleeper and have a stuffed animal, musical mobile, and rattle in the crib. IV with D5W running at 7 mL/hr. Vitals: HR = 100 beats/minute, RR = 35 breaths/minute, temperature = 37.3°C, O_2 saturation = 98%
Preschool scenario	Hospital room with a child in a bed: Aunt is sitting in a chair at the bedside. The HPS is wearing a hospital gown and has a teddy bear and coloring book. He should be pale with dark circles under his eyes, his lips should look dry and cracked, and there should be a few bruises on his legs and a scab on his knee. There should be syringes, cups, favorite juice, and stickers to support fluid intake. Vitals: Pain = 8/10, HR = 75 beats/minute, RR = 26 breaths/minute, temperature = 37.1°C, O_2 saturation = 99%
Adolescent scenario	Hospital room with an adolescent in the bed and her dad is sitting at the bedside. Her mom is standing against a far wall. The HPS should have pink hair and a recent manicure or pedicure. She should have an iPad, cell phone, magazines (with diabetic positive role models), diabetic camp brochures, TV, insulin pen in the room. Vitals: HR = 70 beats/minute, RR = 16 breaths/minute, temperature = 37.0°C, O_2 saturation = 100%

HPS, human patient simulator; HR, heart rate; IV, intravenous; RR, respiratory rate.

Instructor Interventions

The role of the instructor or facilitator is to act as the voice of the human patient simulator (HPS), set the tone during briefing, and facilitate student reflection and knowledge acquisition during debriefing.

Evaluation Criteria

Use Exhibit 23.7 to develop a checklist for required actions during the hands-on-care phase of the simulation.

Have students complete an evaluation of their simulation experience. The facilitator should spend time reflecting on and evaluating the simulation and his/her facilitation skills.

Exhibit 23.7	Expected/Required Student Assessments/Actions
All scenarios	Washes hands upon entering the room. Introduces self to the child in a developmentally appropriate manner. Introduces self to parent(s) and describes role. Develops a therapeutic relationship before starting the physical assessment. Completes a developmentally appropriate physical assessment including the family when appropriate. Ensures child and family are comfortable before leaving the room.
Infant scenario	Asks about intake, output, and activity level of the infant. Completes assessment moving from least invasive to most invasive. Asks mother what is normal behavior for the infant.

(continued)

Exhibit 23.7	Expected/Required Student Assessments/Actions *(continued)*
	Asks mother how she is coping with her daughter's illness.
	Asks how grandma is coping with child care requirements.
	Includes mother during the assessment.
	Asks mother whether there is anything special she wants us to know about the child and family.
	Asks mother what she feels is most concerning about her child's illness and listens to the health/illness story.
Preschool scenario	Asks the aunt whether there is anything special she wants us to know about the child and family and listens to the health/illness story.
	Completes a physiological assessment in an opportunistic manner.
	Assesses intake and output.
	Completes a developmentally appropriate pain assessment.
	Asks Noah and his aunt what words he uses for pain. What does he normally do when he is in pain?
	Develops a relationship before trying to get Noah to drink.
	Makes drinking fun for Noah.
	Has a nonjudgmental attitude regarding how uninterested Noah's aunt appears to be.
Adolescent scenario	Asks Melissa and family about the need for social work support.
	Asks Melissa whether she would like her parents in the room when you do your assessment.
	Asks Melissa about her life and friends. Does she have any peers with diabetes?
	Establishes trust based on shared interests and then asks about illness. What is it like for her?
	Listens to Melissa's story, does not provide solutions, does not give advice unless asked.
	If Melissa did ask for advice, student used principles of teaching and learning and kept the conversation professional.
	Links Melissa's change in the management of diabetes to her parent's separation and her body image during debriefing.

G. DEBRIEFING GUIDELINES

Issues to Consider

Knowledge acquisition should focus on developmentally appropriate assessment of the infant, pre-school child, and adolescent; developmentally appropriate communication; and relational practice with children and families.

Student Questions

Reaction: In these scenarios, the following two questions are used only for the students who provide hands-on-care to the HPS.

1. What do you feel you did well?
2. What would you like to do differently next time?

Analysis: During this phase, questions for the students assigned to the observer role could center around how the plan of care is similar or different to what occurred in the simulation suite.

1. What was your first impression of the child and family when you entered the room? How did this change, based on the conversations you had with them?
2. What do you feel helped you make a therapeutic connection with the patient and family? What went well and what would you do differently next time? Why?
3. How did you feel your developmentally supportive assessment went? What went well and would you do anything differently? Why?
4. How did you feel your communication strategies went? Were you able to communicate effectively with each developmental stage? Why or why not?
5. Do you feel you were able to provide atraumatic care when completing your assessments and interventions? Why or why not?

Summary

1. How do you think your experience today will help you when you are in the clinical setting?
2. What are some of the nursing care similarities and differences between the adults you have cared for and the HPS you cared for today?

Classroom Observers Questions/Roles

The observers do not watch the simulation live; instead they focus on completing a pen-and-paper nursing care plan. Students who provide hands-on care to the HPS engage in a quick, facilitated debriefing using the reaction questions listed earlier. This debriefing occurs in the simulated suite off camera. All students then meet in the debriefing room. Students watch a condensed recording of the scenario and write their thoughts about what they feel went well, what did not go so well, and any questions they may have. Debriefing begins after the scenario has been watched. Questions from the analysis and summary phases are used in this debriefing session. We debrief the recorded scenario as well as the care plans developed by the observers.

H. SUGGESTIONS/KEY FEATURES
TO REPLICATE OR IMPROVE

These scenarios could be easily modified to include cultural aspects, an interprofessional focus, or an illness focus. The age of the children and the complexity of illness can change based on the learning needs of the students. The use of a standardized patient to act as the family or adolescent patient could enhance psychosocial assessment and add to the realism of this scenario. Students tire when they are engaged in an all-day simulation, so frequent breaks; flexibility; responsiveness to the students' situation; and lively, engaging discussion helps to keep energy levels high. If all three scenarios are used in 1 day, then at the end of the day, discussion of the similarities and differences between the care of each age group can be beneficial for student learning.

I. RECOMMENDATIONS FOR FURTHER USE

If the focus is on changes from infancy to adolescence following the cycle of human growth and development, the infant scenario should come first.

A more traditional role, such as watching the scenario live, could be assigned to the observers if time is limited.

J. HOW SIMULATION-BASED PEDAGOGY HAS CONTRIBUTED TO IMPROVED STUDENT OUTCOMES

Following the simulation experience, students appear to be less anxious and more comfortable when communicating with families and children in the clinical setting. As a result, less time is spent in clinical experience simply gaining comfort with the environment, thereby freeing up more time for learning.

K. EXPERT RECOMMENDATIONS AND WORDS OF WISDOM

It is tiring to complete three scenarios in one day. Students do, however, find this day beneficial as afterward they see an improvement in their skills, can compare different approaches with nursing care dependent on development and family form, and become more comfortable in the simulated environment.

If the simulated patient says something humorous (which children often do in the clinical setting) this can decrease student anxiety during the hands-on care of the HPS.

The use of an experienced pediatric faculty member for the voice of the HPS enhances the student experience. It also enables the facilitator to point to his or her own mistakes. For example, not sounding like a child or answering a question incorrectly. This helps the students to share their experience, and reframe mistakes as a normal part of learning.

L. EVALUATION OF BEST PRACTICE STANDARDS AND USE OF CREDENTIALED SIMULATION FACULTY

The UFV Health Studies Simulation committee has developed a simulation scenario template based on the INACSL *Standards of Best Practice: Simulation*[SM] (INACSL, 2013/2016). This template helps to ensure that there is consistency in simulation design across the program and that scenario development, implementation, and evaluation are informed by evidence. Faculty in the School of Health Studies have the opportunity to engage in simulation professional development each year.

REFERENCES

American Association of Colleges of Nursing. (2008). *The essentials of baccalaureate education for professional nursing practice.* Washington, DC: Author. Retrieved from http://www.aacnnursing.org/Portals/42/Publications/BaccEssentials08.pdf

College of Registered Nurses of British Columbia. (2015). *Competencies in the context of entry level registered nurse practice in British Columbia.* Vancouver, BC, Canada: Author.

International Nursing Association for Clinical Simulation and Learning. (2013, updated 2016). INACSL standards of best practice: Simulation. Retrieved from https://www.inacsl.org/i4a/pages/index.cfm?pageID=3407

Megel, E. M., Black, J., Clark, L., Carstens, P., Jenkins, L. D., Promes, J., & Goodman, T. (2012). Effect of high-fidelity simulation on pediatric nursing students' anxiety. *Clinical Simulation in Nursing, 8*(9), e419–e428. doi:10.1016/j.ecns.2011.03.006

National Council of State Boards of Nursing. (2016). NCLEX-RN examination: Test plan for the National Council Licensure Examination for Registered Nurses. Retrieved from https://www.ncsbn.org/RN_Test_Plan_2016_final.pdf

Oermann, M. H., & Lukomski, A. P. (2001). Experiences of students in pediatric nursing clinical courses. *Journal of the Society of Pediatric Nurses, 6*(2), 65–72.

CHAPTER 24

Care of an Older Adult With Congestive Heart Failure

Alison Kris

A. IMPLEMENTATION OF SIMULATION-BASED PEDAGOGY IN YOUR INDIVIDUALIZED TEACHING AREA

Because geriatrics content is typically offered during the second year of the baccalaureate program, elementary simulations allow faculty to introduce foundational content essential to the care of older adults. Examples of content reinforced through the use of scenarios has included (a) differentiating delirium, dementia, and depression and (b) distinguishing normal from abnormal changes of aging.

At Fairfield University, faculty have also been able to participate in a faculty learning community (Shea, Campbell, & Miners, 2013), which facilitated discussions about the goals and expected outcomes associated with simulations. In addition, there was discussion of the pedagogical theory supporting the use of simulations to enhance the delivery of nursing content.

B. EDUCATIONAL MATERIALS AVAILABLE IN YOUR TEACHING AREA AND RELATED TO YOUR SPECIALTY

The Fairfield University School of Nursing's Robin Kanarek Learning Resource Center is a state-of-the-art facility that presents realistic patient care scenarios. It comprises a simulation room, a control room, and an adjacent classroom enabling classes of up to 35 students to view the ongoing scenario as it progresses. A high-fidelity human patient simulator (HPS) allows students to assess the typical vital signs (VS) and lung sounds of a nursing home resident with an acute exacerbation of congestive heart failure (CHF). In the following scenario, students may use an actual computer interface to access patient lab values and history. If such technology is not available, sample charting materials can be provided.

C. SPECIFIC OBJECTIVES OF SIMULATION USAGE WITHIN A SPECIFIC COURSE AND THE OVERALL PROGRAM

This scenario is intended for students enrolled in Geriatric Nursing, a second-year course in a 4-year baccalaureate nursing program. The course focuses on the nursing care of older adults living in long-term care settings. Building on skills developed in a previous course in health assessment, normal physiological changes of aging and related assessment skills are incorporated into this course. Management of common geriatric care problems is emphasized. Because geriatric nursing is the first clinical course in the nursing curriculum, students will also be provided with the opportunity to develop an understanding of how the nursing role merges with life goals, philosophy, and meaning and to use those values to develop professional behaviors consistent with these aspects of life. In our curriculum, students have studied pharmacology before geriatric nursing coursework. This scenario allows for the reinforcement of pharmacology content, and reviews the side effects of diuretics.

D. INTRODUCTION OF SCENARIO

Setting the Scene

The simulation will take place in a nursing home. The resident will be in bed in his or her room. A certified nursing assistant (CNA) will provide a report on the resident.

Technology Used

This simulation will make use of a medium- or high-fidelity HPS with the capacity to transmit respiratory sounds, a video-recording device, simulated oxygen, pulse oximeter, blood pressure (BP) cuff, stethoscope, electronic health record, water pitcher, call light, and ID bracelet. The patient should be wearing a diaper.

Objectives

Nursing students will be required to evaluate and manage the complex and dynamic hydration status of the older adult nursing home patient suffering from CHF. This simulation will include evaluating the nursing home resident for signs and symptoms of both dehydration and overhydration. The scenario will test decision-making skills regarding the administration of diuretic medications and the evaluation of key laboratory values and will require communication with other nurses, physicians, and the patient's family members.

Description of Participants

One or two students; an instructor to act as the voice of the resident, Mrs. Fertal; a "CNA" to deliver the patient report; and a "physician" to whom students may report change of condition

E. RUNNING OF THE SCENARIO

The initial settings for the HPS for parts 1 to 3 are (a) BP: 130/85 mmHg, P: 75 beats/minute, respiratory rate (RR): 17 breaths/minute, temperature: 97.5°F; (b) oxygen saturation (O_2 sat) settings should be set to 90%; (c) place notecards on the legs of the HPS indicating that she has +1 pitting edema to her ankles; (d) lung sounds with slight crackles bilaterally; (e) atrial fibrillation; (f) resident is sitting in bed in a high Fowler position; and (g) place a reddened area on the patient's coccyx indicating a stage 1 pressure ulcer (use a model when available/appropriate).

F. PRESENTATION OF COMPLETED TEMPLATE

Title

Care of an Older Adult With Congestive Heart Failure

Scenario Level

This simulation is used within a geriatric course given during the second-semester sophomore year of a baccalaureate program or first-semester freshman year of an associate degree program.

Focus Area

This scenario is geared toward sophomore-level geriatric nursing students practicing in long-term care settings.

Scenario Description

One or two students will receive a report from a CNA working nights, and some key data will be missed and/or misinterpreted (e.g., weight gain). An instructor will act as the voice of Mrs. Fertal, and a physician will be available (either by phone in the control room or physically present) for students to report changes of condition.

Nursing students will be required to evaluate and manage the complex and dynamic hydration status of the older adult nursing home patient, including evaluating the patient for signs and symptoms of both dehydration and overhydration in light of the diagnosis of CHF. The scenario will test decision-making skills regarding the administration of diuretic medications and the evaluation of key laboratory values and will require communication with other nurses, physicians, and patient family members.

Scenario Objectives

1. Introduce self.
2. Check ID band.
3. Check VS, including pulse oximeter.
   a. Note low pulse oximeter reading.
   b. Note that decreased temperature is a common and normal finding in the older adult.
4. Conduct a head-to-toe assessment.
   c. Note rales in bilateral bases.
   d. Note pedal edema.
   e. Note reddened area on coccyx.
   f. Note atrial fibrillation.
5. Check the compressor to ensure that it is working and delivering the correct amount of oxygen to the patient.
6. Assess mental status for signs of acute confusion and signs of depression.
7. Student documents relevant findings: color, position, breath sounds, heart sounds, VS, weight, change in activity level, presence of a stage 1 pressure ulcer. While charting, student checks back to compare the current weight with the previous weight. Student checks the chart for relevant lab values.
8. Student notes that abnormal labs indicate hypovolemia: decreased blood urea nitrogen (BUN) and decreased hematocrit.
9. Student contacts the physician and reports relevant findings in a cohesive way. This may be done via phone in the simulation room, which connects him or her to faculty in the control room acting as the nurse practitioner and physician.

The scenario allows students to practice key elements from the National Council Licensure Examination for Registered Nurses (NCLEX-RN®) test plan (National Council of State Boards of Nursing, 2015), including: *Physiological integrity*: Basic care and comfort (nutrition and oral hydration, rest, and sleep), *Pharmacological and parenteral therapies* (expected effects/outcomes, pharmacological agents/actions), *Reduction of risk potential* (laboratory values, system specific assessments, VS), *Physiological adaptation* (hemodynamics, fluid and electrolyte imbalances, pathophysiology).

Setting the Scene

Patient: Mrs. Irma Fertal
Age: 89 years
Allergies: Penicillin, codeine
Weight: 177.2 pounds
Physician: Dr. Newman
Major diagnoses: CHF, chronic obstructive pulmonary disease (COPD), diabetes, hypothyroidism, atrial fibrillation, osteoarthritis of the left hip
Medications and orders:
Fluticasone propionate (Advair discus) 250/50
Furosemide (Lasix) 20 mg by mouth daily
Levothyroxine (Synthroid), 50 mcg by mouth daily
Predisone (Deltasone), 10 mg by mouth daily
Wafarin (Coumadin), 5 mg by mouth daily
Neutral protein Hagedorn (NPH) insulin, 25 U each morning and each evening
Codeine, 2 tabs every 4 hours as needed
Oxygen, 2 L continuous flow
Oxygen saturation reading each evening
Lab values: Instructor may place a lab value sheet in an electronic medical record or in the HPS, indicating that all lab values are within normal range with the exception of decreased BUN and decreased hematocrit.

Scenario Part 1

Part 1: Setting the Scene

Patient history: Mrs. Fertal is an 89-year-old resident of White Oak Nursing Home, where she has lived for 5 years. She is a heavyset woman with a round, pleasant face. Her white hair has grown a bit longer than it should be kept. Her nightstand and overbed tables are cluttered with all sorts of items: the TV remote, tissues, a cordless phone, used cups, packets of artificial sweetener, and a basket of other assorted necessities. She has a walker that sits in the corner of the room and a bedside commode next to the TV. On the wall at the foot of the bed there is a bulletin board that has some photos of her family.

Recently, she has experienced increasing shortness of breath. Although normally able to ambulate to the bathroom with minimal assistance, she recently has had more difficulty with ambulation. She is on oxygen 2 L via nasal cannula (NC), which is delivered by a compressor that also sits next to her bed.

CNA report: The CNA reports to you that Mrs. Fertal is refusing to get out of bed today because she is too tired. The CNA reports that she was surprised to find that Mrs. Fertal had gained almost 10 pounds since her last weight check, despite the fact that she has not been eating very well. When you arrive, you find Mrs. Fertal sitting in bed.

Subjective report from patient: "I just don't feel much like getting out of bed today. I'm too tired."

Part 1: Scenario Implementation

Required student assessments and actions:

___Introduce self.
___Check ID band.
___Check VS, including pulse oximeter.
___Note low pulse oximeter.
___Note that decreased temperature is a common and normal finding in the older adult.
___Conduct a head-to-toe assessment.

__Note rales in bilateral bases.

__Note pedal edema.

__Note reddened area on coccyx.

__Note atrial fibrillation.

___Check the compressor to ensure that it is working and delivering the correct amount of oxygen to the patient.

___Assess mental status for signs of acute confusion and signs of depression.

___Document relevant findings: color, position, breath sounds, heart sounds, VS, weight, change in activity level, presence of a stage 1 pressure ulcer. While charting, student checks back to compare the current weight with the previous weight. Student checks the chart for relevant lab values.

___Note that abnormal labs indicate hypovolemia: decreased BUN and decreased hematocrit.

___Contact the physician and report relevant findings in a cohesive way. This may be done via phone in the simulation room, which connects the student to faculty in the control room acting as nurse practitioner and physician.

At the conclusion of the scenario, the physician gives the order to "monitor" the patient.

Part 1: Debriefing

What did the students do correctly?

Are the students forgetting anything, or was anything done incorrectly?

What are the students' concerns about Mrs. Fertal?

What is the cause of the concern, and why might this be a cause for concern?

What actions do you need to take? What are the priorities?

What is Mrs. Fertal experiencing?

Why might she have developed a pressure ulcer?

Scenario Part 2

Part 2: Setting the Scene

Mrs. Fertal is once again sitting in bed in a high Fowler position.

CNA report: The CNA reports to you that Mrs. Fertal has gained 32 pounds since her last weight check 1 month ago. "That is so strange," says the CNA. "She really has not been eating very well." The CNA then states, "I guess that is what happens when you get old."

Subjective report from patient: "My feet look like footballs. I'm so tired. I just can't seem to catch my breath."

Part 2: Scenario Implementation

Initial settings for the HPS:

BP: 160/90 mmHg, P: 85 beats/minute, RR: 23 breaths/minute, temperature: 97.2°F

Bounding pulse

Oxygen saturation settings should be set to 88%

Place notecards on the legs of the HPS indicating that she has +3 pitting edema to her thighs

Lung sounds with loud crackles bilaterally

Atrial fibrillation

Resident is sitting in bed in a high Fowler position

Place a reddened area on the patient's coccyx indicating a stage 2 pressure ulcer

Simulated distended neck and peripheral veins

Simulated blue–purple lips.

Required student assessments and actions:

___Introduce self.
___Check ID band.
___Check VS, including pulse oximeter.
  __Note low pulse oximeter.
  __Note increase in RR.
___Conduct a head-to-toe assessment.
  __Note rails in bilateral bases.
  __Note pedal edema.
  __Note stage 2 pressure ulcer.
  __Note atrial fibrillation.
  __Note significant weight gain.
___Check the compressor to ensure that it is working and delivering the correct amount of oxygen to the patient.
  __Adjust the compressor as ordered.
___Recognize the need to humidify oxygen when delivered above 2 L/minute.
___Assess mental status for signs of acute confusion and signs of depression.
___Document relevant findings: color, position, breath sounds, heart sounds, VS, weight, change in activity level, presence of a stage 2 pressure ulcer. While charting, check back to compare the current weight with the previous weight. Check the chart for relevant lab values.
___Note that abnormal labs indicate hypovolemia: decreased BUN and decreased hematocrit.
___Contact the physician and report relevant findings in a cohesive way.

Part 2: Debriefing

What did the students do correctly?
Are the students forgetting anything, or did they do anything incorrectly?
Why might have Mrs. Fertal's pressure ulcer worsened?
What are your concerns about Mrs. Fertal now?
What is the cause of the concern, and why might this be a cause for concern?
What actions do you need to take? What are the priorities?
What is Mrs. Fertal experiencing?
What do you think about the comment of the CNA? How might you address this?

Scenario Part 3

You receive a call back from Dr. Newman, who gives you the following order: "Increase Lasix to 80 mg twice a day (BID), increase oxygen as needed (PRN) to maintain O_2 saturation more than 92%." Mrs. Fertal has been on this new Lasix regimen for 3 days.

Part 3: Setting the Scene

Mrs. Fertal is once again sitting in bed in a high Fowler position. She is wearing two diapers.

CNA report: The CNA reports to you that Mrs. Fertal said she started feeling very dizzy when being transferred into her shower chair. She states that Mrs. Fertal is usually an "easy transfer" but that today her legs were weak and she almost fell.

Subjective report from patient: "I am just so dizzy...my head is spinning. I feel like I might pass out."

Lab values: All labs are within normal range with the exception of an elevated BUN, elevated BUN creatinine ratio, and a decreased potassium level. Hematocrit is higher than previously noted, although still within the normal range.

Part 3: Scenario Implementation

Initial settings for the HPS:

BP: 90/60 mmHg, P: 110 beats/minute, RR: 20 breaths/minute, temperature: 99.2°F
Weight: 150 pounds
Oxygen saturation settings should be set to 94%
Legs are now without any edema
Lung sounds are clear
Atrial fibrillation
Resident is sitting in bed in a high Fowler position
Place a reddened area on the patient's coccyx indicating a stage 2 pressure ulcer
Place two diapers on the resident

Required student assessments and actions:

___Introduce self.
___Check ID band.
___Check VS, including pulse oximeter.
  __Check for orthostatic hypotension.
  __Note increased temperature as a sign of dehydration.
___Conduct a head-to-toe assessment.
  __Note condition of mucous membranes.
___Check the compressor to ensure that it is working and delivering the correct amount of oxygen to the patient.
___Document relevant findings: color, position, breath sounds, heart sounds, VS, weight, change in activity level, presence of a stage 2 pressure ulcer. While charting, check back to compare the current weight with the previous weight and note discrepancy. Check the chart for relevant lab values.
___ Note that abnormal labs indicate hypovolemia: increased BUN, increased BUN creatinine ratio, increased hematocrit. In addition, note hypokalemia.
___Contact the physician and report relevant findings in a cohesive way. Note the lab abnormalities and ask about holding the next dose of Lasix. The physician gives the order for 0.9% of normal saline (NS) at 150 mL per hour × 3 L.

G. DEBRIEFING GUIDELINES

Student Questions

What are your concerns about Mrs. Fertal?
What is the cause of the concern, and why might this be a cause for concern?
What actions do you need to take? What are the priorities?
What is Mrs. Fertal experiencing?
Why might Mrs. Fertal have two diapers on? How might you handle this, and what might you say to the CNA?
What is missing from the physician orders? Does Mrs. Fertal need anything else?

H. SUGGESTIONS/KEY FEATURES
TO REPLICATE OR IMPROVE

Faculty may wish to review the pathophysiology of common causes of shortness of breath in the older adult, such as CHF, COPD, and pneumonia. Facilitate discussion among students about how these diseases may present differently from each other as well as how they may present in atypical ways in the older adult.

Faculty may also wish to review Starling's Law (Grossman & Porth, 2014), the concepts of cardiac preload and afterload, and how each of these concepts applies in this particular case. A discussion about the issues related to the use of furosemide (Lasix) in the older adult may naturally follow.

I. RECOMMENDATIONS FOR FURTHER USE

There are several different ways this scenario can be modified depending on the content area and audience. A unit on communication may have the student contact a worried daughter and communicate the resident's change in health or may center on how to improve communication between CNAs and other nursing staff. A student in a clinical nurse leader track may wish to explore the multiple quality-of-care issues (e.g., development of a pressure ulcer) that arise in this case and devise ways to improve the process of care.

J. HOW SIMULATION-BASED PEDAGOGY
HAS CONTRIBUTED TO IMPROVED STUDENT OUTCOMES

Because this simulation is carried out in front of the class, students may be more motivated to arrive to class prepared. This method can also help students make the sometimes-difficult leap of translating the theory they read in their textbooks into clinical practice. Instructors may tailor simulations to mimic those situations that students are likely to encounter on their clinical units in order to enhance clinical performance.

K. EXPERT RECOMMENDATIONS
AND WORDS OF WISDOM

This scenario can be modified in many ways to create a different focus throughout the simulation. Communication of key findings to physicians and other members of the health care team is an essential component of this scenario. Instructors may want to highlight different communication strategies (i.e., situation, background, assessment, recommendations [SBAR]) in communicating this information (Thomas, Bertram, & Johnson, 2009). Second-year baccalaureate students may need additional support in recognizing key findings from a physical assessment, whereas more advanced students should be allowed to complete physical assessments with a greater degree of independence.

L. EVALUATION OF BEST PRACTICE STANDARDS
AND USE OF CREDENTIALED SIMULATION FACULTY

Our experiences have shown us that the most critical component to any simulation is debriefing (Standard VIII of the International Nursing Association for Clinical and Simulation Learning

[INASCL] guidelines; Lioce et al., 2015). However, because the debriefing tends to occur near the end of the scenario, it is often likely to be cut short because of time constraints. Faculty may wish to review INASCL Criterion VIII for additional guidance on this key standard.

ACKNOWLEDGMENT

This case was developed from data gathered from a research grant provided by the John A. Hartford Foundation. The discussion questions were adapted from the Carnegie Foundation (2007).

REFERENCES

Carnegie Foundation. (2007). Integrative teaching at its best: Study of nursing education. Retrieved from http://www.carnegiefoundation.org/programs/sub.asp?key=829&subkey=2309&topkey=1829

Grossman, S., & Porth, C. (2014). *Pathophysiology: Concepts of altered health states*. Philadelphia, PA: Wolters Kluwer Health/Lippincott Williams & Wilkins.

Lioce, L., Meakim, C. H., Fey, M. K., Chmil, J. V., Mariani, B., & Alinier, G. (2015, June). Standards of best practice: Simulation standard IX: Simulation design. *Clinical Simulation in Nursing, 11*(6), 309–315. doi:10.1016/j.ecns.2015.03.005

National Council of State Boards of Nursing. (2015). NCLEX-RN examination: Test plan for the National Council Licensure Examination for Registered Nurses. Retrieved from https://www.ncsbn.org/RN_Test_Plan_2016_Final.pdf

Shea, J. M., Campbell, S. H., & Miners, L. (2013). Faculty learning communities: An innovative approach to faculty development. In S. H. Campbell & K. M. Daley (Eds.), *Simulation scenarios for nursing educators: Making it real* (2nd ed., pp. 25–31). New York, NY: Springer Publishing.

Thomas, C. M., Bertram, E., & Johnson, D. (2009). The SBAR communication technique: Teaching nursing students professional communication skills. *Nurse Educator, 34*(4), 176–180.

FURTHER READING

Azad, N., & Lemay, G. (2014). Management of chronic heart failure in the older population. *Journal of Geriatric Cardiology, 11*(4), 329–337. doi:10.11909/j.issn.1671-5411.2014.04.008

The Older Adult in an ICU With Acute Respiratory Failure: Critical Care Nursing Senior-Year Elective

Sheila C. Grossman

A. IMPLEMENTATION OF SIMULATION-BASED PEDAGOGY IN YOUR INDIVIDUALIZED TEACHING AREA

This three-credit course is a fourth-year last-semester elective in a baccalaureate program called "Critical Care Nursing." The course combines theory and clinical laboratory courses that are offered concurrently with the students' transition-to-professional-role course. This transition course has the student paired with a nurse preceptor for 165 hours in the inpatient clinical setting. The students taking critical care nursing are working with their preceptor on critical care units, step-down units, and acute care medical and surgical units.

This course is an introduction to critical care nursing. The nursing diagnoses and management of patients focus on cardiovascular, pulmonary, gastrointestinal, renal, neurological, and multisystem alterations. Common problems of critical care patients, such as sleep, pain, nutritional and psychosocial difficulties, are also discussed. Palliative care issues are also described in each of the systems mentioned. Frequently used medications and relevant nursing implications are addressed. Basic EKG interpretation is covered and significant nursing interventions are addressed.

The students gain many of their skills in the college laboratory practice sessions and then apply their knowledge from class, clinical rotations, and work experience in carrying out simulated case scenarios. They volunteer for one of the simulation scenarios, such as the respiratory care case discussed in this chapter, and work in a group of four students practicing the case. Then each group carries out the scenario for the class. The students welcome the challenge of working with simulated critically ill case scenarios given the difficulty level of the skills, high patient acuity, and need for expanded theory compared to what the students have received in their medical and surgical courses, and in most situations, they lack clinical experience with the critically ill patient and with providing palliative care to critically ill patients. This process of learning by reading assigned text and articles related to the topic, listening and participating in class regarding application of the knowledge to case studies, seeing demonstrations and practicing specific skills on models in the college laboratory, obtaining firsthand clinical experience in rotations if possible, maintaining a reflective practice log on patient experiences, and participating and observing simulated case scenarios allows maximum critical thinking and problem solving for the students to gain as much new knowledge as possible.

B. EDUCATIONAL MATERIALS AVAILABLE IN YOUR TEACHING AREA AND RELATED TO YOUR SPECIALTY

This simulation experience can be made to fit the long-term subacute facility or even the home setting, as many patients who are not able to be weaned are on a ventilator outside of the critical care area. It is important that there are enough students and/or faculty to assume the roles of nurse, family member(s), and intensivist so that there can be a collaborative discussion as well as health teaching with the family members. Perhaps the most difficult aspect of this scenario is the communication between the wife and children regarding the patient's do-not-resuscitate/do-not-intubate (DNR/DNI) status. Using the critical care area of the learning resource center at the Fairfield University School of Nursing makes it easy to carry out the critical care scenarios as monitor, bed, oxygen and suction equipment, ventilator, and all types of intravenous (IV) lines and medications are already set up. The high-fidelity human patient simulator (HPS) is handled by a teaching assistant who is able to run the controls and software. This handler has already been apprised by the faculty of the appropriate EKG tracing, respiration rate (RR), blood pressure (BP), and pulse parameters to have displayed on the monitor during the various aspects of the scenario. All of the equipment, as stated previously, has been checked and labeled for the students involved in the scenario. There is even a telephone and area for the family/significant others to sit in while waiting for their 10- to 20-minute visit in the intensive care unit.

This scenario also covers a palliative care focus for the students, and this DNR/DNI information could be extracted and applied to a patient with respiratory difficulty who is facing death if she or he is not intubated. Setting this up as a less acute experience would also be beneficial for the students to practice talking about death with members of the health care team, patient, and family/significant others. There are multiple resources for the palliative care focus available from the American Association of Colleges of Nursing (AACN) End-of-Life Nursing Education Consortium (ELNEC) website (www.aacn.nche.edu/elnec); The Palliative Care of Dying Critically Ill Patients' Algorithm (Grossman, 2013) also assists nurses in steps to follow when providing palliative care.

C. SPECIFIC OBJECTIVES OF SIMULATION USAGE WITHIN A CRITICAL CARE NURSING ELECTIVE COURSE AND THE OVERALL PROGRAM

Overall Course Objectives

The overall purpose of the course is for students to gain increased knowledge, clinical reasoning, clinical skills, case management, and awareness of their communication skills in an ICU. The goals for this complex scenario are for students to gain experience in managing the care of a patient on a ventilator, as the students do not get this opportunity in the clinical area, as well as to experience collaborating with the physician, other nurses, and family regarding the patient's needs related to comfort and satisfaction with the end life.

Student Learning Activities

Many students voice serious anxiety about suctioning, airway maintenance, working with a patient on a ventilator, and caring for someone who is terminal and may die during the students' assigned time with the patient. Perhaps the most important outcome from this practice of skills is the self-confidence one usually achieves after performing well in the scenario, and this increased confidence in clinical skill performance was demonstrated with simulation by Fisher and King (2013).

D. INTRODUCTION OF SCENARIO

Setting the Scene

This scenario was developed for final-semester senior baccalaureate nursing students. They have completed their medical and surgical, pediatric, geriatric, mental health, and women's health specialty courses. They are concurrently taking their Public Health and Transition to Professional Role course. The following is the scene for this end-stage chronic obstructive pulmonary disease (COPD) patient.

Eighty-one-year-old Mr. Whisper is ventilated and attempting to talk around his endotracheal (ET) tube. He is Irish, married, and a retired judge with a strong Catholic faith. He has three grown children and 12 grandchildren who all come to visit regularly. His current diagnosis is COPD exacerbation secondary to emphysema with bilateral lower lobe pneumonia, dyspnea, a long history of atrial fibrillation, aortic valve replacement, coronary artery disease (CAD), hyperlipidemia, and hypertension. He receives lisinopril (Zestril) 10 mg, metoprolol (Lopressor) 100 mg, hydrochlorothiazide 12.5 mg, tiotropium (Spiriva) inhaler qd, levofloxacin (Levaquin), warfarin (Coumadin), and fluoxetine (Prozac). He receives morphine sulfate (MS) 2 to 10 mg IV as needed for anxiety. This is his fifth admission to the hospital in 3 months, and his children have brought up the option of DNR/DNI with him. His wife has been against this option until this admission, but now she is in agreement with their children that Mr. Whisper should not be intubated again. He is having multiple high-pressure alarm problems because of his emphysema pathology and large amount of mucus plugging from the pneumonia.

Technology Used

The scenario takes place in the critical care area; the patient is a high-fidelity HPS lying in a bed connected to a ventilator and cardiac/hemodynamic monitor and there is also an area where the wife/family can sit. A phone is nearby in case the nurse wants to call for help or discuss an issue with the respiratory therapist or physician or another nurse. An electronic health record is in front of the bed for the student to use for charting or to find any patient information.

Objectives

After completing the scenario simulation exercise the students are able to do the following:

1. Communicate with the patient and his wife about the patient's condition regarding his palliative care measures.
2. Communicate with the nurse giving the previous shift report, along with other health care team members.
3. Demonstrate oral, closed, and open endotracheal (ET) suctioning and hyperventilation on a ventilated patient.
4. Assess breath sounds on a COPD patient with pneumonia.
5. Assess and manage premature ventricular contractions (PVCs) on the patient's cardiac monitor.
6. Troubleshoot a ventilated patient with high-pressure alarm problems.
7. Administer MS to an anxious patient according to evidence-based protocols.
8. Facilitate the wife's participation with her three children in preparing for a palliative care family meeting and revise the patient's advance directives to reflect his wishes.
9. Manage the IV, being sure to have two access sites and to monitor fluid intake.
10. Assist with insertion of a central line and follow evidence-based protocols before using the newly established line.

Description of Participants

Mr. Whisper: He is generally a simulated manikin, but a student or faculty member could perform this role.

Mrs. Whisper: She could be a faculty member or a student. It seems the student gains much from being in this role and having to handle the family and patient regarding DNR/DNI.

Nurse assigned to Mr. Whisper: This student is responsible for performing the care; assessing the patient; collaborating with the health care team and family about DNR/DNI issues; and talking to the patient, who is intubated. A magic slate or a pad and pencil are used.

Nurse going off shift: A student can do this role easily and still participate in the rest of the scenario by moving to the side and noting any concerns or mistakes she or he sees. This student can offer this information in the debriefing.

Experienced nurse: This is a student who acts more comfortable in the ICU setting and assists the assigned nurse in caring for the patient when necessary.

ICU intensivist: A student generally takes this role and has to participate in talking with Mrs. Whisper and Mr. Whisper regarding his plan of care.

Teaching assistant: This person runs the simulator from the control room.

A faculty member is observing in the critical care area of the learning resource laboratory during the scenario to be best able to evaluate the student's performance, but does not offer any hints or assistance until the students join the rest of the class for debriefing after the scenario.

E. RUNNING OF THE SCENARIO

Students have read the required materials on caring for acute care respiratory patients, had a class discussion regarding this same topic, and have accomplished the ventilator demonstration laboratory module. They also completed all of the undergraduate ELNEC components and reviewed The Palliative Care of Dying Critically Ill Patients' Algorithm (Grossman, 2013); at least two of the students have worked with a ventilated patient in clinical. All the students have also worked in the critical care area of the learning resource center for skill practice, so they are familiar with working with the monitor, bed, oxygen, and the suction.

The equipment set up on a bedside table consists of a central line kit, central line dressing kit, bedpan, toilet paper, suction catheter, sterile gloves, tray, stethoscope, gloves, and saline solution. All medications, syringes, and needles needed are in the medication Pyxis machine next to the patient. The patient is connected to two IV lines, the ventilator, monitor, and oxygen, and suction is available in the adjacent wall.

This is a 20-minute scenario planned for class presentation by four students. Students have practiced as a group three times and even once with their instructor, so they are prepared to present the scenario to the class.

F. PRESENTATION OF COMPLETED TEMPLATE

Title

The Older Adult With Acute Respiratory Failure in an ICU

Scenario Level

Senior baccalaureate nursing students

Focus Area

Critical care nursing, therapeutic communication, health assessment, medical–surgical nursing, palliative care

Scenario Description

Patient history: This scenario takes place in the medical ICU where the patient, Mr. Whisper, has been intubated and on a ventilator for some time. He is not doing well and is requesting a change in his DNR/DNI status. His wife is in the process of agreeing with this change now, and their children have supported their father's wishes. A meeting is planned with his family to make some plans for his death. The scenario involves the difficult suctioning and runs of premature ventricular contractions (PVCs) that occur with people who have end-stage COPD who are on ventilators, but who are not progressing to recovery. Mr. Whisper is quite anxious, dislikes all of the ventilator and cardiac alarms, and has prolonged periods of dyspnea when he has mucus plugs. This causes his wife also to be very upset. Students participate in this scenario for communication, critical care, and palliative care experience.

    Health assessment results: Physical assessment reveals the following significant findings:

Skin: thin with multiple abrasions, decreased turgor, decreased moisture of oral mucosa
Heart: displaced point of maximum impulse (PMI), atrial fibrillation
Respiratory: barrel chest, unequal chest excursion, scattered rhonchi throughout, rales and decreased breath sounds in lower lobes

    Medication record: He receives lisinopril (Zestril) 10 mg, metoprolol (Lopressor) 100 mg, hydrochlorothiazide 12.5 mg, tiotropium (Spiriva) inhaler qd, levofloxacin (Levaquin), warfarin (Coumadin), and fluoxetine (Prozac). He receives morphine sulfate (MS) 2 to 10 mg IV as needed for anxiety.

Scenario Objectives

Key Elements From NCSBN

Since the last edition of this book a landmark study through the National Council of State Boards of Nursing (NCSBN) by Hayden, Smiley, Alexander, Kardong-Edgren, and Jeffries (2014), found that up to 50% of clinical hours of the undergraduate programs could be substituted by simulation pedagogy, and in 2015 the "NCSBN Simulation Guidelines for Prelicensure Nursing Programs" was published (Alexander et al., 2015). The National Council Licensure Examination for Registered Nurses (NCLEX-RN®) test plan categories and subcategories (NCSBN, 2015) addressed in the simulation are as follows:

Safe and effective care environment: *Management of Care, Safety and Infection Control*; **Health promotion and maintenance; Psychosocial integrity; physiological integrity:** *Basic care and comfort, Pharmacological and parenteral therapies, Reduction of risk potential, Physiological adaptation.*

Key Elements From BSN Essentials

The AACN (2008) has created nine BSN Essentials that are used as a guide to developing curriculum for baccalaureate nursing programs. The Essentials document states "Simulation experiences augment clinical learning and are complementary to direct care opportunities essential to assuming the role of the professional nurse"(p. 4). The Essentials that are addressed in this simulation by objective are listed as follows:

Essential II: Basic Organizational and Systems Leadership for Quality Care and Patient Safety
Knowledge and skills in leadership, quality improvement, and patient safety are necessary to provide high-quality health care. The students must be leaders in advocating for their patients as well as provide high-quality and safe care to all, especially the terminally ill.
Essential III: Scholarship for Evidence-Based Practice
Professional nursing practice is grounded in evidence-based practice. Students follow these protocols with Mr. Whisper regarding the ventilator, oxygenation, suctioning, and palliative care.
Essential IV: Information Management and Application of Patient Care Technology

Knowledge and skills in information management and patient care technology are critical in the delivery of quality patient care. Students use electronic documentation and Pyxis.

Essential V: Health Care Policy, Finance, and Regulatory Environments

Health care policies, including finances and regulations, influence the nature and functioning of the health care system, and therefore are important considerations in professional nursing practice. Preparing and changing advance directives are part of professional nursing practice.

Essential VI: Interprofessional Communication and Collaboration for Improving Patient Health Outcomes

Communication and collaboration among health care professionals are critical to delivering high-quality and safe patient care. Students collaborate with all members of the health care team to deliver care to patients such as Mr. Whisper.

Essential VIII: Professionalism and Professional Values

Professionalism and the inherent values of altruism, autonomy, human dignity, integrity, and social justice are fundamental to nursing. Students are dealing with life-and-death issues with patients and their families.

Essential IX: Baccalaureate Generalist Nursing Practice

The baccalaureate graduate nurse is prepared to practice with patients, including individuals, families, groups, communities, and populations across the life span and across the continuum of health care environments. The baccalaureate graduate understands and respects the variations of care, the increased complexity, and the increased use of health care resources inherent in caring for patients.

Setting the Scene

Equipment Needed:

HPS to be the patient; critical care area with bed, oxygen, ventilator, cardiac monitor, suction, BP cuff and stethoscope, alcohol wipes, gloves, and Pyxis machine with medications; IV lines, central venous line setup and dressing, bedpan, suction and oxygen equipment; and electronic record

Resources Needed

Critical care textbook, medical–surgical textbook, procedures textbook

Simulator Level

Mid- to high-fidelity HPS

Participants Needed

Student nurses to play nurse, intensivist, and family roles; an HPS; and a person to run and/or observe the scenario

Scripted Lines for Student Participant Involved in the Scenario

The nurse is given report from the nurse going off shift. The reporting nurse **says:** "I was busy every minute and did not have time to get Mr. Whisper suctioned in the last 3 hours. He needs some help now that he is agitated with the ET and his high-pressure alarm has been triggered several times recently. I am not having success communicating with him and his wife, and they are dissatisfied with the care. She was in last evening and was complaining to the 3-to-11 nurse, who told me the wife and children are going to have a family meeting regarding changing the DNR status soon. He has not had MS for longer than 6 hours. The only peripheral IV line is questionably patent and running erratically. He is having loose stools and is on the buzzer 24/7."

After the report, the nurse checks the medication documentation and prepares the MS for administration.

The nurse introduces self to patient, who is trying to talk around his ET tube. The nurse gives him a pad/pen and some effective communication transpires.

Nurse assesses Mr. Whisper and determines how much MS he should receive and administers it. He should receive 4 mg via IV push.

Nurse sees that he needs immediate suctioning as the high-pressure alarm is triggering every 2 to 3 minutes and the airway pressure is greater than 40 cm H_2O.

Nurse preoxygenates the patient via the ventilator with 100% O_2 and begins closed suctioning but is unsuccessful in suctioning enough of the mucus to shut off the alarm. Nurse stops and decreases the FiO_2 back to 40% O_2 as it was previously set at the 100% setting for the suctioning.

Nurse auscultates Mr. Whisper's lungs and determines decreased breath sounds in the left lower lobe (LLL) and rhonchi. (This is a deterioration as previously he was clearing in both the left and right lung fields.) Nurse notices PVCs on the monitor and the sat O_2 saturation decreases to the low 80s from 91% during the suctioning and remains lower after suctioning. The PVCs spontaneously stop.

Now the nurse determines that the patient is agitated and is trying to talk around his ET, his RR is 36 breaths/minute, he is fighting the ventilator, and the high-pressure alarm is almost constantly alarming because the airway pressure is around 30 cm H_2O.

The wife arrives and becomes hysterical about her husband's inability to relax and his constant triggering of the ventilator and the alarms. She **says:** "My husband is a judge and he needs to be treated with utmost dignity. He cannot be allowed to feel he cannot catch his breath. What are you doing? You look so unprepared to take care of my husband. Do you know what you are doing? I am going to get a more experienced nurse to help you who knows what to do. You are just unfit to work with him and you do not know anything. Why hasn't the doctor called me about his worsening condition?"

The more experienced nurse comes in and takes Mrs. Whisper away from the bedside and discusses the situation with her and their plan to remove the mucus plug so he will stop triggering the pressure alarm and be able to rest. She also broaches the subject of DNR status for the upcoming family visit.

The original nurse explains to the patient their plan of removing him temporarily from the ventilator to suction him. The intensivist comes in and says she will help the nurse remove the mucus plug. She starts to hyperventilate the patient with 100% O_2 and large deep breaths × 3. They suction the tube 3 times and procure the plug and lots of loose mucus. They note that there are quite a few PVCs occurring during the suctioning time and some are three in a row. They start a lidocaine drip at 3 mg per minute and reattach him to the ventilator. His O_2 saturation was in the 60s during the suctioning and now it is up to 85% and the PVCs are slowing.

The intensivist emphasizes the need for frequent suctioning and orders mucolytics and more MS. The nurse prepares and administers another 4 mg of MS and documents this on his flow sheet. The lidocaine is decreased to 1 mg per minute. The peripheral line is noted to be sluggish and so the intensivist says a central line would be prudent as there is potential for the peripheral line to fail.

The intensivist explains to Mr. Whisper that they are putting in a central line to assist with making him feel more comfortable and he agrees and signs for the procedure. The nurse has the central line equipment ready and assists the intensivist in inserting the line into the subclavian vein. An x-ray is called to confirm the placement before being able to use the line.

The experienced nurse brings Mrs. Whisper back into the room; she appears more subdued and pleasant. She sits with her husband as they await the family discussion meeting.

The experienced nurse talks with the intensivist and other nurse regarding Mrs. Whisper's reluctant agreement to change her husband's advance directive to what he has requested. This is his last admission and it is hoped he will be able to be extubated or go home on his ventilator to die. There will be no more intubations after this. Owing to the advance directive, the physician has to insert the central line as Mr. Whisper has no other access for medication administration if the interventions are to continue. If the DNR/DNI is accepted for Mr. Whisper by the family, then the central line can be removed as the only medication will be given subcutaneously.

Scenario Implementation

Initial Settings

If the clinical laboratory does not have a critical care area one can develop a unit with one bed and wall suction, oxygen, and cardboard monitor that depicts changes in vital signs (VS) by just putting stickers up as the scenario transpires. Perhaps a huge appliance box could be made to resemble a ventilator if an outdated respirator cannot be obtained from an affiliating hospital.

Expected/Required Student Assessments and Actions

Final-semester senior baccalaureate students have completed all required clinical skills as well as leadership, management, and communication courses. They are prepared to manage challenging issues such as advance directives and high-acuity patients. The faculty should be confident that the students can demonstrate all skills safely and effectively. Students have had multiple case study analyses and should be able to practice developing a script themselves. Subsequently, they should have a rehearsal with the faculty, who should assist them in polishing the script. After the designated time, they should accomplish the scenario objectives, be able to self-critique their performance, receive constructive feedback from the class, and identify their strengths and weak areas.

Instructor Interventions

The faculty need to develop the objectives for the learning experience and share a case with the students. The background information given, along with the objectives for the student learning, is then molded into a script. It is up to the senior students to practice and perfect the scenario and then obtain feedback from the faculty. More practice is suggested until the students feel comfortable and confident to perform the script independently for the 20-minute time frame in front of their classmates. The faculty need to keep the students to the time frame by holding up cards notifying them of the time still left. The debriefing session is held with the whole class, and the faculty lead the discussion, being sure to evaluate the students' performance and answer questions that may come up. On the basis of the objectives for this scenario the following evaluative criteria need to be measured.

Evaluative Criteria

___Obtains report from previous nurse and develops plan for next half hour with priorities.
___Performs hand hygiene.
___Introduces self to patient/family.
___Communicates clearly with patient/family/health care team members.
___Demonstrates professional dress/behavior.
___Assesses patient's status with ventilator, performs appropriate troubleshooting with high-pressure alarm.
___Interprets VS and ventilatory status of patient.
___Inquires about loose bowels with physician, develops a plan.

___Asks pertinent questions about the family meeting and palliative care plan: Will the patient be extubated or be discharged to home/hospice on a ventilator?

___Asks questions in a manner that the patient can understand and allows alternative communication because patient is intubated.

___Performs focused physical examination in logical order.

___Uses appropriate medications for anxiety and dysrhythmia.

___Acknowledges patient's concerns and feelings, teaches about ventilator, explains what procedures are being performed and why.

___Collaborates appropriately with health care team members.

___Is able to state normal and abnormal pressure alarm ranges and O_2 saturation levels.

___Seeks assistance when necessary.

___Assists physician with central line insertion.

___Is able to discuss advance directives in a professional manner.

G. DEBRIEFING GUIDELINES

Issues to Consider

Students need to receive immediate feedback after the simulated scenario. As long as the scenario was developed along sound objectives, the students prepared and studied diligently, and there were measurable evaluative criteria, debriefing is very matter of fact. Generally, it is a good idea to ask the participants to give their own self-evaluation using the recorder's notes so they can stay organized. Subsequently, it is important to obtain the classmates' feedback. Be sure that the classmates are aware that they need to prepare for this scenario as if they were going to be participating. In this way they can be more a part of the evaluation process. Once the students realize they are going to be called on either by the faculty or the scenario participants for feedback or asked a question regarding the case, they prepare thoroughly.

Student Questions

Senior students generally have no difficulty discussing and sharing their ideas in the debriefing session. The faculty should limit the time to no more than 30 minutes, and if students are not asking appropriate questions the faculty should steer the discussion toward the evaluative criteria.

Classroom/Observer Questions

Some questions that may assist the class to get started on the discussion are:

1. Would you have done anything differently at any time? Give a rationale.
2. How would you see the role of the nurse regarding collaborative communication?
3. Did the nurse manage the priorities first?
4. What model do you use to determine what the priority for a given patient situation is?

H. SUGGESTIONS/KEY FEATURES TO REPLICATE OR IMPROVE

This scenario is focused on gaining experience with suctioning and caring for a patient with acute respiratory failure on a ventilator, along with seeking a change in advance directives. Some additional components that could spin off this same case scenario for a different group of students could include the following:

- Have Mr. Whisper go into ventricular tachycardia during his suctioning and then have a full-blown cardiac arrest with a code
- Follow up on the diarrhea with Mr. Whisper—either have him also have a feeding tube that needs to have a change of feeding supplement or have him be impacted, after which he could experience a vagal syncope episode
- Have Mr. Whisper progress to acute respiratory distress syndrome and then systemic inflammatory response syndrome and manage these deteriorating conditions

I. RECOMMENDATIONS FOR FURTHER USE

Given that this present scenario is already 20 minutes in length, it seems long and complex enough to hold the students' attention and maximize multiple learning gains. However, many additional problems could be added regarding the family, staff, or a legal problem. For example, Mr. Whisper could have his son or daughter unplug him from the ventilator without bothering to change the advance directive. A family member could become "emotionally upset" seeing his or her father connected to so many machines, gasping for air, and complaining of discomfort. Or the staff might all be intolerant of Mrs. Whisper, who seems to have a negative personality and wants to blame everything on the nurses.

Perhaps a most important recommendation would be to keep the scenario at 20 minutes, have no more complications arise and share important clinical hints for assessment when caring for difficult-to-wean ventilator patients. This simulation offers great potential for students to be exposed to situations they might not have experienced in traditional clinical environments and can serve to impact students' clinical reasoning ability, which is identified as a potential outcome of debriefing (Fomeris, 2015).

J. HOW SIMULATION-BASED PEDAGOGY HAS CONTRIBUTED TO IMPROVED STUDENT OUTCOMES

It is most important that students have an opportunity to volunteer for the scenarios they want to participate in and to be responsible for teaching the content to their colleagues. In addition, faculty need to be sure the students feel comfortable with their upcoming performance. By having small-group practices and demonstrations of complex skills, students feel more confident in their abilities.

It is important to establish a culture in the simulated laboratory that indicates it is fine to stay as long as one wants to practice and to even videotape oneself so that it is easy for students to do a self-evaluation. Certainly one's most honest critique will be from oneself. So, faculty need to allow enough practice time, privacy, quiet, and someone who is available to demonstrate skills, correct skill performance if necessary, and to discuss questions one might have. Our simulation director has started the use of videotaping and self-reflection with all simulations and she even records the simulation before class and faculty upload these to the class, so they can visualize the simulation before class. This affords more class time for debriefing and more participation from the class. Faculty are in the process of becoming certified in simulation and a new simulation laboratory is under construction. With the additional challenges in obtaining clinical sites, the increased student enrollment, and the ability to provide classic patient experiences via simulation to all students, the pedagogy of simulation is being integrated fully into all baccalaureate courses.

K. EXPERT RECOMMENDATIONS
AND WORDS OF WISDOM

Readers can refer back to the previous sections as these recommendations are integrated throughout.

L. EVALUATION OF BEST PRACTICE STANDARDS
AND USE OF CREDENTIALED SIMULATION FACULTY

Dealing with critically ill patients, such as Mr. Whisper, who are in the process of obtaining a DNR/DNI advance directive offers students a challenge they might not have experienced in a traditional clinical experience. Evidence suggests that simulation experience can improve one's competence in caring for the terminally ill (Lippe & Becker, 2015). The International Nursing Association for Clinical Simulation and Learning (INACSL) developed the INACSL Standards of Best Practice: Simulation (INACSL, 2013/2016), which are very helpful with designing and revising simulations and can be accessed at www.inacsl.org/i4a/pages/index.cfm?pageid=3407. For example, Standard II Professional Integrity of Participant(s) (Gloe et al., 2013), emphasizes the importance of maintaining a scenario as close to reality as possible during the simulation, and delineates many good ideas on doing this.

REFERENCES

Alexander, M., Durham, C., Hopper, J., Jeffries, P., Goldman, N., Kardong-Edgren, S., & Tillman, C. (2015). NCSBN simulation guidelines for prelicensure nursing programs. *Journal of Nursing Regulation, 6*(3), 39–42.

American Association of Colleges of Nursing. (2008). *Essentials of baccalaureate education for professional nursing practice.* Washington, DC: Author. Retrieved from http://www.aacnnursing.org/Portals/42/Publications/BaccEssentials08.pdf

Fisher, D., & King, L. (2013). An integrative literature review on preparing nursing students through simulation to recognize and respond to the deteriorating patient. *Journal of Advanced Nursing, 69*(11), 2375–2388.

Fomeris, S. (2015). Enhancing clinical reasoning through simulation debriefing: A multisite study. *Nursing Education Perspectives, 36*(5), 304–310.

Gloe, D., Sando, C. R., Franklin, A. E., Boese, T., Decker, S., Lioce, L.,…Borum, J. C. (2013). Standards of best practice: Simulation standard II: Professional integrity of participant(s). *Clinical Simulation in Nursing, 9*(6S), S12–S14.

Grossman, S. (2013). Development of the palliative care of dying critically ill patients' algorithm: Implications for critical care nurses. *Journal of Palliative and Hospice Nursing, 15*(6), 355–359.

Hayden, J. K., Smiley, R. A., Alexander, M., Kardong-Edgren, S., & Jeffries, P. R. (2014). The NCSBN National Simulation Study: A longitudinal, randomized, controlled study: Replacing clinical hours with simulation in prelicensure nursing education. *Journal of Nursing Regulation, 5*(2S), 1–66.

International Nursing Association for Clinical Simulation and Learning. (2013, updated 2016). INACSL standards of best practice: Simulation. Retrieved from https://www.inacsl.org/i4a/pages/index.cfm?pageID=3407

Lippe, M. P., & Becker, H. (2015). Improving attitudes and perceived competence in caring for dying patients: An end-of-life simulation. *Nursing Education Perspectives, 36*(6), 372–378.

National Council of State Boards of Nursing. (2015). NCLEX-RN examination: Test plan for the National Council Licensure Examination for Registered Nurses. Retrieved from https://www.ncsbn.org/RN_Test_Plan_2016_Final.pdf

CHAPTER 26

Communication With an Elderly Client

Lillian A. Rafeldt, Heather Jane Bader, and Suzanne Turner

A. IMPLEMENTATION OF SIMULATION-BASED PEDAGOGY IN YOUR INDIVIDUALIZED TEACHING AREA

Simulation and guided reflection are used throughout the curriculum at Three Rivers Community College (TRCC). Role-playing in the classroom and nursing laboratory helps students make meaning of clinical content for proficiency in examinations and clinical practice. Students learn to collect cues, process information, consider alternative actions, and implement and evaluate outcomes. Reflective writing through carefully crafted prompts and directed questions strengthens the practice (Rafeldt et al., 2014). Faculty strive to remove obstacles of fear and inflexibility so that critical thinking becomes clinical reasoning. It is easy to carry out rote procedures rather than assessing and "thinking out" what to do in a situation. When students learn how to use broad concepts, they can perform procedures long after graduation (Nosich, 2008). Currently, standardized patients and static and high-fidelity human patient simulators (HPSs) are the "patients" in actual and video nursing simulation exercises.

Under the leadership of previous nursing directors, simulation has grown. Edith Ouellet, RN, MSN, now leads the work in which all faculty have been trained in debriefing, scenario, and equipment use. Two faculty members, Suzanne Turner, RN, MSN, and Joan Graham, RN, MSN, participated in a National League for Nursing simulation grant. Joan is completing her dissertation work in student simulation outcomes. Students complete dedicated simulation days with gerontologic, postpartum, and medical–surgical patients, reporting increased confidence and ability to practice in clinical. A multifaceted approach in the creation of laboratory classwork, independent study material, clinical experiences, and presentation of theory supports increased retention rates without depleting resources.

B. EDUCATIONAL MATERIALS AVAILABLE IN YOUR TEACHING AREA AND RELATED TO YOUR SPECIALTY

Some of the first successful simulation experiences included students who demonstrated clinical reasoning ability while caring for clients with orthopedic conditions. After completing the learning unit, students signed up in groups of three to four to care for "Mr. Bili Rubin," who had a right total hip replacement. He had one of eight complications; the students had to identify the complication correctly and then implement appropriate care. Because there were eight possible complications, students could not listen to "the grapevine" to prepare their actual care. Critical thinking skills within the moment in the discipline of nursing were required. Students rated this experience as an extremely positive activity. Now simulation activities are used in lab and active learning within the classrooms.

Another successful simulation experience included students who were returning or transferring into the program at varying levels. Simulation exercises were constructed to include outcomes from previous program levels. Students completed the simulations with laboratory staff, and were debriefed and evaluated by faculty to determine course placements. Simulation was not the only criterion for placement level.

Simulation and reflection in nursing education provide a foundation for knowledge, skill performance, collaboration, clinical reasoning, and development of self-confidence. Dewey (1944), an educational reformer, suggested that activity with purposeful reflection supports learning as a "moving force" toward positive change. In this simulation scenario, communication with an elderly client, students have the opportunity to reinforce previously learned content and explore principles used in communication with the older adult. Vygotsky (1978) defined *scaffolding* as an instruction technique whereby scaffolds facilitate a student's ability to build on previous knowledge and internalize new information. Reflection and *scaffolding* approaches enrich the following scenario.

C. SPECIFIC OBJECTIVES OF SIMULATION USAGE WITHIN A SPECIFIC COURSE AND THE OVERALL PROGRAM

Nurses assess, interview, examine, and gather data to develop plans and implement and evaluate care. Nurses of the 21st century use critical thinking when communicating with elders—the most rapidly expanding group of the population. Development of expert skills in communication facilitates efficient client-centered care, resolution of illness, and promotion of health. This scenario focuses on communication with an elderly client in the hospital. A generalist nurse provides direct and indirect care.

The scenario can be used in an introduction-to-nursing or gerontologic nursing course or as a tutoring tool for students who desire reinforcement of learning to support clinical practice. It may be used as an individual or group exercise. This scenario builds on previous learning, using the principles of scaffolding while focusing on achievement of new outcomes. Standard nursing behaviors when interacting with a client are expected in each scenario; new outcomes are added. The scenario can be enhanced in advanced nursing courses when the client becomes deaf, aphasic, or visually impaired, or is diagnosed with dementia. The scenario can be extended to develop nursing diagnoses and plans of care.

D. INTRODUCTION OF SCENARIO

Students enter a "nursing lab." Evaluators can predetermine whether a uniform or any other equipment from home is required to care for the client. At the bedside, the student or students will find Mrs. Anderson, as described in the scenario description that follows. Choices are provided for high-fidelity or live role-play scenarios. Consider 20 students entering the lab: Five students could be assigned to act as the "active scenario participants," while the other 15 students could be assigned to be observers using the evaluative checklists. The student observers could watch the scenario within the same room or in an observation classroom, depending on the constructed environment. Principles of teamwork can be fostered. Multiple simulations are required throughout a semester, so roles can be rotated. The simulations can be recorded and used as tools in active learning classrooms. For specifics regarding setting the scene, technology used, and description of participants with their roles and scripts, see Exhibit 26.1.

Exhibit 26.1	Scenario Progression Outline			
Timing	**Mrs. Anderson**	**Expected Actions**	**Prompts, Questions, Teaching Points**	**Other Prompts/Cues**
Frame 1: First 5 minutes	Temp. 99°F A: Sinus tachycardia: 90 beats/minute BP: 140/88 mmHg	Verify orders. Wash hands.	Is environment conducive for interview—light, background noise, private, warm?	
	Monitor controls: SpO$_2$: 98% RR: 22 breaths/minute Auscultation sounds: Lungs: Clear Heart: S1S2 Bowel: Normative	Introduce self; faces client, uses normal tone. Turns lights on.	Is the student speaking face to face with the client, not off to the side, with hands away from face, and not chewing gum?	Understands that presentation of disease in an elderly client may be atypical; falls may indicate infection.
	Use microphone or put in program as handlers (SimMan).	Identify client by ID band and ask client name, DOB, where she is, and why.	Is the student speaking in a normal way, not shouting? Is time given for conversation?	A temperature of 99°F may indicate a fever in an elderly client.
Can go to third frame if the client is not acknowledged or no appropriate response to patient's complaint of pain is given.	"My name is Mrs. Anderson. I'm here to feel better. I've been tired and wetting myself. It is so embarrassing. I never wet myself."	Provide privacy for client in semi-Fowler position. IVF and site; assess and match to order. Assess and document VS.	Did the student use a three-item recall screening technique? Needed? No cognitive impairments seen. Does student acknowledge client's suffering? Does the student use open-ended questions when gathering information?	Incontinence is abnormal in the normal aging process.
		Answer client questions.	Does the student's nonverbal and verbal comunication convey a sense of caring?	

(continued)

Exhibit 26.1	Scenario Progression Outline	*(continued)*		
Timing	**Mrs. Anderson**	**Expected Actions**	**Prompts, Questions, Teaching Points**	**Other Prompts/Cues**
	Whispering, "I'm sorry I'm here. I'm not sure what will happen to me. My mouth hurts."	Determine that pain may interfere with assessment and that an intervention is available.	Does the student recognize that pain may interfere with communication?	
Frame 2: Next 10 minutes, from minute 6 to minute 15	A: Sinus tachycardia: 100 beats/minute BP: 140/90 mmHg Monitor controls: SpO$_2$: 96% RR: 24 breaths/minute Auscultation sounds: Lungs: Clear Heart: S1S2 Bowel: Normative	Validate ciprofloxin and Mycostatin order; prepare and administer using safe medication practices.	Does student explain medications to client and validate understanding?	Reinforce previous learning of safe medication administration.
Can go to the third frame if no action taken in response to client not understanding instructions or stating she is wet.	Use microphone or put in program as handlers (SimMan): "My name is Mrs. Anderson, I was born on March 7th." "What do you want me to do with that medicine? Did you say 'ish is outh'?"	Document: Explains procedure, places bed in high position, collects urine specimens. Returns bed to lowest position. Label and place specimen in bag for delivery to lab.	Does the student enunciate instructions clearly: "Swish this around your mouth"? Consonants are not heard as well. Is the student using a low-pitch voice? High-pitch sounds are the first sounds an elderly client may not hear.	This represents scaffolding or building on previous learning to increase the complex dimensions of a student.
	"Some of the urine wet my bed. I don't want to talk anymore."	Clean client, remove wet underpad, and replace with dry pad. Wash hands.	Does the student change linen, providing comfort to the client before continuing the assessment?	
	"Thank you, I feel better. I'm tired. Can you come back later?"		Does the student complete the assessment or let the client sleep? What is the rationale given by the student?	

(continued)

Exhibit 26.1	Scenario Progression Outline *(continued)*			
Timing	Mrs. Anderson	Expected Actions	Prompts, Questions, Teaching Points	Other Prompts/Cues
Frame 3: Occurs if no nursing intervention for pain, lack of understanding by nurse, or client is left wet.	Temp: 99.8°F A: Sinus tachycardia: 130 beats/minute BP: 150/98 mmHg Monitor controls: SpO$_2$: 92% RR: 28 breaths/minute Auscultation sounds: Lungs: Clear Heart: S1S2 Bowel: Normative Use microphone or put in program as handlers (SimMan): Moaning, "This is horrible. Help me."	Recognize intervention was required.	Does student identify that client may exhibit distress when communication is not effective?	

BP, blood pressure; DOB, date of birth; RR, respiratory rate; VS, vital signs.

E. RUNNING OF THE SCENARIO

Frames within high-fidelity simulation can be used to assist progression of the simulation. Student actions can drive progression toward new frames, or check boxes completed by the controller can be used. The controller would identify "done," "not done," or "done with prompt" within the program. The use of evaluative checklists by multiple observers encourages assessment, reflection, and professional growth for all participating in the process. Complexity in feedback and active learning can be embraced by using evaluative checklists for primary objectives as well as for standard nursing behaviors when interacting with a client.

F. PRESENTATION OF COMPLETED TEMPLATE

Title

Communication With an Elderly Client

Scenario Level and Focus Area

First-year nursing course or gerontology course

Scenario Description

An 85-year-old woman is admitted to a medical–surgical unit with a suspected urinary tract infection. She is a widow of 3 years, was married for 62 years, has three adult children, and lives in her own home with an unmarried son. She has a history of two incidents of congestive heart failure (CHF) 4 years ago, a total hysterectomy 22 years ago, a left total knee replacement (LTK) 15 years ago, and situational depression when her husband passed away. The "nurse" or participant in this scenario will practice principles of communication with the elderly woman.

The woman presents with the following vital signs (VS): blood pressure (BP): 140/88 mmHg, pulse (P): 90 beats/minute, respiratory rate (RR): 22 breaths/minute, and temperature (T): 99°F. She complains of falling into her chair at home, dribbling when trying to get to the bathroom, fatigue, and not being hungry for 1 week. Her physician evaluated her urine (urinalysis [UA]) and complete blood count (CBC) with differential and recommended admission to the hospital for further evaluation and treatment. She is 5 feet, 5 inches tall and weighs 160 pounds.

The scenario starts with the "nurse" entering the room.

Scenario Objectives

The National Council of State Boards of Nursing National Council Licensure Examination for Registered Nurses (NCLEX-RN®) test plan categories and subcategories (NCSBN, 2015) included in this scenario are as follows:

Safe and effective care environment: *Management of care* (client rights), *Safety and infection control* (safe use of equipment); **Health promotion and maintenance:** *Aging process*; **Psychosocial integrity:** *Therapeutic communications*; **Physiological integrity:** *Basic care and comfort* (elimination, personal hygiene), *Pharmacological and parenteral therapies* (dosage calculation, medication administration, parenteral/intravenous therapies), *Reduction of risk potential* (potential for complications from surgical procedures and health alterations, vital signs), *Physiological adaptation* (illness management).

For this scenario, the American Association of Colleges of Nursing's (AACN; 2008) *Essentials of Baccalaureate Education for Professional Nursing Practice* items addressed include:

Essential II: Basic Organizational and Systems Leadership for Quality Care and Patient Safety
Essential IV: Information Management and Application of Patient Care Technology
Essential VI: Interprofessional Communication and Collaboration for Improving Patient Health Outcomes
Essential VIII: Professionalism and Professional Values

Learning Method

Active learning is used within the cognitive, psychomotor, and affective domains through high-fidelity simulator, standardized patient, role-play, or case study.

Primary Learning Outcomes

During and after completing the simulation experience, the student will be able to do the following:

1. Identify intrinsic and extrinsic factors that affect communication with an elderly client
2. Identify, perform, and discuss strategies that can increase communication with an elderly client
3. Identify client conditions that can contribute to impaired communication
4. Perform and discuss therapeutic communication skills in phases of the nurse–client relationship
5. Discuss how attitudes affect behavior and propose changes that could be made in future interactions with elderly clients.

Student Preparation for the Simulation

Required Readings and Websites to Explore

Required readings relate to communication and the elderly in your curriculum. Chapters from a fundamentals of nursing or gerontology text or a journal article would be listed.

Websites: John A. Hartford Foundation (2016),
　　Refer to med–surg text.
　　Urinary tract infection (University of Maryland, 2012),
　　umm.edu/health/medical/reports/articles/urinary-tract-infection

Materials to Prepare

Completed medication sheet/card: Information sheet/card for ciprofloxin 200 mg (IV) every 12 hours, nystatin (Mycostatin) 400,000 U orally once a day, furosemide (Lasix) 60 mg orally once a day, potassium supplement (K-Dur) 40 mEqs orally once a day, digoxin (Lanoxin) 0.25 mg orally once a day.

　　Review of standard nursing behaviors when interacting with a client: Verification of client orders and plan of care, identification of client, introduction of self and explanation of reason there, asepsis as appropriate, preparation and gathering of equipment/supplies needed, maintenance of privacy and Health Insurance Portability and Accountability Act (HIPAA) standards, appropriate ergonomic/body mechanics when assessing or performing care, maintenance of a safe environment (bed position, call bell, and equipment placement), and documentation. Use of the evaluative criteria for standard nursing behaviors when interacting with a client (as shown later in this chapter) succinctly identifies the behaviors.

　　Completion of survey: Beliefs about the elderly—answer the following statement with a yes or no. Bring this to the simulation. Highlights will be discussed in debriefing.

1. Most old people are sick.
2. Most old people are in nursing homes.
3. Most old people are retired.
4. Most old people would like to live in a warm climate.
5. Most old people live in poverty.
6. Most old people cannot learn as easily as when they were young.
7. Most old people are hard of hearing.
8. Most old people have no interest in sex.
9. Most old people are more religious than young people.

Setting the Scene

Equipment Needed

____ Female wig on head
____ Peripheral IV in left arm (nondominant)—IV catheter, tape, ordered IV fluid on infusion pump
____ Female genitalia
____ Sequential compression devices (SCDs), bilaterally on lower extremities
____ Equipment to measure VS (thermometer, stethoscope, sphygmomanometer)
____ Hospital gown
____ ID bracelet with name, age, physician, medical record number, and allergies
____ Collection container for routine UA and culture and sensitivity test
____ Curtain or ability to create private assessment area
____ Oxygen available via nasal cannula tubing
____ Medication administration tools: drug handbook or personal digital assistant with medication program, measuring cup, intravenous piggyback (IVPB) tubing, simulated ordered medications, water pitcher with glass
____ Client medical record that includes orders, history and physical, medication administration record, input and output (I&O) record, and progress documentation forms
____ Telephone (for access to admitting nurse and physician)

Participants Needed

1. Transfer assistant (if needed)
2. Lab member (if role-play used)
3. Voice of admitting nurse (can be simulation controller, other student, or preprogrammed handler)
4. Voice of physician (can be simulation controller, other student, or preprogrammed handler)
5. Simulation controller (if high-fidelity HPS is used)
6. Mrs. Anderson (other prepped student nurse)
7. Observers to participate in debriefing (if used as a group exercise)

Scenario Implementation

Expected run time is 15 to 20 minutes. The "nurse" is given a report from the admitting nurse via the telephone as the client is transported to the unit via stretcher. The medical record is brought to the unit with the client. Another student can assist with transfer, or this step can be eliminated by having the client in the bed to begin the scenario.

The report given is as follows: Mrs. Anderson, age 85 years. VS: BP: 140/88 mmHg, P: 90 beats/minute, RR: 22 breaths/minute, T: 99°F. She complained of falling into her chair at home, dribbling when trying to get to the bathroom, being tired, and not being hungry for 1 week. Dr. Smith evaluated a UA and complete blood count (CBC) with differential and recommended admission to rule out sepsis and urinary tract infection. Mrs. Anderson also has a fungal infection within her mouth. She is 5 feet, 5 inches tall and weighs 160 pounds.

Mrs. Anderson is a widow of 3 years, was married for 62 years, has three adult children, and lives in her own home with an unmarried son. She has a history of two incidents of CHF 4 years ago, a hysterectomy 22 years ago, an LTK replacement 15 years ago, and situational depression when her husband passed away.

Physician/provider orders include the following:

Admit to 1 South
Activity level: Bed rest today
Diet: Low NA (sodium), low cholesterol
D5 1/2 NS at 100 mL per hour
UA and urine culture and sensitivity (C/S)
Ciprofloxin 200 mg IVPB stat
SCDs
VS q 4 hr
Oxygen 2 L via nasal cannula titrated to maintain and PaO_2 of 92% prn
Lasix 40 mg PO qd
KDur tab 40 mEqs PO qd
Digoxin 0.25 mg PO qd
Mycostatin 400,000 U qid swish 1/2 of dose in each side of mouth; hold
Tylenol 650 mg PO q 4 h prn for temperature higher than 101°F

The student begins the scenario by transferring Mrs. Anderson from the stretcher to the bed and assessing her. The student will be expected to focus on primary learning outcomes; however, basic principles of safety and infection control as nurse–client behaviors will also be expected.

Three frames are constructed within a high-simulation program. Frame 1 lasts 5 minutes, frame 2 lasts 10 minutes, and frame 3 occurs only if interventions are not done within frames 1 and 2. A microphone can be used during the exercise, or voice handlers can be built into the scenario. Exhibit 26.1 shows the scenario for a high-simulation program (such as SimMan by Laerdal) but can be adapted for role-play.

The simulation controller concludes the scenario and allows the students (and observers of group exercise) to reflect on behaviors within the scenario for 5 to 10 minutes. A 12-item "communication with the elderly" true–false quiz is given and will be self-evaluated by the student(s) in the debriefing.

Evaluative Criteria for Standard Nursing Behaviors When Interacting With a Client

Students will be given feedback based on the degree to which they, in the appropriate order and with or without coaching, perform the actions as listed in Exhibit 26.2.

Evaluative Criteria for Communication With an Elderly Client

Students will be given feedback based on the degree to which they, in the appropriate order and with or without coaching, perform the actions outlined in Exhibit 26.3.

G. DEBRIEFING GUIDELINES

The estimated session time is 30 minutes for groups. A general discussion ensues related to the basic skills performed in this scenario. The evaluative criteria in Exhibits 26.2 and 26.3 are used as the foundation. Questions related to technique are encouraged. If videotape is available, the scenario can be reviewed. This is conducive to participation by all (either by the group; in a circle; or direct, one-to-one seating for an individual and facilitator). The discussion leader is the simulation controller or faculty member. A projector, screen, overhead projector, or computer is used.

Exhibit 26.2	Evaluative Criteria for Standard Nursing Behaviors When Interacting With a Client		
Behavior	**Independent**	**Prompt**	**Comments**
Verifies orders.			
Turns lights on; assess/intervene for safe environment.			
Introduces self/role.			
Washes hands.			
Identifies client by identification band and verbal method.			
Positions ergonomically/provides privacy.			
Identifies IVF, site health; assesses match to order.			
Assesses/documents VS.			
Notifies provider if needed.			
Addresses pain.			
Answers questions.			
Performs interventions appropriately.			
Completes other assessments/interventions.			
Document.			

IVF, intravenous fluid; VS, vital signs.

Exhibit 26.3	Evaluative Criteria for Communicating With an Elderly Client			
Student Speaking/Listening Behavior		**Independent**	**Prompt**	**Comments**
Client sees nurse's face in appropriate light.				
Uses normal volume.				
Allows time for client reflection.				
Uses open-ended questions.				
Sense of caring is conveyed.				
Recognizes that pain interferes with communication.				
Gives explanation related to procedures.				
Enunciates consonants.				
Uses low-pitched voice.				
Addresses physical needs.				
Recognizes communication timing.				

Completed surveys related to beliefs about the elderly are reviewed. This can be done in a number of ways: via individual presentation, surveys handed in before the scenario and tabulated as group data, or automated response anonymous clickers used during the actual discussion. Inferences are solicited about beliefs, assumptions, and resulting behaviors. The discussion leader gives examples of how a belief that "older people are hard of hearing" may lead to shouting or the belief that "older people have no interest in sex" may lead to a disregard in assessment questions. The student or group is guided to focus on positive themes and facts of today's elderly. Stories may be shared as appropriate to objectives and time. The criteria detailed in Exhibit 26.3 are reinforced.

Finally, a review of the 12-item "communication with the elderly" quiz (similar to the survey review style used earlier) is done. Implicit bias is identified and *ageism* is discussed.

1. Shouting is required when speaking with older adults. (F)
2. Elderly people hear high-pitch tones easily. (F)
3. Background noise will enhance hearing ability. (F)
4. Light will promote communication. (T)
5. Fatigue, pain, and physical discomfort will influence communication. (T)
6. Hearing aids may need to be turned on, adjusted, or have the battery changed if communication is impaired. (T)
7. Standing off to the side in a shadow facilitates communication. (F)
8. The three-item recall screening asks the assessor to "tell the client to remember three items: apple, table, and dime. Then, a distracting activity is done, and 2 to 3 minutes later, the assessor asks the client what the three items were." (T)
9. Active listening involves reflecting on what a patient has said while listening. (T)
10. Consonants such as *ch*, *sw*, or *th* are not heard well as one ages. (T)

11. Attitudes and beliefs influence interactions with elders. (T)
12. Asking elderly clients to bring in their medications (prescription and nonprescription)—the "drug bag"—facilitates accurate assessment of medication intake. (T)

The discussion leader facilitates a review of the answers. Rationales are discussed, and participants are encouraged to share what they would continue to do and what they would do differently in future interactions with elderly clients.

Reinforce Standard Nursing Behaviors When Interacting With a Client

These standard behaviors are verification of client orders and plan of care, identification of client, introduction of self and explanation of reason there, asepsis as appropriate, preparation and gathering of equipment/supplies needed, maintenance of privacy and HIPAA standards, appropriate ergonomic/body mechanics used when assessing or performing care, maintenance of a safe environment (bed position, call bell, and equipment placement), documentation.

H. SUGGESTIONS/KEY FEATURES TO REPLICATE OR IMPROVE

Continue to reinforce learning through constructivist methods such as scaffolding. Use of standard nursing behaviors reinforces and develops confidence in student ability. Refer to Exhibit 26.2.

I. RECOMMENDATIONS FOR FURTHER USE

Complexity can increase in this scenario. Students can develop diagnoses and nursing care plans, and peer evaluation can be done in relation to outcome attainment and use of the nursing process.

In senior-level courses this scenario can be adapted for use with clients who have neurologic conditions or any type of progressive dementia. Clients with psychiatric conditions may also use this scenario with specific adaptations.

J. HOW SIMULATION-BASED PEDAGOGY HAS CONTRIBUTED TO IMPROVED STUDENT OUTCOMES

Active learning can promote greater understanding of concepts (Nosich, 2008), higher retention of information (Stice, 1987), and the opportunity to apply knowledge gained through action (Florea, Rafeldt, & Youngblood, 2011). Constructivist learning theory supports simulation in both high and low fidelity. Although debriefing is critical to facilitate desired outcomes, educators must remember that incorporation of surveys, discussion, and the NCLEX style questions will also contribute to efficient internalization of content and resulting practice as a student nurse and future RN.

K. EXPERT RECOMMENDATIONS AND WORDS OF WISDOM

Simulation experiences guide student learning. Particularly important is the creation of a safe environment where students can express their thoughts. All questions are encouraged by facilitators for development and adoption of the RN role. The way in which the facilitator gives feedback fosters students' ability to use medical words, remove their own biases and make connections in new situations. With this experience, some students realize their need to learn more about aging, alternate presentations of disorders, and biases they may have. When those students go into a community senior center they listen to the stories of an older adult with curiosity and joy. Nursing practice becomes holistic, professional, safe, and competent.

L. EVALUATION OF BEST PRACTICE STANDARDS AND USE OF CREDENTIALED SIMULATION FACULTY

The International Nursing Association for Clinical Simulation and Learning (INACSL, 2013/2016) has guided simulation learning and curriculum development at TRCC. Standard II Professional Integrity (of participants) and Standard V Facilitation drove establishment of guidelines for students, participants, and faculty. All educators participate in professional development through company and nurse educator conferences. It has been helpful to have onsight Laerdal workshops for all. Standard III Outcomes and Objectives supported our continued focus on measured experience and curricular outcomes. We have a strong history of curricular development within our college and as a member of the Connecticut Community College Nursing Program. Standard VI Debriefing and Standard VII Participant Evaluation were validated through the clear statements. TRCC developed a foundation in reflective practice through the Connecticut Distance Learning Consortium (CTDLC) and National ePortfolio/Catalyst for Learning grants with Bret Eynon and LaGuardia Community College, New York City, New York.

Areas in which we are growing through the leadership of Edith Ouellet, Joan Graham, and champion super-users from each course are: terminology, Standard I, faculty simulation credentialing, Standard VII, overall assessment and evaluation beyond a specific experience, Standard VIII, interprofessional simulation experiences, and Standard IX, simulation design. Quality review continues through the lens of program outcomes, graduate and employer surveys, and professional organizations such as INACSL.

REFERENCES

Dewey, J. (1944). *Democracy and education.* New York, NY: Free Press.

Florea, M., Rafeldt, L., & Youngblood, S. (2011). Using an information literacy program to prepare nursing students to practice in a virtual workplace. In Information Resource Management (Ed.), *Virtual communities, concepts, methodologies, tools and applications* (pp. 1482–1498). Hershey, PA: Information Science Reference.

International Nursing Association for Clinical Simulation and Learning. (2013, updated 2016). INACSL standards of best practice: Simulation. Retrieved from https://www.inacsl.org/i4a/pages/index.cfm?pageID=3407

John A. Hartford Foundation. (2016). Resources for aging. Retrieved from http://www.johnahartford.org/grants-strategy/current-strategies/age-friendly-hospitals

National Council of State Boards of Nursing. (2015). NCLEX-RN examination: Test plan for the National Council Licensure Examination for Registered Nurses. Retrieved from https://www.ncsbn.org/RN_Test_Plan_2016_Web.pdf

Nosich, G. (2008). *Learning to think things through: A guide to critical thinking across the curriculum* (3rd ed.). Upper Saddle River, NJ: Prentice Hall.

Rafeldt, L., Bader, H., Czarzasty, N., Freeman, E., Ouellet, E., & Snayd, J. (2014). Reflection builds twenty first century professionals. *Peer Review, 16*(1), 19–23.

Stice, J. (1987). Using Kolb's learning cycle to improve student learning. *Engineering Education, 77*(5), 291–296.

University of Maryland. (2012). UTI assessment and treatment. Retrieved from http://umm.edu/health/medical/reports/articles/urinary-tract-infection

Vygotsky, L. S. (1978). *Thought and language.* Cambridge, MA: MIT Press.

FURTHER READING

Rafeldt, L. (2008). Age-related care of older adults. In M. Hogan (Ed.), *Comprehensive review for NCLEX-RN: Reviews and rationales* (pp. 254–268). Upper Saddle River, NJ: Prentice Hall.

CHAPTER 27

Discharge Teaching for an Immigrant Woman With Congestive Heart Failure and Atrial Fibrillation

Mary Ann Cordeau and Leonie Rose Bovino

A. IMPLEMENTATION OF SIMULATION-BASED PEDAGOGY IN YOUR INDIVIDUALIZED TEACHING AREA

Leonie Rose Bovino

In my role as a laboratory instructor, I have developed and implemented simulation experiences using human patient simulators (HPSs) to meet course outcomes.

Mary Ann Cordeau

I have been involved in development and research related to simulation-based experiences (SBEs) since 2006. Drawing on Leonie's knowledge of Jamaican culture and the need to provide students with realistic culturally relevant patient teaching experiences, we paired to develop this scenario.

B. EDUCATIONAL MATERIALS AVAILABLE IN YOUR TEACHING AREA AND RELATED TO YOUR SPECIALTY

The clinical simulation laboratory at Quinnipiac University resembles a hospital unit with five rooms, each with a patient and control area separated by one-way glass. With the appropriate props, rooms can be arranged to mimic an emergency room, community setting, and a home health setting. All five simulation rooms can be used simultaneously and are equipped with an audiovisual system (AVS) for recording, debriefing, and streaming real-time scenarios to any other classroom in the building. There are three adult HPSs, one pediatric and one newborn HPS, and a maternity HPS. The rooms are large enough to hold group clinical simulation experiences— the glass doors to each simulation room can be closed for private SBEs.

C. SPECIFIC OBJECTIVES FOR SIMULATION USAGE WITHIN A SPECIFIC COURSE AND THE OVERALL PROGRAM

SBEs begin in the fall semester of the third year. Students have SBEs in most content areas; they are increasingly being used to meet clinical course outcomes when clinical experiences are limited. This

321

scenario is designed for third- and fourth-year baccalaureate (RN) students who have completed or are concurrently in a medical–surgical nursing course and have had cultural competence and patient teaching content. This scenario is delivered in a course that focuses on preparing students to meet the provider-of-care role, the designer/manager/coordinator-of-care role, and member-of-a-profession role (American Association of Colleges of Nursing [AACN], 2008). AACN's (2008) *Essentials of Baccalaureate Education in Professional Nursing* were used to develop course outcomes. Key elements from the National Council of State Boards of Nursing (NCSBN, 2015)—National Council Licensure Examination for a Registered Nurse (NCLEX-RN®) detailed test plan were used in developing this scenario. International Nursing Association for Clinical Simulation and Learning (INACSL, 2013/2016) INACSL Standards of Best Practice were used for scenario design and implementation. On completion of the course, the student should be able to:

1. Demonstrate expected proficiency in the application of knowledge and performance of clinical skills related to community and public health nursing.
2. Demonstrate expected proficiency in the application of pharmacotherapeutic knowledge and the performance of related clinical skills.
3. Demonstrate expected proficiency in the application of knowledge and performance of clinical skills related to health teaching and health counseling.
4. Demonstrate expected proficiency in the application of knowledge and performance of clinical skills related to health promotion and wellness.

D. INTRODUCTION OF SCENARIO

Setting the Scene and Technology Used

The scene takes place on a cardiac telemetry unit of a hospital. A simulated patient is used. If available, a system for recording and viewing the SBE can be used for debriefing. If not, no special technology is used in this scenario.

Scenario Objectives

INASCL Standards of Best Practice for Participant Objectives (Lioce et al., 2013) were used when developing scenario outcomes. After participating in this SBE, the learner is able to:

1. Assess patient and family understanding of self-care management for congestive heart failure (CHF) and atrial fibrillation (AF).
2. Assess patient and family ability to follow discharge instructions and comply with the prescribed treatment regimen.
3. Provide clear, culturally sensitive, holistic, evidence-based, and patient-preference instructions to patient and family about self-care and management of CHF and AF.
4. Identify and communicate available resources for self-care management of CHF and AF.

The NCLEX-RN test plan categories and subcategories (NCSBN, 2015) addressed in this scenario include the following:

Safe and effective care environment: *Utilize information resources to enhance the care provided to a client* (evidenced-based research, information technology, policies, and procedures), *Recognize the need for referrals and obtain necessary orders, Identify community resources for the client,* **Health Promotion and Maintenance:** *Provide care and education for the adult client ages 65 through 85 years and over, Identify risk factors for disease/illness* (age, gender, ethnicity, lifestyle), *Educate the client on actions to promote/maintain health and prevent disease* (diet), *Evaluate client understanding of health* *promotion behaviors/activities* (weight control, exercise actions), **Psychosocial Integrity:** *Cultural aware-ness/cultural influences, Assess the importance of client culture/ethnicity when planning/providing/evalu-ating care, Recognize cultural issues that may impact the client's understanding/acceptance of psychiatric diagnosis, Incorporate client cultural practice and beliefs when planning and providing care, Respect cultural background/practices of the client* (does not include dietary preferences), **Therapeutic Communication:** *Assess verbal and nonverbal client communication needs, Respect the client's personal values and beliefs, Allow time to communicate with the client, Use therapeutic communication techniques to provide client sup-port, Encourage the client to verbalize feelings* (fear, discomfort), *Evaluate the effectiveness of communi-cations with the client,* **Pharmacological and Parenteral Therapies:** *Adverse effects/contraindications/ side effects/interactions, Assess the client for actual or potential side effects and adverse effects of medica-tions* (prescribed, over-the-counter, herbal supplements, preexisting condition), *Provide information to the client on common side effects/adverse effects/potential interactions of medications and inform the client when to notify the primary health care provider,* **Pharmacological and Parenteral Therapies:** *Medication administration, Educate client about medications, Educate client on medication self-administra-tion procedures, Participate in medication reconciliation process,* **Reduction of Risk Potential:** *Changes/ abnormalities in vital signs, Apply knowledge needed to perform related nursing procedures and psycho-motor skills when assessing vital signs, Apply knowledge of client pathophysiology when measuring vital signs, Laboratory values, Educate client about the purpose and procedure of prescribed laboratory tests,* **Physiological Adaptation:** *Illness management, Apply knowledge of client pathophysiology to illness management, Educate client regarding an acute or chronic condition, Educate client about managing illness* (chronic illnesses).

The AACN *Essentials of Baccalaureate Education for Professional Nursing Practice* (AACN, 2008) addressed in this scenario include:

Essential VII: Clinical Prevention and Population Health, Objectives 3, 4, 5
Essential IX: Baccalaureate Generalist Nursing Practice, Objectives 3, 4, 5, 7, 10, 16, 17

Description of Participants

The simulated patient is a 78-year-old Jamaican woman of mixed race (Black, White, and Asian) who presently resides in the United States, but has lived in Jamaica for most of her life. One RN student who has been briefed on his or her role serves as a daughter/son scenario role player. The patient's child was also born in Jamaica but started living in the United States after marrying a U.S. citizen at the age of 22 years. Another student serves as the RN caregiver and is expected to prepare for the scenario in advance by reading about the pathophysiology of CHF and AF, the medical and nursing management of patients with these common and often comorbid conditions, and Jamaican cultural practices.

Although English is the official language of Jamaica, Patois, which is a combination of English and some African languages, is commonly spoken. Most Jamaicans are of partial African descent. Families are close-knit and usually provide both emotional and economic support to each other. Jamaicans typically distrust those in authority and place faith in those they know well. Religion is important to Jamaican life and the majority are Christians as evidenced by the fact that Jamaica has the highest number of churches per capita in the world. Jamaicans typically address people by their official title (Mr., Mrs., or Ms.) until a personal relationship is established. They are also typically reserved until they get to know someone. They can be direct communicators and tend to say what they think. They expect others to be equally direct. Herbal medicines are popular; when traditional herbs fail, modern medi-cine is tried. A large number of herbs are used to cure a variety of illness and maintain good health. Jamaican cuisine consists of many unprocessed foods, smaller portions of meats and a high content of starches, beans, and vegetables. It includes a mixture of dishes from the indigenous people (Arawaks), the Spanish, British, Africans, Indian, and Chinese who lived on the island.

E. RUNNING OF THE SCENARIO

Before running the scenario, a facilitator-led briefing session emphasizing patient education and culturally relevant care should be conducted with all participants (Lioce et al., 2015). The Discharge Teaching for an Immigrant Woman with CHF and AF rubric should be reviewed with the participants before participation in the SBE. The facilitator may also serve as the simulated patient. Following the briefing, the simulated patient and scenario role player enter the hospital room, the simulated patient gets in the hospital bed, and the scenario role player sits on a bedside chair. The RN has been briefed that he or she has been caring for the patient the entire shift and has performed his or her vital signs and physical assessment; vital signs are stable, lung sounds are normal, and the patient has little to no dependent edema. The RN is informed that the patient is ready for discharge and needs discharge instructions. The RN is expected to implement the discharge teaching.

F. PRESENTATION OF COMPLETED TEMPLATE

Title

Discharge Teaching for an Immigrant Woman With CHF and AF

Scenario Level

Third- and fourth-year RN students

Focus Area

Patient education, culturally relevant care

Scenario Description

This scenario involves providing culturally relevant patient education to an elderly Jamaican woman and her child. The patient is sitting on bed in a hospital room in a cardiac telemetry unit. She is talking with her son/daughter (scenario role player) who is at the bedside. A discharge order has been written for the patient to be discharged to home. The RN provides discharge teaching to the patient who is an elderly Jamaican woman (Mrs. Brown) with a past medical history of CHF and AF. Mrs. Brown is currently in day 3 of her hospital stay and has been diagnosed with CHF exacerbation and AF with rapid ventricular response. Ms. Brown was initially treated in the emergency department (ED) and moved to the cardiac telemetry unit. Her medication regimen for hypertension was adjusted to control her elevated blood pressure. She was anticoagulated with warfarin (international normalized ratio [INR] goal 2–3). She is currently therapeutic at an INR of 2.9.

Mrs. Brown's hospital care was coordinated with a multidisciplinary team. The RN caregiver noted that when performing medication reconciliation, she asked about the use of herbal supplements. Mrs. Brown's daughter informed her that her mother started to drink white periwinkle tea sent to her a month ago by her sister in Jamaica as a remedy for hypertension (Clement, 2011). The RN caregiver expressed concern about Mrs. Brown's use of periwinkle tea as an herbal remedy because when she conducted a literature review about periwinkle tea she discovered that cardiac ischemia was listed as a side effect (Moudi, Go, Yien, & Nazre, 2013). Therefore, this may have contributed to the exacerbation of her CHF and to the rapid AF that led to this hospitalization.

Description of Patient

Name: Beverly "Bev" Brown *ID number:* (Insert ID number) *Gender:* F

Age: 78 years

Race: Black

Weight: 163 pounds (74 kg)   *Height:* 5 feet, 2 inches   *Marital status:* Widowed

Religion: Pentecostal

Major support: Daughter   *Phone:* 888-999-9999

Allergies: Sulfa (sulfonamide antibiotics)   *Attending physician:* Dr. Payne

Patient history: Beverly Brown is a Jamaican immigrant who presented to the ED with complaint of shortness of breath starting gradually over the last week, accompanied by wheezing. She was found to be in AF with a rapid ventricular rate. She was also noted to have an elevated blood pressure (180/ 87 mmHg). She thinks her symptoms may have been precipitated by hypertension, as her blood pressure has remained elevated over the past 2 months despite taking her prescribed medications.

Past medical history: Mrs. Brown has chronic AF, hyperlipidemia, hypertension, constipation, macular degeneration, peripheral edema, and peripheral vascular disease. She never smoked and denies illicit drug use.

Social history: Mrs. Brown is a widow and lives with her daughter, who works full time. Mrs. Brown has been living in the United States for 11 years and therefore is only eligible for minimal Medicare benefits.

Medication Record

Simvastatin (Lipitor) 10-mg tablet, metoprolol (Lopressor) 100-mg immediate release tablet, amlodip-ine (Norvasc) 5-mg tablet, polyethylene glycol (Miralax) 17-g packet, quinapril (Accupril) 20-mg tablet, furosemide (Lasix) 20-mg tablet, potassium chloride (Klor-Con) 100-mEq extended release (ER) tablet, warfarin (Coumadin) 2-mg tablet

Setting the Scene

Equipment Needed

_____Simulated patient wearing a hospital gown, identification bracelet

_____Hospital bed, overbed table, chair, book, flowers

_____Medical record (electronic or paper)

_____Pen

Resources Needed

_____Discharge instructions

_____Teaching materials—patient information on diet, medications, herbal remedies

_____Signed prescription for Lopressor (metoprolol)

_____Evaluation of discharge teaching for an immigrant woman with CHF and AF rubric

Participants Needed

Three individuals, one simulated patient (who may also be the facilitator), one scenario role player playing the son/daughter role, and one RN student to perform discharge teaching are needed for this scenario.

Scenario Implementation

The patient is ready for discharge and the RN is expected to implement the discharge teaching. The RN will have all of the necessary discharge teaching materials/paperwork with him or her on entering the patient room to begin the teaching. Expected simulation run time: 30 minutes, expected guided reflection time: 30 to 60 minutes depending on the participant needs.

After-Visit Summary: Beverly Brown **MRN:** xxxxxxx

If you have questions between now and your scheduled follow up, please contact:

1. Your primary provider during your hospitalization—Dr. Payne
2. Primary care provider—Dr. Peabody

Follow-Up Information

1. **Follow up with Peabody, Sam, MD. Schedule an appointment as soon as possible for a visit in 2 week(s).** Specialty: Internal Medicine: Address: _____ Phone: _____
2. **Follow up with Kites, Steven, MD. Schedule an appointment as soon as possible for a visit in 1 week(s).** Specialty: Cardiovascular Disease: Address: _____ Phone: _____

Hospitalization Summary

About Your Hospitalization

You were admitted on: [Insert date]. You were discharged on: [Insert date].

Problem List for Hospitalization

AF, CHF exacerbation

Discharge Instructions

Discharge Diet Orders: Heart-healthy diet. Limit fluids to 1,500 mL/d

Discharge Activity Orders: Activity as tolerated

Contact Your Doctor if: If you have temperature (fever) higher than 101°F; if you have trouble breathing; fast or slow heartbeat; dizziness that does not go away after resting for 15 minutes; if you have weight gain of 2 to 3 pounds or more a day or worsening swelling in your ankles, legs, or abdomen. Weigh yourself daily.

Medication Schedule

You should always bring this list to your next doctor's appointment. Please update the list if you stop taking any of these medications or you start taking any new medications, including over-the-counter medications and herbal remedies.

Exhibit 27.1 provides a list of instruction for medications and Exhibit 27.2 provides specifics related to warfarin dosing.

Allergies: Sulfa (sulfonamide antibiotics)

Additional Information

Heart Failure and AF

Many people have both heart failure and AF. They usually have one of these conditions at first, but this condition weakens the heart, causing the other to happen.

Heart Failure

Heart failure is a condition in which your heart does not pump as well as it should. As a result, blood is not moved very well throughout the body and fluid can back up in the feet and lungs. This can result in the swelling of your feet, trouble breathing, and feeling tired.

Exhibit 27.1 Discharge Instructions

Change How You Take This Medication	Instructions	Morning	Noon	Night	Bedtime	Other
Metoprolol (Lopressor) 100-mg immediate release tablet Last dose, time: [Insert time] 100 mg on [Insert date] 9:42 a.m.	Take one tablet (100 mg total) by mouth 2 (two) times daily. Quantity: 180 tablet, refills: 2	√		√		

Continue Taking These Medications	Instructions	A.m.	Noon	P.m.	Bedtime	Other
Simvastatin (Zocor) 10-mg tablet Last dose, time: [Insert time] 10 mg on [Insert date] 9:42 p.m.	Take one tablet (10 mg) by mouth nightly.				√	
Amlodipine (Norvasc) 5-mg tablet Last dose, time: [Insert time] 5 mg on [Insert date] 9:42 a.m.	Take 2 tablets (10 mg total) by mouth daily. Quantity: 30 tablet, refills: 11	√				
Polyethylene glycol (Miralax) 17-g packet Last dose, time: [Insert time] 17 g on [Insert date] 9:42 a.m.	Take 17 g by mouth daily. Mix in eight ounces of water, juice, soda, coffee, or tea before administration.	√				
Quinapril (Accupril) 20-mg tablet Last dose, time: [Insert time] 20 mg on [Insert date] 9:42 a.m.	Take one tablet daily. Quantity: 90 tablets, refills: 1	√				

(continued)

Exhibit 27.1 Discharge Instructions (*continued*)

Change How You Take This Medication	Instructions	Morning	Noon	Night	Bedtime	Other
Furosemide (Lasix) 20-mg tablet Last dose, time: [Insert time] 20 mg on [Insert date] 9:42 a.m.	Take 1 tablet (20 mg total) by mouth daily. Quantity: 30 tablets, refills: 0	√				
Potassium chloride (Klor-Con) 10 mEq one tablet ER tablet Last dose, time: [Insert time] 10 mEq on [Insert date] 9:42 a.m.	Take 10 mEq by mouth daily	√				
Warfarin (Coumadin) 2-mg tablet Last dose, time: [Insert time] 2 mg on [Insert date] 6:00 p.m.	Take as directed according to INR per MD orders. Quantity: 90 tablets, refills: 0			√		

ER, extended release; INR, international normalized ratio.

Exhibit 27.2	Recent Warfarin Dosing			
Recent Warfarin Dosing	**Latest Ref. Range**	**[Insert Date]**	**[Insert Next Consecutive Day]**	**[Insert Next Consecutive Day]**
INR	INR 0.90–1.18	2.4 (H)	2.6 (H)	2.46 (H)

INR, international normalized ratio.

Symptoms of heart failure can include feeling tired or weak, having trouble breathing, swelling in the feet, and sudden weight gain.

Atrial Fibrillation

AF involves a problem with the heart's rhythm. In people with AF, the electrical signals that control the heartbeat are abnormal, resulting in the top two chambers not pumping effectively. As a result, all of the blood does not move out of these chambers with each heartbeat. Blood can collect in these chambers and can start to form clots. These clots can travel to the brain through the blood vessels and cause strokes. The signs of stroke include uneven face, arm is weak, and speech strange.

Symptoms of AF can include feeling like your heart is racing or skipping beats; having mild chest discomfort, tightness or pain; feeling dizzy or lightheaded, or like you are going to pass out.

Warfarin

I Understand

Warfarin increases the risk of bleeding, so it is important to take my warfarin as instructed and monitor its effects with scheduled INR blood draws.

Certain foods can affect the INR level in my blood. It is important to consume a consistent amount of food with vitamin K, and to notify my doctor before making any changes to my diet.

An appointment has been scheduled for me at discharge. I should follow up with my primary care provider within 1 week for warfarin monitoring.

Warfarin increases the risk of bleeding, and medications can affect the INR level in my blood, so it is important that I do not take or discontinue any prescription or over-the-counter medication, except on the advice of my primary care provider.

Using Herbs and Supplements

I Understand

Although herbs or "bush teas" are natural medicines, they can also have harmful side effects on my body, especially when taken in large amounts.

Herbal products can affect some of the medicines that have been prescribed for me. I need to tell my primary care provider about all the herbal products I am taking.

I Understand

Regular activity within limitations is important for my health. I should report changes in my ability to do all the things I normally do.

I should look for changes in my breathing. It is important to report to my primary care provider if I cough more than usual, use more pillows than usual to sleep at night, and get out of breath doing things I normally do without a problem.

Eating a low-fat, low-salt, and low-cholesterol diet with plenty of fruits and vegetables can reduce my chance of worsening heart failure.

Weighing myself daily and reporting a gain of 2 to 3 pounds a day and/or 5 to 6 pounds a week to my primary care provider is important.

It is important to take my medicines as directed to reduce the chance that AF will cause a stroke.

If any of my symptoms worsen, I will contact my primary health provider, or go to the nearest ED.

A copy of these discharge instructions was given to and reviewed with the patient/or patient representative before leaving the hospital.

Patient/Parent/Guardian Signature: _____ Date: _____

Attending Electronic Signature: *Payne, Frank, MD*

Suggested Scripts for Simulated Patient and Scenario Role Player

Scenario Role Player—Patient's Son/Daughter

1. States that Bev's sister currently living in Jamaica found that periwinkle tea was very effective in lowering her blood pressure when she drank it two times every day.
2. Assesses mother's radial pulse following instructions from the student nurse.
3. Describes the nature of CHF and AF after instruction.
4. Describes symptoms that may indicate recurring heart failure after instruction.
5. States that she will not be able to afford home health care, but had other family members available to assist in her mother's care.
6. Describes the therapeutic regimen, including medications, awareness of potentially negative effects of herbal supplements, diet, and recommended activity levels after instruction.
7. States time and date of follow-up appointments after instruction.
8. States understanding of community resources after instruction.

Simulated Patient

1. Asks for clarification of a "heart healthy" diet
2. Correctly demonstrates radial pulse assessment after instruction
3. Responds to patient teaching by asking questions related to illness management, cues student if necessary
4. Describes pertinent health-promotion activities (e.g., perform prescribed exercises balanced with rest periods, daily weights at the same time with the same clothes) after patient teaching has occurred
5. Describes a daily exercise program she participates in at her Pentecostal church and that she loves to plant her vegetable and herb garden
6. Describes signs and symptoms that she must report immediately to the primary care provider—after patient teaching has occurred
7. Describes the interaction between periwinkle tea and cardiac ischemia after patient teaching (Herrmann et al., 2016)
8. Expresses thanks for the information on how to manage her condition
9. States she appreciates the excellent care she has received at the hospital

Evaluative Criteria

This SBE is designed for formative assessment. The Discharge Teaching for an Immigrant Woman with CHF and AF rubric can be used to guide assessment during debriefing. This rubric (Appendix A) should be completed by the simulated patient/facilitator or facilitator who observed/participated in the SBE.

G. DEBREFING GUIDELINES

Debriefing takes place immediately after the scenario ends. All participants participate in the debriefing. INASCL Simulation Standard VI is used to guide debriefing (Decker et al., 2013; Appendix A).

K. EXPERT RECOMMENDATIONS AND WORDS OF WISDOM

Initially HPSs were used as patients in patient teaching SBEs, but after running several patient education SBEs, we found their use limits or prohibits physical and psychological fidelity (Meakim et al., 2013). Student evaluations of SBEs support the use of simulated patients for increasing physical and psychological fidelity.

L. EVALUATION OF BEST PRACTICE STANDARDS AND USE OF CREDENTIALED SIMULATION FACILITY

The authors noted in each section above where best practice standards were incorporated in the preparation of scenarios, faculty, and the simulation program.

REFERENCES

American Association of Colleges of Nursing. (2008). *The essentials of baccalaureate education for professional practice*. Washington, DC: Author. Retrieved from http://www.aacnnursing.org/Portals/42/Publications/BaccEssentials08.pdf

Clement, Y. (2011). Limited clinical evidence to support the integration of Caribbean herbs into conventional medicine. *Focus on Alternative and Complementary Therapies, 16*(4), 289–292.

Decker, S., Fey, M., Sideras, S., Caballero, S., Rockstraw, L., Boese, T., . . . Borum, J. C. (2013). Standards of best practice: Simulation standard VI: The debriefing process. *Clinical Simulation in Nursing, 9*(6S), S27–S29. doi:10.1016/j.ecns.2013.04.008

Herrmann, J., Yang, E. H., Iliescu, C. A., Cilingiroglu, M., Charitakis, K., Hakeem, A., . . . Marmagkiolis, K. (2016). Vascular toxicities of cancer therapies: The old and the new–an evolving avenue. *Circulation, 133*(13), 1272–1289.

International Nursing Association for Clinical Simulation and Learning. (2013, updated 2016). INACSL standards of best practice: Simulation. Retrieved from https://www.inacsl.org/i4a/pages/index.cfm?pageID=3407

Lioce, L., Meakim, C. H., Fey, M. K., Chmil, J. V., Mariani, B., & Alinier, G. (2015, June). Standards of best practice: Simulation standard IX: Simulation design. *Clinical Simulation in Nursing, 11*(6), 309–315. doi:10.1016/j.ecns.2015.03.005

Lioce, L., Reed, C. C., Lemon, D., King, M. A., Martinez, P. A., Franklin, A. E., ... Borum, J. C. (2013, June). Standards of best practice: Simulation standard III: Participant objectives. *Clinical Simulation in Nursing, 9*(6S), S15–S18. doi:10.1016/j.ecns.2013.04.005

Meakim, C., Boese, T., Decker, S., Franklin, A. E., Gloe, D., Lioce, L., . . . Borum, J. C. (2013). Standards of best practice: Simulation standard I: Terminology. *Clinical Simulation in Nursing, 9*(6S), S3–S11. doi:10.1016/j.ecns.2013.04.001

Moudi, M., Go, R., Yien, C. Y., & Nazre, M. (2013). Vinca alkaloids. *International Journal of Preventive Medicine, 4*(11), 1231–1235.

National Council of State Boards of Nursing. (2015). NCLEX-RN detailed test plan for the National Council Licensure Examination for Registered Nurses. Retrieved from https://www.ncsbn.org/2016_RN_DetTestPlan_Educator.pdf

APPENDIX A

Discharge Teaching for an Immigrant Woman With CHF and AF Rubric

Student Name: _____   Date_____

Intervention	Y	NI	N
Introduced self.			
Performed hand hygiene.			
Verified provider orders.			
Identified patient using two identifiers.			
Assessed for pain and/or discomfort.			
Assessed patient's beliefs about illness.			
Assessed daughter/son beliefs about illness.			
Assessed patient's knowledge deficits.			
Assessed daughter/son knowledge deficits.			
Demonstrated radial pulse assessment.			
Assessed return demonstration of radial pulse assessment.			
Identified existing and potential barriers to self-care and management.			
Addressed existing and potential barriers to self-care and management.			
Provided written discharge instructions and signed prescription(s).			
Reviewed written discharge instructions with patient and family.			
Informed patient and family about homecare service recommendation.			
Identified community resource(s) for patient and family.			
Provided clear evidence-based information on herbal supplements related to CHF and AF and included content on potentially harmful effects to patient from cardiac glycosides identified in the periwinkle plant.			
Assessed for diet preferences and provided appropriate information on diet.			
Evaluated patient and family understanding of discharge teaching.			
Answered patient and family questions using evidence-based information.			

(continued)

(continued)

Intervention	Y	NI	N
Obtained signature from the patient verifying an understanding of the discharge instructions.			
Provided culturally sensitive care.			
Provided evidence-based information.			
Provided information with clarity.			
Treated patient and daughter/son with courtesy and respect.			
Documented care provided.			

AF, atrial fibrillation; CHF, congestive heart failure; N, not done/done incorrectly; NI, needs improvement/ needed cue; Y, completed competently.

CHAPTER 28

End-of-Life Scenario With Limited-English-Proficiency Patients

Desiree A. Díaz and Lynn Allchin

A. IMPLEMENTATION OF SIMULATION-BASED PEDAGOGY IN YOUR INDIVIDUALIZED TEACHING AREA

The introduction and discussion of end-of-life concepts are easily incorporated into lectures and clinical conferences. The actual experience of caring for a dying patient, or one who has died, may not actually occur during the students' academic tenure. Providing a simulation scenario that enables each student to experience a patient death and then be able to discuss their thoughts and feelings is essential to providing the best nursing education has to offer.

Considering the use of International Nursing Association for Clinical Simulation and Learning (INACSL) "Standards of Best Practice: Simulation[SM]" (INACSL, 2013/2016), a needs assessment should be done. The needs assessment identifies gaps in the curricula that may exist related to the content of dying and death. A deeper delve into the gap guides the design of the simulation-based education (SBE) activity. This also guides the level of fidelity within the simulation as well.

This simulation scenario is based on the fact that in every health care setting and in every patient population, death can occur. Even happy environments, such as labor and delivery and the newborn nursery, have the occasional death of a mother, baby, or both. Each nurse must accept that at some point in their career the nurse will be faced with the loss of a patient through death. Creating a caring and empathetic environment via simulation can assist students to identify areas they personally need to develop (Díaz, Maruca, Kuhnly, Jeffries, & Grabon, 2015). It is essential that at some point during a nurse's education, end-of-life concepts are introduced, discussed, and, we hope, experienced.

B. EDUCATIONAL MATERIALS AVAILABLE IN YOUR TEACHING AREA AND RELATED TO YOUR SPECIALTY

In a hospital or acute care setting that is dedicated to an end-of-life patient, there is an importance for it to resemble a home environment. Moulage or props should be included in the environment that make it appear more comfortable and home-like. It is relatively easy to add homemade blankets and pillows to accent the environment for a realistic feel. A radio or television is useful to promote a soothing environment.

C. SPECIFIC OBJECTIVES FOR SIMULATION USAGE WITHIN A SPECIFIC COURSE AND THE OVERALL PROGRAM

Program objectives include the following:

1. Comparing and contrasting advanced directives and do not resuscitate orders (DNR)
2. Identifying important report information
3. Therapeutic communication with distraught family members
4. Postmortem care

In addition, critical thinking when entering an acute care end-of-life/hospice room is essential. Students must use all senses to assess the atmosphere, which may be charged with emotions such as anxiety, anger, or fear on the part of the patient and/or family members. Many learners are unfamiliar with the process of caring for a patient who is actively dying.

This simulation has been used with prelicensure baccalaureate students in traditional and accelerated nursing programs in an attempt to raise awareness of patient and family needs during the transition period at the end of life. Group discussion and vicarious learning are key to engaging learners.

This scenario helps to address many National Council Licensure Exam (NCLEX®) identified areas of learning, including, but not limited to error prevention, end-of-life care, collaboration with interdisciplinary team, advanced directive, loss, and grief.

D. INTRODUCTION OF SCENARIO

Ms. Garcia, 54, was admitted into the acute care setting to the hospice room again yesterday with uncontrolled pain and the inability to care for herself. She has a history of stage IV cervical cancer, diagnosed 10 months ago, and has recently experienced progression of her disease while on chemotherapy. She seems to be giving up, she's tired and in pain. Her children, although not happy, understand she is suffering and does not want to go on. Her cousin, on the other hand, believes Ms. Garcia needs to fight to stay alive.

This simulation takes place in a typical hospice room in an acute care setting. The simulation lasts approximately 15 minutes. It may be a little longer or shorter. Remember, the facilitator/instructor and the observer are not allowed to talk to the group during the simulation unless specified on the role play instructions.

The human patient simulator (HPS) or confederate is lying in the bed and is nonverbal. This may also be a student role. The radio is playing spiritual music quietly. The patient's head is turned to face the music. There is a Welcome to Hospice packet near the bedside. The room includes an intravenous (IV) pole and pump, chair for a visitor, and a bedside table. Added realism includes a robotic stuffed animal as a pet on the bed with the patient.

E. RUNNING OF THE SCENARIO

The scenario is meant to be a hybrid, with use of role play and the simulator. The objectives for the learners are the same if used as a regular scenario. The goal is for the learners to understand the complexities of caring for an end-of-life patient within a family dynamic. It is important to keep in mind the facilitator role within each type of application of this scenario. The facilitator should be cognizant of the type of scenario and the potential emotions that may be elicited with an end of life patient. Criterion II: Simulation Best Practice Facilitation (Franklin et al., 2013) encourages the use of cues and discussion before the simulation. For a realistic and meaningful experience, it is imperative that the participants understand the role they are assigned and their level of active engagement. A participant who overly engages in the role assigned hinders the learning environment for other participants.

Simulation role assignment includes the possibility of eight student participants. This facilitates an entire clinical group. The scenario has roles for eight students but can fit for more or less as necessary. A simple way to assign roles is to cut the simulation role page into individual slips and have each student randomly pick one slip that will be his or her scenario role. Students may share only their role title: float nurse, aide, and so on. No other information about the specific role should be shared. The facilitator should allow participants to practice as they would in a live situation.

During the simulation, the facilitator/instructor ideally does not speak to the students. Best practice related to running the scenario (Standards of Best Practice: Facilitator IV) encourages the simulation to continue and be minimally interrupted (Franklin et al., 2013). If necessary, a yes or no answer may be enough to keep the scenario moving forward. When the facilitator/instructor thinks the scenario objectives have been met, usually after 15 minutes, the facilitator will call out, "The simulation has ended" so that all participants know to stop their role-playing. If participants have not met the scenario objectives after 15 minutes or so, the simulation needs to come to a stop. If participants take the simulation off course, the facilitator/instructor may need to stop the scenario and let the participants regroup. This can then be used as part of the debriefing/discussion.

Debrief/discussion as a group should always begin with a positive comment to the participants: "You did fine." "You picked up on some missing elements." "Exhale, I know that can be a tough scenario."

F. PRESENTATION OF COMPLETED TEMPLATE

Title

End-of-Life: The Acute Care Setting

Scenario Level

Nursing: Prelicensure, accelerated degree, degree completion

Focus Area

Medical–Surgical/Hospice

Scenario Description

Ms. Garcia, 54, was admitted again yesterday with uncontrolled pain and inability to care for herself. History of stage IV cervical cancer, diagnosed 10 months ago, recently experienced progression of her disease while on chemotherapy. She states she is giving up; she's tired and in pain. Her kids are on board, not happy but understand she is suffering. Her cousin, on the other hand, believes Ms. Garcia needs to fight to stay alive.

Ms. Garcia had a total abdominal hysterectomy (TAH), bilateral salpingo-ophorectomy (BSO), and lymph node dissection (LND) followed by four cycles of chemotherapy with progression of her disease. Chemotherapy drugs were changed; she had two cycles with progression of her disease.

Ms. Garcia has been an administrative assistant for the last 20 years. She has never married. She does have three adult children living in the state. She lives alone and had been very social at the local center. She has smoked one pack of cigarettes per day for 25 years and drinks three to four glasses of wine per week.

Scenario Objectives

In accordance with Criterion 3 of Standards of Best Practice: Participant Objective III (Lioce et al., 2013), it is important to keep the simulation within the overall program objectives. A more global view of program objectives includes the national exam. One area of specific objectives for this simulation is taken from the National Council Licensure Examination for Registered Nurses (NCLEX-RN®) test plan categories (National Council of State Boards of Nursing, 2015).

This end-of-life simulation includes the following NCLEX-RN test categories:

Safe and effective care environment: (advance directives, ethical practice, legal rights and responsibilities, collaboration with interdisciplinary team, continuity of care), **Safety and infection control:** (error prevention), **Psychosocial integrity:** (end-of-life care, grief and loss, support systems, therapeutic communications), **Physiologic integrity:** (palliative/comfort care), **Pharmacological and parenteral therapies:** (parenteral/intravenous therapies, pharmacological pain management, expected effects/outcomes).

Setting the Scene

Equipment Needed

Throw blanket, throw pillows, local newspaper and/ or magazine, coffee mug, and pictures or framed picture with HPS next to bedside.

Participant Roles

Simulation roles (eight roles)

Primary RN: Ms. Garcia (54 years old) is well known to you as she has been in and out of the hospital and palliative care unit five times in the past 4 months. This is the worst you have seen her. During her previous admissions, she has spoken to you about how she is ready to go to heaven. The pain and chemotherapy have made her miserable. She is tired and wants relief. She has made her wishes known to her children; her cousin is the person who does not want her to die and thinks Ms. Garcia should have more surgery and a new kind of chemotherapy.

You went on your lunch break reporting to the float RN, as you return to the unit you see people running into Ms. Garcia's room. You know of Ms. Garcia's wishes and the do not resuscitate (DNR) order in the chart.

Float RN: The primary nurse reported to you because she is going to lunch. You do not really know Ms. Garcia except that she has widespread cervical cancer and has a morphine drip for pain control. You are called to Ms. Garcia's room by loud screaming from her visitor. You find the patient without pulse or respirations. You call a code and begin cardiopulmonary resuscitation (CPR). The patient's visitor encourages you to do CPR; "Maria is not ready to die," the visitor says.

Cousin: You are heartbroken that your cousin is…well, very sick (you do not accept the fact that she cannot be cured of her widespread cervical cancer). You are visiting and your cousin stops breathing. You FREAK OUT and scream for HELP. When help arrives you **say:** "Keep her alive, she is not ready to die! Help! Help! Help her!" and "Do CPR; save her!" You want to stay in the room as the health care team arrives.

Recorder: You are to take notes on the sequence of events. You may not say anything to the students in the "roles" or direct them in any way. Your notes do not have to be neat and you are not graded on spelling, grammar, and so forth. We just want a record of the events.

Code Team: There are two of you who respond to the "Code Blue" in this room. You run into the room and cannot understand why the visitor is still in the room. You are yelling for the chart and want a history from the float RN about this patient. You ask the float nurse about diagnosis, allergies, code status, primary physician, vital signs, and so forth.

Hospital Chaplin: You were visiting another patient when you heard the scream from Ms. Garcia's room. You see everyone running into the room and go in to see whether you can help in any way. You see the patient's cousin (she is screaming and distraught) and realize the patient has died, but the code team is there. You approach the cousin and try to offer comfort.

Nursing Assistant: You were in the room (straightening the sheets) with the patient and her cousin when the patient stopped breathing. You do not know what to do, this is only your first week on the job. Your anxiety gets the better of you and you **say:** "Save her, save her," and wring your hands saying again and again: "SAVE HER, SAVE HER."

Scenario Implementation

Expected/Required Student Assessments/Actions

Students will:

__ Demonstrate proper patient identification.
__ Demonstrate RN to RN report that may have lacked detail regarding DNR status.
__ Synthesize documentation to properly distinguish living will status and code status.
__ Collaborate with family for proper care considerations.
__ Discuss postmortem care.
__ Discuss the role of chaplain and what to do with the frantic family member.

Instructor Interventions

The instructor or facilitator should not intervene if possible. The students should be briefed as to the roles before the start of simulation.

__ Collaboration with health care team members, therapeutic communication, and critical elements was demonstrated.
__ Proper hand hygiene used within the home.
__ Patient was properly identified.
__ DNR orders were properly identified and adhered to.
__ Therapeutic communication with families that are not coping well was demonstrated.
__ Health assessment were demonstrated within the scenario.
__ Simulation ends when the DNR order is found and CPR ends or 15 to 20 minutes has lapsed

G. DEBRIEFING GUIDELINES

As debriefing after simulation is a vital part of the learning process, specific questions for discussion are included. However, it is recognized that the debriefing process is dynamic and fluid, and other areas of discussion may be brought up by the student participants and/or the simulation leader. This end-of-life scenario includes the following as a guideline for debriefing:

1. How did you feel entering the room?
2. Why do you think this happened?
3. How could some/any of this been prevented from happening?
4. What is the role of a DNR/allow natural death (AND) order?
5. What is the role of advanced directives?
6. Does an individual need both or just one?
7. How can the nurse/health care worker help a distraught family member? What actions can be taken?

8. Describe the role of the hospital chaplin.
9. Discuss the idea that dying comes before death, just like loss (or thoughts of impending loss) comes before grief.
10. What is postmortem care?
11. How might this scenario have been different (or the same) if it had taken place in the cousin's home?

H. SUGGESTIONS/KEY FEATURES TO REPLICATE OR IMPROVE

A key feature of this simulation scenario is that all students are introduced to a patient who is dying and succumbs to death during their "shift." Within the scenario are major concepts of dying and death: end-stage disease, cultural implications, family dynamics, pain and pain management, ethical and legal aspects of end-of-life care, advanced directives, code status, and postmortem care. The end-stage disease that the client has is the focus of the didactic portion that the student is studying. Cultural awareness can be reflected in the scenario. Every nurse at some point in his or her career works with someone who is dying. Although, not all students are fortunate enough to experience dying and death during a clinical rotation when an instructor and/or staff nurse are close by to lend help either physically or emotionally.

The scenario creates an engaging learning environment in which to discuss certain procedures that may not be assigned in the clinical setting, such at postmortem care. Many hospital settings use the unlicensed professional to do postmortem care and mummy-wrap the patient. This can be an unsettling interaction, especially if the student has never seen rigor mortis. The participant can also discuss feelings of how to interact with the family, which is often still in the room when this occurs.

The scenario can also be used with English as a second language or with a hearing- or vision-impaired patient or family member. This would increase the complexity of the scenario and perhaps be more suited to last-term students. Incorporating varying religious views of death and dying could also be included to potentially change the participant objectives as well.

I. RECOMMENDATIONS FOR FURTHER USE

This particular simulation "patient" lends herself to progressive simulation. For example, Ms. Garcia's first simulation can be placed within a fundamentals-of-nursing course when students are learning to take health histories and complete basic physical assessments. As a postoperative patient, Ms. Garcia can be taught basic skills such as using an incentive spirometer, splinting, self-administration of pain medication, safe ambulation, medication teaching, and diet/nutrition teaching. Ms. Garcia may later appear in a wound-dehiscence and infection simulation, either at the end of a fundamentals course or at the beginning of an adult health course. Skills for students would include wound assessment, wound packing/wound vac application, patient teaching for home care, medication teaching, sterile/clean technique, and nutrition instruction for wound healing. Finally, Ms. Garcia is seen in the end-of-life simulation scenario during an adult health course.

This end-of-life simulation can also take place in the home setting, which would add another level of complexity with students having to assess the home environment as well as the patient and family. Being a guest in a patient's home as a visiting nurse is also quite different than having full access to a patient in the acute care setting. Being the only health care professional in the home can take courage as other health care professionals are not readily available for questions and help. A scenario that is set in the community does not require a large amount of space. Creativity is the key in providing a realistic space. The end-of-life scenario does require a sofa, bed, or recliner as the patient is at the end of life and wants to remain comfortable. This scenario can be used in a faculty lounge as an alternate setting area as well. This has been done to facilitate home care scenarios when space is limited.

Additional discussions related to end-of-life home care settings include the following: What is ethical practice? How do you manage family that is arguing over care? What is the legal responsibility of the nurse in pronouncing death? How do you manage grief and loss as the nurse? What are pain management strategies? What assisted medical death laws related to dying and pharmacology and related to polypharmacy in this setting?

J. HOW SIMULATION-BASED PEDAGOGY HAS CONTRIBUTED TO IMPROVED STUDENT OUTCOMES

In a study conducted with fifth/sixth-term/junior-level nursing students who had cared for a dying person during their clinical experience (Allchin, 2006), students reflected on the, complex care they provided. There was also an overlap between their student experience and their personal experience of loss, grief, dying, and death. Having this experience with the support of an instructor and staff nurse was important to the 12 study participants. They felt eased into the situation and not thrown in. As not all students have the opportunity to care for a dying patient and family, this simulation can help provide students of all levels the knowledge and skills, both physically and emotionally, to care for those who are experiencing loss, grief, dying, and death. Students and nurses can experience end-of-life situations in any health care setting and, as stated previously, this simulation can take place in any setting (home hospice, acute care, intensive care, emergency department, skilled nursing facility, etc.) with some physical modifications.

When students have a safe way to experience difficult situations, such as simulation, and an opportunity to discuss, as during debriefing, their thoughts and feelings, learning is enhanced. One specific simulation scenario, such as end-of-life care, can influence a student both professionally and personally as she or he progresses through school and as a graduate nurse. Reflection of important end-of-life concepts does not end with the one scenario or clinical experience. Self-reflection and discussion continues within the classroom and clinical settings.

K. EXPERT RECOMMENDATIONS AND WORDS OF WISDOM

The best way to use this simulation is if you had a live person in the bed as Ms. Garcia. We have done it both ways. We have found that students bend down to the eye level of the patient if it is a real human versus the HPS. We have also used a static manikin to imply that death has already happened. The manikin does absolutely nothing. It was important to allow the participants to continue as they thought the manikin was alive. In the debriefing we were able to discuss the actual simulation and steps of nurse death pronouncement.

Moulage and props also facilitate realism in this simulation. For instance, if a naturopathic practitioner is added to the scenario, a box of props would increase the realism of the scenario. This included spices, herbs, lace cloths, and religious medallions. Students have gone as far as lighting real matches to cleanse the air.

Facilitation of roles is conducted before the start of the scenario. Passing out roles one by one is best. We have taken students individually into the hall and given them a role. This allows them to ask questions and receive direction.

L. EVALUATION OF BEST PRACTICE STANDARDS AND USE OF CREDENTIALED SIMULATION FACULTY

This scenario has been run by both Certified Healthcare Simulation Educator (CHSE)-prepared and National League for Nursing (NLN) Simulation Innovation Resource Center (SiRC)-prepared nurse educators. A basic understanding of simulation pedagogy is needed when dealing with complex emotions attached to the death of a patient or loved one. Many participants have not been in this particular situation and may feel unprepared or isolated. A trained educator can use facilitation strategies to embrace varying and potentially opposing views. It is important to understand the basic principles of suspending disbelief in this scenario and allowing students the freedom to explore how they think the roles should respond to the situation. This is also true for nurse educators/facilitators, as this can bring up feelings in them too; so, being sensitive all around is important. This can be discussed before the running of the scenario and can be handled in a professional development workshop. This option may be good for faculty and nursing staff who may not have had this kind of gentle introduction in school and may have been scarred/traumatized by some of their professional experiences.

REFERENCES

Allchin, L. (2006). Caring for the dying: Nursing student perspectives. *Journal of Hospital Palliative Nursing, 8*(2), 112–119.

Díaz, D. A., Maruca, A., Kuhnly, J., Jeffries, P., & Grabon, N. (2015). Creating caring and empathic nurses: The lived experience of a simulated ostomate. *Clinical Simulation in Nursing, 11*(12), 513–518. doi:10.1016/j.ecns.2015.10.002

Franklin, A. E., Boese, T., Gloe, D., Lioce, L., Decker, S., Sando, C. R.,...Borum, J. C. (2013). Standards of best practice: Simulation standard IV: Facilitation. *Clinical Simulation in Nursing, 9*(6S), S19–S21.

International Nursing Association for Clinical Simulation and Learning. (2013, updated 2016). INACSL standards of best practice: Simulation. Retrieved from https://www.inacsl.org/i4a/pages/index.cfm?pageID=3407

International Nursing Association for Clinical Simulation and Learning Standards Committee. (2016a). Standards of best practice: Simulation: Facilitation. *Clinical Simulation in Nursing, 12*(S), S16–S20. doi:10.1016/j.ecns.2016.09.007

International Nursing Association for Clinical Simulation and Learning Standards Committee. (2016b). Standards of best practice: Simulation: Simulation design. *Clinical Simulation in Nursing, 12*(S), S5–S12. doi:10.1016/j.ecns.2016.09.005

Lioce, L., Reed, C. C., Lemon, D., King, M. A., Martinez, P. A., Franklin, A. E.,...Borum, J. C. (2013). Standards of best practice: Simulation standard III: Participant objectives. *Clinical Simulation in Nursing, 9*(6S), S15–S18.

National Council of State Boards of Nursing. (2015). NCLEX-RN test plan. Retrieved from https://www.ncsbn.org/RN_Test_Plan_2016_Final.pdf

FURTHER READING

International Nursing Association for Clinical Simulation and Learning Standards Committee. (2016a). Standards of best practice: Simulation: Facilitation. *Clinical Simulation in Nursing, 12*(S), S16–S20. doi:10.1016/j.ecns.2016.09.007

International Nursing Association for Clinical Simulation and Learning Standards Committee. (2016b). Standards of best practice: Simulation: Simulation design. *Clinical Simulation in Nursing, 12*(S), S5–S12. doi:10.1016/j.ecns.2016.09.005

CHAPTER 29

QSEN CAROUSEL for First-Year Nursing Students

Lillian A. Rafeldt

A. IMPLEMENTATION OF SIMULATION-BASED PEDAGOGY IN YOUR INDIVIDUALIZED TEACHING AREA

In this chapter, readers consider an approach used with concepts, tasks, and skills in a freshman nursing course. A Quality and Safety Education for Nurses (QSEN) framework orients students to a systems approach when evaluating quality so that "blame" is not a focus and professional accountability is developed. Burnhas, Chastin, and George (2012) describe a just understanding of safety. Removal of fear is critical in learning and practice. The International Nursing Association for Clinical Simulation and Learning (INACSL, 2013/2016) has developed the INACSL Standards of Best Practice: Simulation^{SM}, an evidence-based framework to guide simulation design. Standard VI speaks of planned debriefing, which promotes reflective thinking (Decker et al., 2013). Simulation with directed prompts for reflection provides the tools and pedagogy for development of prelicensure QSEN behaviors. A simulation laboratory is a unique setting in which to introduce and develop QSEN competencies. In Chapter 26, the growth of simulation-based pedagogy is discussed. The foundation for simulation as a learning approach throughout the curriculum is practiced by full-time and adjunct faculty.

B. EDUCATIONAL MATERIALS AVAILABLE IN YOUR TEACHING AREA AND RELATED TO YOUR SPECIALTY

In addition to the simulation resources described in Chapter 26, technology resources include online and in-person librarian access to evidence-based data search engines, such as Cumulative Index of Nursing and Allied Health Literature (CINAHL), and electronic charting tools that allow for real-world experience in electronic documentation.

C. SPECIFIC OBJECTIVES OF SIMULATION USAGE WITHIN A SPECIFIC COURSE AND THE OVERALL PROGRAM

QSEN is an initiative promoting commitment to quality and safety recommendations from the Institute of Medicine. The *Health Professions Education: A Bridge to Quality* (IOM, 2003) discussed an overhaul and transformation of the education system. Joint gap analyses by faculty and clinical

Table 29.1	QSEN Competencies
Competency	**Definition**
Patient-Centered Care	Recognizes the patient or designee as the source of control and full partner in providing compassionate and coordinated care based on respect for patient's preferences, values, and needs.
Evidence-Based Practice	Integrates best current evidence with clinical expertise and patient/family preferences and values for delivery of optimal health care.
Safety	Minimizes risk of harm to patients and providers through both system effectiveness and individual performance.
Teamwork and Collaboration	Functions effectively within nursing and interprofessional teams, fostering open communication, mutual respect, and shared decision making to achieve quality patient care.
Informatics	Uses information and technology to communicate, manage knowledge, mitigate error, and support decision making.
Quality Improvement	Uses data to monitor the outcomes of care processes and uses improvement methods to design and test changes to continuously improve the quality and safety of health care systems.

QSEN, Quality and Safety Education for Nurses.

partners guided curricular development, strengthening experiences (Fater, 2013; Ouellet et al., 2012). Competencies include ability to provide patient-centered care, effectively work in interprofessional teams, understand evidence-based practice, measure quality of care, and use health information technology, as defined in Table 29.1 (QSEN, 2014). These competencies were developed with and demonstrate a basic skill set that includes cognitive knowledge, psychomotor skills, and professional nursing values and attitudes (Kantor, 2010). Introducing these competencies and skill sets in an introductory nursing course promotes a systems-based foundation for critical thinking and professional accountability in nursing (Lambton & Mahlmeister, 2010).

D. INTRODUCTION OF SCENARIO

Previous studies suggested students travel through a series of stations using a circular approach to learn and achieve desired outcomes (Florea & Rafeldt, 2005; Florea, Rafeldt, & Youngblood, 2011). Standardized patients and high- and low-fidelity simulations with individual workstations for online CINAHL searches and electronic record charting are used throughout the rotations. The term *CAROUSEL* is an acronym used to identify and translate the QSEN focus of each station. C = commitment to safe practice; A = achieving an "A" in practice by considering knowledge, skills and professional nursing values, asking about and evaluating care within systems; R = role play, simulation, and activities; O = consideration of others and patient-centered care; U and S = taking care of yourself so that you can be an effective team member; E = finding evidence-based practice resources using technology; and L = legal and ethical implications for documentation using technology.

The QSEN CAROUSEL approach can be used with any concept or skill within the curriculum. These activities also introduce students to the effective use of simulation and reflection. Many students then learn to practice in the laboratory on their own and with peers. Tables 29.2 and 29.3 list a sampling of approaches with first-year nursing students.

Table 29.2	Developing Safe and Competent Practice in Mobility, Critical for Health
Immobility, Fall Risk, and the Need for Mobility	**Station Learning Activity**
C—Commitment to safety	Review practice guidelines for evaluating patients using fall-risk tools, pre- and postambulation vital sign assessement, and implementing safety plans
A—Achieving an "A" in practice	Knowledge—Practice guidelines for transferring a patient from bed to wheelchair and reverse, ambulating a patient
Considering knowledge, skills, and professional nursing values	Psychomotor skills—Completing the transfers with and without Hoyer, Seralift, and Sam Haul Turner, turning aids; ambulating the patient with and without gait belts
Asking about and evaluating care within systems	Affect and professional values—Feelings related to using mechanical lifts, what to use if gait belt cannot be found, what if patient falls, and how to translate into safe practice; participating in root-cause analysis to ask about and evaluate care using a systems approach
R—Role play and actual simulation	Transfer of patient from floor to bed, varying use of Hoyer lift, inflatable lift, or two-person assist
O—Other considerations and patient-centered care	Consider age and disease/surgical condition variations in risk parameters—Vulnerabilities related to orthostatic hypotension; effects of a low hemoglobin and hematocrit; pain, multiple patient care tubes, orthopedic, neurologic, cardiac conditions Consider the effects of immobility.
U and S—Taking care of yourself so that you can be an effective team member	Are you using ergonomic principles in care and preventing occupational vulnerabilities from becoming reality?
E—Finding evidence-based practice resources and using technology	Use CINAHL and/or search engine to find an evidence-based practice scholarly article related to prevention of falls and the value of mobility in aging populations; share and discuss
L—Legal and ethical implications for documentation and using technology	Reinforce need for risk assessment each shift, use of preventive devices, and documentation of falls; review use of an incident report

CINAHL, Cumulative Index of Nursing and Allied Health Literature.

E. RUNNING OF THE SCENARIO

These simulation experiences can be completed in multiple 7.5-hour clinical labs, half-day clinical labs, or individual sessions.

Faculty structure the development of critical thinking with transparency in learning to facilitate application of theory to practice. Station learning activities can be discussion based—debriefing sessions, actual live or human simulator experiences, or individual work centers. Crafted prompts reinforce retention. Consideration related to student/faculty ratio, contact time for the experience, and early preparation of the student are some of the variables that influence the design.

Table 29.3	Developing Clinical Decision-Making Behaviors in Basic Nutritional Safety
Collecting, Interpreting and Implementing Nutritional Support and Safety for Patients	**Station Learning Activity**
C—Commitment to safety	Reviewing practice guidelines working collaboratively with provider, nursing staff, dietary, and speech and occupational therapists as needed Review swallow guidelines Review how to approach patients who are not eating prescribed diet Review how to assess and evaluate advancing the diet from NPO to clear liquids in a postsurgical patient
A—Achieving an "A" in practice Considering knowledge, skills, and professional nursing values Asking about and evaluating care within systems	Knowledge—Differentiating what is recorded for I&O, entering the percentage of meal eaten by the patient, differentiating when to enter percentage and actual foods for calorie count by dietitian Psychomotor skills—Completing an actual I&O or nutrition form Affect and professional values—Feelings related to nurses' role in assessing nutrition, valuing own contributions in clinical settings, novice advocacy for changes in patient's diet
R—Role play and actual simulation	Feeding a patient—Varies in each group (opening containers—setup, verbal cueing, feeding with no adaptive devices, feeding with adaptive devices, mixing liquids with Thicket to varying consistencies) Assess for signs and symptoms of nutritional health and malnutrition Interpret nutritional laboratory values of serum albumin and prealbumin and their uses in clinical practice
O—Other considerations and patient-centered care	Consider age and cultural variations in nutritional parameters Identify what to do if families bring in food for patient and where it is stored
U and S—Taking care of yourself so that you can be an effective team member	Are you planning for your own meal during clinical? Are you reporting off to the nurse, CNAs/PCTs, and instructor when going to lunch/dinner?
E—Finding evidence-based practice resources and using technology	Use CINAHL and/or search engine to find and identify implications of dysphagia in patients and how an NPO order over time affects patient outcomes
L—Legal and ethical implications for documentation and using technology	Reinforce need for dietary order and assessment of the order with action as needed and documentation

CINAHL, Cumulative Index of Nursing and Allied Health Literature; CNAs, certified nursing assistants; I&O, intake and output; NPO, nothing per os; PCT, patient care technician.

F. PRESENTATION OF COMPLETED TEMPLATE

Title

QSEN CAROUSEL in Collecting, Interpreting, and Acting on Patient Vital Signs

Scenario Level and Focus Area

First year of nursing study

Scenario Description

First-year nursing students rotate through stations in their clinical or classroom groups as they are introduced to the QSEN concepts and an area of content knowledge. Table 29.4 describes the specifics. At each station, a faculty member guides them through the station, providing brief feedback that they bring to the end-of-day group discussion. In a full-day session, students begin at different "letters" and rotate through the lab. In a half-day experience students might begin with the A, U to S, E, and C, and follow with R, O, and L. Students could also be assigned preparation stations before coming to the clinical laboratory experience.

Scenario Objectives

Learning Method

Active learning within the cognitive, psychomotor, and affective domains through standardized patients, high- and low-fidelity simulators, role play, individual workstations, and large-group debriefing promotes retention and subsequent application in clinical settings. INASCL Standard IV states facilitators use multiple methods to facilitate the learning needs of the participants (Franklin et al., 2013) Variations in the carousel approach may be needed after assessment of the learners. Reflective pedagogy reinforces the foundation for learning and development of plans for personal success in learning, clinical reasoning, and professional accountability. Reflection on action promotes development of clinical decision making in new situations (Dreifuerst, 2015).

Primary Learning Outcomes

During and after completing the simulation experience, the students are able to do the following:

1. Identify the QSEN principles as they relate to vital signs (VS) assessment, interpretation, and resulting actions.
2. Demonstrate safe, effective practice when assessing VS and act on the assessed data.
3. Use standardized patients or human patient simulators (HPSs) for growth in learning.
4. Use information from the patient's medical record such as orders, history and physical with baseline VS, medication administration, and progress documentation records.
5. Chart VS data in the electronic record and discuss implications of real-time charting.
6. Effectively use CINAHL to find evidence-based articles and answers to VS questions.
7. Identify own professional accountability and plan for success in knowledge, skill, and affect.

The National Council of State Boards of Nursing National Council Licensure Examination for Registered Nurses (NCLEX-RN®) test plan categories and subcategories (NCSBN, 2016) included in this scenario are as follows:

Safe and effective care environment: *Management of care* (client rights and establishing priorities), Safety and infection control (safe use of equipment and medical and surgical asepsis standard/transmission based other precautions); **Health promotion and maintenance:** *Aging process, techniques of physical assessment;* **Psychosocial integrity:** *Therapeutic communications;* **Physiological integrity:** *Basic*

Table 29.4	Developing Safe, Effective Assessment, and Practice
Collecting, Interpreting and Acting on Patient Vital Signs	**Station Learning Activity**
C—Commitment to safety	Review adult and elderly practice guidelines, use the two step palpation method for BP, differentiate normal and abnormal patient parameters, identify the correct BP, T, P, R, O_2 saturation meter readings Consider the relation of VS to oxygenation and perfusion in the body
A—Achieving an A in practice Considering knowledge, skills and professional nursing values Asking and evaluating care within systems	Knowledge—When to take VS, what do you do if a patient is on contact precautions and you must take his or her VS? Psychomotor skills—Break down the BP into component skills, demonstrate proficiency, differentiate apical and radial pulse; work in pairs and compare assessments Affect and professional values—Identify extrinsic and intrinsic motivation to own practice in the lab; using a Plan, Do, Study, Act approach, consider how knowledge of the VS at the start of the shift promotes safe patient practice.
R—Role-play, actual simulation	Introduce self and use manual equipment appropriately with the patient. Obtain VS that are not within the normal parameters and act on the results—are nurse and instructor notified in a time-appropriate manner? Does the student recognize the need for a PRN (when needed) order of acetaminophen (Tylenol) if appropriate? Is the student able to recognize and count atrial fibrillation? Can the student identify basic abnormal lung sounds and resulting actions? What does the student do if a pulse oximeter reading of 88% is obtained?
O—other considerations and patient centered care	Consider age and cultural variations in parameters and identification of vulnerable groups for hypertension. Use low-fidelity simulators as an elderly patient with a temperature of 96°F, 98.8°F, 99.6°F, and 101.4°F. Interpret and debrief presentation of illness in an elderly patient.
U and S—Taking care of yourself so that you can be an effective team member	Use simulators to answer: How is your hearing, vision? What is your anxiety level with a new skill? What is your plan in clinical when working together with limited equipment?
E—Finding evidence-based practice resources and using technology	Use CINAHL and/or search engine to find an evidence-based practice scholarly article related to VS. What is the difference in sounds when using the bell or diaphragm of the stethoscope? What may abnormal breaths sound like on postop day one compared to postop day eight mean?
L—Legal and ethical Implications for documentation and using technology	Reinforce need to take VS at start of shift and document VS on the electronic medical record or board. Discuss time entry for data; no predocumentation/back-documentation, document in real time.

BP, blood pressure; CINAHL, Cumulative Index of Nursing and Allied Health Literature; VS, vital sign.

care and comfort (mobility/immobility), *Pharmacological and parenteral therapies* (expected effects/outcomes), *Reduction of risk potential* (vital signs and system-specific assessments), *Physiological adaptation* (illness management).

For this scenario, the American Association of Colleges of Nursing's *Essentials of Baccalaureate Education for Professional Nursing Practice* (AACN; 2008) items addressed include:

> Essential II: Basic Organizational and Systems Leadership for Quality Care and Patient Safety
> Essential III: Scholarship for Evidence-Based Practice
> Essential IV: Information Management and Application of Patient Care Technology
> Essential VI: Interprofessional Communication and Collaboration for Improving Patient Health Outcomes
> Essential VIII: Professionalism and Professional Values

Student Preparation for the Simulation

Required Readings and Websites to Explore

Required readings relate to VS and the age groups in your curriculum. List chapters from a fundamentals-of-nursing text or a journal article. Link American Heart Association: www.heart.org and QSEN: www.qsen.org to preparation and review.

Materials to Prepare

> VS equipment, including oxygen saturation meter
> Computer stations, laptops, or mobile devices as needed
> *Completed medication sheet/card:* PRN Tylenol 650 mg PO (per os) PRN (as needed) for temperature more than 101°F

Setting the Scene

Equipment Needed

1. Multiple stations with standardized patients and/or low- and high-fidelity HPSs
2. Computer stations, laptops, or mobile devices for electronic documentation and CINAHL searches
3. Equipment to measure VS (thermometer, stethoscope, sphygmomanometer, and pulse oximeter)
4. ID bracelet with name, age, physician, and/or medical record number as Health Insurance Portability and Accountability Act (HIPAA) and agency appropriate; and allergy bracelet
5. Curtain or ability to create private assessment area
6. Available oxygen via nasal cannula tubing
7. Telephone (for access to admitting nurse and physician)
8. Quiet areas for feedback and discussion

Participants needed

Students can perform multiple assessments at a time. Observers can also provide feedback to colleagues.

Scenario Implementation

Expected run time for each station is 45 to 50 minutes. There is a 45-minute lunch included in a full day with over an hour for total group debriefing at the end of the day. The INACSL (2013/2016) has guided simulation learning and curriculum development at Three Rivers Community College (TRCC). Particularly important in this QSEN CAROUSEL approach are Standard VI: The Debriefing Process and Standard VII: Participant Assessment and Evaluation. Students use checklists, discussion, and facilitator feedback to discover new learning, professionalism, and 21st-century nursing practice. Teaching, learning, and assessment are connected for both students and faculty. The debriefing guidelines later give specifics.

G. DEBRIEFING GUIDELINES

Gather the entire group at the end of the day for a group debriefing. The group has received small-group feedback and now the students come together to enhance their learning through social pedagogy. Review QSEN competencies using the knowledge, skills, and attitude approach. Reinforce cognitive knowledge in VS as needed. Recommend continued psychomotor skills practice. Have each group present an "a-ha" they had from the various stations, compare and contrast "a-ha"s. Ask members of the group how simulation can help their individual learning. Use reflective pedagogy techniques; ask questions such as, "What was your main goal while going through the stations? What were your strengths and areas for improvement? How you use what you learned today in future experiences?" Help students make the connections of theory to application in clinical settings. Reinforcing repetitive practice with reflection and discussion promotes development of clinical reasoning skills and success in patient care (Lasater, 2007).

Reinforce Standard Nursing Behaviors When Interacting With a Patient

The following behaviors need to be reinforced: verification of patient orders and plan of care, identification of patient, introduction of self and explanation of reason there, asepsis as appropriate, preparation, and gathering of equipment/supplies needed, maintenance of privacy and HIPAA standards, appropriate ergonomic/body mechanics when assessing or performing care, maintenance of a safe environment (bed position, call bell, and equipment placement), and documentation, and be tested in the simulation lab, clinical setting, and theory exams. Students begin to understand the need to retain previous learning.

H. SUGGESTIONS/KEY FEATURES TO REPLICATE OR IMPROVE

If student nurses see the transparency in teaching and learning they improve in their own learning, as well as become better teachers for their own patients, so it is important to continue to reinforce learning through reflection and constructivist methods such as scaffolding and stacking of principles (Ireland, 2008). Take the time to reinforce with freshman students the standard nursing behaviors when interacting with patients. Use this clinical day not only to refine specific clinical skills and reinforce core values and behaviors, but also to develop students' confidence in their ability to care for patients. A checklist helps a novice learner practice safely. A confident learner can keep the checklist in his or her pocket.

I. RECOMMENDATIONS FOR FURTHER USE

Movement in learning supports student engagement and can also be used in a classroom. This QSEN CAROUSEL approach can be used with senior-level concepts, diseases, and disorders. For instance, students could differentiate safe, effective care for a patient who has had a hemorrhagic stroke as compared with a patient who has clot-based pathology through practice guidelines in both the emergent and rehabilitation phases of care. The CAROUSEL learning activity can also be applied with other core values and concepts besides QSEN with other creative acronyms. Rotation through planned simulation/stations is the key.

J. HOW SIMULATION-BASED PEDAGOGY HAS CONTRIBUTED TO IMPROVED STUDENT OUTCOMES

Novice nursing students focus on tasks when they begin their nursing education. Many students state, "I gave my first injection; now I am a nursing student." New approaches to teaching content provide students with a comprehensive overview of safe, system-based initiatives. Use of integrated QSEN concepts within a clinical simulation day promotes holistic, systems thinking for the learner of professional nursing practice. Making the teaching and learning transparent helps students develop personal learning of the multitude of behaviors and skills required of a flexible nurse, an important step in professional accountability. Rodgers (2002) describes reflection as social pedagogy for personal growth that is systematic and disciplined. It promotes the integrated learning that is necessary to develop clinical reasoning and actualization of the QSEN behaviors. Simulation, in varying formats, prepares freshman students to engage in the professional nursing role through transparency, reflective feedback, and use of a holistic approach.

REFERENCES

American Association of Colleges of Nursing. (2008). *The essentials of baccalaureate education for professional nursing practice.* Washington, DC: Author. Retrieved from http://www.aacnnursing.org/Portals/42/Publications/BaccEssentials08.pdf

Burnhas, L. D., Chastin, K., & George, J. L. (2012). Just culture and nursing regulation: Learning to improve patient safety. *Journal of Nursing Regulation, 2*(4), 43–49.

Decker, S., Fey, M., Sideras, S., Caballero, S., Rockstraw, L., Boese, T., . . . Borum, J. C. (2013). Standards of best practice: Simulation standard VI: The debriefing process. *Clinical Simulation in Nursing, 9*(6S), S27–S29. doi:10.1016/j.ecns.2013.04.008

Dreifuerst, K. T. (2015). Getting started with debriefing for meaningful learning. *Clinical Simulation in Nursing, 11*(5), 268–275.

Fater, K. H. (2013). Gap analysis: A method to assess core competency development in the curriculum. *Nursing Education Perspectives, 34*(2), 101–105.

Florea, M., & Rafeldt, L. (2005, January). *Information literacy for nurses.* Presentation given at the North East American Library Association Conference, Boston, MA.

Florea, M., Rafeldt, L., & Youngblood, S. (2011). Using an information literacy program to prepare nursing students to practice in a virtual workplace. In Information Resource Management (Ed.), *Virtual communities, concepts, methodologies, tools and applications* (pp. 1482–1498). Hershey, PA: Information Science Reference.

Franklin, A. E., Boese, T., Gloe, D., Lioce, L., Decker, S., Sando, C. R., . . . Borum, J. C. (2013). Standards of best practice: Simulation standard IV: Facilitation. *Clinical Simulation in Nursing, 9*(6S), S19–S21. doi:10.1016/j.ecns.2013.04.011

International Nursing Association for Clinical Simulation and Learning. (2013, updated 2016). INACSL standards of best practice: Simulation. Retrieved from https://www.inacsl.org/i4a/pages/index.cfm?pageID=3407

Institute of Medicine. (2003). *Health professions education: A bridge to quality.* Washington, DC: National Academies Press.

Ireland, M. (2008). Assisting students to use evidence as a part of reflection on practice. *Nursing Education Perspectives, 29*(2), 90–93.

Kantor, S. A. (2010). Pedagogical change in nursing education: One instructor's experience. *Journal of Nursing Education, 49*(7), 414–417.

Lambton, J., & Mahlmeister, L. (2010). Conducting root cause analysis with nursing students: Best practice in nursing education. *Journal of Nursing Education, 49*(8), 444–448.

Lasater, K. (2007). High-fidelity simulation and the development of clinical judgment: Students' experiences. *Journal of Nursing Education, 48*(7), 388–394.

National Council of State Boards of Nursing. (2016). NCLEX-RN examination: Test plan for the National Council Licensure Examination for Registered Nurses. Retrieved from https://www.ncsbn.org/RN_Test_Plan_2016_Final.pdf

Ouellet, E., Graham, J., Bader, H., Morse, H., MaCauley, P., & Rafeldt, L. (2012, April). *Gap analysis nursing education and practice*. Paper presented at Connecticut League for Nursing meeting, Wallingford, CT.

Quality and Safety Education for Nurses. (2014). QSEN competencies. Retrieved from http://qsen.org/competencies/pre-licensure-ksas

Rodgers, C. (2002). Defining relection: Another look at John Dewey and reflective thinking. *Teachers College Record, 104*(4), 842–866.

FURTHER READING

Center for Patient Safety. (2016). Just culture. Retrieved from http://www.centerforpatientsafety.org/just-culture

Assessing a Patient With a Mood Disorder

Audrey M. Beauvais and Joyce M. Shea

This chapter presents a simulation activity that incorporates the students' knowledge of psychiatric illness and risk assessment with a focus on mood disorders and substance abuse. The simulation exercise builds on skills in therapeutic communication, lethality assessment, and recognition of signs and symptoms of major depression and alcohol abuse. Postscenario discussion can assist in clarifying issues in documentation, patient rights, and legal requirements of mental health nursing practice.

A. IMPLEMENTATION OF SIMULATION-BASED PEDAGOGY IN YOUR INDIVIDUALIZED TEACHING AREA

Faculty in baccalaureate nursing programs face many difficulties in their efforts to connect theory to practice for students. In a mental health nursing course, the difficulties can be compounded by the abstract nature of the content and the students' potential discomfort with the unique processes associated with mental health nursing care. Taking a broad-based approach to simulation allows the mental health nursing instructor to incorporate a variety of highly interactive strategies, many of which have traditionally been used to set the stage for the students' entrance into clinical sites. For example, I have frequently relied on role play exercises to sharpen communication techniques and build confidence in students as they prepare for their initial exposure to acute care psychiatric patients. The creative use of case studies has also provided a means for students to demonstrate their skill in comprehensive and interdisciplinary care planning. As mental health nursing students need to integrate multiple sources of information on a patient, including observations on affect (e.g., facial expression) and speech (e.g., tone, rate, patterns, etc.), creation of a high-fidelity simulation using a human patient simulator (HPS) may not be the most effective teaching strategy. The following scenario has been created for use with a standardized patient (SP)—a human actor, paid or volunteer—who brings the situation to life and challenges the students to draw on diverse areas of theoretical knowledge as the interaction progresses. Students can also be assigned auxiliary roles, such as that of a family member, employer, or roommate.

B. EDUCATIONAL MATERIALS AVAILABLE IN YOUR TEACHING AREA AND RELATED TO YOUR SPECIALTY

The scenario can be run in a number of settings and requires minimal preparation or setup. At the Fairfield University Marion Peckham Egan School of Nursing and Health Studies (SONHS) Robin Kanarek Learning Resource Center there is a home health area designed for simulations in mental health or community/public health care. Accessories include a twin bed, a table with lamp, an upholstered chair, a throw rug, a floor lamp, and a phone. If students in the mental health nursing course have the opportunity to conduct psychiatric home visits, the scenario may be run in this setting as a mobile outreach, with roles for family members or friends to be involved in the interaction; otherwise, the scenario may be run as an interaction in an employee health clinic, a walk-in clinic, or the urgent care section of the emergency department (ED). The setting for these situations requires either two chairs and a desk, or an examination table and a chair or stool for the nurse conducting the assessment interview. Blood pressure (BP) cuffs, a breathalyzer machine, and a "clinic" phone should be available. Intake forms (including mental health assessment), substance use screening forms, depression screening forms, and a suicide lethality scale should also be present. There are substance use (Ewing, 1984a, 1984b) and depression screening (Zung, 1965) forms available on the web, as well as a sample suicide lethality scale, as shown in Appendix A.

C. SPECIFIC OBJECTIVES OF SIMULATION USAGE WITHIN A SPECIFIC COURSE AND THE OVERALL PROGRAM

The main objective of the scenario is accurate assessment of psychiatric symptoms and risk factors for self-harm. The nursing process is used to identify priorities among patient needs and an evidence-based plan of care is established. Students at SONHS who are taking mental health nursing are either in the second semester of the second year of the baccalaureate program or in the first semester, third year of their baccalaureate program. Before this course, students would have completed chemistry, anatomy and physiology, and pathophysiology/pharmacology. In addition, they have taken or will be concurrently taking courses in health assessment, developmental psychology, and microbiology. Students are beginning to work on the integration of content across courses, particularly in the areas of communication and health assessment. The simulation activity presented in this chapter specifically helps students to meet objectives for the mental health nursing course in the following areas: identifying risk factors for psychiatric disorders, developing therapeutic communication skills and planning appropriate evidence-based care for psychiatric patients, recognizing ethical and legal issues as they present in patients with psychiatric illness, and understanding the role of the nurse based on the American Nurses Association (2014) standards of practice for psychiatric–mental health nursing.

D. INTRODUCTION OF SCENARIO

A human actor plays a 28-year-old female who presents to the employee health clinic with complaints of a migraine headache and fatigue. The nursing students are responsible for conducting the initial intake and assessment. They are given the standard forms used for routine clinic visits and are told that they may also make use of any other equipment present in the examination room. The students' goal is to complete an initial assessment and establish a plan of care based on the data collected within 15 minutes. They are evaluated on their skills in conducting the interview, their ability to gather necessary information, and to determine the priority of needs at this time, their appropriate use of equipment/supplies, and the establishment of a comprehensive plan of care for the patient. Additional roles for students may include a coworker or supervisor, family member, or friend.

E. RUNNING OF THE SCENARIO

Before running the scenario, the human actor playing the SP is given details about the patient's background, including medical and psychiatric history, work and school history, current stressors, and behavioral patterns. She is instructed to provide minimal information until prompted by the student. There is no past medical record available. Students are given access to a phone to allow for contact with other health care providers (e.g., mental health care crisis workers) or a hospital ED as needed. In addition, students can use their personal digital assistants (PDAs) to access information on evidence-based practice related to depression and substance abuse. Although they are unable to access/communicate with the instructor or other students during the scenario, they are given the opportunity to identify additional sources of information they would have liked to use on completion of the interview (e.g., family members).

F. PRESENTATION OF COMPLETED TEMPLATE

Title

Assessing a Patient With a Mood Disorder (for second semester, sophomore year or first semester, junior year baccalaureate students in Nursing 305—Mental Health Nursing)

Focus Area

Psychiatric/mental health nursing, health assessment, risk assessment

Scenario Description

Tina Hall is a 28-year-old, single, African American female who comes to the employee health clinic complaining of a migraine headache and fatigue. She has been an employee in the information technology department for the past 6 years, having started immediately after graduating with honors from college. She is currently working as an interim department manager while her supervisor is on medical leave. She lives alone in her own apartment and recently became engaged. Although she has experienced migraines on occasion in the past, they are now happening more frequently (1–2 per week) and are becoming more severe (7/10 self-report of pain accompanied by nausea and light sensitivity). She has been feeling extremely stressed and fears being unable to cope with the responsibilities of her job. She has had several recent conflicts with the employees under her supervision. She is having increasing trouble sleeping and has recently begun to have two or three glasses of wine before going to bed every night. She feels edgy and distressed, and wants to be given "something like Ativan" to help calm her nerves and get her through the day. She has no other medical problems and no known allergies.

Scenario Objectives

Students who successfully complete this scenario exercise have demonstrated their ability to do the following four tasks: (a) communicate effectively with a distraught client, (b) recognize the signs and symptoms related to a mood disorder, (c) conduct a lethality assessment using scale in Appendix A, as well as a substance use assessment with the CAGE scale (Ewing 1984a, 1984b), and (d) offer some appropriate nonpharmacologic interventions to reduce the client's level of stress.

Successful completion of the simulation activity would also allow the student to meet several of the revised American Association of Colleges of Nursing (AACN; 2008) *Essentials of Baccalaureate Education*, including:

Essential I (objectives 2, 3, 5)
Essential II (objectives 1, 2, 7, 8)
Essential III (objectives 1, 6)
Essential VI (objectives 2, 6)
Essential VIII (objectives 1, 2, 4, 6, 9, 10)

Areas of the 2016 National Council Licensure Examination for Registered Nurses (NCLEX-RN°) test plan categories that are covered in the exercise include (National Council of State Boards of Nursing, 2015):

Safe and effective care: *Management of care* (advocacy, establishing priorities); **Health promotion and maintenance:** (health screening, high-risk behaviors); **Psychosocial integrity:** (behavioral interventions, chemical and other dependencies/substance use disorder, coping mechanisms, crisis intervention, cultural awareness/cultural influences on health, mental health concepts, stress management, support systems, therapeutic communication, and therapeutic environment).

Setting the Scene

Equipment Needed

Examination table, chair or stool for nurse, BP cuff, breathalizer machine, phone, intake and assessment forms, and patient information brochures on anxiety and depression. Students are informed that they will be allowed to use a PDA to access information on evidence-based practice related to the treatment of depression and associated risk factors such as suicide (American Psychiatric Association [APA], 2010; University of Michigan Health System, 2011; U.S. Preventive Services Task Force, 2014, 2016). The SP and the student are the only required participants, but additional roles may be developed for a coworker, family member, or friend.

Scenario Implementation

The SP was instructed to present with a moderate level of agitation and to focus on physical complaints and her sense of being overwhelmed. All other information would be divulged only in response to students' questions. Students are required to respond appropriately to the level of agitation displayed by the SP, use effective communication techniques, conduct a thorough health history (physical as well as psychological), perform a lethality assessment and alcohol abuse assessment to determine priorities for care, and implement a short-term plan of action to meet identified needs. The instructor facilitated the students' learning through the debriefing process on completion of the scenario.

Evaluation Criteria

Students are evaluated on the basis of their effective integration of theory with practice (i.e., their ability to elicit the necessary information, gain a thorough understanding of the client's needs, determine the priorities for care, and establish a reasonable plan based on clinical evidence). Their ability to conceptualize the main issues is captured in their efforts to present a plan of care to the client.

Checklist of Interventions and Assessments

___Introduces self
___Establishes therapeutic relationship with patient
___Demonstrates therapeutic communication skills

___Uses skills to reduce patient agitation
___Obtains information on chief complaint
___Obtains information on past medical history
___Conducts mental status assessment
___Evaluates symptoms of depression
___Conducts lethality assessment
___Evaluates pattern of substance use
___Presents patient with nonpharmacological alternatives for stress reduction
___Establishes appropriate plan of care with patient

G. DEBRIEFING GUIDELINES

A critical component of simulation is to debrief the experience to promote reflective thinking (Decker et al., 2013; Lavoie, Pepin, & Boyer, 2013). At Fairfield University SONHS, the International Nursing Association for Clinical Simulation and Learning (INACSL) Standards of Best Practice: Simulation[SM] are used (Decker et al., 2013). In other words, debriefing is facilitated by an individual who is competent in the process of briefing and occurs in a safe learning environment. The facilitator observes the simulated experience and uses a structured framework for debriefing. Although the optimal time and duration of debriefing is flexible, the facilitator allows at least 15 minutes for debriefing and discussion (Decker et al., 2013). The facilitator focuses the debriefing on the stated outcomes and objectives (Decker et al., 2013). The instructor may choose to debrief the student individually at first, asking him or her to reflect on the following questions:

1. Did you prepare for this scenario in any way and, if so, how?
2. What were you thinking and feeling during the simulation?
3. How did your skills improve?
4. What would you do differently?
5. Do you need additional knowledge, information, or skills?

In addition, the instructor can ask questions based on observed actions and results. For example, the facilitator can say "It looks to me like ... "
The following questions may be posed to the larger class:

1. What specific communication techniques were used?
2. What additional areas of assessment needed to be addressed?
3. What additional patient needs could be identified?
4. What would you do if the patient indicated that she was intending to commit suicide?
5. What information should/must be included in the employee's health record?
6. How much information can/should be shared in a referral for mental health care?
7. In what ways has your understanding of the role of the baccalaureate-prepared nurse increased?

H. SUGGESTIONS/KEY FEATURES
TO REPLICATE OR IMPROVE

The key features of communication and assessment can be replicated in scenarios with patients who have various diagnoses, ages, comorbidities, and risk factors. The scenario, as is, can be implemented only if the students have completed background reading on stress, mood disorders, suicidality, substance abuse, and therapeutic communication. In addition, students benefit from having completed the first several weeks of the mental health clinical practicum before attempting the scenario.

I. RECOMMENDATIONS FOR FURTHER USE

This simulation could be developed with a focus on an elderly client in the home setting or a crisis situation in the community. Additional legal and ethical issues, such as competency and involuntary hospitalization, could be introduced. The simulation activity described here can easily be modified for graduate psychiatric nurse practitioner students by having the student play the role of an outpatient clinician who is performing an intake assessment, and requiring him or her to develop a plan of care that includes pharmacologic as well as cognitive-behavioral interventions.

J. HOW SIMULATION-BASED PEDAGOGY HAS CONTRIBUTED TO IMPROVED STUDENT OUTCOMES

A simulation-based pedagogy may seem initially to have limited usefulness in a mental health nursing class, but the impact could at least equal that achieved in any other class, if approached in the right way. Case studies and role play have long been deemed appropriate methods to help bridge the gap between theory and practice for baccalaureate students. The use of an SP and integration of a well-designed scenario could lead to tremendous opportunities for significant learning to take place. Students are more likely to be active participants if the class activity is interesting to them, and the debriefing period allows for a sharing of thoughts and reactions that makes the learning process personal and memorable. The student who takes on the main role in the scenario will have a solid experience on which to build his or her understanding of psychiatric assessment, suicide risk, substance abuse, and stress response and reduction. Basing the scenario in a location other than an inpatient psychiatric unit also promotes a greater understanding of the application of mental health nursing principles across settings.

K. EXPERT RECOMMENDATIONS AND WORDS OF WISDOM

Although the simulation has worked well, some modifications have been made over the past few years. In particular, we have added a prebrief before the simulation that allows an opportunity to establish an environment of trust, integrity, and respect. During the prebrief, students are oriented to the simulation environment and provided ground rules. Facilitators are encouraged to ask questions such as: "What are your resources?" "Will you walk me through what you plan to do?" and "What do you expect to see?" The prebrief is intended to prepare students for the upcoming simulation in an effort to promote their ability to meet the objectives and actively participate (Jeffries, McNelis, & Wheeler, 2008).

L. EVALUATION OF BEST PRACTICE STANDARDS AND USE OF CREDENTIALED SIMULATION FACULTY

Fairfield University SONHS is in the process of becoming a Society for Simulation in Healthcare (SSH) Accredited Program. As such, efforts have been made to implement the new INACSL standards to help ensure that all faculty have the knowledge, skills, and abilities to provide quality health care simulation activities. Knowing that faculty expertise in simulation is imperative, the SONHS has supported six faculty members in receiving simulation training and to sit for the certification examination. All faculty are encouraged to attend conferences and share the information with the full faculty. The SONHS provides faculty development programs, many of which have focused on simulation. For example, this past year we hosted a well-received 6-hour debriefing and facilitation training program for faculty and adjuncts. Fairfield University SONHS values simulation education as a link between classroom learning and real-life clinical experience and thus continues to explore ways to strengthen our program.

REFERENCES

American Association of Colleges of Nursing. (2008). *The essentials of baccalaureate education for professional nursing practice*. Washington, DC: Author.

American Nurses Association. (2014). *Psychiatric-mental health nursing: Scope and standards of practice* (2nd ed.). Silver Spring, MD: Author.

American Psychiatric Association. (2010). *Practice guideline for the treatment of patients with major depressive disorder* (3rd ed.). Arlington, VA: American Psychiatric Publishing. Retrieved from https://www.guide lines.gov/content.aspx?id=24158

The Crisis Call Center. (2012). Suicide lethality scale. Retrieved from http://036beb2.netsolhost.com/wordpress1/wp-content/uploads/2016/04/Suicide-Lethality-Scale.pdf

Decker, S., Fey, M., Sideras, S., Caballero, S., Rockstraw, L., Boese, T., . . . Borum, J. C. (2013). Standards of best practice: Simulation standard VI: The debriefing process. *Clinical Simulation in Nursing, 9*(6S), S26–S29.

Ewing, J. A. (1984a). CAGE questionnaire. Retrieved from http://www.integration.samhsa.gov/images/res/CAGEAID.pdf

Ewing, J. A. (1984b). Detecting alcoholism. The CAGE questionnaire. *Journal of the American Medical Association, 252*(14), 1905–1907.

Jeffries, P. R., McNelis, A. M., & Wheeler, C. A. (2008). Simulation as a vehicle for enhancing collaborative practice models. *Critical Care Nursing Clinics of North America, 20*(4), 471–480.

Lavoie, P., Pepin, J., & Boyer, L. (2013). Reflective debriefing to promote novice nurses' clinical judgment after high-fidelity clinical simulation: A pilot test. *Dynamics, 24*(4), 36–41.

National Council of State Boards of Nursing. (2015). *NCLEX-RN examination for the National Council Licensure Examination for Registered Nurses*. Chicago, IL: Author.

U.S. Preventive Services Task Force. (2014). Screening for suicide risk in adolescents, adults, and older adults in primary care: U.S. Preventive Services Task Force recommendation statement. *Annals of Internal Medicine, 160*(10), 719–726. doi:10.7326/M14-0589

U.S. Preventive Services Task Force. (2016). Screening for depression in adults: U.S. Preventive Services Task Force recommendation statement. *Journal of the American Medical Association, 315*(4), 380–387.

University of Michigan Health System. (2011). Depression. Retrieved from http://www.guideline.gov/content.aspx?id=34406

Zung, W. W. K. (1965). Zung Self-Rating Depression Scale. Retrieved from http://library.umassmed.edu/ementalhealth/clinical/zung_depression.pdf

APPENDIX A

Suicide Lethality Scale

Risk Level	Details	Mental Health	Precipitating Event	Person's Disposition	Action
Low	– Person states he or she is feeling suicidal. – No suicide plan developed. – Person not in immediate danger (i.e., the means to carry out the plan are not present, intent is not immediate).	– May or may not have received counseling in the past. – May or may not have received mental illness diagnoses/treatment.	– Recent crisis or string of crises	– Primary need seems to be someone to talk to who will listen. – Person is open to and active in developing a positive plan of action. – Person has a basic support system available.	– Explore primary issues. – Discuss short- and long-term plans of actions. – Contract with person to fulfill positive plan of action. – Contract with person to reach out for help again if the suicidal feelings return.
Medium	– Person states he or she is feeling suicidal. –Person has a plan. –Means to carry out the plan are available but not readily accessible. – Means are available but not immediately lethal. – Intent is not immediate.	– May have family history of suicide and/or mental illness. – May have chronic mental illness diagnosis.	– Likely feels that negative life events have been ongoing for years. – May resist the idea of "here and now."	– Person may seem uncertain about prospect of future happiness/wellness. – Person still willing to reach for help and develop a positive plan of action.	– Explore primary issue. – Discuss short- and long-term plans of action, including the possibility of mental health assessment. – Contract with person to fulfill a positive plan of action. – Contract with person to reach out for help again if the suicidal feelings return.

(continued)

(continued)

Risk Level	Details	Mental Health	Precipitating Event	Person's Disposition	Action
High	– Person states he or she is feeling suicidal. – Plan developed. – Intent is immediate or within near future. – Means are lethal and accessible. – Likely to have attempted before, and has probably felt suicidal for a long period of time.	– Presence of chronic mental illness is likely, whether or not it has been diagnosed. – Likely has family history of mental illness/suicide.	– Recent crisis likely in addition to ongoing crisis/distress.	– Person states intent to die. – Resistant to open communication/alternatives. – Disillusioned with helping system, strong feelings of hopelessness and diminished fear in the face of death. – You believe the person will harm him- or herself.	– If suicide is in progress, call 911 to dispatch emergency services. – Contract with person to seek immediate assistance from a mental health professional; follow up to make sure this was done. – Contract with person to reach out for help again if suicidal feelings return.

Source: The Crisis Call Center (2012).

CHAPTER 31

Diabetes Management: Nurse Practitioners

Kellie Bryant

A. IMPLEMENTATION OF SIMULATION-BASED PEDAGOGY IN YOUR INDIVIDUALIZED TEACHING AREA

Nurse practitioner (NP) instructors are finding it increasingly challenging to evaluate students in the clinical area because of an increase in nursing school enrollment, nursing faculty shortage, and difficulty in evaluating students in the clinical setting because of the Health Insurance Portability and Accountability Act's (HIPAA) privacy rules. Although the need for clinical evaluations is not eliminated, nursing instructors can use simulation to evaluate student's clinical performance in a safe learning environment using standardized clinical scenarios. Faculty can schedule an evaluation of a large number of students in one central location versus traveling to different clinical sites. Simulation has been found to improve knowledge, skills, and attitudes in undergraduate students; however, more research is needed to evaluate the benefits of simulation for NP students (Rutherford-Hemming, Nye, & Coram, 2016).

Simulation- based pedagogy has been implemented in the Common Health Problems of Adults and Older Adults course as a method of teaching/learning to prepare NP students for their first clinical rotation. This course is designed to enable students to develop the necessary knowledge base and problem- solving skills for practice as an NP in the management of common health problems such as hypertension and diabetes. The goal of the diabetes management scenario is to allow students an opportunity to complete a comprehensive patient encounter in the context of a modified objective structured clinical examination (OSCE) format. A group of three to four students rotate through five stations that represent each component of a patient encounter. These stations include patient history taking, physical examination, ordering of a diagnostic test, development of a diagnosis and treatment plan, and discussion of treatment plan with the patient. Each group is allowed 15 minutes at each station and instructors provide feedback during the simulation. This formative simulation experience enhances assessment, critical thinking, teamwork, and communication skills.

B. EDUCATIONAL MATERIALS AVAILABLE IN YOUR TEACHING AREA AND RELATED TO YOUR SPECIALTY

New York University (NYU) Meyers College of Nursing's Clinical Simulation Learning Center (CSLC) is designed to simulate the hospital and outpatient environment for both undergraduate and graduate students. Our cutting-edge simulation center is larger than 10,000 square feet and consists of 21 simulation rooms to simulate medical–surgical rooms, outpatient examination rooms, and the home environment—all with video-recording capability. Each week, more than

100 simulation sessions are conducted at the CSLC for more than 1,200 undergraduate BS and graduate MS students. The CSLC allows students to enhance their clinical skills and nursing knowledge in a safe learning environment.

The CSLC is currently equipped with close to 30 human patient simulators (HPS), including SimMan 3G, Birthing Noelle, mid fidelity HPSs, and five pediatric HPSs. In addition to the HPSs, the CSLC has a database of more than 20 diverse standardized patients (SPs) that are used for almost all graduate simulations and selected undergraduate simulation sessions.

The scenario can take place in either a simulation room or an OSCE room. The rooms contain either a bed or examination table, laptop for charting, a medical and diagnostic headwall. The role of the patient can be represented by a faculty member or an SP.

C. SPECIFIC OBJECTIVE FOR SIMULATION USAGE WITHIN A SPECIFIC COURSE AND THE OVERALL PROGRAM

The Common Health Problems of Adults and Older Adults course enables students to use their knowledge base and clinical skills to manage simulated patients in the simulation center, as well as real patients in their assigned clinical placement. The scenario was designed for all NP students who are scheduled to begin their first clinical rotation. All students enrolled in the course have completed pathophysiology and advance health assessment courses.

Student Learning Activities

1. Review diabetes management.
2. Complete a history on a patient with diabetes mellitus, type 2.
3. Perform a complete physical assessment.
4. Order appropriate diagnostic test.
5. Develop a comprehensive plan of care based on findings.

D. INTRODUCTION OF SCENARIO

Setting the Scene

The setting is an outpatient primary care clinic. The patient is seated in a chair in the NP's office. The medical assistant has taken the patient's vital signs and has written them on the assessment form.

Technology Used

A medium- or high-fidelity HPS or SP can be used for this scenario. The HPS is wearing a patient gown, a female wig, and female genitalia are applied. The vital signs are programmed as follows: heart rate (HR): 84 beats/minute, respiratory rate (RR): 14 breaths/minute, and blood pressure (BP): 144/84 mmHg, temperature: 98.7°F. If using an SP, a programmable BP cuff and thermometer can be used.

Objectives

1. Obtain a patient history based on patient's chief concern
2. Perform a focused physical assessment based on patient presentation
3. Order appropriate diagnostic test based on history and physical examination
4. Develop a diagnosis based on clinical findings
5. Create a treatment plan based on evidence-based practice
6. Demonstrate effective techniques in providing patient education

Description of Participants

Mrs. Roberta Johnson is a 62-year-old African American female who presents to the clinic because she is feeling "tired" and thinks she has a "bladder infection" because of an increase in urination. She is a regular patient at the clinic and was last seen by another primary care NP 5 months earlier for her annual physical checkup. She has a history of hypertension and diet-controlled type 2 diabetes mellitus. Her last hemoglobin A_{1c} (HbA_{1c}) was done 5 months ago and was 6.8%.

E. RUNNING THE SCENARIO

The students are divided into groups of three to four and assigned times to begin the scenario. The students rotate through each of the five stations starting with station 1: history taking, station 2: physical examination, station 3: diagnostic test ordering and interpretation of results, station 4: diagnosis and development of treatment plan, and station 5: review treatment plan with the patient. Each group is staggered 15 minutes apart to allow each group 15 minutes to complete each station. All five stations are clearly labeled. Each group is given a one-page subjective objective assessment plan (SOAP) format form to be used for charting the patient encounter. An instructor or SP plays the role of the patient and is seated across from the four students at the first station. The second station has an HPS or SP seated on an examination table. At this station the students are expected to complete a focused assessment. A programmable BP cuff, thermometer, and stethoscope are used for the SP. If an HPS is used, an instructor is at the station to provide assessment findings that cannot be elicited by the HPS. At station 3 an instructor or staff member is seated across from the students and provides lab reports requested by the group. The person at station 3 is assigned to be the time keeper and resets the timer every 15 minutes. The fourth and fifth stations are located in the second room. At station 4, students complete the treatment plan as a group using available resources such as Epocrates Essential, Cochrane Reviews, or UpToDate. At the fifth station the students discuss the treatment plan with the patient (instructor), who has returned to the clinic 3 days later for results.

F. PRESENTATION OF COMPLETED TEMPLATE

Title

Diabetes Management

Scenario Level

This scenario is used as a formative evaluation of graduate students in the clinical course titled Common Health Problems of Adults and Older Adults. Students must complete 30 hours of lecture followed by 120 clinical hours.

Focus Area

NP students

Scenario Description

Patient: Roberta Johnson
Age: 62 years
Allergies: No known drug allergies
Race: African American woman
Height: 5 feet, 4 inches. *Weight:* 175 pounds

Reason for visit: The patient presents to her primary care provider stating that she has been "very tired" the past month and thinks she has a "bladder infection" because of her frequent urination.

Past medical history: Patient has a history of diabetes mellitus type 2 for the past 2 years that has been controlled with diet. She did not receive a blood glucose monitoring machine at the time of diagnosis. She has a history of hypertension for the past 10 years.

Medications: Lisinopril 20 mg PO (per os) daily and hydrochlorothiazide 25 mg PO daily.

Surgical history: Has not had any surgeries.

Social history: Married, has two adult children. She is a retired Post Office worker. She denies alcohol, drug use, or cigarette use.

Physical assessment:

HR: 84 beats/minute, RR: 14 breaths/minute, temperature (T): 98.7°F, BP: 144/84 mmHg

Head, ears, eyes, nose and throat (HEENT): Unremarkable, normal fundus examination

Respiratory: Lungs clear bilaterally

Cardiovascular: Normal rate and rhythm; no murmurs

Integument: Clean, dry, and intact

Abdomen: Bowel sounds present; all 4 quadrants; soft, no masses or bruits

Extremities: Pulses 2+, no edema or abnormalities noted, no loss of sensation during monofilament test

Scenario Objectives

1. Students obtain a focused patient history. The focused patient history should include questions about current symptoms, review of past medical history, blood glucose monitoring, current medications, level of exercise, and diet. Students should ask the patient whether she has any signs and symptoms of a urinary tract infection (UTI) and/or hypothyroidism.

2. Perform a physical assessment based on patient presentation and history. The focused physical examination should include examination of the heart, lungs, extremities, and eyes.

3. Order appropriate test based on clinical findings and patient history. The group should order a complete blood count (CBC), comprehensive metabolic panel, lipid panel, urine dipstick, urinalysis, HbA_{1c}, EKG, and microalbumin test.

4. Analyze laboratory results and identify abnormal findings (McKulloch, 2015).

5. Develop an appropriate diagnosis and an appropriate treatment plan based on evidence-based practice. The group should order Metformin 500 mg by mouth daily with meals (McKulloch, 2015). Provide education on lifestyle changes, including blood glucose monitoring, diet, and exercise.

This scenario also allows graduate students the opportunity to practice essential skills as outlined by the American Association of Colleges of Nursing (AACN); *Essentials of Master's Education in Nursing* (AACN, 2011).

Essential I: Background for Practice from Sciences and Humanities, Objectives 1, 5

Essential V: Informatics and Healthcare Technologies, Objective 5

Essentials VIII: Clinical Prevention and Population Health for Improving Health, Objective 5

Essential IX: Master's Level Nursing Practice, Objectives 1, 2, 7, 12, 13

Setting the Scene

Equipment Needed

The HPS or SP seated on examination table, video recording equipment (optional), BP cuff, timer, stethoscope, a hard copy of lab results for each group, picture of normal fundus of eye (if using HPS), and 10-gauge nylon monofilament. The scenario requires five stations that are spaced far enough apart to avoid noise distraction among the groups. The patient history station requires a chair for the patient and four additional chairs circled in front of the patient. The physical examination station is an examination table where the SP or instructor is seated. The monofilament, ophthalmoscope, and a picture of a normal retinal fundus examination are located beside the HPS. The diagnostic test station has a seat for the person distributing lab results, folders containing copies of lab results, and four chairs for the students. The diagnosis and treatment plan station can be in a separate room that contains chairs, a desk, and a computer with Internet connection. The fifth station has chairs for the patient and each student.

Resources Needed

Computer access for Epocrates Plus, UpToDate, and Cochrane Reviews

Simulator Level

SP or medium- or high-fidelity HPS; SP or instructor is needed at the stations for history taking and physical examination.

Participants Needed

A minimum of four people are needed for this scenario. An instructor or SP is needed to play the role of the patient at the history-taking station. Each "patient" is provided with a script of standardized responses to history questions. An SP or instructor is needed at station 2 for the physical examination. If an HPS is used, the instructor must provide students with assessment findings that the HPS cannot elicit such as sensation from the monofilament test. A third person (can be nonfaculty person) is needed at the diagnostic test station to distribute test results based on the labs ordered by the group. Lastly, an instructor is needed at the fifth station to play the role of the patient returning to the clinic for results and a treatment plan.

Scenario Implementation

Initial Settings for HPS

- HPS is seated on the examination table with a patient gown, a female wig, and female genitalia.
- Bedside table has a picture of a normal fundal examination of eyes and 10-gauge nylon monofilament.
- BP cuff and stethoscope are at HPS bedside.
- HPS vital signs programmed as follows: HR: 84 beats/minute, RR: 14 breaths/minute, temperature: 98.7°F, BP: 144/84 mmHg

Resources Needed

- Lab reports: CBC (all values within normal limits)
- Complete metabolic panel: fasting glucose level 254 mg/dL (all other values within normal limits)
- Lipid panel: (all values within normal limits)
- Urine dipstick: +2 glucose
- Urinalysis: +2 glucose
- HbA$_{1c}$: 7.8%
- 12-lead EKG: normal sinus rhythm
- Microalbumin: 11.8 μg/mL
- SOAP format form with vital signs written on the form

Required Student Assessments and Actions

Station 1: History

___ Introduce self to patient
___ Ask patient's purpose of visit
___ Elicits information on concerns
___ Obtains patient's medical history
___ Obtains surgical history
___ Obtains medication history
___ Obtains information on family history
___ Asks patient about social history, including alcohol, cigarette use, and drug use
___ Asks patient about current diet
___ Asks patient about level of exercise

Station 2: Physical Examination

___ Auscultates heart sounds
___ Auscultates lung sounds
___ Examines lower extremities
___ Performs a monofilament test
___ Performs a retinal examination

Station 3: Diagnostic Test

___ Orders CBC, comprehensive metabolic panel, HbA_{1c}, microalbumin, lipid panel, urinalysis, EKG, and thyroid-stimulating hormone (TSH)

Station 4: Diagnosis Development of Treatment Plan

___ Analyzes lab work for abnormalities
___ Develops treatment plan as a group based on evidence-based practice

Station 5: Discussion of Treatment Plan With Patient

___ Explains the results of laboratory results with patient
___ Discusses the need to start metformin
___ Explains proper use and side effects of medication
___ Discusses proper diet with patient
___ Encourages weight loss
___ Encourages patient to exercise
___ Discusses the need for blood glucose monitoring at least once a day
___ Orders education on blood glucose monitor by RN
___ Explores patient's questions/concerns
___ Asks patient to repeat treatment plan

Instructor Interventions

The SP or instructors at stations 1, 2, and 5 will be allowed to provide feedback during the last 5 minutes of the rotation. If a key element of the history or physical examination was missed, the SP/instructor can cue the students in order to make sure that they have key necessary information needed to develop a treatment plan. Students are not allowed to discuss the simulation with other groups and are not allowed to repeat stations.

Exhibit 31.1	Standardized Patient Script
Student Questions	**Standardized Response**
How are you feeling today?	*I have been feeling tired. I have been urinating almost every 1 to 2 hours, which is interfering with my sleep.*
Do you have any burning when you urinate? Any fever? Back pain? Cloudy urine?	*No*
Have you noticed any hair loss, weight gain/ loss, constipation, or any other signs of hypothyroidism?	*No*
How long have you had diabetes and high blood pressure?	*Diabetes 2 years, high blood pressure 10 years*
How would you describe your sleep habits?	*Tired everyday, however, sleeping 7 to 8 hours each night*
What meds are you on?	*Lisinopril 20 mg every day, HCTZ 25 mg daily*
Do you take any herbs or OTC medications?	*Baby aspirin every day*
Do you drink, smoke, or use drugs?	*No*
Describe your diet?	*Southern diet, which includes fried meats (pork chops), rice and peas, macaroni and cheese, candied yams, vegetables cooked with pork*
Do you check your blood sugar?	*No, I was never given a machine*
Do you exercise?	*I walk the dog a couple of blocks twice a day*
Past hospitalizations?	*Two normal deliveries*
Past surgeries?	*None*
Stress level?	*Denies any stressful events in her life*

HCTZ, hydrochlorothiazide; OTC, over-the-counter.

Station 1: SP/instructor playing the role of the patient must review and memorize the SP responses (Exhibit 31.1) before the simulated experience. In addition, all instructors must attend a rehearsal of the scenario before implementation.

Station 2: If an HPS is used, the instructor gives the group a picture of the retinal examination when prompted. The instructor provides patient response to monofilament test by stating that the patient can feel the monofilament when pressed against the HPS's foot.

Station 4: An instructor or other staff member is seated at a desk and has copies of each lab result. The group should only receive a copy of the specific lab that has been requested.

Station 5: The instructor should play the role of the patient and ask questions regarding the treatment plan.

In addition to the checklist for each group, instructors are also taking general notes on the positive behaviors witnessed as well as areas of improvement needed for the groups. Each group is given a copy of their checklist after the exercise is completed. The class is debriefed as a group at the completion of the simulation or during class.

Exhibit 31.2	Evaluation of Expected Student Behaviors

Station 1: History	**Completed**	**Not Completed**
Introduces self to patient.		
Asks patient purpose of visit.		
Elicits information on complaints of frequent urination and fatigue.		
Obtains patient's medical history.		
Obtains surgical history.		
Obtains medication history.		
Obtains information on family history.		
Asks patient about social history, including alcohol, cigarette use, and drug use.		
Asks patient about current diet.		
Asks patient about level of exercise.		

Station 2: Physical examination		
Auscultates heart sounds.		
Auscultates lung sounds.		
Examines lower extremities.		
Performs a monofilament test on HPS's feet.		
Performs a retinal examination.		

Station 3: Diagnostic test		
Orders CBC.		
Orders comprehensive metabolic panel.		
Orders hemoglobin A_{1c}.		
Orders microalbumin.		
Orders lipid panel.		
Orders urinalysis.		
Orders TSH.		

Station 4: Diagnosis development of treatment plan		
Determines HA_{1c} is elevated.		
Prescribes metformin 500 mg by mouth daily.		
Determines patient's need to monitor blood glucose a minimum of at least once a day.		

Station 5: Discussion of treatment plan with patient	**Completed**	**Not Completed**
Establishes rapport with patient.		
Explains the results of blood test with patient using nonmedical terms.		
Discusses the need to start metformin.		
Explains proper use and side effects of medication.		

(continued)

Exhibit 31.2	Evaluation of Expected Student Behaviors	*(continued)*	

Station 5: Discussion of treatment plan with patient	**Completed**	**Not Completed**
Discusses proper diet with patient.		
Discusses the importance of weight loss.		
Encourages patient to exercise.		
Discusses need for blood glucose monitoring at least once a day.		
Orders education on blood glucose monitor by RN.		
Explores patient's questions/concerns.		
Asks patient to repeat treatment plan.		
Arranges for a follow-up appointment.		

CBC, complete blood count; HbA$_{1c}$, hemoglobin A$_{1c}$; HPS, human patient simulators; TSH, thyroid-stimulating hormone.

Evaluative Criteria

The instructors at stations 1, 2, and 5 complete their assigned section of the checklist in Exhibit 31.2. The instructor marks either "completed" or "not completed" beside each expected student behavior.

G. DEBRIEFING GUIDELINES

Issues to Consider

Patient history: The need to differentiate between UTI and polyuria associated with hyperglycemia. It is important to rule out hypothyroidism as cause of fatigue.

Physical examination: What would you include as part of the focused examination for this patient? Why is it important to perform a monofilament test?

Diet: How can you recommend a diet that reflects the patient's culture?

Diagnostic test: It is important to order only necessary tests to reduce wasteful spending. Which labs are essential based on the patient's presentation and physical examination?

Discussion with patient: What are some of the key aspects of providing effective patient education?

Questions to Ask the Students

1. How are you feeling right now?
2. What do you think of the care you provided to this patient?
3. What were some of the positive aspects of the care you provided to this patient?
4. What would you do differently if you were given another chance to complete this simulation?
5. What were some of your differential diagnoses based on the patient's history?
6. What were some of your challenges?
7. What did you learn today that you can incorporate into clinical practice?

Classroom/Observers Questions/Roles

This simulation should be conducted in a simulation center. The SPs provide brief feedback to the students in regard to their experience as a patient and the student's performance.

H. SUGGESTIONS OR KEY FEATURES
TO REPLICATE OR IMPROVE

The scenario was initially used to evaluate 110 NP students during a 1-day session. The scenario required two large rooms and five instructors to assist with the implementation of the simulation. Based on the feedback from instructors and students, I would make the following suggestions:

- Students should be given instructions before the scheduled simulation session, which includes time, group number, room location, equipment to bring, and uniform. I recommend distributing the schedule to students before the simulation. Students should arrive at least 15 minutes early and they should not be allowed to participate if they arrive late in order to stay on schedule.
- Assign students to review diabetes management and physical assessment information before the simulation. It may also be helpful to assign students a diabetes case study using a slightly different clinical situation in order to help prepare them for the simulation experience.
- I suggest requiring instructors to participate in a dry run of the scenario at least 1-week before the scheduled simulation day. Although a scenario may look perfect on paper, it is always helpful to run the scenario to determine whether any revisions need to be made.
- To avoid instructor fatigue, I recommend limiting each SP/instructor to a 3- to 4-hour session.
- Owing to the number of students we needed to evaluate in 1-day, we decided the best method was to set up OSCE style stations. The simulation can also be implemented as an evolving scenario in which one group of students completes all five stations in one room using one instructor and an HPS.
- If available, use an electronic health record (EHR) system to store the patient's past lab results and earlier notes from the last visit. Students can also document their notes into the EHR, which can be reviewed by the instructors after the simulation session.
- Have students complete an evaluation at the end of the simulation. I find students have great suggestions for improvement and I have often incorporated student suggestions into subsequent simulations.

I. RECOMMENDATIONS FOR FURTHER USE

The diabetes management simulation can be converted into an OSCE and used as a summative evaluation for NP students. Before using the simulation as a summative evaluation, the scenario needs further testing for reliability and validity. The simulation experience can be videotaped allowing an opportunity for the students to review their performance and allow instructors an opportunity to evaluate at a later time.

J. HOW SIMULATION-BASED PEDAGOGY
HAS CONTRIBUTED TO IMPROVED STUDENT OUTCOMES

Simulation is a creative teaching/learning method used to meet the learning outcomes of a course. The simulation serves as a great bridge between didactic content and clinical practice. This scenario gave students the opportunity to enact the role of an NP in the context of a simulated simulation experience. Students were able to complete a comprehensive patient encounter, including history taking through discussion of the treatment plan with the patient. Although a formal evaluation was not completed, instructors could evaluate the performance of their students and determine whether learning outcomes have been met. The informal feedback from the students indicated that they enjoyed the learning experience and felt the experience helped prepare them for their first clinical experience.

K. EXPERT RECOMMENDATIONS AND WORDS OF WISDOM

Organizing this simulation session requires many moving pieces and can be complicated to implement. It is important that there is a key-point person who ensures all stations are prepared, students are scheduled, labs are printed, SPs have been trained, faculty have been trained, and all equipment is available before the session. A dry run with all faculty is essential in order to work out any logistical issues and ensure everyone is prepared for the simulation session.

L. EVALUATION OF BEST PRACTICE STANDARDS AND USE OF CREDENTIALED SIMULATION FACULTY

The International Nursing Association for Clinical Simulation and Learning (INACSL) Standards of Best Practice (2013/2016) were used to create this simulation activity. The professional integrity of participants was incorporated into the simulation by requiring the students to maintain confidentiality of the content of the simulation. The scenario has well-defined objectives that are measurable and can be achieved within the allocated time frame. The objectives were created to be obtainable for the level of the learner. Feedback is theoretically based and provided at every station to help participants meet the learning objectives. The facilitators and SPs are all experienced and were provided training on the standards of best practice in simulation. Debriefing is completed at the end of the history, physical assessment, and treatment plan stations, which includes reflective thinking from the learner. The simulation is a formative assessment that allows students the opportunity to improve on their cognitive, affective, and psychomotor skills.

REFERENCES

American Association of Colleges of Nursing. (2011). *The essentials of master's education in nursing.* Washington, DC: Author. Retrieved from http://www.aacnnursing.org/Portals/42/Publications/ MastersEssentials11.pdf

International Nursing Association for Clinical Simulation and Learning. (2013, updated 2016). INACSL standards of best practice: Simulation [Electronic version]. Retrieved from http://www.inacsl.org/ i4a/pages/index .cfm?pageID=3407

McKulloch, D. K. (2015). Initial management of blood glucose in adults with type 2 diabetes mellitus. In D. M. Nathan (Ed.), *UpToDate.* Retrieved from http://www.uptodate.com/contents/ initial-management-of-blood-glucose-in-adults-with-type-2-diabetes-mellitus

Rutherford-Hemming, T., Nye, C., & Coram, C. (2016). Using simulation for clinical practice hours in nurse practitioner education in the United States: A systematic review. *Nurse Education Today, 37,* 128–135.

CHAPTER 32

Assessment and Differential Diagnosis of the Patient Presenting With Chest Pain

Nancy A. Moriber

A. IMPLEMENTATION OF SIMULATION-BASED PEDAGOGY IN YOUR INDIVIDUALIZED TEACHING AREA

The use of simulation in nurse anesthesia training has been an integral part of the educational process for many years. Low-fidelity simulators and static manikins have been utilized to teach basic psychomotor skills and critical decision making with much success. However, with the addition of high-fidelity simulation, nurse anesthesia education has moved to an entirely new level through the incorporation of a simulation-based pedagogy into the nurse anesthesia curriculum. High-fidelity simulation scenarios are used in the student's clinical orientation and throughout all five clinical practicums in order to facilitate the progression from novice to competent anesthesia care provider. Students are given the opportunity to use increasingly complex critical decision-making skills in the anesthetic management of their patients. In addition, students are introduced to situations that are rarely encountered in the clinical setting, but in which expertise is essential for safe practice. Students are therefore able to "experience" rare and complex clinical situations before entering into practice so that the first time they care for these types of patients is not in a crisis situation. The following scenario demonstrates the use of simulation in increasingly complex situations and will be applicable to senior-level undergraduate and entry-level advanced practice students (master's and doctoral preparation).

This chapter focuses on the assessment, differential diagnosis, and initial management of the patient who presents to the emergency department (ED) with complaints of crushing substernal chest pain. The student is required to conduct a rapid history and physical; develop an initial diagnosis; initiate lifesaving therapy; and use effective communication techniques with the patient, family, and members of the interdisciplinary health care team in order to successfully meet the objectives of the scenario. The scenario can be modified for use in the primary care, intensive care, medical–surgical, or the perioperative setting as required to meet the specific needs of the students.

B. EDUCATIONAL MATERIALS AVAILABLE IN YOUR TEACHING AREA AND RELATED TO YOUR SPECIALTY

The Fairfield University Egan School of Nursing and Health Sciences (SON) will be moving into a new building and state-of-the-art simulation center on the Fairfield University campus in the fall of 2017. This facility embraces the simulation-based pedagogy adopted by the SON and has been designed to foster the development of psychomotor, cognitive, and affective clinical skills in the students enrolled in all programs. It will be equipped with two fully functional operating rooms, as well as critical care, acute care, and primary care facilities to facilitate simulation across programs. Simulation space is also available to mirror other hospital environments such as a preoperative holding area or postanesthesia care unit (PACU) in order to run scenarios in other locations where anesthesia care providers are required to manage patients. Control rooms are adjacent to the simulation rooms and are designed to allow separation of the facilitators from the students participating in the scenarios to increase fidelity. The control rooms are equipped with and capable of recording and transmitting to adjacent classrooms in real-time running scenarios in order to facilitate effective debriefing.

In addition to the high-fidelity simulation rooms, independent skills labs have been incorporated to house the low-fidelity simulators and static trainers, which can also be used to supplement learning within the high-fidelity simulation environment. A stand-alone 20-bed graduate health assessment lab with integrated audiovisual capabilities for recording and debriefing is also available for use. Faculty have the ability to use recorded sessions for both formative and summative evaluation of student performance within the health care setting.

C. SPECIFIC OBJECTIVES FOR SIMULATION USAGE WITHIN A SPECIFIC COURSE AND THE OVERALL PROGRAM

The overarching objectives of this scenario are threefold and are consistent with both the program essentials for undergraduate, graduate, and doctoral education as delineated by the American Association of Colleges of Nursing (AACN; 2006, 2008, 2011). This scenario will enhance the student's ability to do the following:

1. Collaborate with peers, patients, health care professionals, and other members of the health care team in the assessment, planning, implementation, and evaluation of health care.
2. Use critical thinking skills and current scientific evidence in clinical decision making.
3. Prioritize patient care to optimize outcomes.
4. Communicate effectively in order to provide appropriate patient-centered care.

This scenario is designed for undergraduate nursing students who have completed their basic medical–surgical experience and are participating in transitional experiences in critical care settings during their senior year. It can also be used at the graduate level as part of the advanced-practice nursing curriculum in the advanced health assessment or advanced physiology and pathophysiology courses in both master's and doctoral entry-into-practice programs.

This scenario addresses the following *Essentials of Baccalaureate Education for Professional Nursing Practice* (AACN, 2008):

Essential II: Basic Organizational and Systems Leadership for Quality Care and Patient Safety, Objectives 1, 2, 5 to 8
Essential VI: Interprofessional Communication and Collaboration for Improving Patient Health Outcomes, Objectives 2 to 6
Essential VII: Clinical Prevention and Population Health, Objective 9
Essential VIII: Professionalism and Professional Values, Objectives 1 and 2
Essential IX: Baccalaureate Generalist Nursing Practice, Objectives 4, 12, and 14

This scenario addresses the following *Essentials of Master's Education in Nursing* (AACN, 2011):

Essential I: Background for Practice From Sciences and Humanities, Objectives 1 and 2
Essential II: Organizational and Systems Leadership, Objectives 1 and 2
Essential III: Quality Improvement and Safety, Objective 1

Eseential IV: Translating and Integrating Scholarship Into Practice, Objectives 1, 2, and 5
Essential VII: Interprofessional Collaboration for Improving Patient and Population Outcomes, Objectives 3, 4, and 6
Essential IX: Master's-Level Nursing Practice, Objectives 3 and 11.

This scenario addresses the following *Essentials of Doctoral Education for Advanced Nursing Practice* (AACN, 2006):

Essential I: Scientific Underpinnings for Practice, Objectives 1 and 2
Essential II: Organizational and Systems Leadership for Quality Improvement and Systems Thinking, Objectives 1 and 2
Essential VI: Interprofessional Collaboration for Improving Patient and Population Health Outcomes, Objectives 1 to 3
Essential VIII: Advanced Nursing Practice, Objectives 1 to 4

D. INTRODUCTION OF SCENARIO

Setting the Scene

This scenario takes place in the ED. The patient has just walked into the waiting room with her husband and tells the nurse at the triage desk that she has had crushing substernal chest pain that has been radiating to her back for the past 2 hours and it has not been relieved by rest. She was out for dinner with her husband at their favorite local Italian restaurant before the onset of symptoms. She states that she feels "terrible." Her husband is very anxious and insistent that something be done for his wife immediately. The patient is placed in a room with a monitored bed, where the ED nurse (student) who will be caring for her is waiting.

Technology Used

In order to run this scenario, a high-fidelity human patient simulator (HPS) is required to allow the student to visualize hemodynamic and EKG changes that will be implemented as part of the scenario. If one is not available, an actor can be substituted, but the instructors will need to be creative with displaying hemodynamic changes. In addition, a training program for simulated patients would need to be developed to ensure that appropriate patient characteristics and actions are displayed during the scenario. Access to patient records, either in electronic or paper format, will also be necessary as they allow for greater fidelity. Audiotaped recordings of the common sounds in the ED should be incorporated into the scenario to simulate the noisy and hectic emergency environment. Finally, video-recording equipment will be required to tape the scenario so that it can be evaluated and discussed during debriefing sessions. The facilitator should make sure that consent for videotaping is obtained from all participants.

Objectives

At the completion of this scenario, the student will be able to do the following:

1. Discuss the differential diagnosis of "life-threatening" chest pain, including alternative diagnoses, such as noncardiac (gastroesophageal reflux disease) and vascular causes
2. Conduct an immediate targeted physical assessment and health history
3. Initiate intravenous fluid therapy
4. Discuss the initial treatment of acute coronary syndrome (ACS), including the drugs, dosages, and adjuvant treatment modalities
5. Apply the advanced cardiac life support (ACLS) ACS algorithm

6. Interpret common laboratory and diagnostic tests used in the differential diagnosis of ACS, including cardiac enzymes, troponin levels, and the EKG.
7. Develop skills as a team leader, patient advocate, and effective communicator.

This scenario addresses the following National Council Licensure Examination for Registered Nurses (RN®) test plan categories and subcategories (National Council of State Boards of Nursing [NCSBN], 2015):

Safe and effective care environment: *Management of care* (case management, collaboration with interdisciplinary team, consultation, establishing priorities, ethical practice, resource management), *Safety and infection control* (handling hazardous and infectious equipment, safe use of equipment, standard precautions), **Health promotion and maintenance:** (techniques of physical assessment), **Psychosocial integrity:** (crisis intervention cultural diversity, family dynamics, situational role changes, support systems, therapeutic communication); **Physiological integrity:** *Pharmacological and parenteral therapies* (dosage calculations, expected effects/outcomes, medication administration, parenteral/intravenous therapies, pharmacological agents/actions), *Reduction of risk potential* (diagnostic tests, laboratory values, potential for alterations in body system, therapeutic procedures), *Physiological adaptation* (alterations in body systems, hemodynamics, medical emergencies, pathophysiology).

Description of Participants

A total of five or six participants will be required to run this scenario. If the scenario is run with undergraduate students, then the student to be evaluated will take the role of the ED nurse assessing the patient. This student will also be assigned the role of team leader and will be required to delegate tasks and coordinate interdisciplinary discussion and activities. An assessment form may be given to the student to help guide the scenario, if deemed appropriate by the instructors. If the scenario is being run with graduate students, then the student evaluated will take on the role of an advanced practice registered nurse (APRN) and an additional participant will be required to take on the role of ED nurse. The graduate student will serve as the team leader, as outlined earlier.

An additional student or actor can take on the role of the nursing technician (or the equivalent). This individual is included to carry out tasks as directed by the team leader, such as sending blood to the lab, obtaining equipment, or assisting with procedures. The purpose is to assess the student's ability to delegate and work as a member of the health care team.

An actor (or student) will be needed to serve as the patient's husband. This individual should be provided with a short script so that he can effectively portray the anxious husband. This individual should not offer any information about the patient unless specifically asked. The husband is included to facilitate communication and activation of support systems.

Example of Husband's Script

The scene: Mr. Hart brings his wife, Mrs. Hart, to the ED with complaints of crushing substernal chest pain that radiates to her back and has lasted more than an hour. The couple was out for dinner at their favorite local Italian restaurant before the onset of the symptom, and they consumed a very heavy meal. Mr. Hart is extremely anxious and is demanding that his wife be seen immediately. He is yelling at the nurses and ancillary staff and is being disruptive to other patients in the waiting room.
  Suggested dialogue:

a. If Mr. Hart's needs are not addressed:
  i. "My wife needs help, and I want it now!"
  ii. "Somebody do something now, or I'll take her inside myself!"
  iii. "Don't tell me to calm down! You don't have any idea how I feel right now."

b. If intervention is appropriate (provision of reassurance and activation of family support services):
   i. "Oh, thank you so much. I knew somebody would care."
   ii. "You are all so wonderful, I know my wife is in good hands!"
   iii. "Will you keep me informed of what is going on? We've been together for 40 years, and I don't know what I would do without her."

Finally, two faculty members will be required to facilitate the scenario. One faculty member will run the simulation and act as the voice of the patient, and the other will serve as the ED physician and will be imbedded in the scenario. If a second faculty member is not available, a student or an actor can be used, but it is necessary to realize that no one will be available to help facilitate movement and guide the student through the scenario should this become necessary. The purpose of the ED physician is to act as a collaborating member of the health care team. The scenario can be modified if desired and the ED physician portrayed in a confrontational fashion, thereby allowing assessment of the student's abilities to handle stressful situations, resolve conflict, and improve communication. If there are no additional participants available to play the role of the physician, the individual running the scenario could portray the physician using a telephone-consult format. This could help refine the student's communication skills, with attention paid to confirming the accuracy of understanding among scenario participants.

E. RUNNING OF THE SCENARIO

Prior to running the scenario, all participants should have completed the didactic module on the care of the patient with ACS and should have a solid foundation in physiology, pathophysiology, and pharmacology, including pharmacokinetics, pharmacodynamics, and drug side effects. The student must also have completed a basic health assessment course, received before training on initiating intravenous therapy, must have completed content on the interpretation of basic laboratory and diagnostic tests, and participated in a discussion of the management of ACS as outlined in the ACLS professional provider's manual (American Heart Association, 2016). The students should be made aware of the general purpose of the scenario—the differential diagnosis of chest pain— before attending the simulation session. In addition, the students should be provided with an ED health history and nursing record in order to familiarize themselves with the documentation. If an electronic database is available, the students must be trained in the proper use of the system so that troubleshooting the electronic record does not become the focus of the scenario. All necessary equipment should be in the simulation room, including a stethoscope, EKG machine, defibrillator, medication cart, all necessary "mock" oral and intravenous medications, oxygen therapy, and all materials for initiation intravenous fluid therapy. All participants should be readily available but not at the patient's bedside so that the student's ability to mobilize resources can be assessed. The scenario will begin when the triage (the instructor) nurse informs the ED nurse that Mrs. Hart is being admitted to bed #5.

F. PRESENTATION OF COMPLETED TEMPLATE

Title

Assessment and Differential Diagnosis of the Patient Presenting With Chest Pain

Focus Area

Advanced health assessment and critical care nursing

Scenario Description

Mrs. Hart is a 54-year-old female who presents to the ED of a major cardiac center complaining of crushing substernal chest pain that radiates to her back. Pain began approximately 1 hour before admission and has not been relieved with rest. She was out for dinner with her husband at their favorite local Italian restaurant before the onset of symptoms. Her husband, who is extremely anxious and is demanding that his wife be seen immediately, accompanies her.

Her past medical history is significant for hypertension × 3 years that has been well controlled as well as noninsulin-dependent diabetes mellitus. Her medications include metoprolol (Lopressor) 50 mg PO (per OS) twice a day, lisinopril (Prinivil, Zestril) 10 mg PO once a day, and metformin (Glucophage) 500 mg PO twice a day. She has no known drug allergies. Surgical history is positive for a tonsillectomy and adenoidectomy as a child.

Scenario Objectives

At completion of the scenario the student will be able to:

1. Discuss the differential diagnosis of life-threatening chest pain, including alternative diagnoses, such as noncardiac (gastroesophageal reflux disease) and vascular causes.
2. Conduct an immediate targeted physical assessment and health history.
3. Initiate the treatment of ACS.
4. Apply the ACLS ACS algorithm.
5. Interpret common laboratory and diagnostic tests used in the differential diagnosis of ACS.
6. Develop skills as a team leader, patient advocate, and effective communicator.

Setting the Scene

Equipment Needed

High-fidelity simulator; video recording device; patient monitor; blood pressure (BP) cuff; EKG machine; pulse oximeter; oxygen flow meter; nasal cannula and face mask; intravenous line; intravenous insertion kit; intravenous pole; blood-drawing equipment; medications, including morphine, aspirin, nitroglycerine, and heparin; and ED patient record (medical)

Resources Needed

Laboratory reports, including complete blood count (CBC) and troponin levels and computer access if laboratory reports are to be posted within a database; ACLS provider manual

Simulator Level

High-fidelity simulation

Participants Needed

Emergency room nurse or APRN (student role), nursing technician (student/actor) ED physician (faculty member imbedded in the scenario), faculty member to operate high-fidelity simulator, actor to play patient's anxious husband; a small part should be scripted for the role of the husband if the actor is a nonfaculty member

Scenario Implementation

Initial Settings for High-Fidelity Simulator

BP: 168/90 mmHg, heart rate (HR): 110 beats/minute, respiratory rate (RR): 28 breaths/minute, oxygen saturation: 98%

Required Student Assessments and Actions

____ Reassures husband, identifies staff member/hospital representative to attend to his needs
____ Monitors and supports ABCs (airway, breathing, circulation). Checks vital signs, including BP, HR, and RR; evaluates oxygen saturation
____ Obtains a 12-lead EKG
____ Implements immediate ED general treatment
    ____ Begins oxygen at 4 L/min if SaO$_2$ less than 90%
    ____ Administers aspirin 160 to 325 mg, nitroglycerine sublingually, morphine via intravenous (IV) line if discomfort not relieved by nitroglycerine
____ Completes concurrent ED assessment (less than 10 minutes):
    ____ Establishes IV access
    ____ Performs brief, targeted history and physical examination
    ____ Completes fibrinolytic checklist and checks contraindications (Exhibit 32.1)
    ____ Obtains initial cardiac markers, electrolytes, and coagulation studies
    ____ Orders portable chest x-ray
____ Reviews EKG, identifies ST-elevation myocardial infarction (STEMI)
____ Recognizes symptoms in less than 12 hours and identifies need for fibrinolytic therapy and reperfusion therapy (percutaneous coronary intervention [PCI])
____ Activates appropriate consults for transport to cardiac catheterization lab
____ Notifies husband of patient's condition

Instructor Interventions

The instructor running the simulator will act as the voice of the patient and will answer all questions posed by the student in the scenario. In addition, this faculty member will be required to "run" the simulator and make the appropriate responses, both verbal and hemodynamic, in response to student behaviors. The instructor imbedded within the scenario is there to facilitate performance and provide guidance in accordance with the terminal objectives of the scenario.

Exhibit 32.1	Contraindications to Fibrinolytic Therapy

- Systolic blood pressure >180–200 mmHg or diastolic blood pressure >100–110 mmHg
- Right versus left arm systolic blood pressure difference >15 mmHg
- History of structural CNS disease (i.e., cerebral aneurysm or AVM)
- Significant closed head/facial trauma within the previous 3 months
- Stroke >3 hours or <3 months
- Recent (within 2–4 weeks) major trauma, surgery or GI/GU bleed
- Any history of intracranial hemorrhage
- Active bleeding, clotting disorder, or patient on anticoagulants
- Pregnancy
- Serious systemic disease (advanced cancer, sever liver or renal disease)

AVM, arteriovenous malformation; CNS, central nervous system; GI/GU, gastrointestinal/genitourinary.

Evaluation Criteria

Student performance in this scenario will be evaluated using the rubric shown in Exhibit 32.2, based on the degree to which students perform, in appropriate order with or without coaching, the actions outlined earlier. The effectiveness of this simulation as an overarching learning tool can be assessed using a program's existing course evaluation tools. It is also essential to make sure that information regarding the students' overall impression of the simulation, including what worked well and where improvement or change might be beneficial, is obtained. This information can be used to improve the simulation experience within your individual programs.

Exhibit 32.2	Evaluating Student Criteria in a Nursing Simulation Scenario		
Behavior	**Independent**	**Prompted**	**Appropriate Order**
Reassures husband.			
Monitors and supports ABCs and checks VS.			
Obtains a 12-lead EKG.			
Establishes IV access.			
Implements immediate ED general treatment: – Oxygen at 4L/min if SaO_2 <90% – Administers aspirin 160–325 mg, nitroglycerine sublingually, morphine IV if discomfort not relieved by nitroglycerine			
Completes concurrent ED assessment (<10 mins): – Establishes IV access. – Performs brief, targeted history and physical examination. – Completes fibrinolytic checklist and checks contraindications. – Obtains initial cardiac markers, electrolytes, and coagulation studies. – Orders portable chest x-ray.			
Reviews EKG, identifies STEMI.			
Obtains 12-lead EKG.			
Recognizes symptoms in <12 hours and identifies need for fibrinolytic therapy and reperfusion.			
Activates appropriate consults for transfer to cardiac catheterization lab.			
Notifies husband of patient's condition.			

ABC, airway, breathing, circulation; ED, emergency department; IV, intravenous; STEMI, ST-elevation myocardial infarction; VS, vital signs.

G. DEBRIEFING GUIDELINES

Debriefing is an essential part of the simulation experience and, in many instances, it is the most important learning tool used in this teaching or learning pedagogy. In order to get the most out of this experience, it would be beneficial for the scenario to be recorded and then critically examined individually by the students as well as by the class as a whole. Students should be provided with the evaluation criteria outlined earlier before viewing the taped simulation. Questions that can be used by the instructor to facilitate discussion should include:

1. Overall, how do you think the scenario went? What do you think could have been done differently? What would you do the same?
2. What is the underlying pathophysiology of ACS?
3. What are the diagnostic criteria for ACS?
4. Do you think the management of the patient with ACS in this scenario was appropriate? How could it have been improved or done differently?
5. How can you (as the ED nurse) facilitate communication and collaboration among members of the interdisciplinary health care team?
6. How did the presence of the patient's husband alter the care provided to the patient?
7. Do you think the husband's needs are a priority in this situation? Why or why not? Whose responsibility is it to see that they are met?
8. What are some of the other possible causes of chest pain in this patient? How do you make the differential diagnosis?

H. SUGGESTIONS/KEY FEATURES TO REPLICATE OR IMPROVE

Understanding the physiologic principles and key aspects of the ACLS ACS algorithm before the execution of this scenario is essential. As patient scenarios become more advanced and incorporate a multitude of physiologic and pharmacologic principles, additional key processes could be added to the required content to enhance learning. Careful review of the ACLS ACS algorithm is also essential during the debriefing phase of the simulation to reinforce the importance and proper order of required actions.

I. RECOMMENDATIONS FOR FURTHER USE

This scenario can be modified and the differential diagnoses changed to further enhance the student's health assessment skills. For example, in the scenario outlined earlier, the patient presenting with chest pain could have had a dissecting thoracic aneurysm, severe esophagitis, or pleuritic chest pain. Although each condition would present with similar symptoms, there are key differences that could be explored in the scenario, thereby sending the student down a different path. Obviously, the objectives and evaluation criteria would need to be revised in order to address the new goals of the scenario.

In addition to changing the differential diagnoses, the role of the participants can also be modified to address cultural and gender issues. For example, the patient could be changed to a non–English-speaking individual, requiring the practitioner to address the language barrier, or the patient could be of a different faith, requiring the student to address religious implications of health care. The possibilities are truly endless. By allowing students to explore different diagnoses, they will be able to improve both their physical assessment skills and their ability to use clinical evidence in the decision-making process.

J. HOW SIMULATION-BASED PEDAGOGY HAS CONTRIBUTED TO IMPROVED STUDENT OUTCOMES

Students enjoy using simulation as a learning tool. It provides them with the opportunity to develop psychomotor, cognitive, and affective skills in a less-threatening and safe environment. It also enables educators to expose students to a greater repertoire of clinical situations than would normally be encountered during the course of education and training. Adopting a simulation-based pedagogy and incorporating simulation throughout the curriculum enables educators to expose students to a variety of complicated and challenging situations that can only improve the quality of care provided by graduates. In addition, as methods of evaluating student performance improve, simulation can be used to guide clinical remediation and even clinical advancement. The opportunities are endless. It only takes motivation, creativity, and a commitment to improving the quality of education provided to our students.

K. EXPERT RECOMMENDATIONS AND WORDS OF WISDOM

Regardless of the practice setting the need to appropriately manage acute crisis situations occurs. Rapid response is essential to ensure the best possible outcomes for our patients. However, when faced with these situations, not all practitioners possess the fundamental knowledge or skill to manage them appropriately. Even practitioners who are certified in basic life support (BLS) and ACLS struggle when faced with crisis situations because they have either not been faced with them in the clinical setting or have not had the responsibility of assuming the leadership role. It is therefore recommended that nurses at all levels of clinical training and expertise participate in simulations that target these crisis situations.

L. EVALUATION OF BEST PRACTICE STANDARDS AND USE OF CREDENTIALED SIMULATION FACULTY

Early recognition and successful management of ACS and cardiac arrest are known to save lives. ACLS training has long incorporated the use of simulation in order to teach basic skills and then evaluate performance before awarding ACLS certification to participants. Current evidence demonstrates that the integration of high-fidelity simulation in ACLS training not only decreases time to the initiation of cardiopulmonary resuscitation, but improves overall performance (Langdorf et al., 2014). In addition, simulation is associated with improved confidence in the ability to perform required skills as well as improved satisfaction with the learning experience (Davis, Strorjohann, Spiegel, Beiber, & Barletta, 2013). Therefore, it is recommended that high-fidelity simulation be used to complement the didactic education given to health care providers.

The Fairfield University Egan SON recognizes the importance of high-fidelity simulation in education and has begun the process to become a Society for Simulation in Healthcare (SSH) Accredited Program. The school is currently using the International Nursing Association for Clinical Simulation and Learning (INACSL) best practice standards (2013/2016) across programs and disciplines as a framework to confirm that our faculty have the knowledge, skills, and abilities to facilitate quality health care simulation activities. In order to promote faculty expertise in simulation, the SON has supported comprehensive simulation training for all faculty interested in developing expertise in this area and has encouraged faculty to sit for the certification examination. Faculty members across disciplines have been invited to participate in university-sponsored debriefing and facilitation training and are given the opportunity to attend outside regional/national simulation conferences. The Fairfield University Egan SON sees simulation as an integral component of the educational pedagogy linking the classroom to the clinical practice arena.

REFERENCES

American Association of Colleges of Nursing. (2006). *Essentials of doctoral education for advanced nursing practice*. Washington, DC: Author. Retrieved from http://www.aacnnursing.org/Portals/42/Publications/DNPEssentials.pdf

American Association of Colleges of Nursing. (2008). *Essentials of baccalaureate education for professional nursing practice*. Washington, DC: Author. Retrieved from http://www.aacnnursing.org/Portals/42/Publications/BaccEssentials08.pdf

American Association of Colleges of Nursing. (2011). *The essentials of master's education in nursing*. Retrieved from http://www.aacnnursing.org/Portals/42/Publications/MastersEssentials11.pdf

American Heart Association. (2016). *Advanced cardiovascular life support: Professional provider manual*. Dallas, TX: Author.

Davis, L. E., Storjohann, T. D., Spiegel, J. J., Beiber, K. M., & Barletta, J. F. (2013). High-fidelity simulation for advanced cardiac life support training. *American Journal of Pharmaceutical Education, 77*(3), 59.

International Nursing Association for Clinical Simulation and Learning. (2013, updated 2016). INACSL standards of best practice: Simulation. Retrieved from https://www.inacsl.org/i4a/pages/index.cfm?pageID=3407

Langdorf, M. I., Strom, S. L., Yang, L., Canales, C., Anderson, C. L., Amin, A., & Lotfipour, S. (2014). High-fidelity simulation enhances ACLS training. *Teaching and Learning in Medicine, 26*(3), 266–273.

National Council of State Boards of Nursing. (2015). *NCLEX-RN examination for the National Council Licensure Examination for Registered Nurses*. Chicago, IL: Author.

CHAPTER 33

Abdominal Pain in a Woman of Childbearing Age: A Trauma-Informed Care Approach

Suzanne Hetzel Campbell and Jenna A. LoGiudice

A. IMPLEMENTATION OF SIMULATION-BASED PEDAGOGY IN YOUR INDIVIDUALIZED TEACHING AREA

In a typical gynecology setting, a common chief concern is lower abdominal discomfort. As the advanced practice nurse obtains the history of present illness (HPI) and assesses a woman with this concern, the patient will often point to her pelvic area as the source of discomfort. In fact, pelvic pain is one of the chief concerns that women's health practitioners will manage (Hacker, Gambone, & Hobel, 2016). Many possible etiologies for pelvic pain exist; therefore, a simulation-based scenario with this chief concern allows students to use strong analytic skills to work toward making a diagnosis. The possible life-threatening diagnoses of appendicitis, ectopic pregnancy, and pelvic inflammatory disease (PID) are often first to be ruled out (Kruszka & Kruszka, 2010). Other common causes of pelvic pain in a woman of reproductive age include adnexal torsion or ovarian cyst (intact or ruptured; Kruszka & Kruszka, 2010). All of these diagnoses are usually at the forefront of a student's thought process as potential etiologies for pelvic pain. However, in our experience, it is also important for students to work through combining both physical assessment and HPI skills to arrive at the etiology of undiagnosed pregnancy in preterm labor as a cause of abdominal pain in a reproductive-aged woman, which this scenario portrays. This diagnosis requires the advanced practice nurse to think outside of the box; display accurate physical assessment skills; and complete a thorough history, with particular attention to the woman's gynecologic, menstrual, and obstetric histories. About one half of all pregnancies in the United States are unintended; therefore, ruling out pregnancy in reproductively aged women is essential (Hacker et al., 2016).

A preterm birth is a birth occurring before 37 completed weeks (37 weeks, 0 days) gestation (American College of Obstetrics and Gynecology [ACOG], 2016). The burden to families and society at large from the fetal outcomes of prematurity and from the cost of preterm births is important to note. The March of Dimes Foundation (2015) reported that the preterm birth rate in the United States was 9.6% in 2015 and that African American women disproportionately experience preterm birth. Further, preterm birth costs over $26 billion in health care spending each year (Behrman & Butler, 2006). Low socioeconomic status, previous preterm birth, urinary tract infections, bacterial vaginosis, smoking, multifetal pregnancy, and lack of prenatal care are all associated with preterm birth (Kiran, Ajay, Neena, & Geetanjaly, 2010). Recent research found that maternal binge drinking also contributes significantly to preterm birth and low birth weight and differs across socioeconomic groups (Truong, Reifsnider, Mayorga, & Spitler, 2013). ACOG's (2016) most recent practice bulletin, No. 171, on the management of preterm labor, is an excellent resource for faculty and students alike when debriefing this case.

This scenario has been enhanced for use with family nurse practitioner (FNP) master's and doctor of nursing practice (DNP) students. Before this simulation, students learn how to conduct gynecological examinations on task trainers and perform their first pelvic and breast examinations on teaching-model patients as part of their health assessment class. The task-trainer activities are introduced in the beginning of the semester, but the hands-on learning culminates with simulation-based patient scenarios at the end of the semester, once the content has all been taught consistently with the International Nursing Association for Clinical Simulation and Learning (INACSL) best practice standards, specifically, Standard IX: Participant Evaluation (Lioce et al., 2015).

This abdominal pain scenario is based on a real patient situation and represents one of the most common presentations of female patients of childbearing age—pelvic or abdominal pain. For FNP students, the diagnostic skills necessary to differentiate appendicitis from ectopic pregnancy or PID are critical to patient safety, given some of these presentations are life threatening. The twist in this scenario is that the patient has an unknown pregnancy and is in preterm labor. It takes a careful identification of patient risk factors (e.g., African American race, irregular menstrual history, previous preterm birth), review of systems (ROS), HPI, and assessment for the FNP student to arrive at the proper diagnosis and treatment.

Since the development of this scenario, which is expected to take place in a clinic or emergency department (ED), many other scenarios were developed and used during the course of the FNP program. For the Adult Health II course, which includes a women's health component, the students have a simulated gynecologic annual well-woman visit, as well as primary care simulations with standardized patients in which they see multiple patients during one simulation environment to mimic a real clinical practice day. Students have 15 minutes per patient to gather the history; assess, diagnose, and order labs treat, and prescribe before moving on to the next patient. Overall, students have been incredibly enthusiastic about the experiences they have gained with the use of simulation at the Fairfield University Marion Peckham Egan School of Nursing and Health Sciences graduate program.

B. EDUCATIONAL MATERIALS AVAILABLE IN YOUR TEACHING AREA AND RELATED TO YOUR SPECIALTY

Currently, the abdominal pain scenario is run in the acute-care setting using a high-fidelity human patient simulator (HPS), but it can easily be adapted to a gynecology or primary care office-based setting. The current setup for the simulation involves a control room with mirrored glass looking into the simulation room. Typically, to run this scenario one or two faculty are needed, one to be the voice of the patient and one to manage the vital signs (VS) and laboratory values. The faculty members running the simulation are able to talk to the students in the simulation room via a microphone into the room, a microphone from the high-fidelity HPS, and a telephone. The telephone communication allows the faculty to call with results as a doctor, certified nurse midwife (CNM), or laboratory technician, or for students to call another health care provider, the lab, the operating room, and so on. An electronic health record system is also available for use by the students in the simulation room. The simulation room also has the capacity to video-record the scenario with student permission for later viewing and evaluation.

In addition, if this scenario is run as a flipped-classroom experience, for the students in the classroom who are active observers, the scenario can be projected live via a 360-degree camera into one of two classrooms (with seating capacity for 35 and 120+ students, respectively). This setup allows the students in the classroom to work through the diagnosis as well and to recognize the strengths and areas for improvement of their classmates' patient assessment skills. Finally, the students participating in the scenario can return to their classmates, who watched the simulation for a debriefing (INACSL Standard VI) with the entire class (Decker et al., 2013).

C. SPECIFIC OBJECTIVES OF SIMULATION USE WITHIN A SPECIFIC COURSE AND THE OVERALL PROGRAM

The primary objective of this scenario is to assess the student's ability to use a trauma-informed care approach to conduct a thorough examination and assessment of a childbearing-age woman with abdominal pain, to recognize abnormal findings, and to determine a plan of action to enhance patient safety and emotional stability. This scenario was initially designed as a flipped-classroom, advanced-level simulation for third-year BSN students. This was a high-level simulation for BSN students and is leveled more approximately for the master's and DNP FNP students we currently run it with during Adult Health II. These students have completed health assessment, pathophysiology, pharmacology, and Adult Health I. In their health assessment course, they have all performed their first pelvic and breast examinations on teaching-model patients. This simulation allows for students to think broadly, use physical assessment skills, and understand the importance of a detailed HPI to arrive at the diagnosis.

Student Learning Activities

- Perform an assessment of a reproductive-aged woman with abdominal pain.
- Review and practice obtaining the chief concern, ROS, and HPI (with particular attention to obstetric, gynecologic, and menstrual history).
- Educate patients regarding potential tests, considerations, and findings.
- Provide trauma-informed care.

D. INTRODUCTION OF SCENARIO

Setting the Scene

The setting can be either acute care or primary care, depending on the student needs.

When this simulation is run with undergraduate students, an ED setting at a hospital of a tertiary-level institution at change of shift is appropriate. In this setting, the students receive a report from the night nurse and are told a CNM is available on call.

For FNP students, either the ED setting listed previously (with a report from the nurse practitioner who worked over night) or a primary care setting may be appropriate. In a primary care setting (private practice or clinic), the patient would present for an episodic visit on the FNP's schedule for today.

Technology Used

The medium-fidelity HPS is a female (wig and female genitalia in place), running manually, with the following initial VS: blood pressure (BP), 116/76 mmHg (up to 186/110 mmHg); O_2 sat, 86% (up to 94%); pulse (P), 88 beats/minute; respiratory rate (RR), 20 breaths/minute; temperature (T), 98.1°F/36.72°C; and pain level 10/10, but these do not show on the monitor, and the pulse oximeter is not in place. The patient is in mild distress and is anxious. She has an obese abdomen. She does not have an intravenous (IV) line in place. She is wearing a panti-liner that has light vaginal bleeding on it (water and red food coloring can be used). A wristband identifies the patient as "Ms. Mary Small." Stethoscopes, gloves, O_2, nasal cannula, and a pulse oximeter are placed nearby for student use, as well as an IV start tray and tubing and IV fluids (choices of 1,000 mL D5NS [potassium chloride in 5% dextrose and sodium chloride injection], Ringer's, or normal saline [NS]). Routine and as-needed (PRN) medications are available: Dilaudid 1 to 2 mg IV push PRN for pain q (every) 4 hours.

Objectives

1. Describe the assessment of a reproductive-age woman with abdominal pain
2. Obtain a history to determine the potential causes of abdominal pain
3. Examine menstrual history to determine chance of pregnancy
4. Perform an accurate assessment of a reproductive-age woman with abdominal pain
5. Educate patient regarding her status and your findings
6. Incorporate and provide emotional support and trauma-informed care to the woman throughout

Description of Participants

Ms. Mary Small: 23-year-old African American woman. She is 5 feet, 2 inches and weighs 200 pounds. Her obstetric history includes gravida 1, term 0, preterm 1, abortions 0, living 1. Her son was born vaginally at 34 weeks, 2 days gestation and is now 2 years old and healthy. She reports her menstrual history as "very irregular menses" and is unsure of her last menstrual period (LMP). She reports she "only has a few menses a year." She has a history of sexual assault as a child and reports "a very difficult time" with vaginal examinations. Patient states that only her CNM, Sarah Jones, has checked her and everything was "fine" at her annual examination last year.

E. RUNNING OF THE SCENARIO

Students enter the simulation room and are given the aforementioned patient history. In addition, they are told by either the nurse or nurse practitioner giving report that the patient is experiencing intermittent abdominal pain with scant vaginal bleeding and is requesting pain medication.

F. PRESENTATION OF COMPLETED TEMPLATE

Title

Abdominal Pain in a Woman of Childbearing Age

Scenario Level

Designed as an in-class, advanced-level simulation for BSN students and graduate nursing FNP students. For use in Nursing 314: Maternal and Newborn Nursing, a specialty clinical course in obstetrics for second-semester third-year or first-semester fourth-year baccalaureate students, and Nursing 643: Adult Health II, a clinical course for graduate FNP students.

Focus Area

ED nursing, gynecology, obstetrics, midwifery

Scenario Description

Patient: Mary Small (M. S.)   *Age:* 23 years
Race: African American   *Gender:* Female
Date of birth: 4/23   *Height:* 5 feet, 2 inches *Weight:* 200 pounds
Allergies: No known drug allergies (NKDA)
Past medical history (PMHx): Obesity
Past surgical history (PSHx): Appendectomy at age 7 years

Exhibit 33.1	Medication Record
Patient: Ms. Mary Small	DOB: 4/23/1994
Notes: none	
Medication list: none	Time given:
PRN List: Dilaudid 1–2 mg IV push PRN for pain q 4 hr	Time given: not administered
Allergy: NKDA	Medical provider: Sarah Jones, CNM

CNM, certified nurse midwife; DOB, date of birth; IV, intravenous; NKDA, no known drug allergies; PRN, as needed.

Social history: Denies tobacco, ethanol, street drugs; reports sexual abuse age 9 to 11 years
LMP: Unknown
History: Gravida 1, term 0, preterm 1, abortions 0, living 1. Her son was born vaginally at 34 weeks, 2 days gestation and is now 2 years old and healthy. She reports that since last evening at approximately 11 p.m. (23:00) she has had severe lower abdominal pain that has been increasing in strength and occurs about every 5 minutes with scant vaginal bleeding. She further reports her menstrual history as "very irregular menses" and is unsure of her LMP. She reports she "only has a few menses a year." She also reports nausea/vomiting and anorexia. She denies fever/chills. She has been passing a few small clots vaginally but denies passing any tissue. The patient has no appetite and has been unable to keep down solid food for the past 12 hours. She has a history of sexual abuse as a child and reports "a very difficult time" with vaginal examinations. She states that only her CNM, Sarah Jones, has checked her and everything was "fine" at her annual examination last year.

When students enter the room, this is what they find:

The patient is now experiencing more cramps diffusely in her abdomen, but the pain is intermittent. Her vital signs are as follows: BP, 116/76 mmHg; O_2 sat, 86%; P, 88 beats/minute; RR, 20 breaths/minute; T, 98.1°F/36.72°C; pain level 10/10; obese abdomen; no IV access. M. S. is in mild distress and anxious. Exhibit 33.1 provides the medication record available to the students.

Scenario Objectives

1. Students introduce themselves to the patient, wash hands, check her name band, get information about present status, and explain the examination to be performed.
2. Obtain a history to determine the cause of abdominal pain. Potential causes of abdominal pain in a reproductive-age woman include but are not limited to ovarian cyst (ruptured or intact), adnexal torsion, ectopic pregnancy, spontaneous abortion, pregnancy, premature labor, full-term labor, appendicitis, PID, or endometriosis. (Important point for debriefing: This patient has an unknown LMP—you should always rule out pregnancy.)
3. Perform an accurate assessment of patient, including VS, abdominal examination, and vaginal examination (describe any signs of erythema, discharge, or lesions).
4. Identify necessary laboratory tests or imaging, such as quantitative pregnancy test for human chorionic gonadotropin (HCG) and abdominal ultrasound (students should be informed of ultrasound results revealing a viable fetus measuring 30 weeks, 1 day gestation).
5. Educate patient regarding her status, provide accurate information, offer an opportunity to ask questions.
6. Determine religious preference (e.g., are blood transfusions permitted should they become necessary?).
7. Assess for current safety related to her history of sexual abuse (trauma-informed care).

8. Given the findings of preterm labor, evaluate more closely for potential preterm delivery:
   a. Monitor rate and quality of respirations
   b. Monitor fetal heart rate (FHR)
   c. Monitor frequency and duration of contractions
   d. Compare blood pressure (BP) to baseline (increased to 186/110 mmHg from 116/76 mmHg)
   e. Assess for cervical dilation (most likely done by CNM when called to evaluate patient, but nurses and nurse practitioners with the knowledge of cervical dilation assessment should evaluate)
   f. Evaluate level of pain.

The scenario also allows students to practice key elements from the National Council of State Boards of Nursing (2015) National Council Licensure Examination for Registered Nurses (NCLEX-RN®) test plan, including:

Safe and effective care environment: *Management of care* (advocacy, collaboration with interdisciplinary team, establishing priorities); **Health promotion and maintenance:** (ante/intra/postpartum and newborn care, techniques of physical assessment); **Psychosocial integrity:** (abuse, crisis intervention, mental health concepts, therapeutic communications); **Physiological integrity:** *Pharmacological and parenteral therapies* (parenteral/intravenous therapies, pharmacological pain management, non pharmacological comfort interventions), *Reduction of risk potential* (laboratory values, potential for alterations in body systems, potential for complications from surgical procedures and health alterations, system-specific assessments, vital signs), *Physiological adaptation* (hemodynamics, medical emergencies, pathophysiology).

For this scenario, the American Association of Colleges of Nursing (2008) *Essentials of Baccalaureate Education for Professional Nursing Practice* items addressed include the following:

Essential I: Liberal Education for Baccalaureate Generalist Nursing Practice, Objectives 2, 5, and 7
Essential II: Basic Organization and Systems Leadership, Objectives 1, 7, and 8
Essential IV: Information Management and Applications of Patient Care Technology, Objectives 1 and 6
Essential VI: Interprofessional Communication and Collaboration for Improving Patient Health Outcomes, Objectives 2, 4, and 6
Essential VIII: Professionalism and Professional Values, Objectives 6 and 9
Essential IX: Baccalaureate Generalist Nursing Practice, Objectives 3 and 12

For this scenario, the American Association of Colleges of Nursing (2011) *Essentials of Master's Education in Nursing* items addressed include the following:

Essential I: Background for Practice From Sciences and Humanities, Objectives 1, 4, and 5
Essential III: Quality Improvement and Safety, Objective 7
Essential V: Informatics and Health Care Technologies, Objective 1
Essential IX: Master's-Level Nursing Practice, Objectives 1, 2, 3, 4, 13, and 15

Setting the Scene

Equipment Needed

Medium-fidelity HPS (or high-fidelity HPS) on hospital bed, video-recording device (optional), projection screen (optional), pulse oximeter, patient ID bracelet, gloves, IV setup with the options of 1,000 mL D5NS, lactated ringers, or NS, BP cuff, and stethoscopes.

Resources Needed

Medication record (see additional digital materials); student activity checklist

Participant Roles

1. Handler (person in control room or managing the high-fidelity HPS) to change settings in response to student actions and speak for the patient in response to student questions
2. Night nurse or nurse practitioner delivering report
3. Nurse or nurse practitioner getting the report and assuming care of the patient
4. Nurse in the nurse practitioner scenario (optional)
5. Faculty member who serves as CNM on call for the patient during the day shift who can create orders and assist with care of patient; a faculty member will also need to facilitate the debriefing session

Scenario Implementation

Initial Settings

___Apply wristband
___Have a printout of medications available to students on request
___Simulate facial grimacing, diaphoresis on human HPS
___Panti-liner/pad with scant bloodstain (red food coloring and water) on HPS with gauze underwear
___IV setup available
___VS initially set at BP: 116/76 mmHg (up to 186/110 mmHg), O_2 sat: 86% (up to 94%), P: 88 beats/minute, RR: 20 breaths/minute, T: 98.1°F/36.72°C, pain level: 10/10, with trend to change BP to 186/110 mmHg, O_2 sat to 94%, and RR to 16 breaths/minute over the first 5 minutes of students entering the room.

Required Student Assessments and Actions

___Reflect on the causes of abdominal pain in a reproductive-age woman
___Wash hands
___Introduce self
___Check name band
___Assess general condition
___Assess VS
___Apply pulse oximetry
___Check capillary refill
___Start IV
___Notice patient's complaints of increasing pain
___Don gloves to do abdominal and external vulvar/vaginal examination
___Ask patient when her LMP was
___Assess patient for potential for pregnancy
___Blood test for pregnancy (HCG quantity)

If BSN student:	If FNP student:
___Assess patient's pad	___ Perform vaginal examination
___ Call CNM for vaginal examination and ultrasound	___ Perform/order ultrasound
___ Get pain medication order	___ Order pain medication
___Transport patient to labor and delivery	

Instructor Interventions

The instructor acts as a CNM and helps students recognize an obstetric medical emergency and directs their care.

Evaluation Criteria: Checklist of Interventions and Assessments

___Washes hands
___Checks name band
___Asks about pain level on a 1-to-10 scale
___Checks for IV access/starts IV
___Notices patient's complaints of increasing pain
___Assesses patient for potential for pregnancy
___Assesses VS: __BP __P __RR __T
___Dons gloves
    Perform abdominal examination

___Introduces self
___Asks how the patient is doing
___Notices that the patient is anxious
___Apply pulse oximeter
___Asks patient when her LMP was
___Blood test for pregnancy (HCG quantity)

If BSN student:
___Assesses patient's pad
___Calls CNM for vaginal examination and ultrasound
___Gets pain medication order
___Counsels the patient about finding that she is pregnant and in preterm labor
___Transports patient to labor and delivery

If FNP student:
____ Performs vaginal examination
____ Performs/orders ultrasound
____ Orders pain medication

G. DEBRIEFING GUIDELINES

Issues to Consider and Student Questions

1. What challenges did you face?
2. What would you do differently next time?
3. Identify diagnoses/problems for this patient (e.g., anxiety related to sudden changes in health status, knowledge deficit regarding pregnancy).
4. Outline a plan of care for this patient.
5. Is there other information that you needed to adequately care for this patient?
6. How did you feel identifying and informing this woman that she was pregnant?
7. What it was like to care for this patient knowing that she was a childhood survivor of sexual abuse?

H. SUGGESTIONS/KEY FEATURES TO REPLICATE OR IMPROVE

This scenario was of a high level for baccalaureate students, given the need to diagnose a woman with an unknown pregnancy in preterm labor. Therefore, this scenario has now been used in the graduate program only. This scenario is an important learning experience for the FNP students. They use theory content about abdominal and pelvic pain and its potential etiologies to match the vaginal bleeding, intermittent pain, and unknown LMP with the most common differential diagnoses: appendicitis, ectopic pregnancy, PID—and of course, preterm labor, which is often a surprise. During the lecture on pelvic pain with this group, the importance of always ruling out pregnancy in a reproductive-aged woman is stressed. This scenario is rewarding to implement, and it is especially fulfilling to work through the debriefing. Throughout the process, the students are reviewing patient symptomology as well as their own physical examination and lab findings to determine the cause for pain in a woman of reproductive age.

I. RECOMMENDATIONS FOR FURTHER USE

An ideal situation would be to perform this scenario with both baccalaureate and nurse practitioner students simultaneously, each in their own role, to enhance the opportunity for interprofessional care, delegation of tasks, and team-based communication practice. Multidisciplinary team training in the simulation of obstetric emergencies improves knowledge, skills, and communication in the clinical setting (Merién, Ven, Mol, Houterman, & Oei, 2010). The FNP students would demonstrate an ease with regular patient care and, it is hoped, the ability to prioritize, which would provide an excellent learning experience for the BSN student. Having BSN students and FNP students work together during the debriefing after viewing the simulation together in real time would be a wonderful learning opportunity as well. In addition, Fairfield University will be opening a nurse midwifery specialty within the DNP program in the fall of 2017 and the goal will be to incorporate CNMs in the simulation to consult on this patient.

J. HOW SIMULATION-BASED PEDAGOGY HAS CONTRIBUTED TO IMPROVED STUDENT OUTCOMES

Jenna LoGiudice was one of Suzanne Hetzel Campbell's undergraduate BSN students when simulation was first introduced at Fairfield University in 2004. Participating in simulation as a student fostered the importance of this learning experience and has informed Jenna's teaching pedagogy. We feel strongly that students must come to simulation readily prepared and understand the key concepts from theory. The goal is for the student to gain confidence during the simulation in both assessment skills and patient communication; therefore, prebriefing the simulation is important to foster these positive student learning outcomes (Page-Cutrara, 2014).

K. EXPERT RECOMMENDATIONS AND WORDS OF WISDOM

Jenna's trajectory of research focuses on the gynecologic and childbearing experiences of survivors of sexual abuse. When debriefing this case, discussing with students what it was like for them to care for Mary knowing she was a childhood survivor of sexual abuse is highly recommended. Did the students ask Mary about this history? Did they recognize that she may have a difficult time with having a vaginal examination given her history (LoGiudice & Beck, 2016)? Developing this simulation with Mary as a survivor of sexual abuse is intentional to begin to open the dialogue with students about the importance of screening women for current or past history of sexual abuse in all encounters and the importance of using trauma-informed care: An adaptive approach to care that focuses on patient control in the context of the health care relationship and approaches all patient interactions with the thought "what has happened in your life?" instead of "what is wrong with you" (Substance Abuse and Mental Health Services Administration, [SAMHSA], 2015; The Trauma Informed Care Project, 2014). Trauma-informed care centers around four Rs: *realizing* the effects of trauma for a patient, *recognizing* the signs of trauma in patients and their families, *responding* by integrating knowledge about trauma in to nursing care, and preventing *retraumatization* of the patient (SAMHSA, 2015). An additional resource for incorporating trauma-informed care into nursing curricula can be found in the work of LoGiudice and Douglas (2016).

Finally, the use of a standardized patient would be extremely beneficial in this scenario, especially to practice discussing a sexual abuse history with a patient.

L. EVALUATION OF BEST PRACTICE STANDARDS AND USE OF CREDENTIALED SIMULATION FACULTY

The use of the standards of best practice in simulation has been woven throughout this simulation. Terminology Used (Standard I; Meakim et al., 2013), Professional Integrity (Standard II; Gloe et al., 2013), and Participant Objectives (Standard III; Lioce et al., 2013) are all used in the prebrief phases of the simulation. Facilitation and Facilitator (Standards IV and V; Boese et al., 2013; Franklin et al., 2013) are conducted by our Fairfield University Director of Simulation, International Nursing Association for Clinical Simulation and Learning (INACSL) Sim Fellow, and National League for Nursing (NLN) Sim Lead Fellow, Anka Roberto. Debriefing is streamlined using Debriefing for Meaningful Learning as a standard debriefing technique (Standard VI; Decker et al., 2013). The facilitator has 4 years' experience in full-time simulation education and is working toward Certified Healthcare Simulation Educator (CHSE) certification. Participants are all evaluated using a Survey Monkey app (Standard VII; Sando et al., 2013). Given the Interprofessional Education focus of the simulation Standard VIII is represented (Decker et al., 2015), and the simulation design follows INACSL's recommendations for Standard IX (Lioce et al., 2015).

REFERENCES

American Association of Colleges of Nursing. (2008). *The essentials of baccalaureate education for professional nursing practice*. Washington, DC: Author.

American Association of Colleges of Nursing. (2011). *The essentials of master's education in nursing*. Washington, DC: Author.

American College of Obstetrics and Gynecology. (2016). Management of preterm labor (Practice Bulletin No. 171). *Obstetrics and Gynecology, 128*(4), e155–e164. doi:10.1097/AOG.0000000000001711

Behrman, R. E., & Butler, A. S. (Eds.). (2006). *Preterm birth: Causes, consequences, and prevention*. Washington, DC: Institute of Medicine of the National Academies Press.

Boese, T., Cato, M., Gonzalez, L., Jones, A., Kennedy, K., Reese, C., . . . Borum, J. C. (2013). Standards of best practice: Simulation standard V: Facilitator. *Clinical Simulation in Nursing, 9*(6S), S22–S25.

Decker, S. I., Anderson, M., Boese, T., Epps, C., McCarthy, J., Motola, I., . . . Lioce, L. (2015). Standards of best practice: Simulation standard VIII: Simulation-enhanced interprofessional education (Sim-IPE). *Clinical Simulation in Nursing, 11*(6), 293–297.

Decker, S. I., Fey, M., Sideras, S., Caballero, S., Rockstraw, L. R., Boese, T., . . . Borum, J. C. (2013, June). Standards of best practice: Simulation standard VI: The debriefing process. *Clinical Simulation in Nursing, 9*(6S), S27–S29. doi:10.1016/j.ecns.2013.04.008

Franklin, A. E., Boese, T., Gloe, D., Lioce, L., Decker, S., Sando, C. R., . . . Borum, J. C. (2013). Standards of best practice: Simulation standard IV: Facilitation. *Clinical Simulation in Nursing, 9*(6S), S19–S21.

Gloe, D., Sando, C. R., Franklin, A. E., Boese, T., Decker, S., Lioce, L., . . . Borum, J. C. (2013). Standards of best practice: Simulation standard II: Professional integrity of participant(s). *Clinical Simulation in Nursing, 9*(6S), S12–S14.

Hacker, N. F., Gambone, J. C., & Hobel, C. J. (2016). *Hacker and Moore's essentials of obstetrics and gynecology* (6th ed.). Philadelphia, PA: Saunders, Elsevier.

Kiran, P., Ajay, B., Neena, G., & Geetanjaly, K. (2010). Predictive value of various risk factors for preterm labor. *Journal of Obstetrics and Gynecology of India, 60*(2), 141–145.

Kruszka, P. S., & Kruszka, S. J. (2010). Evaluation of acute pelvic pain in women. *American Family Physician, 82*(2), 141–147.

Lioce, L., Meakim, C. H., Fey, M. K., Chmil, J. V., Mariani, B., & Alinier, G. (2015, June). Standards of best practice: Simulation standard IX: Simulation design. *Clinical Simulation in Nursing, 11*(6), 309–315. doi:10.1016/j.ecns.2015.03.005

Lioce, L., Reed, C. C., Lemon, D., King, M. A., Martinez, P. A., Franklin, A. E., . . . Borum, J. C. (2013). Standards of best practice: Simulation standard III: Participant objectives. *Clinical Simulation in Nursing, 9*(6S), S15–S18.

LoGiudice, J. A., & Beck, C. T. (2016). The lived experience of childbearing from survivors of sexual abuse: "It was the best of times, it was the worst of times." *Journal of Midwifery & Women's Health, 61*(4), 474–481.

March of Dimes Foundation. (2015). Premature birth report card. Retrieved from http://www.marchofdimes.org/materials/premature-birth-report-card-united-states.pdf

Meakim, C., Boese, T., Decker, S., Franklin, A. E., Gloe, D., Lioce, L., . . . Borum, J. C. (2013). Standards of best practice: Simulation standard I: Terminology. *Clinical Simulation in Nursing, 9*(6S), S3–S11.

Merién, A. E., van de Ven, J., Mol, B. W., Houterman, S., & Oei, S. G. (2010). Multidisciplinary team training in a simulation setting for acute obstetric emergencies: A systematic review. *Obstetrics and Gynecology, 115*(5), 1021–1031.

National Council of State Boards of Nursing. (2015). NCLEX-RN examination: Test plan for the National Council Licensure Examination for Registered Nurses. Retrieved from https://www.ncsbn.org/RN_Test_Plan_2016_Final.pdf

Page-Cutrara, K. (2014). Use of prebriefing in nursing simulation: A literature review. *Journal of Nursing Education, 53*(3), 136–141.

Sando, C. R., Coggins, R. M., Meakim, C., Franklin, A. E., Gloe, D., Boese, T., . . . Borum, J. C. (2013). Standards of best practice: Simulation standard VII: Participant assessment and evaluation. *Clinical Simulation in Nursing, 9*(6S), S30–S32.

Substance Abuse and Mental Health Services Administration. (2015). National Center from Trauma-Informed Care. Retrieved from http://www.samhsa.gov/nctic/trauma-interventions

The Trauma Informed Care Project. (2014). Retrieved from http://www.traumainformedcareproject.org/index.php

Truong, K. D., Reifsnider, O. S., Mayorga, M. E., & Spitler, H. (2013). Estimated number of preterm births and low birth weight children born in the United States due to maternal binge drinking. *Maternal and Child Health Journal, 17*(4), 677–688.

FURTHER READING

Karnath, B. M., & Breitkopf, D. M. (2007). Acute and chronic pelvic pain in women. *Hospital Physician, 43*, 20–26.

LoGiudice, J., & Douglas, S. (2016). Incorporation of sexual violence in nursing curriculum using trauma-informed care: A case study. *Journal of Nursing Education, 55*(4), 215–219. doi:10.3928/01484834-20160316-06

Primary Care Patients With Gastrointestinal Problems: Graduate Program Advanced Physiology and Pathophysiology

Sheila C. Grossman

A. IMPLEMENTATION OF SIMULATION-BASED PEDAGOGY IN YOUR INDIVIDUALIZED TEACHING AREA

This three-credit course is mandatory for all graduates of accredited master's programs in nursing. It is commonly referred to as one of the "three Ps" (physical assessment, physiology and pathophysiology, and pharmacology). The course combines theory and case study analyses across the life span and in all health care delivery settings. It is a prerequisite for any of the specialty track courses for nurse practitioners (NPs), midwives, and nurse anesthetists.

The course focuses on the physiological processes central to biophysical and psychopathologic alterations of function across the life span. Analysis of physiologic responses and implications of the genome model to illness are included. Interpretation of laboratory data for patient management of acute and chronic disease is discussed. Students analyze case studies of hospitalized and primary care patient scenarios.

B. EDUCATIONAL MATERIALS AVAILABLE IN YOUR TEACHING AREA AND RELATED TO YOUR SPECIALTY

This simulation experience can be made to fit any type of community health center clinic, hospital emergency department (ED), private practice, long-term subacute facility, or even the home setting. It is important that there are enough students and/or faculty to take the NP, family member(s), and physician roles so there can be a collaborative discussion as well as health teaching with the family members. Using the primary care clinic area of the Learning Resource Center at the Fairfield University School of Nursing makes it easy to carry out the scenarios because an examination table, four primary care curtained-off "rooms," electronic documentation, and mobile vital signs (VS) devices are already set up. The high-fidelity human patient simulator (HPS) is handled by the teaching assistant, who is able to run the controls and software. This handler has already been apprised by the faculty of the appropriate settings for the HPS.

C. SPECIFIC OBJECTIVES OF SIMULATION USAGE WITHIN ADVANCED PHYSIOLOGY AND PATHOPHYSIOLOGY

General Learning Objectives

The overall objectives are for students to gain increased knowledge, pathophysiology rationale for signs and symptoms, clinical reasoning, and some basic clinical skills for a primary care patient. The goals for this complex scenario are for students to be successful in identifying three differential diagnoses and the pathophysiology rationale for each diagnosis.

Student Learning Activities

Students need to be knowledgeable about the risk factors for colon cancer, signs and symptoms, and the pathophysiology of adenocarcinomas. Students need to review the pathophysiology of colon cancer and physiology of the intestines and be able to successfully accomplish the simulation goals.

D. INTRODUCTION OF SCENARIO

Setting the Scene

The following is the scene for students working with this beginning advanced-practice patient with gastrointestinal (GI) complaints:

Background: Mr. Luiz is a 73-year-old Hispanic U.S. citizen from Puerto Rico, who has been one of your patients for the last 3 years. His English is good, although he often speaks quickly in Spanish. He generally comes to the clinic on a bus with his wife. His chief complaint today is abdominal tenderness and distention and a change in bowel habits. He presents with fatigue, anorexia, and blood in his stool, which he says has been going on at least 3 months.

He has been your patient at the Bridgeley Community Health Center and has been in good health. He was adopted and has no known family history and no known drug allergies. In Puerto Rico, he never had much health care and definitely no prevention. His last visit was approximately 1 year ago for his annual physical examination, which was within normal limits. He has a history of benign prostate hyperplasia (BPH) and takes no over-the-counter (OTC) medication. He takes no prescription drugs and does not have any history of street drug or ethanol use. He has Medicare with some supplemental insurance.

Technology Used

Settings for HPS

Settings will remain the same throughout the scenario:

- Pulse oximetry ranging from 92% to 94% over 5 minutes
- Pulse increased from baseline of 70 beats/minute from last visit to 84 beats/minute
- Blood pressure (BP) increased from baseline of last visit of 120/70 mmHg to 150/80 mmHg
- Respiratory rate (RR) ranging from 18 to 24 breaths/minute
- Patient complains of chills and slight sweating, temperature = 100°F
- Patient exhibits no shortness of breath at rest, has tenderness over maxillary and facial sinuses, nasal secretions of thick yellow mucus, nasal congestion hence a nasal voice, nonproductive cough, and postnasal drip
- Lungs are clear
- No pretibial swelling palpated or other signs of heart failure

Objectives

After completing the scenario simulation exercise the students will be able to:

1. Demonstrate knowledge of obtaining patient history
2. Demonstrate cultural awareness in caring for patient and family
3. Demonstrate appropriate communication with patient/family
4. Demonstrate timely and effective assessment of patient's signs and symptoms
5. Identify the three differential diagnoses given this patient's presentation and history
6. Describe the pathology of colon cancer

Description of Participant Roles

Student NP: One student is the NP assigned to work with this patient
Mr. Luiz: A high-fidelity HPS programmed with gastrointestinal (GI) symptoms spoken by the teaching assistant or faculty member
Physician: One student role-plays the physician who is called for a consultation
Mrs. Luiz: One student role-plays the wife
Observer: One student is assigned to document the entire scenario in order to share with the class
Teaching assistant/faculty member: Runs the simulator from the control room

E. RUNNING OF THE SCENARIO

Students have read the required reading on GI disease, had class with discussion regarding this same topic, and have completed the study guide questions regarding GI problems. The students have already had a class on neoplasia earlier in this course. All of the students have also had an opportunity to practice in the Learning Resource Center if they desire. Some students may have already had the advanced assessment course and thus will be familiar with working with the monitor and examination table.

The equipment set up on a bedside table consists of a stethoscope, oximeter, intravenous (IV) and blood-drawing equipment, gloves, K-Y lubricating jelly, guaiac cards, and an anoscope. The patient is sitting up on the examination table at a 60° angle and does not seem to be in pain.

The scenario is planned for 15 minutes and the students have practiced themselves and had an actual run-through of the scenario before presenting it to their classmates independent of the faculty.

F. PRESENTATION OF COMPLETED TEMPLATE

Title

Primary Care Patient With Gastrointestinal Problems

Scenario Level

Graduate nursing students in a graduate nursing program studying advanced practice

Focus Area

Pathophysiology, diagnosis workup

Scenario Description

Students participate in this scenario for experience in obtaining data from the patient and family, records, and patient assessment in order to work up the patient's diagnosis of colon cancer and to identify the etiology of the signs and symptoms obtained (the three differential diagnoses are early-stage colon cancer, benign polyps, and late-stage colon cancer with systemic lymphatic spread and liver metastasis). The scenario takes place in a simulated primary care clinic.

Patient history: Mr. Luiz's chief complaint today is abdominal tenderness and distention and a change in bowel habits. He presents with fatigue, anorexia, and blood in his stool, which he says has been going on at least 3 months. His last visit was approximately 1 year ago for his annual physical examination, which was within normal limits. He has a history of BPH only and takes no OTC or prescription medication.

Health assessment results: Skin assessment shows poor skin turgor and dry oral mucous membranes. Abdominal assessment reveals increased bowel sounds, abdominal distention with wide abdominal girth, mild tenderness with palpation but only mild tenderness over liver with percussion and palpation, enlarged liver span, no splenomegaly. Rectal examination shows loose stool palpated with some discomfort and overt blood noted. No other significant findings.

Medication record: No medications.

SCENARIO OBJECTIVES

Objectives Based on Master of Science in Nursing Essentials

The American Association of Colleges of Nursing (2011) has created nine master's-level Essentials that are used as a guide to developing curriculum for graduate nursing programs. The Essentials addressed in this simulation by objective are:

Essential I: Background for Practice From Sciences and Humanities
Essential III: Quality Improvement and Safety
Essential IV: Translating and Integrating Scholarship Into Practice
Essential V: Informatics and Health Care Technologies
Essential VIII: Clinical Prevention and Population Health for Improving Health
Essential IX: Master's-Level Nursing Practice

Setting the Scene

Equipment Needed

HPS to be the patient, primary care unit in the simulated geriatric clinic, BP cuff and stethoscope, oximeter, alcohol wipes, gloves, anoscope, IV and blood-drawing equipment, and electronic record

Resources Needed

Pathophysiology textbook, patient record, participant's script

Simulator Level

Mid- to high-fidelity HPS

Participant Roles

Student NPs to play NP, physician, and wife role; an HPS, and a person to run and/or observe the scenario. We have recently been using undergraduate students majoring in theater to play the various roles—including the patient—and this has been extremely successful (Fletcher, Justice, & Rohrig, 2015).

NP Script

NP: Hello, Mr. Luiz. How are you feeling?

Mr. L: Not so good, I'm having "fullness in my stomach," no appetite, feel really tired and have no energy. I have been sleeping almost every day approximately 14 hours, and the rest of the time I am going to the bathroom.

Mrs. L: He also has been bleeding down there and leaves a "very stinky" smell in the bathroom.

Mr. L: The bleeding is worse now.

NP: When did you notice the bleeding? [NP tests for hydration and finds poor skin turgor, dry oral mucous membranes, within normal limits (WNL) level of consciousness, no confusion].

Mr. L: It started approximately 3 months ago and I thought it would go away, like a hemorrhoid or something.

Mrs. L: I told him to come see you as soon as he saw the blood. It is a very bad sign, isn't it?

NP: Well, I need to examine you, so can you step out for a minute Mrs. L?

Mr. L: I have to go about eight times a day and it is loose now, with blood every time.

NP: [While doing exam]: Do you have any abdominal pain? Have you ever had a test where they look with a tube through your rectum into your bowels—this is called a *colonoscopy*?

Mr. L: No, not really; it just is tender when you are touching it just about everywhere, no tests like that were ever done.

NP: [Abdominal assessment reveals increased bowel sounds, abdominal distention with wide abdominal girth, mild tenderness with palpation but only mild tenderness over liver with percussion and palpation, enlarged liver span, no splenomegaly.] Can you please turn over so I can do a rectal exam? [Loose stool palpated with some discomfort and overt blood noted.]

NP: Let me recheck your blood pressure—it is about the same as when the tech took it: 90/60 mmHg, pulse is 119 beats/minute, respiratory rate is 18 breaths/minute, temperature is 98.8°F, and your weight is 20 pounds less than at your last visit 1 year ago. I am going to have you lie down and start an IV and ask your wife to come back in. [Asks tech to call ambulance.]

Mrs. L: So, what is wrong? It is cancer, isn't it? I knew he had cancer—he smells like cancer. What is happening, Paul? You look so white in your face.

NP: I am going to admit you to Barry Hospital now and start an IV since you are dizzy and seem to be dehydrated from all the rectal bleeding.

Mr. L: I think I should not go by bus—I feel so dizzy. And my wife does not drive.

Mrs. L: We are going by ambulance, aren't we?

NP: Yes, and I want you to call someone to come down and be with you…why don't you do that now while I draw some bloods and get the IV in.

(NP starts an IV normal saline [NS] @ 150/hr in right antecubital vein [AC]. Blood drawn and sent stat [immediately] to Barry Hospital lab for chemical profile, complete blood count [CBC] with differential, amylase, lipase, transaminases. Writes up short summary for Mr. L's case and arranges transfer to ED via ambulance.)

The next day, the NP gets a report showing multiple tumors in the ascending and descending bowel approximately 3 to 1.5 cm, so Mr. Luiz is scheduled for surgery.

The following day, the surgical report indicates complete large bowel removal and rectum with ileostomy, liver metastasis.

Scenario Implementation

Initial Settings for HPS/Equipment

If the clinical laboratory does not have a primary care clinic area, one can develop a one-patient unit with an examination table. Two other ways to teach this material would be to have the faculty give a demonstration in class of the simulation or show a digital video recording (DVR) of the simulation performed by other students to the entire class. If possible a box of gloves; anoscope; IV and blood-drawing equipment module; and a mobile BP, temperature, oximeter, otoscope, and ophthalmoscope setup could be available.

Expected Student Assessments and Actions

This advanced pathophysiology course may be the first course a master's student takes at the graduate level. More than likely, at least half of the students in the class have probably had simulation experience as an undergraduate or continuing-education student or from their employer. Students may feel more comfortable having some hands-on experience in simulation working with a high-fidelity simulator (HFS) than just having lecture and discussion classes for this course. Introducing the patient to working up a diagnosis should assist the student in seeing the importance of having a strong pathophysiology base. Ebbert and Connors (2004) found that graduate students perceived simulation learning as a realistic, challenging, and positive experience that greatly influenced their education. Students will have had multiple case study analyses in the course, so participating in a few simulations toward the middle to end of the course develops their confidence. Students involved in the actual simulation should assist in creating a script. Next, they should have a rehearsal with the faculty member, who should assist them in polishing the script. After the designated time, they should accomplish the scenario objectives, be able to self-critique their performance, receive constructive feedback from the class, and identify their strengths and weak areas.

Instructor Interventions

The faculty member needs to develop the objectives for the learning experience and share the case with the students. The background information given, along with the objectives for the student learning, is then molded into a script. It is up to the students to practice and perfect the scenario and then obtain feedback from the faculty member. More practice is suggested until the students feel comfortable and confident to perform the script independently for the 15-minute time frame in front of their classmates. The faculty member needs to keep the students to the time frame by holding up cards notifying them of the time still left. The debriefing session is held with the whole class and the faculty member leads the discussion, being sure to evaluate the students' performance and answer questions that may come up. Based on the objectives for this scenario, the following evaluative criteria need to be measured.

Evaluative Criteria

___Reviews patient's chief complaint and VS
___Begins diagnostic reasoning
___Checks electronic record for most recent lab reports and finds they are from 1 year ago
___Begins plan for next 10 minutes with priorities
___Performs hand hygiene
___Introduces self to patient/wife
___Communicates clearly with patient/wife
___Demonstrates professional dress/behavior
___Assesses patient's status regarding hydration level given low BP
___Interprets VS and poor turgor
___Performs a focal assessment regarding GI and cardiovascular (CV) systems, does rectal examination
___Asks pertinent questions about the last few months with regard to the signs and symptoms obtained, determines this patient probably has colorectal cancer at a late stage
___Puts in IV and starts fluid resuscitation, explaining to patient and wife that Mr. Luiz needs to be brought to the ED to have a colonoscopy
___Has medical technologist stay with patient and redo VS and obtain blood specimens (CBC with differential, chem profile with blood sent to hospital lab so reports will be ready once patient is worked up at hospital)
___Tells tech to call ambulance and notify ED of patient's status and expected arrival time
___Explains information to patient/wife, tells wife to call friend or family member to meet them there
___Documents on electronic record for health care workers at hospital (has appropriate differentials along with all supporting data).

G. DEBRIEFING GUIDELINES

Issues to Consider

Students need to receive immediate feedback after each simulated scenario. As long as the scenario was developed using sound objectives, the students are prepared and studied diligently, and there were measurable evaluative criteria, debriefing is very matter of fact. Generally, it is a good idea to ask the participants to give their own self-evaluation using the recorder's notes so they can stay organized.

Student Questions

Next, it is important to obtain the classmates' feedback. Be sure that the classmates are aware they need to prepare for this scenario just like they were going to be participating in it. In this way they can be more a part of the evaluation process. Once the students realize they are going to be called on either by the faculty member or the scenario participants for feedback, or asked a question regarding the case, they will prepare thoroughly.

Classroom Questions

Some questions that may assist the discussion among the class in getting started are listed as follows:

1. What focal assessments were done, and why?
2. What were your differentials besides colon cancer?
3. What were your rationales for your differentials?
4. Describe the pathophysiology of Mr. Luiz's problem.
5. What were your rationales for ordering the labs, and what do you think the lab results were?

Senior students generally have no difficulty discussing and sharing their ideas in the debriefing session. The faculty member should limit the time for the debriefing to no more than 30 minutes and, if students are not asking appropriate questions, should steer the discussion toward the evaluative criteria.

H. SUGGESTIONS/KEY FEATURES TO REPLICATE OR IMPROVE

This scenario is focused on gaining experience with analyzing patients' differential diagnoses and explaining the etiology for each diagnosis. In identifying patient signs and symptoms to determine three differential diagnoses, the students gain much confidence in their reasoning skills. Also, the case provides some application of assessment skills for students to collect data regarding this patient's GI complaints.

I. RECOMMENDATIONS FOR FURTHER USE

Ultimately, each pathophysiology class may include a similar simulation of a diagnostic workup. Future cases could be modeled after this one but with a chief complaint of a specific system. Currently, the students develop individual case studies depicting diagnostic reasoning for the development of three differential diagnoses. Small groups of students could pick one case to use as a simulation and receive a group grade for this. More complex cases could be developed in sequential courses whereby the students who worked a specific simulation, such as that of Mr. Luiz in advanced physiology and pathophysiology, encounter him again in their first specialty track course and add a follow-up of how the patient did postoperatively and the management needed for his care. It is imperative during debriefing that faculty and the involved students have a chance to review their simulation immediately after performing the simulation. In my experience, I have found this to greatly assist the students who were in the simulation to participate fully in the general debriefing with the rest of the class.

Graduate students seem to enjoy simulation (Chikotas, 2008; Harris, Shoemaker, Johnson, Tompkins-Dobbs, & Domian, 2016). The general consensus is that most students feel it is important to practice and bridges the gap between theory and clinical practice. Even though this advanced pathophysiology course is one of the seven core graduate courses that everyone must take, all graduate students, from NPs to nurse anesthetists, rank this course as extremely important. Being able to practice diagnostic reasoning, critical thinking, and working up differential diagnoses are skills that come with knowledge and practice. Therefore, simulation pedagogy allows the student to get a glimpse of what this pedagogy is and, at our institution, allows them the opportunity to practice in a simulated primary care clinic. After getting acclimated to the HFS, students can book time in the simulated clinic to practice their skills as well as time management and interviewing. In fact, students can arrange time to videotape and self-critique their performances. Administrators need to allow funding for necessary resources so these invaluable experiences can happen. Student learning outcomes, as well as their self-perceived confidence in adapting to their new advanced practice role, should improve.

J. HOW SIMULATION-BASED PEDAGOGY HAS CONTRIBUTED TO IMPROVED STUDENT OUTCOMES

Graduate students, with little to much clinical experience as an RN, have shared with the faculty that they enjoy and gain much knowledge and clinical competency from the use of simulation in the NP courses. For example, students in the advanced pathophysiology course have improved their laboratory scores on quizzes and examinations since doing simulation in this course. Most of the students request more simulations, even if they are just group simulations in class. Their rationale is that the process of analyzing the cases, that is (a) identifying three differentials for each patient, (b) describing pertinent pathophysiology for each differential, and (c) discussing specific genetics for each differential assists them in remembering the content they are learning. Preliminary evaluation of student's knowledge retention of this content in the family NP track courses points to improved learning outcomes and less time needed to be spent reviewing laboratory values for the majority of diagnoses that were applied to a simulation in the pathophysiology course.

K. EXPERT RECOMMENDATIONS AND WORDS OF WISDOM

It seems the more simulation that can be used for NP students, the more in depth the teaching and learning can become for the students. Not only does the student assist in creating the case scenario, but also seems to enjoy the "competitive edge" being experienced by all of the students. Everyone wants their case to be the most interesting and to provide "pearls of wisdom" to the class. This seems to motivate everyone to work harder and develop a very challenging scenario for the class. Of course, the faculty needs to review each simulation scenario and add or even, at times, correct content, and, of course, this is labor intensive. However, using simulated scenarios and the Socratic method of questioning has resulted in higher grades on student quizzes and exams as well as, according to student evaluations, more confident, prepared students for clinical practica.

L. EVALUATION OF BEST PRACTICE STANDARDS
AND USE OF CREDENTIALED SIMULATION FACULTY

Many of the ah-ha moments and "Wow, I really get this now" statements are a result of a successful debriefing. The International Nursing Association for Clinical Simulation and Learning (INACSL, 2013/2016) developed the INACSL Standards of Best Practice: Simulation, which are very helpful when designing and revising simulations and can be accessed at www.inacsl.org/i4a/pages/index.cfm?pageid=3407. For example, Standard VI: Debriefing Process, explains various techniques on how to best debrief nursing and other health care professionals after simulation (Chikotas, 2008).

At our school of nursing, some faculty are getting certified in simulation pedagogy and these faculty will serve on the school's Innovative Simulation committee. Under the direction of our new director of simulation we are also integrating interprofessional simulated scenarios into many undergraduate and graduate courses.

REFERENCES

American Association of Colleges of Nursing. (2011). *The essentials of master's education in nursing.* Washington, DC: Author. Retrieved from http://www.aacnnursing.org/Portals/42/Publications/MastersEssentials11.pdf

Chikotas, N. E. (2008). Theoretical links supporting the use of problem-based learning in the education of the nurse practitioner. *Nursing Education Perspectives, 29*(6), 359–362.

Ebbert, D. W., & Connors, H. (2004). Standardized patient experiences: Evaluation of clinical performance and nurse practitioner student satisfaction. *Nursing Education Perspectives, 25*(1), 12–15.

Fletcher, L., Justice, S., & Rohrig, L. (2015). Designing a disaster. *Journal of Trauma Nursing, 22*(1), 35–40; quiz E3.

Harris, J., Shoemaker, K., Johnson, K., Tompkins-Dobbs, K., & Domian, E. (2016). Qualitative descriptive study of family nurse practitioner student experiences using high fidelity simulation. *Kansas Nurse, 91*(2), 12–15.

International Nursing Association for Clinical Simulation and Learning. (2013, updated 2016). INACSL standards of best practice: Simulation. Retrieved from: http://www.inacsl.org/i4a/pages/index.cfm?pageid =3407

CHAPTER 35

Using Simulation to Enhance Emotional Intelligence in Nurse Anesthesia Students

Nancy A. Moriber and Audrey M. Beauvais

Nurse anesthesia programs are faced with the critical challenge of preparing students to practice safely and effectively in the demanding and emotionally charged perioperative environment. The nursing literature has begun to recognize the importance of noncognitive factors, such as emotional intelligence (EI), on clinical performance and decision making. This chapter will focus on the use of targeted simulation as a tool to enhance EI of student registered nurse anesthetists.

A. IMPLEMENTATION OF SIMULATION-BASED PEDAGOGY IN YOUR INDIVIDUALIZED TEACHING AREA

The integration of simulation technology into nurse anesthesia education has become a common practice. Although low-fidelity simulators and static manikins have been used for decades to teach basic psychomotor and critical decision-making skills, the addition of high-fidelity simulation (HFS) has enabled educators to tackle more complex concepts and clinical situations than ever before. Students are encouraged to use increasingly complex critical decision-making skills in the management of patients in the perioperative period. In addition, the program is able to expose students to a wider range of clinical situations, many of which are rarely encountered in clinical practice, but in which experience in management is essential to practice. HFS is incorporated throughout the anesthesia curriculum, beginning in the students' clinical orientation and across all five clinical practicums in order to facilitate the progression from novice to independent anesthesia care providers. Students are exposed to the theoretical concepts in their didactic courses and are then given the opportunity to apply them in the safety of the simulation environment.

Although most anesthesia simulation has focused on developing clinical expertise, program faculty have recognized the importance of noncognitive factors, such as EI, on student success and patient outcomes. *EI* is defined as the ability to reason with and about emotions (Mayer & Salovey, 1997). It includes a set of skills that allows a person to more fully appreciate and adapt to the context of a situation by combining feelings with thinking, and can be described as four related but distinct abilities: (a) perceiving emotions, (b) using emotions, (c) understanding emotions, and (d) managing emotions (Mayer & Salovey, 1997). This chapter focuses specifically on the first EI domain: perceiving emotions.

B. EDUCATIONAL MATERIALS AVAILABLE IN YOUR TEACHING AREA AND RELATED TO YOUR SPECIALTY

The Fairfield University Egan School of Nursing and Health Sciences (SON) will be moving into a new building and state-of-the-art simulation center on the Fairfield University campus in the fall of 2017. This facility has been designed to foster the development of psychomotor, cognitive, and affective clinical skills in the students enrolled in both the graduate and undergraduate programs. It will be equipped with two fully functional anesthesia simulation locations designed to allow for the implementation of high-fidelity simulation across the life span (newborn to geriatric) and health care continuum. Students have access to Laerdal's SimBaby and 3G SimMan, as well as CAE Healthcare's iStan (http://caehealthcare.com/images/uploads/brochures/iStan-brochure.pdf) high-fidelity simulators. Simulation space is also available to serve as a preoperative holding area, postanesthesia care unit (PACU), and intensive care unit in order to run scenarios in other locations where anesthesia care providers are required to manage patients. The simulation rooms will share a control room that will be capable of recording and transmitting in real time running scenarios to adjacent classrooms in order to facilitate effective observation and debriefing. In order to enhance the fidelity of the EI simulation curriculum, students participating in the university's standardized patient initiative will be used.

In addition to the HFS rooms, independent skills labs have been designed to house the low-fidelity simulators and static trainers, which can also be used to enhance the fidelity and supplement learning within the HFS environment. A stand-alone 20-bed graduate health assessment lab with integrated audiovisual capabilities for recording and debriefing will be available for use.

C. SPECIFIC OBJECTIVES FOR SIMULATION USAGE WITHIN A SPECIFIC COURSE AND THE OVERALL PROGRAM

The primary objective of this scenario is to enhance EI skills in entry-level nurse anesthesia students preparing at either the master's or doctoral level. Nurse anesthesia programs are charged with the vital task of preparing students to competently practice in the challenging and emotionally draining perioperative setting. To meet this challenge, educators have focused on the students' ability to meet competencies by presenting theoretical content and ensuring skill acquisition (American Association of Colleges of Nursing [AACN], 2011). Such a focus relies on cognitive thought. However, noncognitive factors, such as EI, are also thought to improve student outcomes (Beauvais, Brady, O'Shea, & Griffin, 2011; Beauvais, Denisco, & Stewart, 2014; Beauvais, Stewart, Denisco, & Beauvais, 2014; Collins, 2013). The concept of EI caught the attention of nursing scholars as some believe EI is at the heart of nursing care (Freshwater & Stickley, 2004). Nursing is a profession that requires the ability to cope with a wide range of human emotions (Freshwater & Stickley, 2004). Nurses are expected to manage their emotional lives while interpreting other people's emotional state (Cadman & Brewer, 2001). In turn, that information is used to make critical decisions.

Thus, the simulation experience outlined in this chapter is designed to incorporate and foster the development of EI skills for nurse anesthesia students. This scenario is intended to enhance the student's ability to:

1. Perceive emotions
2. Use emotions
3. Understand emotions
4. Manage emotions

Nurse anesthesia students who deal with emotionally charged situations could certainly benefit from such exposure. The scenario presented in this chapter is envisioned for anesthesia students in the first year of the anesthesia program, but can be modified for use in undergraduate and graduate programs across disciplines. Other scenarios used to enhance EI skills have been developed for the middle and end of the anesthesia program.

D. INTRODUCTION OF SCENARIO

Setting the Scene

This scenario takes place in the endoscopy suite of a medical facility. A 65-year-old male presents for a colonoscopy under general anesthesia. He has a past medical history that is significant for hypertension (HTN), obstructive sleep apnea (OSA), obesity (body mass index [BMI]: 40), and active gastroesophageal reflux disease (GERD). He is on metoprolol 25 mg twice a day (BID) and uses a continuous positive airway pressure (CPAP) machine at home. You are very concerned about the potential for airway obstruction and aspiration if you anesthetize the patient so you decide to place a secure airway endotracheal tube [ETT]). The patient is placed on the procedure table and attached to standard monitoring equipment, including EKG, blood pressure (BP) cuff, pulse oximeter, and end-tidal carbon dioxide monitoring. The endoscopist enters the suite and on discussion with him regarding the anesthetic plan he or she becomes irate and starts yelling that the patient does not need to be intubated and he or she will do the procedure without anesthesia if you attempt to intubate the patient. The scenario begins when the student must determine how to proceed.

Technology Used

This scenario can be run using either a high-fidelity human patient simulator (HPS) or, if desired, a standardized patient, which would have the advantage of increasing the fidelity because the focus of the scenario is on perceiving emotions. If standardized patients are used it will also be necessary to provide adequate training to ensure that appropriate patient characteristics and actions are displayed during the scenario.

Access to patient records, either in electronic or paper format, should be provided. As most facilities have transitioned to electronic records, access to an electronic format during the simulation would offer greater scenario realism and allow participants (anesthesia and nurses) to chart information as would be appropriate during an actual procedure. Audiotaped recordings of sounds commonly heard in the environment where anesthesia is administered should be incorporated into the scenario to simulate the hectic environment of an endoscopy suite. Finally, audiovisual capabilities are required to allow for recording and debriefing of the scenario. If recording is planned, it is necessary to obtain written permission either at the start of the simulation session or, ideally, on entrance into the training program. A blanket release can be obtained and used to cover all simulation sessions in which a student participates during his or her educational experience.

Objectives

Students who successfully complete this scenario exercise will have demonstrated their ability regarding the following four skills:

1. Understand the first EI domain: perceiving emotions
2. Recognize his or her own feeling as they relate to the situation
3. Understand the feelings of others
4. Identify verbal and nonverbal manifestations of emotions

Successful completion of this simulation activity would also allow the student to meet several of the American Association of Colleges of Nursing's *Essentials of Master's Education in Nursing* (AACN, 2011), including:

Essential I: Background for Practice From Sciences and Humanities, Objectives 1, 3 to 5
Essential II: Organizational and Systems Leadership, Objectives 1 and 2

Essential IV: Translating and Integrating Scholarship Into Practice, Objective 4
Essential VII: Interprofessional Collaboration for Improving Patient and Population Health Outcomes, Objectives 3 and 4
Essential IX: Master's Level Nursing Practice, Objectives 1 to 4

This scenario addresses the following *Essentials of Doctoral Education for Advanced Nursing Practice* (AACN, 2006):

Essential I: Scientific Underpinnings for Practice, Objectives 1 to 3
Essential II: Organizational and Systems Leadership for Quality Improvement and Systems Leadership, Objectives 1 to 3
Essential VI: Interprofessional Collaboration for Improving Patient and Population Health Outcomes, Objectives 1 and 2
Essential VIII: Advanced Nursing Practice, Objectives 1 to 4

Description of Participants

A minimum of four participants will be required to run the scenario. The role of the endoscopist should be played by an actor who is provided with a description of the scenario and a short script so that he or she can effectively portray the physician. Unknown to all other participants, the endoscopist is irate because the last time he or she had a patient who was intubated for a procedure the endoscopist was delayed by an hour and had to cancel office hours. Therefore, unless the anesthesia students' specifically try to identify the reasons for his or her refusal, the endoscopist will continue to hold this position. If the students attempt to identify the underlying reason for his annoyance, then the endoscopist may become amenable to a discussion of the merits of endotracheal intubation in this patient.

The patient can either be portrayed by a standardized patient or high-fidelity simulator, but regardless it is important that the patient reacts to the communication exchange with increasing anxiety. Two students are required to portray the anesthetists assigned to care for the patient during the colonoscopy. If other students are available, one can be scripted into the scenario to play the role of the endoscopy nurse. This individual may be included to carry out tasks as directed by the gastroenterologist.

E. RUNNING OF THE SCENARIO

Before running the scenario, all students must have completed the didactic component required to effectively participate in the simulation. Before the date of simulation, students are provided with an article outlining EI and are then given the opportunity to discuss it as part of the prebriefing with the facilitators. This scenario is run with two faculty facilitators who are present for the briefing and debriefing. During the actual simulation, one facilitator stays with the students observing the simulation via live videostream and the other facilitator provides the voice of Mr. Jones (patient). Students come to the classroom to be briefed with a general description of the scenario. Two students are randomly chosen to participate in the simulation while the other students are tasked with observing the scenario via live videostream in a nearby classroom. The equipment necessary for running the scenario is available in the simulation room. An actor plays the endoscopist in the scenario.

F. PRESENTATION OF COMPLETED TEMPLATE

Title

Perceiving Emotions During the Anesthetic Management of a Patient Presenting for Colonoscopy

Scenario Level

This scenario is designed to run with students enrolled in nurse anesthesia programs at the master's or doctoral level

Focus Area

Nurse anesthesia students in the first year of the program

Scenario Description

Mr. Jones is a 65-year-old male who presents for colonoscopy under general anesthesia. He has a past medical history that is significant for HTN, OSA, obesity (BMI of 40), and active GERD. He is on metoprolol 25 mg BID and uses a CPAP machine at home. You are very concerned about the potential for airway obstruction and aspiration if you anesthetize the patient so you decide to place a secure airway ETT. On discussion with the endoscopist, he becomes irate and starts yelling that the patient does not need to be intubated and he will do the procedure without anesthesia if you attempt to intubate the patient. How do you proceed?

Scenario Objective

At the completion of the scenario the participant will:

1. Understand the importance of perceiving emotions in interprofessional collaboration and conflict resolution
2. Recognize his or her own feeling as they relate to the individual situation
3. Understand the feelings of others
4. Identify verbal and nonverbal manifestations of emotions as they affect communication

Setting the Scene

Equipment Needed

High- (or low)-fidelity simulator; procedure table; standard monitoring equipment, including BP, EKG, pulse oximetry, and end-tidal carbon dioxide measurement; nasal cannula; auxiliary oxygen; medications, including propofol, succinylcholine, ephedrine, and phenylephrine; emergency airway equipment; video-recording device

Simulator Level

High-fidelity simulation

Participants Needed

Four participants required: Two anesthesia care providers (student role), endoscopist (actor), patient (standardized patient or high-fidelity simulator), endoscopy nurse (student) if available

Scenario Implementation

Initial Settings for High-Fidelity Simulator or Patient Monitor

BP: 149/86 mmHg, heart rate (HR): 76 beats/minute, respiratory rate (RR): 18 breaths/minute, SaO_2: 99% (vital signs will gradually rise as patient becomes more anxious during endoscopist/anesthesia care provider exchange).

Required Student Assessments and Actions

Because of the nature of the scenario, assessment of students' ability to meet objectives is determined during the debriefing process through critical reflection and ability to accurately recognize their feelings/emotions, recognize the feelings/emotions of the endoscopist and the patient, and identify verbal and nonverbal manifestations of the feelings/emotions. However, the student is assessed on carry out the following actions:

1. Completes a comprehensive anesthesia history and physical, including airway assessment
2. Explains anesthetic plan of care to the patient
3. Attaches standard monitors and supplemental oxygen
4. Communicates anesthetic plan of care to endoscopist
5. Acknowledges endoscopist's concerns and communicates rationale for plan
6. Attempts to identify underlying issues for endoscopist's emotions
7. Recognizes impact of communication on the patient's emotional state

Evaluation Criteria

___ Student is able to recognize how he or she feels in the scenario.
___ Student understands how and why the endoscopist feels the way he or she does in the scenario.
___ Student recognizes both the verbal and nonverbal manifestations of emotions in all involved parties.
___ Reflective journal is evaluated.

Checklist of Interventions and Assessments

Exhibit 35.1 contains the checklist used to evaluate students in the scenario.

Exhibit 35.1	Evaluation of Required Student Assessments and Actions: Perceiving Emotions During the Anesthetic Management of a Patient Presenting for Colonoscopy		
Student Behavior	**Independent**	**Prompting**	**Not Attempted**
Completes a comprehensive anesthesia history and physical, including airway assessment			
Explains anesthetic plan of care to the patient			
Attaches standard monitors and supplemental oxygen			
Communicates anesthetic plan of care to endoscopist			
Acknowledges endoscopist's concerns and communicates rationale for plan			
Attempts to identify underlying issues for endoscopist's emotions			
Recognizes impact of communication on the patient's emotional state			

G. DEBRIEFING GUIDELINES

An essential element of simulation involves debriefing the experience to encourage reflective practice (Decker et al., 2013; Lavoie, Pepin, & Boyer, 2013). Fairfield University SON uses the *Standards of Best Practice: Simulation Standard VI: The Debriefing Process* (Decker et al., 2013). As such, debriefing is led by faculty who are competent in the process and happens in a safe learning environment. The faculty facilitator watches the simulation and employs a structured framework to debrief while focusing on the stated outcomes and objectives (Decker et al., 2013). For the purposes of this simulation, the ability-based model of EI conceptualized by psychologists Jack Mayer and Peter Salovey (1997) is used. Their four-branch model defines EI as the ability to reason with and about emotions. EI combines feelings with thinking and can be described as four related but distinct abilities: (a) perceiving emotions, (b) using emotions, (c) understanding emotions, and (d) managing emotions (Mayer & Salovey, 1997). As a result, during the debriefing, students are asked to reflect on all four branches of EI. General debriefing questions are provided as follows for each of the branches.

Branch 1: Perceiving Emotions

- What were you feeling during the scenario?
- What do you think the other people in the scenario were feeling?

Goal: The ability to learn to identify and label specific feelings in yourself and others, ability to clearly and directly communicate and discuss these emotions

Branch 2: Using Emotions

- How did your feelings guide you to what is important to think about?
- How did you use your feelings to help you with decisions that were appropriate for you and others involved?

Goal: The ability to use your feelings constructively

Branch 3: Understanding Emotions

- What was the purpose of the emotion you felt?
- What was the purpose of the emotion expressed by others in the scenario?
- What was the relationship between emotions? How and why did they change from one to another?
- How did emotions lead to the behavior in yourself and others?
- What was the relationship between thoughts and feelings?
- What were the causes of your emotion and what is the relationship to your human psychological needs, especially your unmet emotional needs?

Goal: The ability to understand the meaning of emotions and how they can change

Branch 4: Managing Emotions

- How were you able to turn negative emotions into positive learning and growing opportunities?
- How were you able to help others identify and benefit from their emotions?

Goal: The ability to manage emotions for personal and social growth

H. SUGGESTIONS/KEY FEATURES TO REPLICATE OR IMPROVE

The health care literature has demonstrated that high levels of EI are associated with improved problem solving and decision making (McQueen, 2004; Moyer & Wittmann-Price, 2008). For nurse anesthetists in particular, EI may help in preparing students for roles, which will necessitate them working in teams and managing conflict (Collins, 2013). Therefore, the incorporation of simulation to promote the development of EI has the potential to have a significant impact on nursing performance and academic success. However, the use of simulation to enhance EI is in its infancy and there is limited information to define the "ideal" curriculum. The key features of EI can be addressed in any HFS as human interaction does not take place independent of emotion. In fact, when engaged in critical thinking and decision making, emotions help to shape what individuals think about and how they think about it. Therefore, it is recommended that when appropriate, questions targeting students' ability to perceive emotions, use emotions, understand emotions, and manage emotions be incorporated into HFS wherever possible.

I. RECOMMENDATIONS FOR FURTHER USE

Although the scenario provided in this chapter focuses on the nurse anesthesia student in the first year of the program, we would recommend that scenarios such as these be incorporated throughout the program to foster the enhancement of EI skills. We would suggest that four scenarios be incorporated into the program. Each scenario would address all four branches of EI: perceiving emotions, using emotions, understanding emotions, and emotional management. Debriefing questions touch on all areas but one branch would be highlighted during each debriefing session and then in the reflective journaling follow-up.

J. HOW SIMULATION-BASED PEDAGOGY HAS CONTRIBUTED TO IMPROVED STUDENT OUTCOMES

A comprehensive simulation curriculum has become an expected component of a nurse anesthesia program. Students enjoy using simulation as a learning tool because it provides them with the opportunity to develop strong psychomotor, cognitive and affective skills in a safe, nonthreatening environment. With the integration of an EI curriculum, students can now learn to manage and use their emotions to obtain positive outcomes in the perioperative setting. Students are able to see both the positive and negative consequences of their actions on the decision-making process. As a result, they tend to have a better understanding of the impact of emotions on their decisions and the decisions of others. Therefore, they tend to rate their overall educational experiences more positively and request more simulation in their programs.

Given the positive correlations between EI and student outcomes, many scholars, such as Collins (2013), have proposed that nursing education should consistently incorporate EI skills development into the nursing curriculum at all levels. Given the potential significance to nursing education outcomes and assuming simulation positively influences EI in nurse anesthetist students, nursing education will have identified a sustainable, powerful teaching strategy that could potentially increase the performance and success of nurse anesthesia students. The possibilities are limited only by the imagination of educators developing simulation scenarios for integration in nursing education.

K. EXPERT RECOMMENDATIONS
AND WORDS OF WISDOM

Overall, the scenario worked very well and received positive evaluations from students. Aside from offering additional EI scenarios throughout the nursing anesthesia program, our other recommendation would be to provide more information presimulation. We found the students were superficially familiar with the term *emotional intelligence*. However, the experience might be enhanced if students are asked to complete some preliminary exercises to ensure they understand the basic concepts before beginning the scenario. For example, during a presimulation for EI branch one (identify emotions) students could be asked to reflect whether they attend to emotions or whether they consider this piece of information irrelevant. Considering that emotions can be read through facial expressions and interpreted through body language and tone of voice, we would recommend that faculty create some presimulation exercises to see whether students can identify the emotional cues and whether they are accurate in their interpretation.

L. EVALUATION OF BEST PRACTICE STANDARDS
AND USE OF CREDENTIALED SIMULATION FACULTY

Fairfield University SON has initiated the process of becoming a Society for Simulation Health Care (SSH) Accredited Program. We are using the International Nursing Association for Clinical Simulation and Learning (INACSL) standards as a framework to confirm that our faculty have the knowledge, skills, and abilities to facilitate quality health care simulation activities (INACSL, 2013/2016). In order to promote faculty expertise in simulation, Fairfield University has encouraged faculty to receive simulation training and to sit for the certification examination. All faculty members who facilitate simulation-based experiences (SBE) have been formally trained through CAE Healthcare and Laerdal via live and webinar-based workshops on simulation pedagogy. In addition, the director of simulation for the SON is fully trained via INACSL and is currently serving as a National League for Nursing (NLN) Fellow. Faculty have been afforded the opportunity to attend simulation conferences. To help reach as many faculty members as possible, the SON has hosted debriefing and facilitation training programs that have specifically targeted the integration of the INACSL best practice standards into the simulation curriculum across programs. Fairfield University SON views simulation as a valuable method to link classroom learning to real-life clinical experiences.

INACSL Standard IX: Simulation Design, has been used as the specific framework for the development, implementation, and evaluation of simulation scenarios across nursing programs and clinical specialties (2013/2016). Within the nursing anesthesia program, specific aims and measurable objectives that correspond to the student's level of knowledge and experience, and that build on previous mastery of concepts and skills, are identified as the basis for individual SBE development. Faculty members are then embedded in the scenarios to provide support and guidance as needed in order promote attainment of course objectives. Scenarios are recorded with the permission of participants so that they can be used as part of the debriefing process to guide discussion, examine best practices, and promote critical reflection among participants. Overwhelming, both the students embedded in the scenarios and those watching the simulcasts find the experiences have a positive impact on their learning and success in the clinical arena because they provide students with the opportunity to test their critical thinking and examine the impact of their decision making in a safe learning environment.

REFERENCES

American Association of Colleges of Nursing. (2006). *Essentials of doctoral education for advanced nursing practice*. Washington, DC: Author. Retrieved from http://www.aacnnursing.org/Portals/42/Publications/DNPEssentials.pdf

American Association of Colleges of Nursing. (2011). *The essentials of master's education in nursing.* Washington, DC: Author. Retrieved from http://www.aacnnursing.org/Portals/42/Publications/MastersEssentials11.pdf

Beauvais, A., Stewart, J. G., & DeNisco, S. (2014). Emotional intelligence and spiritual well-being: Implications for spiritual care. *Journal of Christian Nursing, 31*(3), 166–171.

Beauvais, A. M., Brady, N., O'Shea, E. R., & Griffin, M. T. (2011). Emotional intelligence and nursing performance among nursing students. *Nurse Education Today, 31*(4), 396–401.

Beauvais, A. M., Stewart, J. G., DeNisco, S., & Beauvais, J. E. (2014). Factors related to academic success among nursing students: A descriptive correlational research study. *Nurse Education Today, 34*(6), 918–923.

Cadman, C., & Brewer, J. (2001). Emotional intelligence: A vital prerequisite for recruitment in nursing. *Journal of Nursing Management, 9*(6), 321–324.

Collins, S. (2013). Emotional intelligence as a noncognitive factor in student registered nurse anesthetists. *American Association of Nurse Anesthetists Journal, 81*(6), 465–472.

Decker, S., Fey, M., Sideras, S., Caballero, S., Rockstraw, L., Boese, T., ... Borum, J. C. (2013). Standards of best practice: Simulation standard VI: The debriefing process. *Clinical Simulation in Nursing, 9*(6S), S26–S29.

Freshwater, D., & Stickley, T. (2004). The heart of the art: Emotional intelligence in nurse education. *Nursing Inquiry, 11*(2), 91–98.

International Nursing Association for Clinical Simulation and Learning. (2013, updated 2016). INACSL standards of best practice: Simulation. Retrieved from https://www.inacsl.org/i4a/pages/index.cfm?pageID=3407

Lavoie, P., Pepin, J., & Boyer, L. (2013). Reflective debriefing to promote novice nurses' clinical judgment after high-fidelity clinical simulation: A pilot test. *Dynamics, 24*(4), 36–41.

Mayer, J. D., & Salovey, P. (1997). What is emotional intelligence? In P. Salovey & D. Sluyter (Eds.), *Emotional development and emotional intelligence: Implications for educators* (pp. 3–31). New York, NY: Basic Books.

McQueen, A. C. (2004). Emotional intelligence in nursing work. *Journal of Advanced Nursing, 47*(1), 101–108.

Moyer, B. A., & Wittmann-Price, R. A. (2008). *Nursing education: Foundation for practice excellence.* Philadelphia, PA: F. A. Davis.

CHAPTER 36

Critical Care/Adult Gerontology Acute Care Nurse Practitioner: Aortic Emergencies

Joshua Squiers and Rose Milano

A. IMPLEMENTATION OF SIMULATION-BASED PEDAGOGY IN YOUR INDIVIDUALIZED TEACHING AREA

The critical care environment is often a difficult and challenging arena in which to provide clinical experiences managing unstable patients for nurse practitioner (NP) students pursuing adult gerontology acute care NP (AGACNP) certification. In most tertiary-level academic critical care centers, students are typically not given the opportunity to independently manage the most unstable critical care patients. Although this may be frustrating for students, this is understandable given the high morbidity and mortality associated with these types of patient encounters. Following graduation, however, many AGACNP students go on to practice in critical care environments where the management of highly unstable patients is commonplace. With this well-documented fact, it becomes necessary for the AGACNP student to become familiar with these types of high-acuity patient care issues before their entry into independent practice. One approach to educating the AGACNP students is to provide them with multiple opportunities to provide care for unstable patients in a high-fidelity human patient simulator (HPS) setting. A simulation curriculum focusing on the independent management of the simulated unstable patient, when paired with clinical rotations in which students are actively managing unstable patients as part of a multidisciplinary team, not only provides the AGACNP student with a diverse learning environment, but also the opportunity to practice what is learned from a clinical practice site in a simulation setting.

When used in conjunction with didactic and clinical curricula, simulation provides unique experiences to improve students' cognitive and psychomotor skills. Ideally, simulation scenarios should focus on a variety of critical care student-specific cognitive outcomes, including distributed cognition, rapid pattern recognition, situational awareness, and cognitive flexibility. Care should be taken when developing critical care simulations to develop both cognitive and clinical objectives for each scenario. In particular, when simulation is used multiple times throughout an NP curriculum, a consistent focus on diagnostics and interventions should provide the foundation throughout the various individual simulations.

Ideally, each single simulation should be constructed to become part of a series of simulations that complement the students' didactic and clinical curriculum. For example, students receive didactic content on ventilator management, including diagnostics and interventions for adult respiratory distress syndrome (ARDS), during their critical care didactic. However, in the critical care clinical rotation it may be that a student would not have the opportunity to manage a patient with ARDS either with the clinical team or independently. A simulated scenario allows students to independently diagnose ARDS (using appropriate diagnostic tools), initiate the appropriate therapeutic interventions, and manage any complications that arise. These simulated learning sessions provide an opportunity for students to independently care for a complex ARDS patient in a risk-free environment while combining knowledge learned in previous didactic and clinical learning sessions. Once the student has mastered this material, further simulation scenarios can expand on ARDS management in patients with more complex comorbidities.

B. EDUCATIONAL MATERIALS AVAILABLE IN YOUR TEACHING AREA AND RELATED TO YOUR SPECIALTY

The Oregon Health and Science University (OHSU) School of Nursing offers a unique AGACNP intensivist program. Its mission is to train AGACNPs for clinical practice in acute care multidisciplinary facilities. AGACNPs specializing in the care of unstable, critically ill patients represent a unique subspecialty of NPs who are routinely required to make highly critical, time-dependent clinical decisions. The overall educational focus for students is in developing cognitive skills that allow for rapid diagnostics and clinical interventions. The AGACNP simulation curriculum revolves around the development of physical and cognitive skills necessary for practice in an acute care environment, including the intensive care unit.

The Collaborative Life Science Building (CLSB) at OHSU was built intentionally to stimulate learning and research across a wide variety of learners. The facility mixes learners and researchers across a variety of health science-related professions. Included in this facility is the 20,000-square foot Simulation Center, which houses the main medical simulation center for the university. This facility contains eight state-of-the-art high-fidelity simulation suites with the ability to be reconfigured into a variety of medical settings, including hospital medical–surgical rooms, operating rooms, emergency department (ED) rooms, ICU suites, a postanesthesia recovery room, and medical consultation rooms. Along with the simulation suites, there are two multipurpose classrooms, seven debriefing suites, eight bed-skills training labs, and 20 clinic rooms for use with standardized patients.

Each simulation suite has separate audio and visual capabilities that allow for projection and recording throughout the CLSB. The separate control rooms, each adjoining a corresponding simulation suite, allow for faculty and a simulation engineer to observe students behind a one-way mirror and to adjust the simulation content depending on student progress. With the size of the room, it is possible to simulate more than one ICU scenario at a time if the faculty wishes to create concurrent scenarios in which multiple complex problems need to be addressed simultaneously. These scenarios allow students to use HPSs as surrogates for live patients while providing a real-world feel to practicing in the ICU. The HPSs are equipped to mimic patients with simulated heartbeats, respirations, bowel sounds, pulses, and the ability to converse with students as the simulation session warrants. In addition to the HPS, critical care monitors display all of the physiologic data typically found in the ICU, and radiographic monitors display tests ordered by students during the simulation. Working ventilators are used for simulations requiring ventilation management. Simulated activities and interactions can be digitally recorded and archived for use by faculty and students to enhance learning.

Partial task trainers are used to provide introductory procedural training, including airway management, arterial line placement, central line placement, chest decompression, and chest tube placement. These skills are then integrated into larger clinical simulations focusing on complex diagnostic reasoning and intervention. Once students are able to master these clinically focused sessions, simulations incorporate trained actors or faculty to expand the scenarios to include patient/family issues and conflict resolution among medical team members. The addition of these situational factors provides students the opportunity to develop interpersonal skills necessary for ICU practice, such as rapid consultation, family and patient interactions, and delivering difficult news to families.

AGACNP faculty are all certified in medical simulation instruction through the Harvard Center for Medical Simulation. This ensures consistency among the faculty regarding the overall approach to objectives, outcomes, and debriefing styles. This is particularly important when simulation is repetitively used, as it provides a consistent educational approach and ensures student outcomes align from simulation to simulation.

C. SPECIFIC OBJECTIVES OF SIMULATION USAGE WITHIN A SPECIFIC COURSE AND THE OVERALL PROGRAM

This scenario is designed as part of a year-long simulation course that runs concurrently with the AGACNP clinical rotations within our academic tertiary-critical care unit. This simulation is considered moderately difficult in the program, as it requires rapid diagnostics and interventions, critical care team interaction, strong medical differential diagnostic skills, the ability to perform rapid sequence intubation, ventilation management, and time-dependent communication with consultative services. This simulation would occur midway through the AGACNP program. All students in the scenario would have had clinical student responsibilities on a critical care team for at least 6 weeks and would have undergone a radiology, advanced airway and ventilator workshop before the simulation.

Student Learning Activities

- Differential diagnosis with identification of primary diagnosis
- Rapid evidence-based interventions
- Identification of the definitive treatment for aortic rupture
- Review of aortic dissection treatment
- Review of aortic rupture treatment
- Review of transfusion strategies for exsanguination

D. INTRODUCTION OF SCENARIO

Setting the Scene

The setting is an ICU hospital room in a tertiary-level medical center. Students are on a critical care team consisting of no more than six students. The provider team has been called to the bedside by the ICU nurse for a new admission, who has just arrived from an outside hospital (OSH) via an emergency service helicopter.

Technology Used

The high-fidelity HPS is a male, running manually, with the following vital signs: heart rate (HR): 116 beats/minute, blood pressure (BP): 128/77 mmHg, pulse oximetry: 100% on 2 L/minute per nasal cannula, respiratory rate (RR): 29 breaths/minute. The HPS has been hooked to basic telemetry, automatic sphygmomanometer (q [every] 15 minutes), and pulse oximetry. The patient has an 18-gauge intravenous (IV) catheter placed at the right antecubital fossa. There is an IV infusion of nitroglycerine running through 25 μg/minute. The HPS is identified by the bedside ICU nurse as "David Johnson" and is dressed in a hospital gown. Stethoscopes, gloves, an airway cart containing intubation equipment, airway adjuncts, a ventilator, and a code cart stocked with advanced cardiac life support (ACLS) medications and medications for rapid sequence intubation (RSI) are available for student use. A screen appropriate to reading radiographs is available for viewing chest x-rays (CXRs) and CT scans. Medications available include IV fluids, inotropes, vasopressors, packed red blood cells, and fresh frozen plasma and platelets. A telephone system is connected to the simulation control center, allowing students the option of "calling" a consultant. A microphone system is connected to the HPS, so it may respond to questions asked by the students.

Objectives

1. Identification of critical care team leader with appropriate distribution of duties among the team
2. Appropriate history and physical examination
3. Differential diagnosis of chest pain (must include aortic dissection/rupture)
4. Appropriate interpretation of chest radiograph
5. Appropriate ordering of CT scan
6. Diagnosis of acute respiratory failure
7. Appropriate airway management with rapid sequence intubation
8. Diagnosis of aortic dissection
9. Appropriate treatment of aortic dissection
10. Diagnosis of aortic rupture
11. Appropriate treatment of aortic rupture
12. Appropriate consultation with vascular surgeon for emergent surgical intervention

Description of Participants

HPS: Mr. Johnson is a 58-year-old gentleman who just arrived from an OSH to be admitted to the ICU. He was seen at the OSH's ED for crushing chest pain and shortness of breath. He has a past medical history (PMH) of hyperlipidemia, arthritis, and prostate hypertrophy. His initial EKG was nonspecific for ischemia and his troponin was negative, but he continued to have significant chest pain. His CXR from an OSH is available and noted to be "mildly abnormal." His pain was treated with as needed (PRN) IV morphine, a nitroglycerin infusion, a single oral dose of aspirin, and oxygen by nasal cannula. He was sent to the ICU for further workup.

AGACNP student critical care team: This team consists of two to six AGACNP students currently training in critical care. A maximum of six students can participate in this scenario. Students should be familiar with the formation of a critical care team for dealing with critically ill patient situations. Ideally, these students have already had critical care team training, airway management, and ventilator management education before participating in this scenario.

Bedside ICU nurse: The bedside nurse is a confederate within the simulation and is available to assist the student team. Ideally, the role of bedside nurse is played by an RN, trained specifically for simulation, teaching, or a simulation engineer trained for the role and has a wireless ear microphone connected to the engineer/faculty within the control room. The bedside nurse is instructed to provide labs or other clinical data as needed throughout the scenario.

Vascular surgery consultant: The vascular surgeon is a confederate within the simulation and should be used for consultation. The surgeon will be available for phone consultation and will be willing to see the patient **only** when students have identified the correct diagnosis (i.e., thoracic aortic rupture) and recommend emergent operation.

E. RUNNING OF THE SCENARIO: PREBRIEFING

Students should be briefed before the simulation with information regarding the simulation setup in general (room, HPS, phone system, etc.), and given adequate instruction to the clinical resources available. In general, we instruct students to assume that they are at an academic medical center with all diagnostic and clinical resources available to them during the simulation.

Before the initiation of the simulation, students are brought to the simulator suite and are read the patient history before entry into the room. They are then introduced to the bedside nurse, and any logistic or HPS-specific questions are answered.

F. PRESENTATION OF COMPLETED TEMPLATE

Title

Critical Care: Aortic Emergencies

Scenario Level

Graduate-level (AGACNP) or doctoral-level critical care specialization master's level AGACNP students (intensivist subspecialty focus)

Focus Area

Intensive care/critical care

Scenario Description

Mr. Johnson is a 58-year-old gentleman who just arrived from an OSH to be admitted to the ICU. He was seen at the OSH's ED for crushing chest pain and shortness of breath. He has a PMH of hyperlipidemia, arthritis, and prostate hypertrophy. His initial EKG was nonspecific for ischemic and his troponin was negative, but he continued to have significant chest pain. His CXR from OSH is available and noted to be "mildly abnormal." His pain was treated with IV morphine, a nitroglycerin infusion, a single oral dose of aspirin, and oxygen by nasal cannula. He is sent to the ICU for further workup.

Past Medical History

Gastroesophageal reflux disease
Hypertension
Hyperlipidemia
Obesity
Migraine headaches
Past surgical history
None

Social History

Marital history: Married
Education: Completed college degree
Employment: Office manager in local business
Denies smoking and illicit drug use

Home Medications

Aspirin 81 mg daily
Lovastatin 20 mg hs (at bedtime)
Lisinopril 20 mg daily
Pepcid 20 mg BID (twice a day)

Allergies

No known drug allergies

Scenario Objectives

1. Identification of critical care team leader with appropriate distribution of duties among the team
2. Appropriate history and physical examination
3. Differential diagnosis of chest pain (must include aortic dissection/rupture)
4. Appropriate interpretation of chest radiograph
5. Appropriate ordering of CT scan
6. Diagnosis of acute respiratory failure
7. Appropriate airway management with rapid sequence intubation
8. Diagnosis of aortic dissection
9. Appropriate treatment of aortic dissection
10. Diagnosis of aortic rupture
11. Appropriate treatment of aortic rupture
12. Appropriate consultation of vascular surgery with recommendation made for emergent surgical intervention

These simulation objectives meet several of the overarching objectives noted within the American Association of Colleges of Nursing's (AACN, 2011) *Essentials of Master's Education in Nursing*. The scenario requires the student to perform two of the core competencies including:

Essential IX: Master's-Level Nursing Practice, Objectives 1, 2, 7

These objectives meet the following overarching objectives noted within AACN's (2006) *Essentials of Doctoral Education for Advanced Nursing Practice:*

Essential VII: Advanced Nursing Practice, Objectives 1, 2

Setting the Scene

Equipment Needed

High-fidelity HPS, video-recording device, medical equipment (e.g., patient monitor, oxygen hookup, airway management equipment, ventilator, pulse oximeter, BP cuff, and stethoscope), and medical record (electronic or paper)

Resources Needed

Contrast chest CT images revealing descending thoracic aortic rupture; students should have had basic airway management (including rapid sequence intubation techniques) and introduction to radiographic imaging before simulation

Simulator nevel

High-fidelity

Participants Needed

AGACNP student critical care team (typically five to six students): This team is formed of AGACNP students currently training in critical care. A maximum of six students can participate in this scenario. Students should be familiar with the formation of a critical care team for dealing with critically ill patient situations. Ideally, these students have already had critical care team training, airway management, and ventilator management education before participating in this scenario.

Bedside ICU *nurse (one confederate):* The bedside nurse is a confederate within the simulation and is available to assist the student team. Ideally, he or she has a wireless ear microphone connected to the engineer/faculty within the control room. He or she is instructed to provide labs or other clinical data as needed throughout the scenario. This role is best played by an RN, trained specifically for simulation teaching, or a simulation engineer trained for the role.

Vascular surgery consultant (one confederate): The vascular surgeon is a confederate within the simulation and should be used for consultation. Initially, he or she is available by phone consultation. The surgeon has received the phone consultation and will be willing to see the patient only when students have identified the correct diagnosis (thoracic aortic rupture) and recommend emergent operation.

Scenario Implementation

For an overview of the suggested simulation timeline, see Table 36.1.

Initial Settings For

HPS: HR: 116 beats/minute (sinus tachycardia), BP: 128/77 mmHg, pulse oximetry: 100% on 2 L/minute via nasal cannula, RR: 29 breaths/minute

Instructor Interventions

This simulation is designed to be experienced without any instructor–student interaction. If students are unable to identify an appropriate diagnosis in the allotted time, the simulation should be stopped and the instructor should discuss potential improvements during debriefing. At that time, it is recommended that the simulation be restarted from the beginning and allowed to proceed.

Evaluation Criteria

Checklist of required interventions:

___Identifies critical care team leader with appropriate distribution of duties among the team.
___Performs appropriate history and physical examination.
___Reaches a differential diagnosis of chest pain (must include aortic dissection/rupture).
___Appropriately interprets chest radiograph.
___Orders a CT scan.
___Diagnoses acute respiratory failure.
___Performs appropriate airway management with rapid sequence intubation.
___Diagnoses aortic dissection.
___Appropriately treats aortic dissection.
___Diagnoses aortic rupture.
___Appropriately treats aortic rupture, including whole-blood transfusion strategy.
___Consults with vascular surgeon with recommendation made for emergent surgical intervention.

G. DEBRIEFING GUIDELINES

Within the AGACNP program at OHSU School of Nursing we generally use the "debriefing with good judgment" approach that has been promoted by the Harvard Institute for Medical simulations (Rudolph, Simon, Dufresne, & Raemer, 2006, p. 49). Critical care simulation instructors within our program are required to

Table 36.1 Suggested Simulation Timeline

Approximate Time (Minutes)	Simulator Actions	Voice Script (Indicating Who Says What)	Anticipated Trainee Actions	Comments/Directions
00:00	HR: 116 beats/minute, BP: 128/77 mmHg, pulse oximetry: 100% on 2 L/minute via NC, RR: 29 breaths/minute.	HPS complains of chest pain of nondescript severe quality.	Should start physical exam and start to get some labs. Ask for the chart and WU from OSH. Look at CXR from OSH. Student should obtain HPI and initiate oxygen, continue drips.	OSH chart have been lost in transport. CXR is the only thing available. Display CXR when requested. CXR reveals mild–moderate widened mediastinum.
02:00			Student should discuss DDX with team.	Robust list of DDX should be developed, including MI, PE, and dissection.
03:00		Patient continues with pain. Lots of moaning.	Administer IV narcotic. Order CT scan. Order labs (hemoglobin and hematocrit [H/H], BMP, type and cross).	Simulation can be paused for patient going to CT scanner.
05:00			Start esmolol for HR control, then nitroprusside for BP control, for suspected aortic dissection.	Goal BP and HR should be discussed. Other appropriate treatments may be used (i.e., labetalol, etc.). Faculty should be familiar with a variety of treatment options.
07:00	RR elevates to 40s. Gasping patient.	Patient gasps from sudden, severe pain. Has difficulty breathing and is unable to speak a few words at once.	Begins rapid sequence intubation.	Patient completes his aortic rupture at this time. If an appropriate airway is not established patient should decompensate to cardiac arrest.
08:00	BP falls to 60/30 mmHg with thready pulse. HR: 100 beats/minute while on esmolol. (HR >140 beats/minute if not on esmolol).		CT scan is available and viewed. Students identify aortic dissection and rupture. Aggressive blood resuscitation initiated. Consider exsanguination protocol with rapid infuser. Consider whole-blood transfusion strategy.	Hct of 17% is reported from lab, if previously ordered.

Time		
11:00	Consult called with vascular surgery.	Student should verbalize HPI and CT findings. Recommend emergent case. If student is unable to succinctly discuss case, consultant should refuse to take to OR and should refuse to see patient until specific diagnosis is identified and appropriate recommendation from the team is made.
14:00	SBP should be maintained less than 90 mmHg, HR <80 beats/minute.	Serial Hgb used to track blood product administration.
16:00		Vascular surgeon arrives to take patient to the OR. He or she requests a bedside discussion with the team for case information and critical care team recommendations.

BMP, basic metabolic panel; BP, blood pressure; CXR, chest x-ray; DDx, differential diagnosis; Hct, hematocrit; Hgb, hemoglobin; HPI, history of present illness; HPS, human patient simulator; HR, heart rate; MI, myocardial infarction; OR, operating room; OSH, outside hospital; PE, pulmonary embolism; RR, respiratory rate; SBP, systolic blood pressure; WU, workup.

complete the Comprehensive Instructor in Medical Simulation workshop through the Harvard Institute for Medical Simulation in order to provide superlative quality and independent high-fidelity simulation instruction. This requirement ensures that instructors are trained to interact appropriately with students following an emotionally charged simulation and have the skills to construct a framework for robust clinically focused debriefing (Decker et al., 2013).

Critical care simulations can be highly stressful and emotionally challenging for many students. Ideally, the initiation into the debriefing session becomes an important step to allow students to decompress emotionally before the clinical portion of the debriefing. In particular, debriefing should be cautiously undertaken when there has been a poor outcome to the HPS related to the students' simulation performance. A typical debriefing session starts with posing the question, "How do you feel?" to the student group collectively. Students are then allowed to openly discuss their feelings and overall opinion of the simulation scenario. During this time the instructor observes the group and, if needed, may guide the students to discuss their reactions to the simulation.

The clinical portion of the debriefing focuses largely on the students' cognitive processes during the course of the simulation scenario. The group is typically queried regarding its differential diagnosis, therapeutic interventions, and overall team management skills. In a complex scenario such as this, it is better to identify one or two single clinical issues for discussion rather than attempting to cover all clinical aspects of the scenario.

Potential clinical points of discussion include the following:

1. Critical care team management
2. Differential diagnosis of chest pain
3. Treatment of aortic emergencies (dissection and rupture)
4. Transfusion strategies for exsanguination
5. Interaction with consultants

H. SUGGESTIONS/KEY FEATURES TO REPLICATE OR IMPROVE

Variations of this simulation have been used over the past 5 academic years, with continued improvements to the clinical debriefing and timing of clinical simulation events. As this simulation is used as part of a simulation curriculum, instructors should be aware that the simulation may need adjustment based on students' needs or issues. For example, if students struggle with the need for rapid differential diagnosis, the scenario may be adjusted to run more slowly with a focus on diagnostics or, if needed, the consultation may be excluded. If students are able to rapidly identify the diagnosis, the simulation can be increased in difficulty by increasing the rate of physiologic decompensation, requiring improved resuscitation efforts, or by inclusion of a hemothorax requiring chest tube insertion during the scenario.

I. RECOMMENDATIONS FOR FURTHER USE

This scenario was developed specifically for AGACNP students who require training in critical care. The scenario itself is of moderate difficulty but has the additional challenge for students of managing their own team while rapidly consulting surgical services to provide definitive surgical intervention. This scenario should be used only for master's- and doctoral-level AGACNP students specializing in critical care. In addition to clinical learning, this scenario provides a robust assessment of student competencies in team management, airway management, aortic emergencies, and requesting consultant services.

J. HOW SIMULATION-BASED PEDAGOGY HAS CONTRIBUTED TO IMPROVED STUDENT OUTCOMES

Critical care simulations can be emotionally stressful and challenging for students. Preparation should be undertaken by simulation instructors to understand the psychological stress placed on students when using high-fidelity experiential simulations before undertaking them with students. Critical care simulations provide the most benefit when used as part of a robust critical care training program that includes didactic, clinical rotations, and simulation experiences. Critical care simulations should have both clinical and cognitive objectives linked to each simulation. Students presented with a robust critical care simulation curriculum build an experiential library for future clinical practice. Simulations that require students to interact with consultants can be used to teach rapid communication skills for critical care practice.

K. EXPERT RECOMMENDATIONS AND WORDS OF WISDOM

- Is it okay to use faculty as the consultant in the simulation? Historically, this simulation has used both faculty and actors in the role of the vascular consultant. Ideally, the consultant should be someone who is unfamiliar to the student because this adds to the realism of the simulation. Typically, when faculty known to the student before the simulation are used as the consultant, students tend to have difficulty deciding whether they are communicating with the "vascular consultant," as in this scenario, or their faculty member in a faculty role.

- What to do if students perform poorly? Following the poor performance, students are debriefed in the standard fashion with a focus on what they might do differently next time. Two potential techniques are then used with the students when they perform poorly during the simulation. The first technique allows the students to immediately repeat the simulation using what they have learned from the first simulation to enhance their performance. This can be helpful in that students have the ability to redeem themselves following a poor performance. The second technique uses a faculty member in the room to facilitate student interaction. During the facilitated simulation, the faculty member can briefly stop the simulation and use teachable moments to improve student performance. Regardless of technique, students should always be allowed to repeat the scenario if there was a poor outcome for the HPS. This allows students to regain clinical confidence and recognize their growing clinical ability.

- What is the ideal size of the student critical care team for use in the scenario? Ideally, the student team should be able to function like an inpatient critical care team, which classically ranges from about two to eight members, depending on the ICU team staffing model. In the simulation, a student identifies as the team leader and assigns roles for the other students (e.g., airway management, patient assessment, recorder, provider to do procedures) as the clinical situation deems appropriate. A team of six provides an appropriate number to facilitate the potential assigned roles but keeps the team small enough to have effective communication and discussion regarding diagnosis and treatment of the HPS during the course of the simulation.

REFERENCES

American Association of Colleges of Nursing. (2006). *The essentials of doctoral education for advanced nursing practice.* Washington, DC: Author. Retrieved from http://www.aacnnursing.org/Portals/42/Publications/DNPEssentials.pdf

American Association of Colleges of Nursing. (2011). *The essentials of master's education in nursing.* Washington, DC: Author. Retrieved from http://www.aacnnursing.org/Portals/42/Publications/MastersEssentials11.pdf

Decker, S., Fey, M., Sideras, S., Caballero, S., Rockstraw, L., Boese, T.,...Borum, J. C. (2013). Standards of best practice: Simulation Standard VI: The debriefing process. *Clinical Simulation in Nursing, 9*(6), S26–S29. doi:10.1016/j.ecns.2013.04.008

Rudolph, J. W., Simon, R., Dufresne, R. L., & Raemer, D. B. (2006). There's no such thing as "nonjudgmental" debriefing: A theory and method for debriefing with good judgment. *Simulation in Healthcare, 1*(1), 49–55.

FURTHER READING

Marino, P. L. (2014). *The ICU book* (4th ed., pp. 195–215). Philadelphia, PA: Lippincott Williams & Wilkins.

Bowen, F., & Dellinger, R. P. (Eds.). (2014). Acute aortic dissection. In J. Parillo & R. P. Dellinger (Eds.), *Critical care medicine: Principles of diagnosis and management in the adult* (4th ed., pp. 576–584). Philadelphia, PA: Mosby Elsevier.

Dries, D. J. (Ed.). (2014). Traumatic shock and tissue hypoperfusion: Nonsurgical management. In J. Parillo & R. P. Dellinger (Eds.), *Critical care medicine: Principles of diagnosis and management in the adult* (4th ed., pp. 409–431). Philadelphia, PA: Mosby Elsevier.

PART III

Interdisciplinary and Interprofessional Scenarios

CHAPTER 37

Placental Abruption After Motor Vehicle Accident: An Interprofessional Simulation

Jenna A. LoGiudice and Anka Roberto

A. IMPLEMENTATION OF SIMULATION-BASED PEDAGOGY IN YOUR INDIVIDUALIZED TEACHING AREA

Central to providing nursing care to pregnant women is the reminder that for low-risk women the goals are empowerment and support of a natural, physiological birth. Having a physiological perspective recognizes that birth is a normal, developmental process in which women benefit from holistic care with as little intervention as possible. This underpinning is at the core of the maternal and newborn nursing curriculum.

However, nurses must also be prepared to quickly recognize and react should an obstetric emergency occur, in order to safeguard maternal and fetal well-being. During obstetric emergencies seconds of time matter. To ensure that the new graduate nurses are poised to provide care in all contexts of birth, they must practice caring for women in emergent scenarios. In the clinical setting, if an obstetric emergency occurs, students become observers and passive learners, given the high-stakes situation in which maternal and fetal lives are at risk. However, in simulation scenarios, students can become actively engaged in making clinical decisions and gain confidence in recognizing the signs and symptoms of obstetric emergencies.

In the case of a placental abruption, both maternal and fetal well-being depend on the ability of RNs, certified registered nurse anesthetist (CRNAs), anesthesiologists, certified nurse midwives (CNMs), and obstetricians (OBs) working together efficiently as a team to identify and treat the situation with emergent delivery of the infant. Placental abruption, when the placenta detaches from the wall of the uterus before the birth of the infant, has many possible underlying causes, including vasospasm related to maternal hypertension or cocaine use, abdominal trauma related to a motor vehicle accident, direct trauma to the abdomen (accidental or purposeful such as in intimate partner violence [IPV]), or other forms of injury during pregnancy (Oyelese & Ananth, 2006). The textbook presentation of a rigid, board-like abdomen with dark-red vaginal bleeding does not always occur if the abruption is partial or concealed, which results in subtler signs and symptoms (Oyelese & Ananth, 2006; Tikkanen, 2011; Tikkanen, Nuutila, Hiilesmaa, Paavonen, & Ylikorkala, 2006). Educating the students to assess pregnant women with pain, bleeding, or symptoms indicating a placental abruption is imperative to maternal and fetal survival.

Student recognition of an obstetric emergency is important, as is the necessity for clear and concise communication with all members of the health care team during this emergency. In the obstetric setting, this involves the RNs, CRNAs, CNMs, and OBs. This high-stakes scenario requires students to quickly assess a pregnant woman and to recognize a placental abruption, as well as to communicate these findings with the health care team. The goal is to get the patient into the operating room (OR) for a cesarean birth as quickly as possible, maintaining patient(s) (mother and infant) safety, and using therapeutic communication with the patient and family members.

The International Nursing Association for Clinical Simulation and Learning simulation Standard IX: Simulation Design (Lioce et al., 2015) is at the core of pedagogy in the development of scenarios for meaningful simulation experiences at the authors' institution. We ensure each participant has a clear plan of what their role will be before entering the simulation environment. Furthermore, we foster a read-through of the scenario to identify key risk factors (in this case a motor vehicle accident [MVA] involving a pregnant patient), to discuss the anticipated patient signs and symptoms, and to outline potential nursing care that the patient may necessitate. This purposeful prebriefing with the course faculty lead and the simulation director is conducted to allow for maintenance of professional integrity and for active and observational learning (Gloe et al., 2013).

B. EDUCATIONAL MATERIALS AVAILABLE IN YOUR TEACHING AREA AND RELATED TO YOUR SPECIALTY

Preoperative Area

Our simulation suite is equipped with a high-fidelity medical surgical room that doubles as a labor and birth (L&B) suite, a pediatric care area, or a long-term care space with a designated control room. A standardized patient (SP) enhances fidelity and humanism in the simulation. A control room with a one-way mirror is adjacent to the simulation room. The control room houses audiovisual equipment, which allows for live streaming of the simulation into the classroom. The use of the new Laerdal LLEAP software is used to control vital signs (VS) of the SP via a patient monitor. A tablet is used to display an electronic fetal heart rate (FHR) using iSimulate, an application that is available for download on an Apple mobile device. A landline is used to communicate to the provider when necessary.

Intraoperative Area

CAE's METIman is used as the high-fidelity human patient simulator (HPS) in our state-of-the-art simulated OR. A placental abruption case was originally developed by Anka Roberto and a CRNA doctoral student in 2014 using the 2013 International Nursing Association for Clinical Simulation and Learning (INACSL) simulation standards. The scenario was piloted in 2014 twice before its implementation. The simulation presented in this chapter was then further augmented and edited by both authors as they began to jointly run the simulation in 2015. Laerdal's PROMPT Birthing Simulator Infant is used during the delivery process. Laerdal's SimBaby is used to exemplify neonatal resuscitation in the immediate postnatal phase. Simulated blood products are used to allow for students to understand the process that takes place for an intraoperative blood transfusion as well as a blood warming unit. A Draeger ventilator is used to allow a rapid sequence induction (RSI) to take place to provide general anesthesia.

Postoperative Area

In the simulation room an SP playing the role of the father is used to allow for therapeutic communication techniques to take place with audiovisual capabilities.

C. SPECIFIC OBJECTIVES FOR SIMULATION USAGE WITHIN A SPECIFIC COURSE AND THE OVERALL PROGRAM

The overarching objective of this simulation is to promote interprofessional education (IPE) between DNP nurse anesthetist students and BSN students. These students will be working together in the clinical setting and the teamwork between these two cohorts is critical, especially in the fast-paced, labor and birth (L&B) setting. Furthermore, recognizing the signs and symptoms of a placental abruption, an obstetric emergency, and quickly and safely generating a plan of care among the health care team is critical to the life of the patient and her neonate.

This scenario was initially designed for Maternal and Newborn Nursing (NS314) as a flipped-classroom, advanced-level simulation. Students enrolled in this course were either second-term, third-year students or first-term, fourth-year baccalaureate students. These students take a medical–surgical course concurrently and have completed pathophysiology, pharmacology, therapeutic skills, and physical assessment courses. This scenario takes place toward the end of the semester, when the students have already had the bulk of their exposure to the maternal and newborn clinical areas. They all have had at least one experience in L&B, the neonatal intensive care unit (NICU) and postpartum and have assessed a pregnant and/or a postpartum woman as well as a newborn. In addition, before entering the maternal and newborn clinical setting, these students spend a full clinical day in the simulation environment providing postpartum assessments on static patients, as well as practicing both newborn assessment and a neonatal resuscitation on Laerdal's SimBaby. Anecdotally, the students have shared how this day prepares them for the clinical setting and helps to enhance their skills and confidence to provide excellent patient care in the hospital environment.

The DNP nurse anesthetist students have already completed their obstetric rotation and serve as content experts in this scenario. Before the start of the simulation these students teach the theory portion of the class on the role of anesthesia and the medical pain management options in labor. All nursing programs at Fairfield University strive to promote holistic nursing care, which is delivered safely and efficiently through all members of the health care team working together.

D. INTRODUCTION OF SCENARIO

Setting the Scene

In the emergency department (ED) of the local hospital, a patient (Mia) arrives to be evaluated. Mia is a G1 P0 and presents s/p (status post) an MVA at 37 weeks, 1 day gestation. Mia, with a history of scoliosis, arrives on a stretcher via ambulance in a lot of pain. She has some vaginal bleeding and is incredibly concerned about her baby. Report is given to indicate that the airbags were deployed after she was rear-ended as the driver. The emergency room (ER) RNs promptly assess her to anticipate a transfer to L&B for the imminent delivery of her newborn. Welcomed by the charge nurse, the L&B RNs assess the patient, obtain VS of both mother and fetus, obtain patient medical history (PMHx), start an intravenous (IV) line, send for blood work, and inform the attending CNM or OB/GYN.

The patient will be admitted for emergent cesarean birth because of placental abruption. The anesthetist assesses the patient recommending general anesthesia because of scoliosis of mother and the emergency condition of placental abruption. After obtaining consent, the anesthetist and the CNM/OB/GYN transfer the patient to the OR. The patient will be transferred to an OR table, anesthesia induction RSI occurs. Time-out will be performed, led by the circulating RN. Surgery will start and the scrub RN will ask for supplies. The infant is delivered not breathing, with a decreased heart rate, cyanotic, little movement, and no audible cry. The infant has an Apgar score of 2 at 1 minute. Neonatal nurses provide appropriate neonatal care following Neonatal Resuscitation Program (NRP) guidelines. The infant is resuscitated, stabilized, and brought to the father in the recovery room; the infant's 5-minute Apgar score is 7.

Technology Used

A classroom with audiovisual capability was used to live stream the recorded simulation into the classroom while the active participants were caring for Mia. The Laerdal LLEAP software is used to control VS of the SP via a patient monitor. A tablet was used to display the electronic FHR using iSimulate. An FHR strip indicating fetal distress was created, in which the FHR drops to 60 beats/minute and does not recover. A landline is needed to call members of the health care team. CAE's iStan is used in the OR. Laerdal's PROMPT Birthing Simulator Infant is used during the birthing process. Laerdal's SimBaby is used for neonatal resuscitation in the immediate postnatal phase. A Draeger ventilator was used to allow for an RSI to take place to provide general anesthesia. In addition, a pulse oximeter, blood pressure (BP) cuff, IV start tray, IV tubing, IV fluids (choices of 1,000 mL D5NS [potassium chloride in 5% dextrose and sodium chloride], Ringer, or normal saline [NS]), vials for blood collection for type and cross, Foley catheter, clippers for surgical prep, a pad with vaginal bleeding (red food coloring and water are used to simulate bleeding), O_2, face mask, Bicitra, Ancef, and external fetal monitors (toco transducer and external FHR monitor). Routine and as needed (PRN) mediations are available.

Objectives

1. Assess a third-trimester patient with abdominal pain and vaginal bleeding
2. Prioritize assessment of the fetus and identify fetal distress through fetal monitoring
3. Use therapeutic communication techniques with patient and family members
4. Maintain patient safety throughout the intraoperative period
5. Communicate efficiently with interprofessional health care team
6. Provide neonatal support and resuscitation using NRP algorithm
7. Recognize one's own limitations in skills, knowledge, and abilities to promote safe and efficient care (Interprofessional Education Collaborative [IPEC] Expert Panel, 2011).

The scenario also allows students to practice key elements from the National Council of State Boards of Nursing (2015) National Council Licensure Examination for Registered Nurses (NCLEX-RN®) test plan, including:

Safe and effective care environment: *Management of care* (advocacy; assignment, delegation and supervision; collaboration with interdisciplinary team; establishing priorities; informed consent), *Safety and infection control* (accident/error/injury prevention; standard precautions/transmission-based precautions/surgical asepsis); **Health promotion and maintenance:** (ante/intra/postpartum and newborn care, techniques of physical assessment); **Psychosocial integrity:** (family dynamics; therapeutic communication); **Physiological integrity:** *Basic care and comfort* (nonpharmacological comfort interventions), *Pharmacological and parenteral therapies* (parenteral/intravenous therapies; pharmacological pain management), *Reduction of risk potential* (changes/abnormalities in vital signs; laboratory values, potential for alterations in body systems, potential for complications from surgical procedures and health alterations, system specific assessments, vital signs), *Physiological adaptation* (hemodynamics, medical emergencies, pathophysiology)

For this scenario, the American Association of Colleges of Nursing (AACN; 2008) *Essentials of Baccalaureate Education for Professional Nursing Practice* items addressed include the following:

Essential I: Liberal Education for Baccalaureate Generalist Nursing Practice, Objectives 2, 7
Essential II: Basic Organization and Systems Leadership, Objectives 1, 7, 8
Essential IV: Information Management and Applications of Patient Care Technology, Objectives 1, 5, 6
Essential VI: Interprofessional Communication and Collaboration for Improving Patient Health Outcomes, Objectives 1, 2, 4, 6
Essential VIII: Professionalism and Professional Values, Objectives 6, 9
Essential IX: Baccalaureate Generalist Nursing Practice, Objectives 3, 5, 12, 21

Description of Participants

Triage RN

Role: As triage RN, you are to maintain patient safety, recognize signs and symptoms of placental abruption, assess patient (Pt.) and fetus (FHR). Obtain past medical history. Make recommendations.

Skills: Obtain VS and PMHx. Start IV and draw labs, including complete blood count (CBC) and type and screen (T&S) blood test. Inform health care provider (OB/GYN or CNM) of obstetrics emergency and give any recommendations.

Labor and Birth RNs

Role: As an L&B RN your role is to maintain patient safety, recognize signs and symptoms of surgical complications, communicate clearly with surgical team, and communicate to NICU team of stat (statim) cesarean birth.

Skills: Recognize the signs of an obstetric emergency. Interpret fetal heart rate patterns.

Charge RN

Role: You are the managing nurse on the OB floor for the shift. You must be aware of and help the new patient throughout the admission.

Skills: Assist where necessary. Assess needs of all involved and determine when you can help. Watch front desk of unit while patient is being attended to. Report any abnormal or pertinent lab reports that are called in.

Circulating RN

Role: As the circulating nurse, you must be aware of patient safety at all times. You must lead surgical time-out and stay vigilant throughout the case, anticipating patient and staff needs, and communicate clearly with the surgical team.

Skills: Grounding Bovie, position patient (L [lateral]), Foley catheter, attend to surgeon and anesthetist needs and supplies. Run OR time-out (stating out loud the patient name, medical record number [MRN], the procedure to be performed, PT drug allergies, antibiotics ordered and given, type of anesthesia, and any anticipated complications).

Neonatal RNs (2)

Role: Assist where necessary and ensure safety of both mother and child. Once born, you must be ready to provide any supportive assistance that the baby may need in the first 10 minutes of life.

Skills: Assist a struggling neonate immediately following birth, including assessment, suctioning/clearing of airway, NRP, provide positive pressure ventilation (PPV) and continuous positive airway pressure (CPAP).

CRNA

Role: Provide safe anesthesia care, including RSI, appropriate anesthetic choice, monitoring of VS, monitoring of input and output (I&O), and communicating clearly with surgical team.

Skills: Assess and consent the patient for surgery and plan for the appropriate anesthesia in the setting of an obstetric emergency. Administer antibiotics. Administer anesthesia and monitor patient as needed. Assess blood loss, assess laboratory values, and intervene as necessary.

CNM/OB (This Role Has Been Fulfilled by the Faculty to Add to the Cohesiveness of the Simulation)

Role: When the RNs on L&B call for a consult of the patient you arrive and receive report. You assess Pt. and diagnose the placental abruption and perform the C-section.

Skills: Use effective communication, request materials (lap pads, Bovie settings to "40/40," etc.), and report the amount of blood loss.

E. RUNNING OF THE SCENARIO

The simulation itself begins with the patient, Mia, arriving on a stretcher via ambulance in the Sim Room, where audiovisual equipment captures the triage process. The observers in the classroom have been given observation roles such as observing for safety, interprofessional communication, communication with patient and family members, patient assessment, and prioritization. The triaging of Mia occurs in the Sim Room (L&B), where nurses must work quickly to assess Mia and recognize that she is experiencing a placental abruption. They are responsible for calling the CRNA and CNM on call using the situation, background, assessment, and recommendation (SBAR) format to communicate the patient's status as well as that of the fetus (Institute for Healthcare Improvement, 2015; Scarrow, 2009). The entire team must then work to quickly and safely get Mia into the OR for an emergency cesarean birth. During this process a time-out is called. After the baby is delivered unresponsive, the neonatal RNs work to resuscitate the infant and communicate with Mia's partner what has occurred.

The simulation is run as a flipped-classroom experience involving the entire class. The simulation is prebriefed to go over expectations, fears, and worries, which allows for psychological safety. Prebriefing also focuses on roles to watch for and best practices in caring for an obstetric patient during an emergency. A presimulation lecture on anesthesia options in the obstetrical environment is given by a CRNA student using visual aides to assist students to understand anatomical consideration for neuraxial anesthesia such as spinals and epidurals. As the scenario is briefed with the students who will be active observers, students do not know exactly what will happen with the case. The briefing with the active observers as well as active participants allows full involvement of all students. As the scenario is running, the active observers watch the simulation live in the classroom, taking notes of opportunities that exemplified teamwork and those that afforded an opportunity for improved communication. After, as debriefing unfolds using Debriefing for Meaningful Learning (Dreifuerst, 2011), the active student participants are given the opportunity to verbalize clinical reasoning and clinical decision making. These decisions are sometimes challenged by the active observers, making for a more robust debriefing.

F. PRESENTATION OF COMPLETED TEMPLATE

Title

Placental Abruption Status Post MVA

Scenario Level

Second-term, third-year students or first-term, fourth-year; second- or third-year DNP nurse anesthetist students

Focus Area

RNs, nurse anesthetists, CNMs

Scenario Description and Objectives

Expected simulation run time: 20 to 30 minutes
Location: Local hospital

Interprofessional simulation learning objectives:

1. Assess a third-trimester patient with abdominal pain and vaginal bleeding
2. Prioritize assessment of the fetus and identify fetal distress through fetal monitoring

3. Use therapeutic communication techniques with patient and family members

4. Maintain patient safety throughout the intraoperative period

5. Communicate efficiently with interprofessional health care team

6. Provide neonatal support and resuscitation using NRP algorithm

7. Recognize one's own limitations in skills, knowledge, and abilities to promote safe and efficient care (IPEC, 2011).

Scenario Implementation

The template for the placental abruption interprofessional simulation is shown in Exhibit 37.1. Exhibit 37.2 outlines the scenario progression, adapted for a flipped-classroom environment.

G. DEBRIEFING GUIDELINES

How did you think the simulation went? Describe the outcomes you were able to achieve. Were you satisfied with your ability to work through the simulation? To Observer/s: Could the team have handled any aspects of the simulation differently? If you were able to complete this scenario again, how could you have handled the situation differently? What did the group do well? What were the key assessments and interventions?

What occurred during the scenario that made you realize you needed assistance from team members from other disciplines? How did communication between disciplines support patient care? How did the contributions of other disciplines impact the care you provided?

H. SUGGESTIONS/KEY FEATURES TO REPLICATE OR IMPROVE

It is key to replicate use of standardized patients each year. Human behaviors require human responses and having an SP, such as Mia and her husband, adds to the reality- of this situation. This simulation could also have improvements surrounding equipment, for example, applying an actual FHR monitor would be beneficial for the students to practice with as currently we use "mock" monitors and an FHR Doppler. Once the students apply the "mock" monitor, we start the iSimulate Electronic FHR (EFHR) tracing for them to interpret. As our new state-of-the-art simulation center will be complete in 1 year, we are hopeful that this simulation continues to improve. Continuing to use the iSimulate FHR via a table is a great investment for this scenario.

In addition, we have found that using a faculty member with expertise in maternal and newborn nursing is essential to fulfill the role of the CNM or the OB/GYN. A faculty member is able to provide cues to help the simulation if needed and adds a level of calmness to a very fast-paced and high-stakes scenario.

I. RECOMMENDATIONS FOR FURTHER USE

Fairfield University will be opening a nurse midwifery specialty within the DNP program in the fall of 2017. The goal is to incorporate nurse midwifery students into the simulation as Mia's provider. Nurse midwives first assist during cesarean birth and will do so in the simulation. The addition of nurse midwives (or medical or physician assistant students if you have a medical school at your university) allows for true conceptualization of the health care team and how the moving parts all work together quickly, safely, and efficiently to promote optimal maternal–fetal outcomes when seconds matter.

Admission Date:

Today's Date:

Brief Description of Client

Name: Mia; **Gender:** F **Age:** 27 **Race:** White

Weight: 77kg (120 pounds) **Height:** 5'7"

Religion: Catholic

Major Support: Partner/husband

Allergies: None

Immunizations: Rubella immune

Attending Physician/Team: Jenna, CNM

Past Medical History: Scoliosis

History of Present Illness: MVA

Social History: Negative ETOH, negative smoking, negative illicit substances; married; works as a middle school teacher

Primary Medical Diagnosis: Pregnant, gestational age 37 weeks, 1 day; placental abruption

Surgeries/Procedures and Dates: no PSHx

Problem List: Pregnant

Medications: Prenatal vitamins, vitamin D

Setting/Environment:

- ER
- Med-Surg
- Peds
- ICU
- OR/PACU
- Women's center
- Behavioral health
- Home health
- Prehospital
- Other _____

Psychomotor Skills Required Before Simulation (by Discipline):

RN

Assessment of pregnant patient

Neonatal resuscitation (NRP)

Fetal-monitoring strip interpretation

IV start

Surgical prep

Nurse Anesthetist:

Intubation

Ordering blood products

Cognitive Activities Required Prior to Simulation:

- CRNA lectures 15 minutes before simulation on obstetric anesthesia options and needs of the laboring/birthing mother.
- The BSN students have had readings and lecture regarding placental abruption and obstetric emergencies. They have also spent an early simulation day practicing NRP.

Terminology: Stat c/s.

Medications and Fluids:

- IV fluids: Lactated Ringer's solution
- Oral meds: Bicitra
- IVPB: Ancef 1 g

Human Patient Simulator/s Needed:

HPS: CAE's METIman/Laerdal SimMan3G, Laerdal's PROMPT Birthing Simulator Infant, Laerdal's SimBaby

Props:

Pad with blood (water and red food coloring); clippers for shaving for surgical prep

Equipment Attached to Simulator:

- IV pump
- O$_2$
- Monitor attached
- ID band on

Equipment Available in Room:

- Bedpan/urinal
- Foley kit

Diagnostics Available:

Labs:

- X-rays (images)
- 12-lead EKG
- Other electronic fetal monitoring: (TOCO and ultrasound)

Documentation Forms:

- Physician orders
- Admit orders
- Flow sheet
- Medication administration record
- Kardex
- Graphic record
- Shift assessment
- Triage forms

(continued)

- o Straight catheter kit
- o Fluids
- o IV start kit
- o IV tubing
- o IVPB tubing
- o IV pump
- o Pressure bag
- o O$_2$ delivery device (type)
- o Crash cart with airway devices and emergency medications
- o Defibrillator/pacer
- o Suction
- o Electric razor
- o Fetal monitor (simulated**)**
- o Fetal monitor strap

- o Code record
- o Anesthesia/PACU record
- o Standing (protocol) orders
- o Transfer orders
- o Discipline-specific documents
- o Other_____

Recommended Mode for Simulation: Manual

Standardized Patients Needed:

Role: Patient (Mia), partner/husband

Age/gender: Reproductive age woman, reproductive age male

Student Information Needed Before Scenario:

- • Has been oriented to simulator.
- • Understands guidelines/expectations for scenario.
- • Has accomplished all presimulation reading and online module requirements.
- • All participants understand their assigned roles.
- • Has been given time frame expectations.

Roles/Guidelines for Roles

- o Primary nurse, secondary nurse
- o Clinical instructor
- o Family member #1
- o Family member #2
- o Observer/s
- o Recorder
- o Physician/CNM
- o Respiratory therapy
- o Anesthesia
- o Pharmacy
- o Lab
- o Imaging
- o Social services
- o Clergy
- o Unlicensed assistive personnel
- o Code team
- o Other: Neonatal RN, CNM, OB/GYN

Important Information Related to Roles:

Understanding psychosocial stressors of childbearing woman and trauma of situation.

Physician Orders:

None at start of simulation given emergency case

Report Students Receive Before Simulation:

In the ED of the local hospital, a patient (Mia) arrives to be evaluated. Mia is a 28-year-old G1 P0 at 37 weeks, 1 day gestation who presents s/p an MVA. She was rear ended while driving and the airbags were deployed. She arrives on a stretcher via ambulance, is in a lot of pain all over, and is incredibly concerned about her baby. She is experiencing some vaginal bleeding. PMHx, scoliosis; PSHx, none. Medications: Prenatal vitamins, vitamin D. She is AOx3 with rapid pulse. VS: BP, 99/56 mmHg; HR, 105 beats/minute; SaO$_2$, 98%, temperature, 99.1°F

Time: 9:30 a.m.

AOx3, aldehyde oxidase 3; BSN, bachelor of science in nursing; CNM, certified nurse midwife; CRNA, certified registered nurse anesthetist; ED, emergency department; ETOH, ethyl alcohol; FHR, fetal heart rate; HPS, human patient simulator; IV, intravenous; IVPB, intravenous piggyback; MVA, motor vehicle accident; PACU, postanesthesia care unit; PMHx, past medical history; PSHx, past surgical history; s/p, status post; stat c/s, immediate cesarean section; VS, vital signs.

Adapted from Child, Sepples, and Chambers (2007). © 2008, National League for Nursing.

Exhibit 37.2	Scenario Progression Outline: Adapted for Flipped-Classroom Environment		
Timing (Approximate)	**Simulator Actions or Standardized Patient Action**	**Expected Interventions**	**May Use the Following Cues**
9:30 a.m.	SP screaming in pain, HR elevated, BP elevated, RR elevated.	Triage RN assesses Pt., obtains PMHx and prenatal Hx, calls the provider.	Role member providing cue: Mia Cue: "Are you not going to do something, I am in so much pain, is my baby going to be okay?"
9:40 a.m.	SP continues to scream in pain and is worrying about her baby.	Charge nurse, labor and birth RN: Assess Pt., obtain VS of mother and fetus, obtain PMHx, start IV and send blood work, communicate with CNM/OB/GYN.	Role member providing cue: Mia Cue: "Where is my midwife? I was supposed to have a natural birth, why is this happening?"
9:45 a.m.	SP and family member are expressing concern about why she needs a c-section.	Anesthesia and CNM/OB/GYN team: Obtain consent for procedure, inform Pt. and family member of situation, transfer to OR.	Role member providing cue: Mia Cue: "I do not understand why this is happening?"
9:50 a.m.	Surgical team is in place and Mia is transferred off of stretcher and HPS used for intraoperative period. SP: Father/family member is escorted to recovery room to wait for his baby to be delivered.	Time-out performed by medical team, surgery starts, critical H&H, order 1 unit PRBCs hung.	Role member providing cue: CRNA Cue: "Did anyone get her crit?"
9:55 a.m. 10:00 a.m. 10:05 a.m.	HPS Sim Baby used for NRP: 0RR, no cry, bradycardia, no movement, cyanosis, flaccid Sim Baby responsive, HR 132, RR 38, shrill cry, acrocyanotic, poor tone SP: Father/family member receives baby in recovery room, nervously awaiting wife to come out.	NICU RNs: NRP, Apgar scoring, PPV and delivery assessment of infant. NICU RNs: Complete cardiovascular and respiratory assessment, obtain first set of VS, communicate Apgar scores to provider. NICU RNs: Communicate clearly and effectively with family member regarding baby's status, inform approximate timeframe to expect infant's mother.	Role member providing cue: OB/midwife Cue: "How is that baby doing over there?" Role member providing cue: OB/midwife Cue: "Everything looking better. What were Apgars?"

BP, blood pressure; CNM, certified nurse midwife; CRNA, certified registered nurse anesthetist; ED, emergency department; H&H, hemoglobin and hematocrit; HPS, human patient simulator; HR, heart rate; Hx, history; IV, intravenous; NICU, neonatal intensive care unit; NRP, Neonatal Resuscitation Program; PMHx, past medical history; Pt., patient; SP, standardized patient; RR, respiratory rate; VS, vital signs.

Adapted from Child, Sepples, and Chambers (2007). © 2008, National League for Nursing.

J. HOW SIMULATION-BASED PEDAGOGY HAS
CONTRIBUTED TO IMPROVED STUDENT OUTCOMES

Simulation pedagogy has engaged our learners to allow for transfer of knowledge into practice. Using Kolb's experiential learning theory (Kolb, 1984; Lisko & O'Dell, 2010) as a framework within our simulation center has allowed the pedagogy to evolve. Students consistently evaluate their simulated learning experiences positively. They identify knowledge translation and the ability to gain the confidence needed to work in teams. Many verbalized their ability to make fast and wise decisions in a safe and effective manner after participating in this simulation. They also prioritize care with ease, perceive that they make sound clinical decisions, and feel positive about their work as a member of an interprofessional team. Students readily mention their overall comfort with speaking to health care providers, which would have otherwise felt intimidating. Most important, students learn how to actively engage family members and use therapeutic communication techniques in a high-stakes simulation.

K. EXPERT RECOMMENDATIONS
AND WORDS OF WISDOM

We have run this simulation with a total of 10 different BSN and DNP CRNA student cohorts (ranging in size from 34 to 50 students each time). What works well in this large flipped-classroom simulation is the engagement of the active observers who are assigned to directly observe for evidence of teamwork and communication. These focused areas have a positive impact during the debriefing phase, which relates to INACSL Standard VI (Decker et al., 2013), and we find all students are engaged and contribute more fully to the debriefing with this assignment.

The scenario can be run without the use of CRNA students by shifting the focus completely to the BSN students' assessment of a pregnant patient in the third trimester who has abdominal pain and bleeding. The element of interprofessional collaboration (Standard IX; Lioce et al., 2015) with the nurse anesthesia students does foster communication across disciplines; however, the simulation can still be a meaningful learning experience for BSN students to recognize the obstetric emergency that is occurring and to respond quickly to prepare the patient for a cesarean birth.

In addition, having run this simulation both with a SimMan patient and a live actor; we found that the live actor facilitated students' comfort with touching the patient and having someone crying out in pain directly in front of them. When Jenna LoGiudice was pregnant she filled the role of Mia, which was serendipitous timing and helpful to the students who had to actually auscultate an FHR on her abdomen. The students continually respond, "That was just so stressful, we had to actually find a fetal heart rate and it was taking so long." They also said, "We were just afraid to touch her [Jenna's] belly because there really was a baby in there, but knew we had to." It adds to this scenario to have a member of the community or standardized pregnant patient act as Mia.

L. EVALUATION OF BEST PRACTICE STANDARDS
AND USE OF CREDENTIALED SIMULATION FACULTY

The standards of best practice in simulation (Sittner et al., 2015) have been woven throughout this simulation (see Chapter 1 for references to the standards). Terminology used (Standard I), professional integrity (Standard II), and participant objectives (Standard III) are all used in the prebrief phases of the simulation. Facilitation and Facilitator (Standards IV and V) are conducted by our Director of Simulation, INACSL Sim Fellow, and NLN Sim Lead Fellow, Anka Roberto. Debriefing is streamlined using Debriefing for Meaningful Learning as a standard debriefing technique (Standard VI). The facilitator has four years' experience in full-time simulation education and is working toward Certified Healthcare Simulation Educator (CHSE) certification. Participants are all evaluated using a Survey Monkey app (VII). Standard VIII is used given the IPE nature of the simulation, and the simulation design (Standard IX) follows INACSL's recommendations.

REFERENCES

American Association of Colleges of Nursing. (2008). *The essentials of baccalaureate education for professional nursing practice.* Retrieved from http://www.aacnnursing.org/Portals/42/Publications/BaccEssentials08.pdf

Child, J. C., Sepples, S. B., Chambers, K. (2007). Designing simulations for nursing education. In P. R. Jeffries (Ed.), *Simulation in nursing education: From conceptualization to evaluation* (pp. 42–58). Washington, DC: National League for Nursing. Retrieved from http://sirc.nln.org

Decker, S., Fey, M., Sideras, S., Caballero, S., Rockstraw, L., Boese, T., . . . Borum, J. C. (2013). Standards of best practice: Simulation standard VI: The debriefing process. *Clinical Simulation in Nursing, 9*(6S), S26–S29.

Dreifuerst, K. T. (2011). Debriefing for meaningful learning: A reflective strategy to foster clinical reasoning. *Clinical Simulation in Nursing, 7*(6), e250. doi:10.1016/j.ecns.2011.09.023

Gloe, D., Sando, C. R., Franklin, A. E., Boese, T., Decker, S., Lioce, L., & Borum, J. C. (2013). Standards of best practice: Simulation Standard II: Professional integrity of participant(s). *Clinical Simulation in Nursing, 9*(6S), S12–S14.

Institute for Healthcare Improvement. (2015). SBAR communication technique. Retrieved from http://www.ihi.org/sites/search/pages/results.aspx?k=sbar

Interprofessional Education Collaborative Expert Panel. (2011). *Core competencies for interprofessional collaborative practice: Report of an expert panel.* Washington, DC: Author.

Kolb, D. A. (1984). *Experiential learning: Experience as the source of learning and development.* Englewood Cliffs, NJ: Prentice-Hall. Retrieved from https://www.learning-theories.com/experiential-learning-kolb.html

Lioce, L., Meakim, C. H., Fey, M. K., Chmil, J. V., Mariani, B., & Alinier, G. (2015). Standards of best practice: Simulation standard IX: Simulation design. *Clinical Simulation in Nursing, 11*(6), 309–315.

Lisko, S. A., & O'Dell, V. (2010). Integration of theory and practice: Experiential learning theory and nursing education. *Nursing Education Perspectives, 31*(2), 106–108.

National Council of State Boards of Nursing. (2015). NCLEX- RN examination: Test plan for the National Council Licensure Examination for Registered Nurses. Retrieved from https://www.ncsbn.org/RN_Test_Plan_2016_Final.pdf

Oyelese, Y., & Ananth, C. V. (2006). Placental abruption. *Obstetrics and Gynecology, 108*(4), 1005–1016.

Sittner, B. J., Aebersold, M. L., Paige, J. B., Graham, L. L., Schram, A. P., Decker, S. I., & Lioce, L. (2015). Standards of best practice for simulation: Past, present, and future. *Nursing Education Perspectives, 36*(5), 294–298.

Scarrow, P. K. (2009). Patient safety in obstetrics and beyond. *Journal for Healthcare Quality, 31*(5), 3.

Tikkanen, M. (2011). Placental abruption: epidemiology, risk factors and consequences. *Acta Obstetricia et Gynecologica Scandinavica, 90*(2), 140–149.

Tikkanen, M., Nuutila, M., Hiilesmaa, V., Paavonen, J., & Ylikorkala, O. (2006). Clinical presentation and risk factors of placental abruption. *Acta Obstetricia et Gynecologica Scandinavica, 85*(6), 700–705.

CHAPTER 38

Interprofessional End-of-Life Care of a Teenager

Mary Ann Cordeau, Darlene Rogers, Dennis J. Brown, Barbara Glynn, Margaret B. Gray, Tania Grgurich, Jennifer L. Herbst, Christine Kasinskas, Meghan A. Lewis, Laura Mutrie, Karen M. Myrick, and Tracy Van Oss

A. IMPLEMENTATION OF SIMULATION-BASED PEDAGOGY IN YOUR INDIVIDUALIZED TEACHING AREA

Mary Ann Cordeau, PhD, RN: My focus is on developing simulation-based education (SBE) to meet the outcomes of a senior-level laboratory course offered during the spring semester.

Darlene Rogers, BSN, RN: I am involved in simulation coordination, faculty development, and faculty training for all levels of SBE at Quinnipiac University.

Dennis J. Brown, MPH, PA-C, DFAAPA: My role in the physician assistant (PA) program has been to enhance the usage of simulation in the educational process of the PA students.

Barbara Glynn, DNP, RN-BC: My focus is on interprofessional simulation, which provides the opportunity to learn how to communicate, collaborate, and experience challenging patient situations as a team of multiple disciplines.

Margaret B. Gray, DNP, MSN, RN-BC: My focus is on the final cumulative debriefing wherein students are provided the ability to pull their experiences together, and reflect and compare their perceptions to those of an actual survivor of the same disease.

Tania Grgurich, DHSc RT(R)(M)(CT)ARRT: I have developed a variety of formative and summative simulation scenarios for radiographic procedures and the radiation exposure laboratory courses that I teach.

Jennifer L. Herbst, JD, M. Bioethics, LLM: I have worked with faculty colleagues in the law and medical schools and across the schools of nursing and health sciences to reenvision the role of law and lawyers in promoting patient and community health.

Christine Kasinskas, PT, DPT: I initiated the use of simulation in the physical therapy (PT) program to introduce and familiarize students with acute care and especially the intensive care unit (ICU) environment.

Meghan A. Lewis, MA, ATC, LAT: My main focus is on incorporating simulation into the emergency management component of the athletic training (AT) profession and to expand into other aspects in the future.

Laura Mutrie, MSW, LCSW: I have worked to incorporate simulated patient experiences into the social work practice curriculum and to develop scenarios for interprofessional and classroom implementation.

Karen M. Myrick, DNP, APRN, FNP-BC, ANP-BC: I am actively involved in interprofessional education (IPE) and working to involve nurse practitioner and nursing students in simulation as a clinically relevant method of education.

Tracy Van Oss, DHSc, MPH, OTR/L, FAOTA: The occupational therapy (OT) department uses simulation as a part of the coursework to teach students to communicate, evaluate, and provide therapeutic interventions.

B. EDUCATIONAL MATERIALS AVAILABLE IN YOUR TEACHING AREA AND RELATED TO YOUR SPECIALITY

The clinical simulation laboratory at Quinnipiac University is a self-contained unit with five acute/chronic/community care rooms, each with a patient and control area separated by one-way glass. The model apartment used in this scenario is a universally designed space for health professionals to learn how an environment can support or inhibit a person of any ability to perform activities of daily living (ADLs). The CT laboratory is a fully energized lab that houses a Toshiba Aquilion 64-slice CT unit. The CT unit is located within a fully shielded room opposite the control room.

C. SPECIFIC OBJECTIVES FOR SIMULATION USAGE WITHIN A SPECIFIC COURSE AND THE OVERALL PROGRAM

At Quinnipiac University, IPE is not attached to a specific course, rather it is currently being offered as a voluntary learning activity for interested students and faculty. IPE began several years ago with the formation of the Interprofessional Simulation Learning and Assessment Committee (ISLAC). This interdisciplinary committee worked collaboratively in the creation of Josh's Journey. Josh's Journey, a Sim-IPE, was developed to promote the ability of participants to work as a team to "cooperate, communicate, and share skills and knowledge" to provide safe and holistic care (Decker et al., 2015, p. 293). Faculty from multiple disciplinary and professional areas worked together to create the Sim-IPE based on "interprofessionality" (D'Amour & Oandasan, 2005, p. 10). A committee has been formed to incorporate the use of Sim-IPE across disciplines. Standards I to IX of the INACSL *Standards of Best Practice: Simulation*[SM] (International Nursing Association for Clinical Simulation and Learning [INACSL], 2013/2016) were used for guiding the scenario development.

D. INTRODUCTION OF SCENARIO

Setting the Scene

This scenario consists of seven scenes involving advanced practice registered nurse (APRN), AT, diagnostic imaging (DI), law, master of social work (MSW), RN, OT, PA, and PT students. Individuals from all professions work together to care for a teenage boy as his illness progresses from a diagnosis of osteosarcoma of the femur discovered after a fall on the basketball court. Josh is a high school student who lives with his parents. Each scene presented is a separate sequential Sim-IPE. Before the start of the Sim-IPE a group prebriefing is held for all participants. The role of each profession is presented. Participants are then assigned to appropriate scenes, which are scheduled over the semester. Participants are engaged in a scenario-related prebriefing and debriefing as well as a culminating debriefing. The entire scenario was filmed and will be used for interdisciplinary educational experiences. Key components of prebriefing stages included learning about end-of-life care, understanding the different interprofessional roles, and feeling comfortable with and safe in the simulation environment.

Technology Used

Depending on the scene, technology used varies and is presented at the beginning of the scene.

Specific Scenario Objectives

- Participate on a patient-centered health care team to respond to the medical and psychosocial needs of a simulated patient from onset of injury to end of life.
- Develop communication skills appropriate for responding to the needs of the patient, the patient's family, and other members of the health care team.
- Gain knowledge and insight into the stages of dying and providing end-of-life care.
- Collaborate in critical decision making and creative thinking in devising patient-centered health care team plans of care throughout the course of an illness.
- Introduce nursing/health sciences students to dispute resolution as potential attorney skillset.

Description of Participants

Prelicensure APRN, AT, DI, Law, MSW, PA, PT, OT, and RN students participate in the appropriate scenes. The simulated patient scenes used are live and students received scene-specific training. Scenario role players used in scenes received scene specific training.

E. RUNNING OF THE SCENARIO

Following a prebriefing , the expected run time for each scene is 20 minutes. The expected time for debriefing is 20 to 40 minutes. Each scene is sequential and conducted as a stand-alone Sim-IPE with appropriate participants.

F. PRESENTATION OF COMPLETED TEMPLATE

Title

Interprofessional End-of-Life Care of a Teenager

Scenario Level

Prelicensure students from a variety of disciplines

Focus Area

Field emergency room (ER) care, diagnostic interventions, acute care, home care, hospice care

Scenario Description

Description of Patient

Name: Joshua Williams
Gender: M
Age: 16
Weight: 160 pounds/73 kg
Height: 5 feet, 8 inches/173 cm
Marital status: Single
Religion: Catholic
Major support: Mother and father
Phone: 203-111-1111
Allergies: None

SCENE ONE: FIELD CARE

Focus Area

This scenario takes place on a basketball court. A simulated patient is laying on the ground moaning in pain.

Patient History

Josh jumped up for the ball, and his opponent crashed into his hip area. As he landed, he heard a sickening crack and felt an extreme pain in his right hip/leg.

Setting the Scene

Equipment Needed

AT kit, vacuum splint bag, an automated external defibrillator (AED), emergency O_2 tank, spine board, Gatorade coolers, radio

Resources Needed

No specific resources

Simulator Level

Simulated patient

Participants Needed

Two AT students, two emergency medical technician (EMT) scenario role players, and one team member scenario role player

Scenario Implementation

The scene begins with Josh laying on the ground moaning. The AT responds and emergency medical service (EMS) is called. A fracture of the right femur is suspected. There is diminished circulation, sensation, movement (CSM); posterior tibialis pulse point and dorsal pedal pulse are absent. Josh is complaining of nausea and light-headedness. Vital signs: blood pressure (BP), 90/70 mmHg; pulse, 134 beats/minute—weak and thready; respiratory rate (RR), 22 breaths/minute and shallow, starting to become labored.

Participant Expectations

The AT participant is expected to check the scene for safety to make sure the play has stopped and it is safe to approach the victim; communicate for someone to contact EMS using the radio; determine level of consciousness; establish airway and assess circulation; calm the athlete down while doing a visual inspection; put on protective equipment; obtain baseline vital signs, signal help to acquire vacuum splint, kit, AED, spine board; communicate with the athlete; advise bystanders to greet the EMTs; apply vacuum splint; treat for shock once leg stabilized; transfer to stretcher once EMS arrives, wheel Josh out of the basketball court en route to the ambulance.

SCENE TWO: EMERGENCY ROOM

Focus Area

Patient assessment and treatment, patient and family teaching and support

Scenario Description

Patient history: During a basketball game, Josh's femur is fractured. He was treated at the scene by an AT and was transferred to the ER via ambulance.

Setting the Scene

Equipment Needed

Computerized patient simulator dressed in sports clothing, identification bracelet, backboard and collar, hare traction, splint on the right leg, cardiac monitor with automated BP, pulse oximetry, intravenous (IV) equipment, normal C-spine (cervical spine) x-ray, fractured midshaft femur x-ray.

Simulator Level

High-fidelity—computerized patient simulator

Participants Needed

APRN/PA student, two RN students, one AT student, one MSW student, and two EMT scenario role players

Scenario Implementation

The scenario starts with Josh on a stretcher in the ER. On arrival at the ER, the AT communicates the facts of the case with the intake team, consisting of a PA/APRN and two RN students. AT remains on site to ensure that the athlete is stable. Josh is complaining of a level-10 pain in his right leg. He has been transported to the ER in full spinal immobilization via ambulance and is being evaluated by the PA/APRN and two RNs. The MSW student is also on the scene to support the patient and the mother, who arrives a few minutes after the scenario begins.

Participant Expectations

APRN/PA: Obtain a history, including past medical history (PMH), medications allergies, social history (SH), last meal; perform secondary trauma survey; work with the nurses to disrobe patient while maintaining appropriate immobilization; order appropriate diagnostics (x-rays, labs, EKG) and interpret the results; order appropriate medications and therapeutics, including forward thinking of possible progression to operating room (OR), therefore, ensuring nothing by mouth (NPO) status, IV, analgesia, and so on.

MSW: Provide emotional support and empathetic calming to the distressed mother.

RN: Assess vital signs; assist team members with disrobing; discuss findings and treatments with other members of the team; receive and verbalize provider orders; documents injuries, evaluations, medications, interventions; administer IV pain medication and oxygen; communicates holistically with patient and mother.

SCENE THREE: ILLNESS DISCLOSURE

Scenario Level

Prelicensure APRN, MSW, OT, PT, RN students

Focus Area

Communication, patient and family teaching, patient family support

Scenario Description

This scenario depicts a patient in the orthopedic unit recovering from a surgical repair of a fractured femur. The patient is lying on the hospital bed with his eyes closed. His mother and father are sitting with him at the bedside. The team comes in to speak to the patient and family about the pathology results of the suspicious lesion found during surgery.

Patient history: Josh is a 16-year-old athlete who fractured his femur as a result of an injury on the basketball court. He underwent an open reduction internal fixation (ORIF) of his femur and, during the procedure, the surgeon saw a suspicious lesion, which was biopsied. Josh is currently in the orthopedic unit. The biopsy results have come back and show that Josh has osteosarcoma. The team will be speaking to Josh and his family today about the diagnosis and treatment options.

Setting the Scene

Equipment Needed

Simulated patient wearing a hospital gown; identification bracelet with patient's name, date of birth, and medical record number. Hospital bed, overbed table, three chairs, call bell, IV pump and 1,000-mL bag of lactated Ringer's solution, posted crutches, gait belt, and long-handle reacher.

Technology Used

No specific technology is needed

Participants Needed

One simulated patient, one MSW student, one RN student, one APRN student, one PT student, one OT student, mother, and father

Scenario Implementation

The scene opens with PT and OT students actively engaged in caring and patient teaching. Mother and father are sitting at the bedside. APRN, MSW, and RN students arrive to give Josh and his family the news of the pathology report and the presence of a tumor. Parents are very upset; Josh is quiet and withdrawn. The APRN is giving facts about what happens subsequently and the MSW is offering support. PT and OT conclude their session, leaving the rest of the group to continue their discussion. The scene ends with an understanding that the oncologist will be in during the afternoon to discuss treatment options.

Participant Expectations

APRN: Discuss the pathology report and answer any questions the patient and family has.
MSW: Offer patient and family the opportunity to reflect and to focus on the present in response to their needs.

OT: Teach Josh to use a long-handle reacher to put on hospital pants.
PT: Teach Josh how to transfer out of bed (OOB) to a chair and to use crutches.
RN: Provide patient teaching and support.

SCENE FOUR: DI CT

Scenario Level

Prelicensure DI and MSW students

Focus Area

Care of a patient undergoing a CT scan, patient support

Scenario Description

Josh is undergoing CT scans to stage his osteosarcoma

Description of Patient

Josh is brought down to CT and he is visibly upset. He states that he is not only overwhelmed and upset by his diagnosis, but he is also worried about what the scans will show. At Josh's request, his social worker has accompanied him to the DI department for moral support.

Patient History

Josh is a 16-year-old athlete who fractured his femur as a result of an injury on the basketball court. He underwent an ORIF of his femur and, during the procedure, the surgeon saw a suspicious lesion, which was biopsied. Josh was diagnosed with osteosarcoma. He has been undergoing chemotherapy and has been receiving nursing care, OT, and PT at home. After biopsy results revealed osteosarcoma, CT scans of Josh's head, chest, abdomen, and pelvis are ordered as part of the staging process.

Setting the Scene

Equipment Needed

One simulated patient wearing a hospital gown; identification bracelet with patient's name, date of birth, and medical record number; wheelchair; and CT scan machine (actual or simulated).

Technology Used

No specific technology is needed

Simulator Level

Simulated patient

Participants Needed

One MSW, two DI students

Scenario Implementation

DI student 1 greets Josh and introduces self. The MSW pushes Josh's wheelchair to the CT room. DI student 1 introduces Josh to DI student 2. In the CT room, DI student 1 explains the procedure and Josh is becoming increasingly apprehensive. The MSW intervenes and talks to Josh to help alleviate his anxiety. Once Josh is more relaxed, he moves to the examination table, where DI student 2 positions him for his CT scan. The scene ends here.

Participant Expectations

DI: Explain the procedure, provide emotional support as necessary, perform the CT scan, and remove Josh from the scanner after the procedure.

MSW: Use relaxation techniques to help Josh manage his anxiety and pain during the imaging procedure.

SCENE FIVE: DISCONTINUATION OF TREATMENT

Scenario Level

Prelicensure law, nursing, PT, and OT students

Focus Area

Emotional and legal aspects of discontinuing care

Scenario Description

OT and PT arrive to Josh's home for a home care visit. Josh's mother greets them at the door and is visibly upset. She explains that she just got off the phone with the provider who told them that the current treatment is not effective and that the cancer has spread. She states Josh's pain is worsening. She states that the provider wants to try a new cocktail of experimental medications. She also states that Josh is increasingly discouraged and is in more pain.

Patient history: Josh is a 16-year-old athlete who fractured his femur as a result of an injury on the basketball court. He underwent an ORIF of his femur and, during the procedure, the surgeon saw a suspicious lesion, which was biopsied. Josh was diagnosed with osteosarcoma. He has undergone multiple chemotherapy and radiation treatments. He has just undergone further testing to see how the cancer is responding to treatment.

Setting the Scene

Equipment Needed

Hospital bed, overbed table, three chairs, posters of basketball in the room, and a cell phone

Technology Used

If available, a system for recording and viewing the SBE can be used for debriefing. If not, no special technology is used in this scenario.

Setting

Home care

Simulator Level

Simulated patient

Participants Needed

One law student, one MSW student, one OT student, one PT student, one RN student, mother

Scenario Implementation

OT and PT are at the bedside working with Josh. His mother calls the home care nurse to discuss what she was told by the provider. The home care nurse tells her that she is on her way along with the social worker. While OT/PT work with Josh, he confides that he does not want to continue treatment for his cancer. During this time, the mom returns and overhears what Josh is saying and becomes very upset and says, "You cannot give up now." A few minutes later the RN arrives at the house with the MSW to assess Josh's pain and discuss the news. They enter the conversation with Josh, his mother, OT, and PT. They are discussing the recent news regarding the chemotherapy not working. While they are talking, there is a knock at the door. Josh tells everyone that he invited his neighbor over (a lawyer) to discuss his desire to stop treatment with his parents. Josh asks everyone to stay for the conversation. The neighbor is a lawyer and family friend of the Williams family (she's probably closer in age to Josh than his parents—but trusted and liked by both parents and Josh). Josh asked the neighbor over as a trusted friend for advice on how to persuade his parents (and/or the health care team) to discontinue chemotherapy and focus on palliative care only going forward. The scene ends when Josh and his parents agree to focus on palliative care only. The MSW, OT, PT, and RN students should remain at the bedside during the conversation.

Participant Expectations

Lawyer: Use negotiation and/or mediation skills to help Josh think through and articulate his wishes to his parents without creating an attorney–client relationship with him (despite Josh's questions about his legal rights to deny treatment).

MSW: Validate Josh's feelings and provide emotional support for the mother.

OT/PT: Listen attentively to what Josh and family members are saying, offer support, and then finally offer family privacy, if they require it.

RN: Offer the patient and family emotional support and education.

SCENE SIX: HOSPICE HOME CARE

Scenario Level

Prelicensure MSW and nursing students

Focus Area

Care of the patient in a hospice home care setting dealing with pain and anxiety; education of the family members regarding change of condition and progression of disease

Scenario Description

Patient history: Josh is a 16-year-old diagnosed with osteosarcoma. He has undergone chemotherapy and radiation treatments, which were not successful. He made the decision to stop all treatment and is now receiving hospice services at home. He is not eating, has difficulty swallowing, and his pain level is increasing. Josh's mother is upset that Josh has not eaten for 2 days. She is becoming increasingly anxious about the changes in his condition. Josh's dad is calm and wants only what Josh wants.

Setting the Scene

Equipment Needed

Bed, three chairs, standardized patient dressed in pajamas, nightstand, cookies on tray, apron for mother, cell phone, and poster with basketball player

Technology Used

If available, a system for recording and viewing the SBE can be used for debriefing. Otherwise, no special technology is used in this scenario

Setting

Home care

Description of Participants

One MSW student, one RN student, mother/father

Simulator Level

Simulated patient

Scenario Implementation

Josh is lying in his bed at home. His mother has requested a visit by the visiting nurse and social worker because she has questions about Josh's pain management and care at home. On arrival, they find Mrs. Williams crying and distressed over the fact that Josh has increasing pain and is eating very little. She states, "Please help my son. I cannot stand seeing him like this! I made him his favorite cookies and he will not eat them!" Mom stands throughout the scenario and Dad is seated in one of the chairs beside the bed.

Participant Expectations

MSW: Validate mother's despair, ensure that she understands what is happening to her son at this moment, offer information related to what may happen later, and respond to her empathically.
RN: Use therapeutic communication skills to assess the situation and devise a plan of care with the MSW to comfort the patient and the parents.

SCENE SEVEN: INPATIENT HOSPICE CARE

Scenario Level

Prelicensure students

Focus Area

Care of the dying patient, care of family members of a dying patient, determination of death, preparing the body for viewing, and care of family members of a patient who has died

Scenario Description

Patient history: Josh is a 16-year-old diagnosed with osteosarcoma. He has undergone chemotherapy and radiation treatments, which were not successful. Josh was transferred to inpatient hospice and is actively dying.

Setting the Scene

Equipment Needed

Hospital bed, two chairs, computerized patient simulator dressed in a hospital gown, identification band, penlight, stethoscope, basin, washcloth, towel, coffee, cookies on tray, and table with chairs for conversation with family

Technology Used

If available, a system for recording and viewing the SBE can be used for debriefing. If not, no special technology is used in this scenario

Simulator Level

High-fidelity computerized patient simulator

Setting

Inpatient hospice unit

Participants Needed

One APRN student, one MSW student, two nursing students, and mother and father

Scenario Implementation

The scenario begins with Josh actively dying. He is laying on his side, flat in bed, no pillow. He is unresponsive, fluid draining from his mouth, agonal breathing. His parents are seated at the bedside, distraught, possibly crying, stating things such as: "I cannot believe this is happening to our Josh." Why is God punishing Josh? Why is God taking Josh away from us? What is happening to Josh's breathing? Why is Josh drooling? Is Josh in pain? How much longer do we have with Josh?"

About 3 minutes into the scene, Josh dies. RN leaves the room to call the APRN and MSW. The other RN remains with Josh's parents to comfort them. The APRN pronounces Josh dead. The APRN and MSW escort Josh's parents out of the room and support Josh's parents while nursing students remain in the room to prepare the body for viewing. The MSW and APRN students are sitting with Josh's parents comforting them and asking them about calling family members, clergy, and so forth. The parents are asking questions related to the removal of Josh's body and other appropriate questions. They may be distraught. Once the nurses have finished preparing the body, the parents are escorted into the room for viewing of Josh's body. Refreshments are in the room. The scenario ends once Josh's parents leave.

Participant Expectations

APRN: Legally and medically determine that Josh has expired, use therapeutic communication to comfort the parents.

MSW: Be present with parents' grief and loss with cultural and spiritual humility, answer questions and ensure that parents have resources needed at this time, provide written information and referrals for future if wanted.

RN: Use therapeutic communication to comfort the parents, prepare Josh for viewing after he has expired, and remain with the parents if they so desire during the viewing.

G. DEBRIEFING GUIDELINES

Important components of the debriefing stages included participants receiving objective feedback and affirmation of their interdisciplinary teamwork, skills, and communication, and participants having the opportunity to reflect on their experience. A culminating debrief offers the students the ability to pull their experiences together and reflect and compare their perceptions to those of an actual survivor of same disease.

I. RECOMMENDATIONS FOR FURTHER USE

It is recommended that a member of the clergy be included in this end-of-life Sim-IPE experience.

J. HOW SIMULATION-BASED PEDAGOGY HAS CONTRIBUTED TO IMPROVED STUDENT OUTCOMES

Students feel that participating in an end-of-life Sim-IPE promotes the development of communication and teamwork skills deemed necessary for patient care. Further evaluation related to each scenario outcome is necessary.

K. EXPERT RECOMMENDATIONS AND WORDS OF WISDOM

It is recommended that multistaged prebriefing and debriefing be implemented in multidisciplinary Sim-IPEs.

L. EVALUATION OF BEST PRACTICE STANDARDS AND USE OF CREDENTIALED SIMULATION FACULTY

The faculty members who participated in this Sim-IPE have had many years of experience in developing, assessing, running, debriefing, and researching clinical simulation scenarios. The use of best practice standards, especially Standard VIII, which relates to interprofessional simulation, led to the use of an appropriate theory to guide the scenario development. In addition, best practices for Sim-IPE related to the incorporation of, "authentic, complex, challenging, reality based activities/scenarios" (Decker et al., 2015, p. 295) led to the development of a scenario that gave students the opportunity to experience end-of-life care, and understand the role of each member of the interprofessional team in end-of-life care.

REFERENCES

D'Amour, D., & Oandasan, I. (2005). Interprofessionality as the field of interprofessional practice and interprofessional education: An emerging concept. *Journal of Interprofessional Care, 19*(Suppl. 1), 8–20.

Decker, S. I., Anderson, M., Boese, T., Epps, C., McCarthy, J., Motola, I.,...Lioce, L. (2015, June). Standards of best practice: Simulation standard VIII: Simulation-enhanced interprofessional education (sim-IPE). *Clinical Simulation in Nursing, 11*(6), 293–297. doi:10.1016/j.ecns.2015.03.010

International Nursing Association for Clinical Simulation and Learning. (2013, updated 2016). INACSL standards of best practice: Simulation. Retrieved from https://www.inacsl.org/i4a/pages/index.cfm?pageID=3407

Interdisciplinary Education in Simulation: Bridging the Gap Between Academic and Career Competencies

Maureen M. Ryan, Anna Macdonald, Brian Farrell, and Darin Abbey

In contemporary health care dialogues about health professional graduates, educators often hear from their clinical associates about the challenges that new professional graduates face when entering the workforce. Moreover, educators of prelicensure health care professionals are challenged to teach to practice in a health care system that appears to be slowly shifting focus from discipline-specific care (e.g., nursing care) to the provision of safe and effective patient care of clinically complex patients. Adding to this shifting landscape is a recent move in Canada toward a business-model approach to health care whereby governmental funding and health care expenditures call for the most effective and the least expensive approach to safe and effective patient care. One might expect that health professional educators may feel overwhelmed by the increasing pressure to provide clinically competent practitioners who are job ready in a constantly changing environment, if they are not set up to compete for resources among each other to deliver their individual health education programs. However, a compelling argument may be made that efficient health care systems rely on collaboration among clinicians working from diverse fields of practice. Thus, we propose that the education of clinicians also rely on the collaboration among educators for student learning opportunities that better prepare them to meet the complexities of patient care provision: interprofessional education (IPE).

A. IMPLEMENTATION OF SIMULATION-BASED PEDAGOGY IN YOUR INDIVIDUALIZED TEACHING AREA

Our nursing students attend the University of Victoria (UVic)'s School of Nursing 4-year baccalaureate program to meet the competencies as outlined by the College of Registered Nurses of British Columbia, including successfully passing the NCLEX-RN. Similarly, medical students must meet competencies as described by the Medical Council of Canada in order to meet their professional licensing objectives (LMCC part I) following completion of the University of British Columbia (UBC)'s Faculty of Medicine Island Medical Program (IMP) located at UVic. In addition, we have other health professional students who practice at the Island Health Authority (IHA) as part of their prelicensure clinical practice education.

Developing an Interprofessional Simulation Center

In 2011, a simulation center in Victoria was envisioned among three partner organizations, the UVic School of Nursing, UBC's Island Medical Program, and the IHA. The idea of simulation education, particularly high-fidelity complex care patient cases, has been on the curriculum agenda for the School of Nursing and the Island Medical Program for several years. Moreover, IHA was investigating new ways to foster staff development, aid in recruitment and retention, and address patient care issues that came to the attention of quality and safety committees' professional practices concerns.

As part of this development, in 2012 a curriculum-working group (CWG) was formed with a faculty lead from the School of Nursing and the Island Medical Program and a lead from the Professional Practice Office at the IHA. The CWG members were trained as simulation trainers through a certificate program at the Centre for Excellence in Simulation Education and Innovation (CESEI), Vancouver, Canada; the Simulation Educator Training (SET) course offered by the Royal College of Physicians and Surgeons; and the Debriefing Assessment for Simulation in Healthcare (DASH) workshop.

Over the following 2 years, the CWG members championed simulation learning at their respective organizations to train as trainers and curriculum revisionists. Each member conducted a needs assessment targeting how simulation would augment current education practices in his or her institution. They piloted simulation projects that followed best practice standards put forth by the *International Nursing Association for Clinical Simulation Learning Standards for Best Practice: Simulation* (International Nursing Association for Clinical Simulation and Learning [INACSL], 2013/2016) with a view to enahncing prelicensure students' preparation to successfully complete the NCLEX-RN alongside the Standards for Accredited Simulation Activities as set the Royal College of Physicians and Surgeons of Canada (2013). Evaluation of the demonstration project for nursing included pre- and posttest questions, an objective assessment via a checklist, and a follow-up survey. At the end of the first year, from the evaluation data we (across discipline facilitators) were asked: "Why are we, students, playing the role of another health professional student during the simulation?" This question was followed by: "We really do not know what the scope of practice is for other health professional students or why they make the decisions they do."

As a result of student feedback, an interprofessional simulation pilot project ensued over the subsequent year led by Drs. Maureen Ryan, RN, PhD (nursing), and Brian Farrell, MD, CCFP (emergency medicine). The pilot project work was informed by the Canadian Interprofessional Health Collaborative (CIHC) National Interprofessional Competency Framework (NICF), which outlines competencies required for effective interprofessional collaboration within six practice domains: role clarification, team functioning, patient/client/family/community-centered care, collaborative leadership, interprofessional communication, and interprofessional conflict resolution (CIHC, 2010). The pilot project focused on role clarification and interprofessional team communication in the debriefing in response to the student questions about roles and how to communicate effectively.

Student volunteers from the health professional schools of respiratory therapy, pharmacy, and nursing attended the medical student and medical resident simulations sessions. The sessions were cofacilitated by nursing and medical faculty from the CWG, and four cases from the UBC-IMP curriculum with a mix of trauma and general medicine were used with attention to how students understood, enacted, and communicated roles (e.g., closed-loop communication). The cofacilitators collected feedback from students following each session debriefing in a face-to-face group setting. The results were analyzed thematically, presented as illustrative case study to key stakeholders across discipline faculty, and presented as a poster at the Simulation Summit sponsored by the Royal College of Physicians and Surgeons Canada in 2013. A decision was made to continue engaging in research projects to formally evaluate the IPE programs.

Developing an Interprofessional Simulation Education Community

Although faculty and organizational leads at the Center for Interprofessional Clinical Simulation Learning (CICSL) recognized the inherent value of IPE, they were also aware of the necessary work needed to reduce discipline-specific educational silos and the concurrent individual and organizational challenges this presents. Hall and Zierler (2015) propose that two organizational challenges must be overcome in order to be successful: the provision of IPE education opportunities and the exposure to clinical settings where IPE is well practiced. Moreover, they suggest that the complexity of scheduling, flexibility of curriculum, competing demands, and the changes that IPE bring to health care often invite organizational resistance. This brings to light the importance of faculty development and the ongoing practice of IPE with students using an IPE competency framework alongside supportive organizational leadership and infrastructures within which faculty and students to teach and learn.

Our organizational leadership supported two independently facilitated workshops that invited members of existing working groups and stakeholders and/or decision makers from each of the partner institutions to participate in shaping the operations of the CICSL.

Two key workshops supported by organizational leadership allowed for interprofessional and interinstitutional contributions to CICSL's core functions. In Exhibit 39.1, we outline the CICSL's vision, mission, and values developed by the group and its commitment to IPE.

Recent publications through the Cochrane Collaboration (Zwarenstein, Reeves, Barr, et al., 2005; Zwarenstein, Reeves, & Perrier, 2005) call for the adoption of a framework to guide IPE efforts, and a decision to continue to use the framework we piloted (NIHC) along with building resources for faculty development necessary to implement the program. As a result, we can now describe two developing research and development programs at the CICSL: The Interprofessional Simulation Educator Pathway, highlighted as one of the innovative approaches to simulation-based faculty development in Chapter 5, and The Interprofessional Communication Curriculum described in the following section.

Introducing an Interprofessional Competency Framework Into Simulation Research and Practice

Using simulation to learn with, from, and about each other is at the heart of the CICSL partnership. In addition, driven by the belief that IPE and collaborative patient-centered practice are central to building effective health care teams and improving the experience and outcomes of patients, in 2010, the CIHC released the NICF. The framework describes the competencies required for effective interprofessional collaboration. Six competency domains highlight the knowledge, skills, attitudes, and values that together shape the judgments that are essential for interprofessional collaborative practice: role clarification, team functioning, patient/client/family/community care, collaborative leadership, interprofessional communication, and interprofessional conflict resolution (CIHC, 2010).

Within each of the domains is a list of competencies that the health professional can self-assess or use to have his or her performance assessed objectively. A full tutorial of the quality indicators within each domain goes beyond the scope of this chapter, interested parties can find more at the CIHC website (CIHC, 2010).

Exhibit 39.1	CICSL's Vision, Mission, and Values	
Vision	**Mission**	**Values**
Improved patient and provider experience	Provide a sustainable, safe, and supportive learning environment	Excellence
Excellence in training and in practice	Foster interprofessional and inter-institutional collaboration	Interprofessionalism
Advanced health education		Patient focus
Leader in research and innovation	Improve simulation education through evidence-informed practice	Integrity
		Innovation
		Collaboration
		Transparency
		Trust

CICSL, Center for Interprofessional Clinical Simulation Learning.

An interprofessional team at CICSL is currently implementing an IPE research project examining safe patient handover within and among interprofessional teams using this framework and a communication curriculum. The communication curriculum is an online module created by Elspeth McDougall and colleagues (including author Maureen Ryan). This module teaches participants the importance of effective interprofessional communication, team functioning, role clarification, collaborative leadership, and interprofessional conflict resolution. The participants are introduced to two patient handover tools—SBAR (situation, background, assessment, recommendations) and IDRAW (identify, diagnosis, recent changes, anticipated changes, what to watch for) to assist them. In Exhibit 39.2, the SBAR template outlines information expected within each of the steps required to communicate information in an urgent or unusual situation. The SBAR is ideal for urgent circumstances such as urgent physician orders, advice required by ICU outreach teams, and when the patient is deteriorating.

Similarly, in Exhibit 39.3, the required steps for patient transfer following the IDRAW method (Hill, 2012) are outlined. The IDRAW is ideal for patient handovers, including changes in the level of care (routine transfer), temporary transfer of responsibility of care to another caregiver (e.g., staff breaks or diagnostic procedures), discharge, and change of shift report.

These tools were adopted into our communication curriculum following a review for applicability by our interprofessional team with the intent to foster safe patient care. Our intent with this project was to answer the call to develop educational strategies that guide safe practices for prelicensure students that would transfer into postgraduate practice (Emanuel et al., 2011; Kohn, Corrigan, & Donaldson, 2000).

In our study, interprofessional teams made up of medical students, nursing students, respiratory therapy students, and pharmacy students in their third year of study take part in emergency-based simulated scenarios before and after taking the online communication curriculum module.

Exhibit 39.2   SBAR—Urgent Communication

Appropriate Assertion/Requiring Action

S Situation

B Background

A Assessment

R Recommendation

Exhibit 39.3   IDRAW—Interactive Handover

INTERACTIVE HANDOVER

Transfer of Accountability

I Identify patient and MRP

D Diagnosis/current problems

R Recent changes (up-to-date vital signs)

A Anticipated changes (next few hours)

W What to watch for

They observed and assessed their communication, teamwork, and handover skills during both simulation sessions to determine whether taking the communication curriculum improves patient handover techniques. Students will also be asked to evaluate themselves, their team, and the curriculum itself following each simulation, and again 3 months after completion. Our aim is to give students an experience of working as part of an interprofessional team and to provide them with skills and knowledge, and a place to practice safe patient handover. This project is a collaboration of Dr. Maureen Ryan (UVic School of Nursing), Dr. Brian Farrell (UBC Island Medical Program), and Dr. Anna Macdonald (CICSL), and is based on the pilot project originally spearheaded by Drs. Ryan and Farrell in 2013.

B. EDUCATIONAL MATERIALS AVAILABLE IN YOUR TEACHING AREA AND RELATED TO YOUR SPECIALTY

In 2015, the CICSL opened with four simulation laboratories, a debrief room, two observation rooms, three clinical skills rooms, and a videoconference space. We also had the aforementioned data from disciplinary and interprofessional pilot projects, which informed our next directions.

C. SPECIFIC OBJECTIVES FOR SIMULATION USAGE WITHIN A SPECIFIC COURSE AND THE OVERALL PROGRAM

One of the logistical issues with creating projects like these is scheduling simulation sessions. Students have competing curricula requirements that can lead to a variety of scheduling conflicts. Furthermore, if simulation sessions are over and above what is required by the curriculum, it can be difficult to get students to commit.

The ways in which we have navigated these issues are twofold. We have ensured that from the beginning, upper level management from each organization is invested in interprofessional collaboration. By making IPE a priority, with top-down support, we are able to build IPE sessions into the different education institution curricula with greater ease. The CICSL Teaching and Learning Committee is also involved, which brings together educators from all three of our partner organizations and provides a platform to discuss ideas and projects together and plan in advance how to make them work.

An example of how the IPE competencies can be addressed in a patient simulation event follows. In this example, we have added the IPE competencies, complete with debriefing questions, to a required simulation learning activity for the third-year medical program. Attending the simulation are third-year medical students, third-year nursing students, respiratory therapy students, and pharmacy students. The simulation event is facilitated by a clinical faculty member from medicine or alternatively cofacilitated with a faculty member from the other disciplines. What we hope to provide here is an example of how the IPE domains and competencies can easily be added to any patient care simulation scenario and in any existing curriculum.

The course in which this patient care scenario resides is Emergency Medicine Resuscitation for Medical Students. The specific learning modules include: respiratory emergency, trauma, poisoning, altered level of consciousness, and the communication curriculum (e-learning on team communication and safe patient handover). In the IMP curriculum, Dr. Afshin Khazei designed four trauma/resuscitation learning modules. The team leadership and communication learning objectives and debriefing guide were developed by Dr. Maureen Ryan, and Dr. Brian Farrell and added to the case scenarios. The teams of interprofessional students progress through the four case scenarios over a 2-hour period; the IPE team objectives are met alongside the medical student course work.

Effective resuscitation of the critically ill patient requires the integration of knowledge, manual/procedural, and team leadership skills, including interprofessional competencies in role clarification, team functioning, interprofessional communication, conflict resolution, and collaborative leadership. To augment the ongoing development of interprofessional competencies for third-year medical students, this seminar also provides an opportunity for team communication in an emergency treatment scenario, including the opportunity to practice safe patient handover. The seminar has nursing students and respiratory therapy students attend as part of their individual curricular learning objectives to increase their knowledge of and practice of interprofessional competencies.

D. INTRODUCTION OF SCENARIO

Setting the Scene and Technology Used

The following scenario requires a high-fidelity human patient simulator (HPS) and the room should be set up with the equipment one would find in a standard emergency department trauma room. For this specific case, the students are required to perform primary and secondary assessments, which include application of a hard collar, obtaining large-bore vascular access, discovery of a pneumothorax requiring needle decompression and insertion of a chest tube, and performance of a bedside ultrasound with a focused assessment with sonography in trauma (FAST) scan positive for free fluid in the abdomen. In addition, investigation, such as EKG blood work, and x-rays, are also to be obtained to help inform ongoing patient care and consultation.

Presimulation Learning-Event Resources

Medical students are asked to review the content in the UBC Emergency Medicine, Undergraduate Core Content Manual, basic life support (BSL) course, advanced cardiovascular life support (ACLS) provider course, advanced trauma life support course, and the communication curriculum. Nursing and respiratory students are asked to review the BLS course, and the communication curriculum.

Student Learning Objectives

1. To apply knowledge about resuscitation in a simulated patient care setting, including cardiopulmonary resuscitation (CPR), identifying and treating arrhythmias using ACLS guidelines and the initial management of shock
2. To apply knowledge about chest trauma in a simulated patient care setting, including primary and secondary assessments, and appropriate interventions and investigations
3. To practice procedural skills of airway maneuvers, insertion of basic airways and preparation for intubation, and postintubation care
4. To apply knowledge and practice in an IPE event, including demonstration of role clarification, team functioning, collaborative leadership, interprofessional communication, conflict resolution
5. To practice safe patient handover

Description of Participants

Prelicensure health professional students who participate as members of the patient care team participate in this scenario. We recommend that the student do not assume the role of another health care professional as this detracts from realism. Two facilitators are ideal: one to focus on the clinical progression of the scenario (e.g., be the voice of the patient) and the other to attend to the team roles and communication.

E. RUNNING OF THE SCENARIO

The team assembles and roles are clarified. The team begins a head-to-toe assessment through delegated acts. The first act is to apply cervical spine (C-spine) precautions.

F. PRESENTATION OF COMPLETED TEMPLATE

Title

Interprofessional Team Approaches to Managing a Motor Vehicle Accident (MVA) Chest Trauma

Focus Area

Respond to trauma-induced hospitalization as a member of an interprofessional team of care.

Scenario Description

This scenario takes place in our simulated trauma room at the CICSL. The HPS is set to resemble a young female MVA victim. The instructor might give report as the emergency first responders or you may include emergency first-responder students practicing patient handover. Either way, the patient is alert, anxious, and quickly decompensates as a result of trauma.

Prebrief (10 Minutes)

Review student learning objectives listed earlier.

- Orient the learners to SimMan 3G and the simulation experience.
- Demonstrate how SimMan 3G works, review resources in the room to support patient care and normal physical exam findings.
- Review roles of participants, including instructors.
- Introduce the debrief and what takes place during debriefing.

Case Scenario (10–15 Minutes)

The student team is informed that a 25-year-old female driver of car is brought in via ambulance. The ambulance attendants say the car was T-boned with ++ intrusion into the driver's side of the vehicle. The jaws of life were used to extract the woman. They report: Ø level of consciousness (LOC), chest pain, left upper quadrant (LUQ) pain, heart rate (HR): 130 mmHg, respiratory rate (RR): 30 breaths/minute, oxygen saturation (SaO$_2$): 92%, blood pressure (BP): 80/40 beats/minute.

Voice of the patient: The patient is talking, asking what happened, wondering where her car is. She can answer all questions and is oriented.

Progression outline: After applying C-spine precautions the team assessment reveals ↓ air entry left side, trachea deviated to right side. The following actions may be: needle thoracotomy or left-sided chest tube gush of air. Change HPS settings to RR: 20 breaths/minute, SaO$_2$ 95%. Further assessment data reveals that the patient is hypotensive and tachycardic with thready pulses. The subsequent step is to insert two large-bore peripheral intravenous (IVs) and run fluids. The choice is 2-L normal saline (NS) bolus, and to order a blood type and crossmatch. Following this the trauma surgeon should be called. The use of SBAR when discussing the care with the trauma surgeon should be seen. The student learner describes the situation at hand, the background, provides an assessment, and negotiates the assessment parameters and resulting recommendations from the trauma surgeon.

The assessment should continue head to toe and log roll, and reveals tender left chest, tender LUQ abdomen with rebound and guarding. A Foley catheter should be ordered and inserted. Further orders include a chest x-ray, which reveals left pneumothorax. If ordered, a pelvic x-ray reveals normal pelvis. A FAST scan is positive for free fluid in the abdomen. Blood work ordered should include complete blood count (CBC), blood type and crossmatch, prothrombin time (PT), partial thromboplastin time (PTT), and an EKG.

The team should reach the diagnosis of left-sided pneumothorax and splenic rupture. The patient is readied for transfer to the operating room (OR). A member of the team (student physician or nurse) calls the receiving member of the OR team and provides the requisite IDRAW information.

G. DEBRIEFING GUIDELINES

The case scenario is debriefed as per the learner objectives either in the simulation room or the attached debriefing room. The facilitator continues to build on the introduction of a safe and supportive environment for learning (in the prebrief) by moving through the phases of debriefing at the learner's pace. Debriefing begins with reactions to the experience and the situation at hand, an analysis of what happened in the scenario, and a summary. The intent of debrief is twofold: (a) to assess and teach clinical judgment and reasoning and, (b) to foster critical self-reflection. Our participants are in third-year prelicensure and this may very well be their first time in an urgent situation working as a team. Following is an in-depth look at how we structure the debriefing of the interprofessional competency.

Role Clarification

The student participants introduce themselves and communicate their role in patient care appropriately throughout the case scenario. Each team member accesses others' skills and knowledge appropriately. Questions you might ask include: Was everyone aware of each other's roles during the scenario? Were you able to enact your role in patient care responsibly and competently? (Elaborate as needed.)

Team Functioning

The student participants facilitate discussions and interactions among team members as required throughout the case scenario. All student members participate, are respectful of each others' participation, and there is evidence of collaborative decision making when required. Questions you might ask include: Do you feel you acted as a respected member of the patient care team? What was needed to strengthen team functioning in this case scenario? (Elaborate as needed.)

Collaborative Leadership

The students understand and can apply shared decision making and individual accountability as part of a collaborative leadership model of patient care. There is evidence of effective team processes and decision making as required throughout the case scenario. Questions you might ask include: How did you cocreate a climate for collaborative practice? How did you facilitate shared decision making (when required)? What might you do differently?

Interprofessional Communication

The students actively communicate as a team using closed-loop communication, call each other by name, and communicate to ensure a common understanding of patient care decisions throughout the simulation experience. Questions you might ask include: What was your experience of how the team communicated? (Positives, things to change in future) What are some of your challenges in communicating during patient care decisions?

Interprofessional Conflict Resolution

The students are able to positively and constructively address disagreements as they arise during the simulation case scenario delivery or in the debrief. Questions you might ask include (as applicable): What do you know or understand about the positive nature of conflict in patient care? How did you see yourself working effectively to resolve disagreements in the case scenario?

H. SUGGESTIONS/KEY FEATURES TO REPLICATE OR IMPROVE

The advantages of having prelicensure students learn alongside each other are multifaceted. Individual program instructors have an opportunity to assess their students' understanding of their professional role contributing to safe patient care and handover of care through demonstrated assessment, interventions, and communications within a simulated environment. Students also have the opportunity to learn about each other and from each other, and this opportunity is not readily available in the clinical practice rotations. We believe the key feature to replicating this scenario is the appropriate matching of student skill, that is, each professional student must have had the theory and practice of the required psychomotor skills before the scenario. We also recommend that students have some introduction to team communication (such as the communication curriculum) before being assessed for team communication.

I. RECOMMENDATIONS FOR FURTHER USE

We are looking forward to the future in solidifying our IPE program for prelicensure students into individual curricula across institutions. Thus, we strongly recommend engaging in research and demonstrating localized evidence that is supported by the wider simulation outcome research but speaks to the representatives from clinical practice and academia in your community. Our community of practice is also the community that we serve in our various roles, and we have found success in putting people together to address common challenges as mentioned, ensuring our students have ample practice opportunities to meet their licensure requirement of interprofessional collaboration.

We are also in the process of integrating validated tools of assessment and observation into our simulation learner events. Examples of such tools include behavioral checklists developed for the communication curriculum and the Mayo High Performance Teamwork Scale (Malec et al., 2007). We have had some success when sharing performance tools among the CICSL partners, for these tools support the development of a shared vocabulary, as well as an increased facilitator understanding of the learner objectives. We are striving toward unified patterns of practice in prebriefing and debriefing, so that our students not only feel safe and supported in their learning, they even have an equitable learning experience with their peers.

After a brief introduction, these tools and others can be used in several ways. During prebriefing, the contents can be shared with simulation participants to assist in setting student goals for the simulation learning event. During simulation, the worksheets can be used by both by-standing participants and faculty alike to provide purposeful and specific observations during debriefing, which helps participants learn about the best practices (in this case teamwork or safe patient handover), and at the same time critically self-reflect on their strengths and future learning goals. We caution that the tools be used judiciously, for we believe it is not a good teaching practice to assess and grade a student performance when students are learning the skill for the first time. Thus, in our third-year project, we observe and teach our student population in debriefing. However, with our medical residents and fourth-year nursing students who have had simulation and practice experience in interprofessional collaboration, our learning objectives are to assess competency.

J. HOW SIMULATION-BASED PEDAGOGY HAS CONTRIBUTED TO IMPROVED STUDENT OUTCOMES

Nursing students use an end-of-semester course evaluation to provide faculty with feedback regarding the use of high-fidelity HPS technology in the laboratory setting. Ongoing feedback echoes the pilot project themes of understanding the differing roles of the patient care team, and learning how to communicate effectively increases the students' confidence in practice.

We are currently collecting data via an observational checklist tool on team performance and in a student self-report survey, which informs us with some evidence of how our approach impacts students.

K. EXPERT RECOMMENDATIONS AND WORDS OF WISDOM

In considering possible words of wisdom that might be shared from our collective experiences at CICSL, we invite simulation educators to engage with us around IPE successes and challenges. Our experience has taught us that continued dialogue about commonalities among disciplines, that is, the desire and responsibility to prepare our students for their entry to practice to the best of our ability, has resulted in ways to approach challenges that we may not have considered had we maintained a singular professional focus. The sharing of expertise and resources has served to create dynamic partnerships among disciplines and between academia and clinical practice partners. We recognize that having simulation champions is a great beginning, and we did this when we started with our curriculum working group, which energetically took on the idea of interprofessional team teaching. We believe that the success of our pilot project occurred in part because of the matching of clinical expertise and academics united in their training in simulation facilitation.

However, experience has taught us that relying on champions or designated faculty is destined to present challenges. We strongly believe that the commitment of organizational leadership in putting simulation pedagogy and practice on the agenda alongside the commitment to funding and creating an infrastructure to support collaborative projects are vital acts.

L. EVALUATION OF BEST PRACTICE STANDARDS AND USE OF CREDENTIALED SIMULATION FACULTY

We noted at the beginning of the chapter how best standards (e.g., INACSL Standards for best practice: Simulation) informed our work. We received funding from the University of British Columbia Faculty of Medicine to evaluate our program and are in the midst of collecting data. We hope to share our results upon study completion.

REFERENCES

Canadian Interprofessional Health Collaborative. (2010). A national interprofessional competency framework. Retrieved from http://www.cihc.ca/files/CIHC_IPCompetencies_Feb1210.pdf

Emanuel, L. L., Taylor, L., Hain, A., Combes, J. R., Hatlie, M. J., Karsh, B., ... Walton, M. (Eds.). (2011). *The Patient Safety Education Program—Canada (PSEP–Canada)* Curriculum. Retrieved from http://www.patientsafetyinstitute.ca/en/education/PatientSafetyEducationProgram/PatientSafetyEducationCurriculum/Documents/05-Plenary%203%20-%20What%20is%20Patient%20Safety.pdf

Hall, L. W., & Zierler, B. K. (2015). Interprofessional education and practice guide No. 1: Developing faculty to effectively facilitate interprofessional education. *Journal of Interprofessional Care, 29*(1), 3–7.

Hill, W. (2012). Handover communication to improve care. Retrieved from https://bcpsqc.ca/documents/2012/12/KGH-ED-Leaders-Team-Work-Communication-background-reading-W-Hill-Feb-1-2013.pdf

International Nursing Association for Clinical Simulation and Learning. (2013, updated 2016). INACSL standards of best practice: Simulation. Retrieved from https://www.inacsl.org/i4a/pages/index.cfm?pageID=3407

Kohn, L. T., Corrigan, J. M., & Donaldson, M. S. (Eds.). (2000). *To err is human: Building a safer health system.* Washington, DC: National Academies Press.

Malec, J. F., Torsher, L. C., Dunn, W. F., Wiegmann, D. A., Arnold, J. J., Brown, D. A., & Phatak, V. (2007). The Mayo High Performance Teamwork Scale: Reliability and validity for evaluating key crew resource management skills. *Simulation in Healthcare, 2*(1), 4–10.

Royal College of Physicians and Surgeons Canada. (2013). Standards for accredited simulation activities. Retrieved from http://www.royalcollege.ca/rcsite/documents/continuing-professional -development/section-3-sap-standards-simulation-e.pdf

Zwarenstein, M., Reeves, S., Barr, H., Hammick, M., Koppel, I., & Atkins, J. (2005). Interprofessional education: Effects on professional practice and health care outcomes (Cochrane Review). *Journal of Continuing Education in the Health Profession, 23*(2), 124–125.

Zwarenstein, M., Reeves, S., & Perrier, L. (2005). Effectiveness of pre-licensure interprofessional education and post-licensure collaborative interventions. *Journal of Interprofessional Care, 19*(Suppl. 1), 148–165.

FURTHER READING

National Council of State Boards of Nursing. (2016). NCLEX-RN examination: Test Plan for the National Council Licensure Examination for Registered Nurses. Retrieved from http://www.ncsbnorg/ testplanshtm

National Steering Committee on Patient Safety. (2002). Building a safer system: A national integrated strategy for improving patient safety in Canadian Health care. Retrieved from http://www.royalcollege .ca/portal/page/portal/rc/common/documents/advocacy/building_a_safer_system_e.pdf

CHAPTER 40

Cardiovascular Resuscitation:
Code Simulation for Health Care Students

Gloria Brummer

A. IMPLEMENTATION OF SIMULATION-BASED PEDAGOGY IN YOUR INDIVIDUALIZED TEACHING AREA

The interprofessional simulation in this chapter is ideal for nursing students in prelicensure baccalaureate, RN-to-BSN students, or graduate programs. It serves pharmacy, respiratory, or medical students and is appropriate for a professional development activity for health care professionals responding to cardiac emergencies. St. John's College of Nursing in Springfield, Illinois, offers this simulation in the baccalaureate program to medical–surgical students during their penultimate semester in the program, after completion of two other medical–surgical courses spiraled in difficulty. The experience is near midterm so that the students can use their acquired knowledge and skills throughout the semester. Interprofessional students include year-three pharmacy students with year-two respiratory care students.

After earlier simulations it became apparent that realism and interprofessional skills, such as teamwork and communication, can be improved on by adding interprofessional students. With the complexity of care that surrounds hospitalized patients, the interprofessional team now often responds to cardiac or respiratory arrests, and these first responders need to be proficient in both basic life support (BLS) and advanced cardiovascular life support (ACLS). When students are prebriefed by faculty and come prepared, having studied assigned algorithms, much learning can be accomplished in the resuscitation simulations. Resuscitation situations for new graduates may be stressful as they often have limited opportunities to practice these skills in the clinical area before graduation. This simulation-based pedagogy allows evidence-based practice in a faculty-supported environment where students can gain confidence and learn from their actions, as well as by observing interprofessional peers.

B. EDUCATIONAL MATERIALS AVAILABLE IN YOUR TEACHING AREA AND RELATED TO YOUR SPECIALTY

St. John's Health Sciences Library and Educational Technology Department is available on campus with student-friendly hours, expert library staff, and many online and printed resources related to ACLS. In preparation for the simulation, nursing students complete a classroom review of basic cardiac rhythms. Then, nursing faculty and students discuss 2 to 3 hours of theory content specifically reviewing the American Heart Association (AHA; 2015) guidelines for cardiac resuscitation and hold a practice code simulation early in the semester. Respiratory care students complete the ACLS provider course before this interprofessional education (IPE) and have additional prereading about cardiovascular resuscitation. Pharmacy students complete prereading, discuss resuscitation with their faculty for 1 hour, view interprofessional videos on BLS and ACLS, and then practice mini scenarios in class. The pocket-sized AHA (2015) *Handbook of Emergency Cardiovascular Care for Healthcare Providers* is organized in a quick-reference format and translates current science to practice. In the 2015 edition, pages 1 to 72 will be most helpful in preparing for cardiovascular resuscitation (AHA, 2015).

The AHA publishes several resources for advanced cardiac care that contain current ACLS guidelines, available through the Channing Bete Company site at http://aha.channing-bete .com. Another resource, the 2015 AHA Guidelines Update for Cardiopulmonary Resuscitation and Emergency Cardiovascular Care Part 1: Executive Summary provides an overview of the science derived from a recent comprehensive review by the International Liaison Committee on Resuscitation (ILCOR). The full report is available online at http://circ.ahajournals.org/content/ 132/18_suppl_2/S313 and discusses current practice evidence (AHA, 2015). An online option for AHA BLS and ACLS courses is available for health care practitioners who desire this method of learning.

In 2011, the Interprofessional Education Collaborative (IPEC) Expert Panel (2011) published *Core Competencies for Interprofessional Collaborative Practice* that directed competencies in four domains, including (a) values/ethics for interprofessional practice, (b) roles/responsibilities, (c) interprofessional communication, and (d) teams and teamwork. With these expectations, a continued need exists to develop and evaluate innovative IPE methods and to disseminate the results (IPEC, 2011).

St. John's simulation laboratory has high-fidelity human patient simulators (HFHPS) from Laerdal, including an infant and a SimMan 3G that has features such as medication recognition, sweating, and cyanosis, and also some low-fidelity HPSs and static manikins. Interprofessional faculty plan the simulation experience with the lab coordinator, who assists with updating scenarios, technological strategies, realism, and provides picture labels of the resuscitation medications.

C. SPECIFIC OBJECTIVES FOR SIMULATION USAGE WITHIN A SPECIFIC COURSE AND THE OVERALL PROGRAM

1. Demonstrate the ability to efficiently care for a client requiring cardiovascular resuscitation.
2. Demonstrate the ability to effectively communicate with other health care professionals during emergency situations.
3. Apply teamwork competencies in a collaborative simulation activity to foster interprofessional team skills necessary to provide patient-centered care.
4. Collaborate with interprofessional partner(s) to promote safe medication administration.
5. Reflect on both individual and team performance improvement.

D. INTRODUCTION OF SCENARIO

Setting the Scene

This simulation represents one of the 12 different scenarios used for the experience with the high-fidelity Laerdal SimMan 3G.

Objectives

Objectives for the experience are listed earlier. In addition, this scenario provides opportunity for students to safely practice key elements from the National Council Licensure Examination for Registered

Nurses test plan (NCLEX-RN®) published in 2015 by the National Council of State Boards of Nursing (NCSBN). Categories and subcategories addressed in the simulation include:

Safe and effective care environment: *Management of care* (advance directives, advocacy, collaboration with interdisciplinary team, continuity of care, delegation, establishing priorities, ethical practice), *Safety and infection control* (accident/error/injury prevention, emergency response plan, error prevention, safe use of equipment/standard precautions); **Health promotion and maintenance:** *Techniques of physical assessment;* **Psychosocial integrity:** *Coping mechanisms, support systems, therapeutic communication, therapeutic environment;* **Physiological integrity:** *Basic care and comfort, Pharmacological and parenteral therapies* (adverse effects/contraindications/side effects/interactions, dosage calculation, expected action/outcomes, medical administration, parenteral/intravenous [IV] therapies), *Reduction of risk potential* (changes/abnormalities in vital signs, diagnostic tests, potential for complications of diagnostic tests/treatments/procedures, system specific assessments), *Physiological adaptation* (hemodynamics, fluid and electrolyte imbalances, illness management, medical emergencies, pathophysiology, unexpected response to therapies).

The landmark report by the Institute of Medicine (IOM) of the National Academies, *The Future of Nursing: Leading Change, Advancing Health*, recommends interprofessional collaboration through joint classroom and clinical education opportunities (IOM, 2010). This interprofessional simulation supports Essential VI: Interprofessional Communication and Collaboration for Improving Patient Health Outcomes from *The Essentials of Baccalaureate Education for Professional Nursing Practice* published by the American Association of Colleges of Nursing (AACN; 2008). Essential VI further states communication and collaboration among health care professionals are critical to delivering high quality and safe patient care (AACN, 2008).

Technology Used

An HFHPS, cardiac monitor, and defibrillator are used. Audiovisual equipment allowed observation from a nearby room that also had a flip chart with scenario information and patient assessment data printed at the front of the room.

Description of Participants

Interprofessional students rotate using the given scenario along with other scenarios that facilitate learning by both participation and observation on audiovisual screen projection in a nearby room. Student participants rotate to different roles within the simulation, ones that they have not done previously. The nursing students maintain roles of code leader as this aligns with practice in our clinical settings. If students are not participating, they are observing. Roles include airway/respiration management, chest compressions, medication administration, cardioversion/defibrillation/pacer, recorder, safety observers, an experienced nurse portrays a family member. Alternating roles allows practice and understanding of each role while facilitating teamwork and communication. Before the scenario, each student is given a card that highlights important role functions. Cards are rotated to the later students as they move to the subsequent role and list pointers such as:

Team leader: Coordinate everyone. Watch patient, monitor, and staff; collaborate with staff asking for confirmation about completed interventions if not communicated by team members.
Recorder: Note age, assessment information, cardiopulmonary resuscitation (CPR) starts and stops, medication, cardioversion and defibrillations settings and clearing.
Defibrillation/cardioversion: Do not delay if defibrillation is needed. Defibrillation uses no "synch."
Medication administration: Open syringe from the bottom; flip yellow caps and screw together; check all medication rights, including right medication for the right patient assessment and algorithm.
Airway and respirations: Perform 30 compressions and two respirations until the advanced airway is inserted; then, deliver 1 breath every 6 seconds. If a pulse returns, check to see whether the patient is breathing. Remove oxygen from the immediate area of defibrillations/cardioversions for fire safety.

Compressions: Perform 100 to 120 compressions per minute if the patient is unresponsive and pulseless. Be alert to assessment changes and when to start and stop CPR.

Safety observer: Note any safety concerns such as cardioversion and defibrillations settings and clearing. Ensure oxygen is moved away during defibrillation.

E. RUNNING OF THE SCENARIO

From a control room, faculty operates the software to control the HFHPS, including voice, heart rate (HR), respiratory rate (RR), pulses, cardiac rhythm, blood pressure (BP), and oximetry (SpO_2). Students are reminded to use closed-loop communication and to collaborate with one another as necessary throughout the scenario using leadership and teamwork skills. Emphasis is given to BLS functions as well as ACLS as science has shown that BLS functions are integral to successful resuscitation. The nurse practitioner faculty actor may periodically enter in and out of the simulation, portraying an advanced practice provider, and ask how the resuscitation is going and collaborate with the team. As nursing students implement the role of the team leader, faculty may let the scenario take an unintended path or cue students in a manner to change the path.

F. PRESENTATION OF COMPLETED TEMPLATE

Title

Cardiovascular Resuscitation: Code Simulation for Health Care Students

Scenario Level

300, 400, or graduate level

Focus Area

Cardiovascular resuscitation

Scenario Description

A new patient arrives in the emergency department (ED), a 75-year-old White male who weighs 70 kg and is approximately 5 feet, 11 inches, who begins to feel "a little dizzy." When the nurse enters the room, he becomes unresponsive and pulseless. The nurse recognizes ventricular tachycardia (VT) on the monitor, which soon converts to ventricular fibrillation (VF), and eventually, sinus rhythm accompanied by hypotension.

Patient: 75-year-old male

Allergies: No known allergies

Medication: Hydrochlorothiazide 25-mg tab once daily and amlodipine 5-mg tab once daily.

Past medical history: Hypertension controlled with medication, no past surgeries or recent illnesses.

Social history: Electronic medical record (eMR) indicates he is White, a retired accountant, and is of the Catholic faith. He does not use illicit drugs and rarely drinks alcohol.

Significant other: Patient's tearful wife is present and states that while her husband was painting the garage, he became "very weak and sweaty." "I am very worried about him; he does not look well," she states. When he is moved to an ED treatment room, he immediately becomes unresponsive, pulseless, and is not breathing. The nurse allows the family the option to be present during resuscitation (Emergency Nurses Association [ENA], 2012).

Setting the Scene

Equipment Needed

___Patient wristband with identification
___HFHPS (static manikin with appropriate monitor/simulator may be substituted)
___EKG monitor and defibrillator
___Oxygen simulation connections
___Ambu bag
___Pulse oximetry
___BP cuff
___Stethoscope
___Medication syringes
___Saline lock set up with appropriate IV drip solutions available
___Hand-hygiene solution
___Audiovisual equipment for recording
___Projector and screen in nearby location
___Flip chart with scenario information to assist observers
___Step stool if needed for individual providing compressions
___Simulated eMR (optional)

Resources Needed

2015 *Handbook of Emergency Cardiovascular Care for Healthcare Providers* (AHA, 2015)
Student activity checklist and rotation schedule

Participants Needed

Approximately eight students are engaged for a 30-minute time frame. As there are approximately twice the number of pharmacy students, the nursing and respiratory students rotate more frequently. Roles are team leader, recorder, one to defibrillate/cardiovert, one to administer medications, one to manage the airway and respirations, one to compress the chest, safety observer, experienced nurse to portray a family member; and a faculty member available for questions.

Scenario Implementation

Instructor Interventions

Initial settings for HPS use a three-waveform layout displaying HR, RR, and BP. When faculty prebriefs the students with important functions and tips of each role before the beginning scenarios, they have time to clarify the roles. Then, as they rotate to the various roles, students can apply the functions and tips on their roles tip card. As leadership is a focus for the simulation outcome, the team leader is instructed to collaborate and coordinate with the rest of the team. It is stressed to learners that the team leader is the individual directing care. Faculty emphasizes that questions about patient care from the interprofessional team are to be directed to the team leader, similar to the clinical practice setting. Faculty feedback is given primarily during debriefing and, if appropriate, during the simulation.

Interprofessional faculty assigns roles while making the schedule. Groups of approximately eight interprofessional students come prepared to learn and rotate until they have performed many of the different roles. Because of the time frame, some students have only one simulation session. Care is given to limit faculty interruptions. In addition, students are alerted that several resuscitation medications, such as amiodarone, atropine, and adenosine, all begin with the letter *a*; therefore it is important to be cautious when verbalizing, selecting, and administering these medications. Exhibit 40.1 provides an outline of the scenario.

Exhibit 40.1	Resuscitation Scenario		
Critical Learner Actions	**Instructor Responses/ Patient Condition Changes**	**Cardiac Rhythm**	**Critical Actions Met/Not Met Comments**
√ Unresponsiveness √ Breathlessness √ Call for AED/defibrillator √ Pulses *(for health care providers is <10 seconds)* Start compressions at lower half of sternum; 30 compressions in no less than 15 seconds and no more than 18 seconds *Push hard at least 100 to 120/minute and @ 2–2.4" depth. Use a backboard or put the bed to CPR position. Allow full chest recoil after compressions* Open airway *(head-tilt chin lift if no evidence of head or neck trauma, after the 30 compressions)* Insert oropharyngeal or nasopharyngeal airway Give 2 breaths *(good seal—each over 1 second with visible chest rise, 100% oxygen)* Resume compressions in <10 seconds; 30:2 compressions is ventilation ratio. Monitor performance of all team members. Ensure high-quality CPR at all times. Minimize interruptions in compressions.	Pt. is unresponsive, has no pulse, and is breathless. A few gasping noises are heard from his upper airway.	Unknown at this time	
Assess rhythm Defibrillate @ 150 J (for our biphasic waveform defibrillator; *do compressions until defibrillation available*). √ Clear before defibrillation Leader oversees the safety of defibrillation, including keeping oxygen source away from immediate defibrillation area.	No pulse, pt. remains in VT.	VT without a pulse	
Team leader monitors effective CPR for 2 minutes and facilitates a change in compressors every 2 minutes to maintain effective compressions.	No pulse, pt. remains in VT.	VT without a pulse	

(continued)

Exhibit 40.1	Resuscitation Scenario *(continued)*		
Critical Learner Actions	**Instructor Responses/ Patient Condition Changes**	**Cardiac Rhythm**	**Critical Actions Met/Not Met Comments**
Assess rhythm. Defibrillate @ 150 J. √ Clear before defibrillation Leader oversees the safety of defibrillation, including keeping oxygen source away from immediate defibrillation area.	No pulse, pt. remains in VT.	VT without a pulse	
CPR resumes for 2 minutes. Direct team to start IV or IO Epinephrine 1 mg IV push (1 mg every 3–5 minutes). Consider advanced airway, capnography.	Pt. remains pulseless, not breathing.	VT without a pulse	
Defibrillate @ 150 J. √ Clear before defibrillation	Rhythm changes to VF.	VF	
CPR resumes for 2 minutes. Administer amiodarone 300-mg IV bolus. Treat reversible causes.	Pt. remains in VF.	VF	
Defibrillate @ 150 J. √ Clear before defibrillation	Pt. remains in VF.	VF	
Present the option of family presence during the resuscitation.	Wife has finished registering her husband and wants to know whether she can be with him. She has a copy of his advanced directives in her purse.		
CPR resumes for 2 minutes. Repeat epinephrine 1-mg IV push (1 mg every 3–5 minutes). Defibrillate @ 150 J. √ Clear before defibrillation	Pt. converts to normal sinus rhythm.	VF to normal sinus rhythm	
Resume CPR for 2 minutes.		Normal sinus rhythm	

(continued)

Exhibit 40.1	Resuscitation Scenario (*continued*)		
Critical Learner Actions	**Instructor Responses/ Patient Condition Changes**	**Cardiac Rhythm**	**Critical Actions Met/Not Met Comments**
Check pulse, respirations, blood pressure.	Pulse present., no spontaneous respirations, BP 60 mmHg/palpation.	Normal sinus rhythm	
Maintain airway, breathing. Administer fluid bolus or dopamine infusion or epinephrine infusion.			
Continue to observe and monitor pt.	Normal sinus rhythm frequent multifocal preventricular contractions (PVCs) BP 90/53	Normal sinus rhythm, frequent multifocal PVCs	
Administer antiarrhythmic, amiodarone, maintenance infusion.		Normal sinus rhythm	
Continue to observe and monitor pt.	Normal sinus rhythm, 100/66, spontaneous respirations	Normal sinus rhythm	

AED, automated external defibrillator; BP, blood pressure; CPR, cardiopulmonary resuscitation; IO, intraosseous infusion; IV, intravenous; Pt., patient; VF, ventricular fibrillation; VT, ventricular tachycardia.
Source: Adapted from American Heart Association (2015).

G. DEBRIEFING GUIDELINES

Student questions are encouraged. Students provide feedback on their experience and their perception of the effectiveness of the activity. Questions that interprofessional faculty ask the interprofessional student group include:

1. What went well?
2. Describe how the team worked together as a group.
3. What would you have done differently if doing it again?
4. Did each member communicate effectively and respectfully to others during the simulation?
5. Did team members use closed-loop communication and convey confidence in their communication?
6. What information could have been clarified in any of the scenarios to prevent misunderstanding in the scenario?
7. Give an example of how team members sought the opinions of others. Were there missed opportunities to collaborate interprofessionally during the scenario?
8. What did you learn from the other professions?

H. SUGGESTIONS/KEY FEATURES TO REPLICATE OR IMPROVE

This scenario can be improved by having the flip-chart information printed on a poster board for ease of viewing and to better follow the scenario in the viewing room. Emphasize to students the best place to stand for best audibility and visibility, which may also assist viewers. Sharing past years' tips with students is helpful such as the importance of recalling the AHA algorithms before the simulation day so that they can be applied in the various situations. A faculty demonstration or video may also serve to reinforce student learning before the simulation day. Timing the scenario at midterm assists students to develop their skills throughout the semester.

I. RECOMMENDATIONS FOR FURTHER USE

Using evidence-based practice guidelines from the AHA allows for repetition in learning that is ideal for an interdisciplinary setting. The report of an expert panel, *Core Competencies for Interprofessional Collaborative Practice*, sponsored by the IPEC (2011), serves as a foundational document for IPE regarding knowledge, skills, and attitudes. This document includes four competency domains, including values/ethics for interprofessional practice, roles/responsibilities, interprofessional communication, and teams and teamwork, which may assist faculty when preparing interprofessional experiences such as this one (IPEC, 2011).

J. HOW SIMULATION-BASED PEDAGOGY HAS CONTRIBUTED TO IMPROVED STUDENT OUTCOMES

Using the Laerdal SimMan 3G high-fidelity technology has given students a dimension not previously attainable, as the HFHPS has more realism when pulses are felt, heart tones and breath sounds are heard, and the patient can exclaim phrases such as, "Doc, I feel like I could die!" and "No, I have no allergies." Interprofessional student feedback via postexperience evaluations reveals themes of better understanding their role and increased effectiveness in teamwork and communication after this experience. Students learn that, with time on task, studying rhythm strips and the AHA ACLS algorithms, they become ready to apply necessary knowledge and skill to resuscitation situations.

An updated systematic review of IPE was conducted involving 15 studies and its effects on professional practice and health care outcomes (Reeves, Perrier, Goldman, Freeth, & Zwarenstein, 2013). Findings in the literature review are important because they put into perspective that evaluation of IPE is in its infancy and more research, both qualitative and quantitative, is needed to fully understand best practices in preparing health care students for collaborative practice.

K. EXPERT RECOMMENDATIONS AND WORDS OF WISDOM

This scenario can be used for a wide variety of professions and educational levels as it is written. Learners must be well matched regarding knowledge. It is important for faculty to identify and to collaborate about the structure of prebriefing for each profession. Experiences must be meaningful for each profession, so each professional group gains a quality experience. It is ideal when there is minimal disruption of the usual schedule of each profession, so the experience does not interfere with other important learning. Tablets are now also being used as monitors to present the patient's cardiac rhythms; this can be a very convenient alternative to bulky, heavy monitors.

L. EVALUATION OF BEST PRACTICE STANDARDS AND USE OF CREDENTIALED SIMULATION FACULTY

Completion of the National League for Nursing (NLN) Simulation Innovation Resource Center (SIRC) series was helpful as faculty prepared student learning experiences with realism and intentionality. Learners had shared goals and worked through complex and challenging scenarios in a safe environment that address regional and national goals for cardiac resuscitation. The IPEC competencies, in addition to the International Nursing Association for Clinical Simulation in Learning Standards of Best Practice: Simulation Standard VIII: Simulation-Enhanced IPE, served as a basis for simulation evaluation by both interprofessional faculty and interprofessional students (Decker et al., 2015). Debriefing was team based, structured, and provided collaborative opportunities. Simulation performance is measured in areas of safety, client assessment, communication, teamwork, critical thinking, and technical skills. A pretest and posttest was administered to each professional group to evaluate cognitive learning.

REFERENCES

American Association of Colleges of Nursing. (2008). *The essentials of baccalaureate education for professional nursing practice.* Washington, DC: Author. Retrieved from http://www.aacnnursing.org/Portals/42/Publications/BaccEssentials08.pdf

Decker, S. I., Anderson, M., Boese, T., Epps, C., McCarthy, J., Motola, I., ... Lioce, L. (2015, June). Standards of best practice: Simulation standard VIII: Simulation-enhanced interprofessional education (Sim-IPE). *Clinical Simulation in Nursing, 11*(6), 293–297. doi:10.1016/j.ecns.2015.03.010

Emergency Nurses Association. (2012). Clinical practice guideline: Family presence during invasive procedures and resuscitation. Retrieved from https://www.ena.org/practice-research/research/CPG/Documents/FamilyPresenceCPG.pdf

Institute of Medicine. (2010). *The future of nursing: Leading change, advancing health.* Washington, DC: National Academies Press.

Interprofessional Education Collaborative Expert Panel. (2011). *Core competencies for interprofessional collaborative practice: Report of an expert panel.* Washington, DC: Author.

National Council of State Boards of Nursing. (2015). NCLEX-RN® examination: Test plan for the National Council Licensure Examination for Registered Nurses. Retrieved from https://www.ncsbn.org/RN_Test_Plan_2016_Final.pdf

Reeves, S., Perrier, L., Goldman, J., Freeth, D., & Zwarenstein, M. (2013) Interprofessional education: Effects on professional practice and healthcare outcomes (update). *Cochrane Database of Systematic Reviews, 2013*(3), CD002213. doi:10.1002/14651858.CD002213.pub.

FURTHER READING

American Heart Association. (2015). *Handbook of emergency cardiovascular care for healthcare providers.* Dallas, TX: Author.

Neumar, R. W., Shuster, M., Callaway, C. W., Gent, L. M., Atkins, D. L., Bhanji, F., ... Hazinski, M. F. (2015). Part 1: Executive summary: 2015 American Heart Association guidelines update for cardiopulmonary resuscitation and emergency cardiovascular care. *Circulation, 132*(S2), S315–S367. doi:10.1161/CIR.0000000000000252

CHAPTER 41

Multiple Patient Medical–Surgical Scenario

Kathleen A. Gordon and Mary S. Cook

A. IMPLEMENTATION OF SIMULATION-BASED PEDAGOGY IN YOUR INDIVIDUALIZED TEACHING AREA

Nurses are required to function in leadership positions and to collaborate interprofessionally very early in their careers. Nurse leaders and nurse educators have identified practice gaps in newly licensed nurses entering the workforce. Some areas identified as needing improvements were prioritization, delegation/teamwork, communication, and problem solving. Clinical experiences in the associate of science in nursing (ASN) degree program do not provide extensive or in-depth opportunities for participation in leadership roles. In addition, nursing students have limited opportunity to collaborate with other health care providers to take verbal or telephone orders, actively participate in multidisciplinary rounds, and give a handoff report to the nonnursing personnel. This lack of experience in these leadership components combined with identified practice gaps was the incentive to develop a leadership scenario. Collaboration between the course faculty and the simulation lab coordinator provided an opportunity to implement simulation-based pedagogy. During this scenario, the second-year, second-semester ASN nursing students were provided an unforgettable introduction to life experience as a graduate nurse, while promoting awareness of practice readiness. Simulation became a way to integrate theory and practice.

B. EDUCATIONAL MATERIALS AVAILABLE IN YOUR TEACHING AREA AND RELATED TO YOUR SPECIALTY

Aultman College of Nursing and Health Sciences, simulation laboratory consists of an open room with a desk that supports the control computers. There is no specific area designated as a control room; therefore, simulation staff are always present in the room. This laboratory room provides instruction for medical–surgical patients, acute and nonacute, as well as obstetrical and pediatric patients. The layout of the room is designed to mimic a patient care area with a nightstand, over bed table, cardiac monitor, real oxygen hookup and suction capabilities, bulletin boards with pain assessment charts, patient bill of rights, get well cards, pictures, flowers, and a visitor's chair. In addition, an area of the lab is arranged as a miniature nurse's station complete with a conference phone and a computer with Internet access. These electronic resources allow the students to make necessary phone calls related to patient conditions and consult electronic resources related to drug compatibilities, diagnostic references, and patient education materials. The lab is equipped with video-recording technology that can record to a DVD or live stream into classrooms. Another conference phone is located in the classroom, which provides an opportunity for the course instructor and remaining students to take on an interactive role by playing primary care providers, ancillary staff, nurse leaders, and family members.

C. SPECIFIC OBJECTIVES FOR SIMULATION USAGE WITHIN A SPECIFIC COURSE AND THE OVERALL PROGRAM

The main objective for the multiple patient scenarios is to assess students' readiness for practice related to prioritization, delegation, teamwork, communication, problem solving, organization, and leadership skills. This scenario was originally designed as an in-class, advanced-level simulation for the second year, second-semester professional role development course but was moved after a curriculum revision to the final medical–surgical course. The scenario takes place at the end of the semester after the students have completed a preceptor clinical rotation.

Prebriefing consists of a worksheet that addresses the following: scope of practice of the RN and the licensed practical nurse (LPN), the role of the charge nurse, leadership and management principles, delegation, confidentiality, and patient rights. Suggested resources for this information include the nurse practice act, professional nursing journals or books, and professional websites. In addition, students are given abbreviated information about the patients so they can begin to develop a patient assignment and formulate a preliminary plan of care.

D. INTRODUCTION OF SCENARIO

Setting the Scene

The simulation lab is one large room, but for this scenario, the room is partitioned into three separate rooms. Each room contains furniture, equipment, and the patient's personal possessions to mimic an actual patient care area. The nurses' station is centrally located in the room. Additional areas are designed as a dirty utility room, clean utility room, and medication room. The students are required to wear official clinical attire. The three patients are: 80-year-old with stroke-like symptoms, a 21-year-old involved in a motorcycle crash, and a 34-year-old having gall bladder surgery.

Technology Used

Three high-fidelity human simulators are used to represent the patients. Each patient has an infusion pump. There is one workstation on wheels (WOW), two conference phones, and videotaping/streaming equipment.

Objectives

1. Identify management/leadership behaviors demonstrated throughout the simulation exercise
2. Recognize the critical thinking and problem-solving skills necessary to care for multiple patients
3. Demonstrate prioritization and organizational skills during the care of multiple patients
4. Communicate appropriately with patient, significant others, and health care personnel
5. Assign appropriate competent individuals to complete specific nursing tasks
6. Evaluate the total experience of caring for multiple patients

Description of Participants

Nursing students are assigned to the roles of charge nurse, staff RN, LPN, unlicensed assistive personnel (UAP), and precepting registered nursing student to provide patient care. Volunteers portray the simulator voices using a provided script but have permission to go off script as necessary to increase the fidelity of the situation. Additional volunteers are recruited to portray significant others, friends, and family members. In addition, the college is fortunate to have the ability to recruit members of the security department, rapid response team, pastoral care, and primary care providers from the affiliate hospital.

E. RUNNING OF THE SCENARIO

All students are prebriefed before the day of simulation. This information is used to develop a patient care assignment and to become familiar with the standard of care for each medical condition. Immediately before the simulation, the students randomly draw roles. Each student wears a name tag designating their role. The students not participating in the simulation are watching from the classroom with the instructor, discussing what they would be doing if they were in the simulation and anticipating what orders to expect from the primary care provider. Personnel from the affiliate hospital (primary health care provider, security officers, pastoral care and rapid response nurses) are contacted earlier in the semester to ensure availability. At the start of the scenario, the students are given a verbal hand-off report. Following this report, the charge nurse determines the priority patient(s), assigns staff, and communicates with other health care members. The team is expected to communicate effectively with a charge nurse and other health care members; work as a team and deliver safe, effective care that includes assessment, checking diagnostic data, performing nursing skills, including medications, and managing crisis situations. Debriefing occurs immediately following the scenario using components from both the Plus Delta (Dusai, 2014) and the Debriefing for Meaningful Learning (Dreifuerst, 2015) methods.

F. PRESENTATION OF COMPLETED TEMPLATE

Title

Multiple Patient Medical–Surgical Scenario

Scenario Level

Prelicensure, second-year, second-semester ASN program

Focus Area

The scenario focuses on principles of leadership and management of patients with the integration of communication skills, problem solving, delegation, organization, prioritization, and professionalism for the second-year, second-semester ASN nursing students.

Scenario Description

The students arrive on the unit for day shift. The charge nurse makes a staff assignment following the report. Two RNs, two LPNs, a UAP, and/or a precepting senior nursing student are assigned to care for the following patients: Mark Johnson (ischemic brain attack resulting in left-sided hemiparesis), Bill Murphy (motorcycle accident), and John York (open cholecystectomy). Students are given patient histories and the night nurse's handoff report for these three simulations.

Patient 1: Mr. Mark Johnson
Age: 80 years, date of birth: 04/14/19XX

History

Patient has allergies to penicillin (PCN) and peanuts. Diabetic for 60 years, controlled with diet and insulin; hypertensive for 30 years, controlled with medication; hypercholesterolemia for 20 years, controlled with medication. Smokes one pack of cigarettes per day but is attempting to quit, Drinks one to two beers per day; weight: 102.3 kg (225 pounds); height: 5 feet, 10 inches; diet: 1,500-calorie diabetic diet. An advanced directive is mentioned on the chart.

Handoff report: This 80-year-old patient of Dr. Neff was diagnosed with ischemic brain attack resulting in left-sided hemiparesis and admitted yesterday. He was not a candidate for tissue plasminogen activator (t-PA); is allergic to PCN and peanuts. Diet: nothing by mouth (NPO) since failing his bedside swallow screen. The health care provider was notified of the failed swallow screen. Bedrest with the head of bed (HOB) elevated 30°. He is high risk for falls with a score of more than 50 on the Morse scale. There is an advanced directive on the chart. Lab work today: activated partial thromboplastin time (APTT), complete blood count (CBC), basic metabolic panel (BMP), and platelets. An ultrasound of the carotid arteries is ordered today. Consultations ordered: physical, occupational, and speech therapy. Last vital signs were: temperature (T): 37.2°C, pulse (P): 88 beats/minute, respiratory rate (RR): 20 breaths/minute, blood pressure (BP): 150/90 mmHg. Appears to be alert and oriented but is difficult to understand when questioned as he slurs his words. Pupils equal, round, reactive to light and accommodation (PERRLA), size 5 mm. Left facial droop with drool draining from the left side of his mouth, has a weak gag reflex and chokes very easily. Left arm and leg strength are moderately weak. Incontinent ×1, missed the urinal. Patient has a 20-gauge over-the-needle catheter in the right forearm with normal saline (NS) infusing at 50 mL/hr via infusion pump. Intravenous (IV) site is clear with dressing intact. No insulin reactions are reported.

Medications

Enalapril (Vasotec) 5 mg twice a day by mouth
Neutral protamine Hagedorn (NPH) insulin (Humulin N) 10 units before breakfast and dinner subcutaneously (SC)
Regular insulin (Humulin R) 5 units before each meal SC
Atorvastatin (Lipitor) 20 mg daily at bedtime by mouth

When the students enter the room, they will find the following:

T: 37.4°C, P: 90 beats/minute, RR: 22 breaths/minute, BP: 200/100 mmHg
Alert and oriented, cannot remember what happened yesterday but can remember past events, cries easily
Short attention span, but does follow commands, complains of (c/o) headache, rating it a 3 on the 0-to-10 scale, has had it since early this morning, nothing makes it better or worse, refuses medication at this time
Pupils: Equal, 6 mm bilaterally, round and reactive to light, c/o some blurred vision
Drool draining from the left side of his mouth with facial droop
Skin: Pale pink, warm, dry, turgor normal for age, reddened area on left hip
NS is infusing via an infusion pump at 50 mL/hr through a 20-gauge over-the-needle catheter in his right forearm
IV site is clear with dressing intact
Lungs: Clear in all lung fields, anterior and posterior, pulse oximeter: 96%
Heart: Normal S1 and S2, regular, capillary refill less than 3 seconds on toes and fingers; nail beds pale pink
Abdomen: Bowel sounds are present in all four quadrants, soft on palpation, no distention

Patient has an observable scar on right lower quadrant, does not remember last bowel movement (BM; wife states it was yesterday), voiding quantity is sufficient as stated by night nurse. Musculoskeletal: Left arm and leg moderately weak, right arm and leg strong, knee-high antiembolic stockings worn on bilateral lower extremities; yellow slipper socks and yellow armband depicting fall risk. An empty urinal and tissue box are on the over bed table.

Diagnostics

Non-contrast CT scan of the head indicated right. hemispheric ischemia, chest x-ray: normal, activated partial thromboplastin time (APTT): 70 seconds, cholesterol: 319 mg/dL, high-density lipoprotein (HDL):

50 mg/dL, very-low-density lipoprotein (VLDL): 35 mg/dL, triglycerides: 170 mg/dL, glycosylated hemo-globin A1C (HbA1C): 7.2%, blood sugar: 130 mg/dL.

Crisis Variation

Patient falls out of bed, while trying to get up to go to the bathroom because of his left-sided weakness. Using a high-fidelity human patient simulator, you must be careful putting him on the floor (might want to think about using a static human patient simulator as it would be easier to pull him out of bed and not have to worry about incurring damage). When the students enter the room, they find the following: Mark lying on the floor calling out for help, P: 160 beats/minute, RR: 24 breaths/minute, BP: 90/50 mmHg, alert and oriented, crying (states he did not hit his head), rubbing his right hip, c/o hurting when mov-ing, rating pain in leg a 7 on a 0-to-10 scale, pain radiates to knee, c/o right wrist pain but able to move it with no increase in pain, 2-inch. abrasion noted on his spine as he slid down the bed when falling.

Diagnostics: An x-ray of the right hip and wrist; the student is expected to notify the health care provider and initiate a variance report form.

Medication record: (see Exhibit 41.1)

Patient 2: Mr. Bill Murphy
Age: 21 years, date of birth: 05/21/1996

History

Allergies: Patient has no known drug, food, or environmental allergies; has been healthy all his life; smokes one pack of cigarettes per day, drinks a six-pack of beer per day, recreational drugs: occasionally uses marijuana; weight: 63.6 kg (140 pounds), height: 5 feet, 8 inches; diet: always hungry, eats most anything but loves McDonalds and potato chips; no advanced directive: patient not interested, laughs about it.

Exhibit 41.1	Medication Record for Patient Mark Johnson

Patient: Mr. Mark Johnson   **Allergies:** Penicillin & peanuts   **DOB:** 04/14/1937

Medical provider: M. Neff

Medication list:		Time given:
Regular Insulin (Humulin R) sliding scale SC		0800, 1000, 1200, 1400, 1600, 1800, 2000, 2400, 0200, 0400, 0600
0–130 BS No insulin	131–200 BS—2 units	201–250 BS—4 units
251–300 BS—6 units	301–350 BS—8 units	>350—call health care provider

Medication record (crisis variation)

PRN medication list:	Time given:
Acetaminophen (Tylenol) 650 mg every 4 hours as needed for pain by mouth (when able to take food);	
meperidine 25-mg IM every 6 hours as needed for pain	

BS, blood sugar; DOB, date of birth; IM, intramuscular; PRN, as needed; SC, subcutaneous.

Handoff report: This 21-year-old is a patient of Dr. Deal who was admitted during the night for observation following a traumatic motorcycle crash. He has no known allergies. Diet as tolerated. Bedrest. He is alert and oriented to person, place, time, and situation. Neurological assessment negative. His vital signs have been stable throughout the night T: 36.8°C, P: 78 beats/minute, RR: 18 breaths/minute, shallow, BP: 120/82 mmHg, c/o pain when takes a breath (rates it a 6 on 0-to-10 scale). Pulse oximeter 91% on room air, oxygen applied at 2 L/nasal cannula (NC). Medicated at 0300 with morphine 1 mg IV with relief. Has road rash and small size bruising all over, states "he hurts all over." IV of 5% dextrose and 0.45 normal saline (D5 1/2NS) running via an infusion pump in left forearm at 100 mL/hr through a 16-gauge over-the-needle catheter, site clear. Cut under his chin (four stitches with a dry dressing) from the helmet strap cutting into it.

Medications

No routine medication is taken. Takes Tylenol for an occasional headache.

When the students enter the room, they will find the following:

Bill is sitting up in bed, wearing a du-rag on his head, with a wide smile. He invites them to sit on his bed. He has a cigarette in his hand plus an ashtray with numerous cigarette butts in it and an empty can of beer on the overbed table. Bill is constantly trying to distract staff with his sexually overt behavior. Oxygen is not running but still plugged into the oxygen outlet (oxygen tubing on the floor); T: 37°C, P: 76 beats/minute, RR: 14 breath/minute and shallow, BP: 116/54 mmHg; alert and oriented, gauze dressing on his chin has slight amount of serosanguineous drainage; pupils: size 4 mm, PERRLA; skin: pink, warm, and dry, road rash, and numerous bruises noted throughout arms, trunk, and legs; IV of D51/2NS running at 100 mL/hr through a 16-gauge over-the-needle catheter via an infusion pump; IV site in left forearm is clear with dressing intact; lungs: shallow breathing, crackles heard in upper lobes, clears with a cough, lower lobes clear anterior and posterior; pulse oximeter 91%; heart: normal S1 and S2, regular, capillary refill less than 3 seconds, nail beds: pink; abdomen: bruises noted throughout approximately 2 to 4 inches in size, bowel sounds present in all four quadrants, slight tenderness on palpation, no distention, last BM was early this morning, voiding with no problems. Musculoskeletal: strong in upper and lower extremities.

Crisis Variation

Bill will have a much larger (6–8 inches) bruise in the left upper quadrant (LUQ) before assessment time. Students have the options to call the rapid response team, pastoral care, and the health care provider for assistance. Mother is at the bedside (mother is of Jehovah Witness faith, although Bill has no religious affiliation). Further testing reveals a tear in the spleen; the physician orders two units of packed red blood cells (RBC) to be given and patient is prepped for a splenectomy. The mother becomes irate when the blood is brought into the room to be initiated. Students need to be able to handle this confrontation or phone for assistance. Bill did sign a consent form for blood, although this is unknown to the mother. When the students enter the room, they will find the following:

P: 120 beats/minute, RR: 24 breaths/minute, BP: 86/60 mmHg, lethargic, hard to arouse, c/o abdominal pain radiating to left shoulder, rating it a 9 on 0-to-10 scale,

Skin: Pale, diaphoretic,

Abdomen: very large bruise in LUQ, diffusely tender and tense on palpation.

Diagnostics

Chest x-ray: normal, CT scan of the chest: no pneumothorax or lacerations, C-reactive protein: 2.5 mg/L, RBC: 4.49 million/mm³, hemoglobin: 14.3 G/dL, hematocrit: 43.5%

Crisis diagnostics: Noncontrast CT scan of the abdomen (reveals laceration of the spleen, no bowel perforation), white blood cells (WBC): 10.80/mm³, RBC: 4.1 million/mm³, hemoglobin: 9.6 G/dL, hematocrit: 36%, type and cross for two units of packed RBCs

Medication record: (see Exhibit 41.2)

Exhibit 41.2	Medication Record for Patient Bill Murphy

Patient: Mr. Bill Murphy　　　　　　　　　　　　　　**Allergies:** NKDA　　**DOB:** 05/21/1995

Medical provider: M. Deal

PRN medication list:　　　　　　　　　　　　　　　　**Time given:**

Morphine sulfate 1 mg every 4 hours IV as needed for pain　0300

Medication record (crisis variation)

Medication list:　　　　　　　　　　　　　　　　　　**Time given:**

2 units of packed RBC with NS infusion

IV, intravenous; NKDA, no known drug allergies; NS, normal saline; PRN, as needed; RBC, red blood cell.

Patient 3: Mr. John York

Age: 34 years, date of birth: 06/01/1983

History

Allergies: No known drug, food, or environmental allergies; diabetic since age 7 years, controlled with diet and insulin; hypercholesterolemia, no other health problems; smokes ½ pack cigarettes per day since age 14 years, would like to quit; drinks an occasional cocktail after work to unwind; no use of street drugs; weight: 136.4 kg (300 pounds); height: 5 feet, 10 inches; diet: 1,200 calorie diabetic diet, but has trouble sticking to it; no advanced directive on chart, wife will bring in.

Present history: For the past 6 months, he has been experiencing localized severe, sharp, steady, suddenly occurring epigastric pain radiating to the right shoulder and lasting up to 5 hours. Feels full even after a small meal, then becomes nauseated and sometimes vomits, especially when he eats pizza, French fries, and other fried foods. He tried antacids and over-the-counter Zantac, took Tylenol and Motrin for the pain, all without success. Attempted unsuccessfully to limit fried foods, but states he loves them too much. Wife talked him into seeing the physician when she thought his eyes looked yellow.

Handoff report: This 34-year-old patient of Dr. Puller's was admitted with cholelithiasis and is day 2 postop after an open cholecystectomy. He has no known allergies. NPO and activity as tolerated. Vital signs have been stable all night, T: 37.9°C, P: 76 beats/minute, RR: 24 breaths/minute and shallow, BP: 128/74 mmHg; the nasogastric tube is connected to low intermittent suction, emptied for 300 ml of a greenish-brown drainage. Lungs have some crackles; patient needs to be encouraged to cough and use the incentive spirometer. The abdomen is slightly firm, hypoactive bowel sounds, abdominal dressing has scant amount of dried sanguineous drainage. Jackson-Pratt drained 10 mL of dark-red drainage. No BM, voiding quantities sufficient. Moves well in bed but reluctant to get up. IV of 5% dextrose with Ringer's lactate (D5RL) with 10 mEq potassium chloride (KCl) running via infusion pump at 125 mL/hr in the left forearm with an 18-gauge over-the-needle catheter. IV site clear, dressing intact. No insulin reaction reported. Medicated for pain at 0200; sleeping at present.

Medications

> Regular insulin (Novolin R) 14 units with each meal SC
> Insulin glargine (Lantus) 20 units at bedtime SC
> Atorvastatin (Lipitor) 40 mg by mouth once a day

When the students enter the room, they will find the following:

John is lying in bed with the HOB slightly elevated, eyes shut and holding his belly. There is an incentive spirometer on his over bed table with a tissue box and a newspaper; T: 37.9°C, P: 74 beats/minute, RR: 24 breaths/minute and shallow, BP: 126/72 mmHg; alert and oriented; pupils: 4 mm, PERRLA, sclera white; skin: pale warm, dry. Mouth dry; IV site in the left forearm is clear with dressing intact; D5RL with 10 mEq of KCl running at 125 mL/hr through an 18-gauge over-the-needle catheter via an infusion pump. Lungs: crackles heard throughout but more so in upper lobes, anterior and posterior; pulse oximeter 93%; heart: normal S1 and S2, regular; capillary refill 3 seconds, nail beds pale; abdomen: bowel sounds absent in all four quadrants, round, slight distention, firm, no flatus; nasogastric tube in left nares connected to low intermittent suction draining greenish-brown fluid with flecks, nares clear. The abdominal dressing has quarter-sized serosanguineous drainage. Jackson-Pratt draining the scant amount of dark-red drainage; c/o incisional pain, rating it a 7 on a 0-to-10 scale; musculoskeletal: strong in upper extremities but reluctant to push on lower extremities; lab value: BS: 203 mg/dL.

Diagnostics

Testing revealed cholelithiasis and surgery was recommended. **Surgical note:** Open cholecystectomy was performed because of the weight of patient and size of the gallbladder. Cholecystectomy with common bile duct exploration and insertion of Jackson-Pratt drainage tube.

Crisis Variation

During a confrontation in the patient's room between the wife and pregnant mistress, Mr. York begins to cough violently which causes his abdominal wound to eviscerate.

When the students enter the room, they will find the following:

Wife and obviously pregnant mistress are arguing; Mr. York is coughing violently, holding his abdomen; c/o a giving feeling in his abdomen and feeling wet; dressing shows a large amount of serosanguineous drainage, when opening the dressing the students will see actual bowel sticking out of the wound, c/o pain in his abdomen rating it an 8 on a 0-to-10 scale; T: 37.7°C, P: 120 beats/minute, RR: 28 breaths/minute, BP: 140/90 mmHg. The students need to cover the bowel appropriately and handle the confrontation between the wife and the mistress. This situation may necessitate notification of security officers to assist with the confrontation. Additional notifications will be the rapid response team to help with the emergency and the surgeon.

Medication record: (see Exhibit 41.3)

Exhibit 41.3	Medication Record for Patient John York

Patient: Mr. John York   **Allergies:** NKDA   **DOB:** 06/01/1983
Medical provider: M. Puller

Medication list:		**Time given:**
Regular insulin (Novolin R) sliding scale SC		0800, 1000, 1200, 1400, 1600, 1800, 2000, 2400, 0200, 0400, 0600
Ceftriaxone, 1 g IV		Every 12 hours 0800 and 2000
<150 BS—no insulin	150–200 BS—2 units	201–250 BS-4 units
251–300 BS—6 units	301–350 BS—8 units	> 350—call health care provider

PRN medication list:	**Time given:**
Morphine sulfate, 2 mg IV, every 6 hours as needed for pain	0200
Ondansetron, 4 mg IV, every 8 hours as needed for nausea	

BS, blood sugar; IV, intravenous; PRN, as needed; SC, subcutaneous.

Scenario Objectives

1. Make an appropriate patient care assignment based on staffing mix and patient acuity.
2. Communicate effectively with health care providers face to face and via phone using the situation, background, assessment, and recommendation (SBAR) format (Eberhardt, 2014).
3. Communicate therapeutically/appropriately with the patient, significant others, and health care personnel while maintaining confidentiality.
4. Initiate assessments based on handoff report and priority patient and reassess as necessary.
5. Interpret diagnostic, laboratory, and/or assessment findings to plan care of the patients.
6. Perform nursing interventions accurately.
7. Delegate and supervise appropriately.
8. Make decisions using problem-solving skills.
9. Display leadership skills.

The scenario also allows students to practice key elements from the National Council of State Boards of Nursing (NCSBN; 2015) National Council Licensure Examination for Registered Nurses (NCLEX-RN®) test plan, including:

Safe and effective care environment: *Management of care* (advocacy, client rights, collaboration with interdisciplinary team, concept of management, confidentiality/information security, continuity of care, assignment, delegation, and supervision, establishing priorities, ethical practice, informed consent, information technology, legal rights and responsibilities), *Safety and infection control* (accident/error/injury/prevention, ergonomic principles, reporting of incident/event/irregular occurrence/variance, safe use of equipment, standard precautions/transmission-based precautions/surgical asepsis, use of restraints/safety devices); **Health promotion and maintenance:** (aging process, health risk behaviors, lifestyle choices, techniques of physical assessment); **Psychosocial integrity:** (behavioral interventions, family dynamics, religious and spiritual influences on health, therapeutic communication, therapeutic environment); **Physiological integrity:** *Basic care and comfort* (elimination, mobility/immobility, nutrition and oral hydration, personal hygiene), *Pharmacological and parenteral therapies* (blood and blood products, central venous access devices, dosage calculations, expected actions/outcomes, medication administration, parenteral/intravenous therapy, pharmacological pain management), *Reduction of risk potential* (changes/abnormalities in vital signs, diagnostic tests, laboratory values, potential for alterations in body systems, potential for complications for surgical procedures and health alterations, systems-specific assessment), *Physiological adaptation* (alterations in body systems, fluid and electrolyte imbalances, hemodynamics, illness management, medical emergencies).

Although this scenario has been used within an ASN program, it could be used in a baccalaureate degree program. The scenario would allow for integration of the following Baccalaureate Essentials (American Association of Colleges of Nursing [AACN], 2008):

Essential VI: Interprofessional Communication and Collaboration for Improving Patient Health Outcomes
Essential IX: Baccalaureate Generalist Nursing Practice

Setting the Scene

Equipment Needed

Human simulators—three high-fidelity (could use mid- or low-fidelity simulators or static manikins) all in hospital beds; video-recording device, streaming capabilities, DVDs, and projector screen (optional); student role status tags; room partitions/dividers (3); room number for each room; patient identification bracelets (3), including allergy and risk for falls; conference phones (2); call bells (3) each with a different sound; vital signs and pulse oximeter equipment; gloves and hand sanitizer (3); intravenous supplies: infusion pumps (3); IV tubing (3); blood tubing (1); secondary IV tubing (2); IV solutions: 1,000 mL NS (2), 1,000 mL D51/2NS, 1,000 mL D5RL with 10 mEq KCl, 500 mL NS; units of blood (2); NS flushes (3 mL and 10 mL); over-the-needle catheters 20 gauge (1), 18 gauge (1), 16 gauge (1); IV dressings (3); urinals (3) and bedpans (optional); oxygen (wall or portable) NC tubing (3); alcohol gauze pads (box); bath supplies: towels, wash cloths, basins; urine volumetric (graduated) (3); operative permits (2) and preoperative checklists (2); syringes: IM, SC, and insulin plus needles; soufflé cups; water pitcher and glasses (1); all medication; and full patient charts (3). See patient-specific resources below for additional equipment needed.

Patient-Specific Resources

Mark Johnson needs red hip (theater make-up), appendectomy scar (fake skin), drool using clear hand lotion or simulator's ability to drool, cotton balls to create drooped left side of mouth, insulin injection pad, fingerstick blood-sugar supplies, meperidine, Tylenol, variance report form, and NPO sign. **Bill-Murphy** needs candy cigarettes, real cigarette package, empty beer can, ashtray, tattoo sleeves, du-rag for the head, a laceration on the chin (fake skin with sutures embedded) covered with a small gauze dressing, theater make-up for bruises and road rash on extremities with a particular focus on the abdomen. **John York** needs nasogastric tube with suction (drainage greenish-brown with flecks), Jackson-Pratt drain (dark-red drainage), dressing supplies: 4 × 4 gauze, abdominal gauze pads 5 × 9 (2), tape, NS for irrigation, two different abdominal wounds (a normal incision and a dehisced wound), incentive spirometer, morphine (IV), ondansetron (IV), regular insulin, ceftriaxone IV, SC injection pad, operative permit, preoperative checklist, and NPO sign.

Additional Resources Needed

Lab data for patient condition changes, drug books, medication compatibility charts, access to hospital policy and procedures, grading rubric, prebriefing worksheet for debriefing, postexperience evaluation form.

Human Simulator Level

Three high-fidelity simulators

Participants Needed

Faculty to play the role of night nurse to give handoff report; hospital personnel to portray all three physicians; actual security officers, rapid response team member, and a member from pastoral care; faculty to role play the mother of Bill Murphy; volunteers to role-play the wife and mistress of John York as well as voices for all the patients using prepared scripts; simulation staff to manage the high-fidelity human simulators, deliver updated diagnostics, and videotape.

Exhibit 41.4	Required Student Assessments and Actions
Perform hand hygiene.	Obtain a handoff report.
Create a patient care assignment using information obtained from the handoff report.	Review patient charts for orders, diagnostics, lab, and medication records.
Reassess the patient(s) after interventions and/or condition change.	Administer ordered medications accurately using the appropriate rights of medication administration.
Document data.	Perform nursing care within the scope of practice.

Scenario Implementation

Initial settings: Arrange the room into three patient areas; place room numbers in each room; apply identification bands to each patient, including allergy and risk for falls; position the nurse's station in the middle of the room; have full patient charts; conference phones (one at the nurses' station and one in the classroom); variance report forms, preoperative checklists, procedure consent forms; prepare an area for clean utility room and medication room with all supplies and medications available; all intravenous solutions in place and running via infusion pumps.

   Mark Johnson: Apply red area on left hip and appendectomy scar; have drool draining from the mouth; initial vital signs: T: 37.4°C, P: 90 beats/minute, RR: 22 breaths/minute, BP: 200/100 mmHg. **Crisis changes:** If the patient falls out of bed: vital signs change to: P: 160 beats/minute, RR: 24 breaths/minute, BP: 90/50 mmHg and c/o pain in his right hip.

   Bill Murphy: Apply du-rag; tattoo sleeves; theater make-up for bruises, road rash, and small dressing on chin; on the overbed table have cigarettes, ashtray and a can of beer; oxygen 2 L NC; initial vital signs are: T: 37°C, P: 76 beats/minute, RR: 14 breaths/minute and shallow, BP: 116/54mmHg. **Crisis changes:** If patient has the tear in the spleen add a bigger bruise to LUQ, vital signs are now: P: 120 beats/minute, RR: 24 breaths/minute, BP: 86/60 mmHg; abdominal pain is rated a 9 on the 0-to-10 scale. Skin is pale; abdomen is distended in the LUQ. Bill becomes lethargic until he becomes nonresponsive. New lab values are faxed.

   John York: Initial vital signs: T: 37.9°C, P: 74 beats/minute, RR: 24 breaths/minute and shallow, BP: 126/72 mmHg; insert nasogastric tube to low intermittent suction, draining greenish brown with flecks; tape a Jackson-Pratt drain under the dressing draining with a small amount blood red; apply the normal abdominal incision with dressing to the simulator; incentive spirometer on the overbed table; have dressing change supplies available. **Crisis changes:** If John dehisces, his vital signs change to: T: 37.7°C, P: 120 beats/minute, RR: 24 breaths/minute, BP: 140/90 mmHg; apply the dehisced incision prior to the scenario but just cover with a dressing until needed.

Precepting Registered Nursing Student Expectations

Communicate therapeutically, maintain confidentiality, assess the assigned patients in order of priority, perform interventions with appropriate supervision, plan care for assigned patients with the assistance of the staff RN.

Instructor Interventions

The simulation lab coordinator acts as a resource within the simulation lab; course faculty remain in the classroom with the nonparticipating students to facilitate the scenario.

Exhibit 41.5	Participant Expectations

Charge nurse: Make outpatient assignment; communicate with the health care providers using SBAR; communicate with significant others while maintaining confidentiality; receive, verify, and transcribe orders; manage crisis situations; make rounds on all patients; delegate appropriately.

Staff RN: Communicate therapeutically, maintain confidentiality, assess the assigned patients in order of priority, supervise and delegate to the LPN and/ or UAP appropriately, perform nursing interventions, plan care for assigned patients, supervise the precepting student nurse.

LPN: Communicate therapeutically, maintain confidentiality, collect data on assigned patients, report findings to the staff RN or charge nurse as appropriate, perform interventions within scope of practice.

UAP: Communicate appropriately, maintain confidentiality, answer call lights, report patient needs to assigned nurse (chain of command), assist patients with personal hygiene.

Evaluation Criteria

A rubric by Lasater (2007) was adapted (with author permission) to allow for comprehensive evaluation of student performance. The rubric evaluates the group's ability to organize, prioritize, utilize problem solving, communicate, perform nursing skills, delegate, and maintain a controlled environment. The rubric contains five sections highlighting the previously detailed activities. Each section identifies the criteria to be met to obtain a rating of one, two, or three for a possible total of 15 points. The course faculty member uses this rubric to evaluate each group. The course faculty member's evaluation is the recorded grade for the group. Students are required to complete a self-evaluation of their group's performance using this rubric. In addition, each student is required to complete a peer evaluation of all other groups. The rationale for the student evaluations is to assist in the development of evaluation skills necessary in practice.

G. DEBRIEFING GUIDELINES

Issues to Consider

Staffing assignment: Experience of personnel plays a role

Conflict management issues: Resources available to the nurse (security officers, health care personnel, rapid response team, pastoral care, primary care provider to assist with conflict

Setting professional boundaries: Discussion of feelings related to sexually overt behavior and possible options for handling these situations

Confidentiality issues: Family calling into the hospital for patient information, what can be told and what should not be communicated, use of a family security code

Prioritization issues: Airway, breathing and circulation; risk potential

Leadership styles: Personal attributes of participants, assigned leader versus informal leader

Problem-solving capabilities: Past experience, resources, and knowledge base

Patient risk factors: Smoking with oxygen, obese diabetic with a wound, latent manifestations of abdominal trauma, and elderly diabetic with impaired mobility and sensation

Organization: Ability to handle unforeseen crises, multitasking requirements of all personnel, ability to handle interruptions, recognize need to make adjustments in the patient care assignment

Student Questions

What were the participants' strengths?

What leadership styles were displayed during the scenario?

Was the patient care assignment appropriate for the patients and the scope or practice for the personnel?

Was the priority patient chosen by the team?

Was the change in priority patient recognized by the participants?

How was the crisis situation handled?

Was confidentiality maintained throughout the scenario? If not, what breaks did you see? How would you handle these in the future?

Were any boundaries crossed?

Was communication therapeutic? If not, how might this be improved?

How were the organizational skills? If not organized, how might these be improved?

What areas of practice have you personally identified as needing improvement before entering professional practice?

What were areas needing improvement?

Did the charge nurse portray the leadership style described or did another leader emerge during the scenario?

Would there be additional options for the patient care assignment?

Did the priority patient change during the scenario?

What changes were noted?

What was the first clue that your patient was going into a crisis situation?

Would you handle the crisis situation the same in the future?

Are there other options for handling conflicts during the scenario (Jehovah Witness religion and wife/mistress)?

We adjusted the scenario to reflect the pregnant mistress and confrontation that leads to the coughing that causes the wound to dehiscence.

What behaviors by the staff were noted in response to the sexually overt behavior? How would you handle this in the future?

Were nursing skills implemented appropriately? If not, how might these be improved?

If you completed the scenario again what would you do differently?

H. SUGGESTIONS/KEY FEATURES
TO REPLICATE OR IMPROVE

This scenario has been used for a number of semesters for continued enhancement. A fourth patient has been utilized in the past to represent a female oncology patient who develops herpes zoster and hypercalcemia. Each human simulator has been preprogrammed. Volunteers (faculty or students) are used to portray the patient voices and are provided a script. Visitor/family roles are: the mother (Jehovah Witness faith) of Bill Murphy, and the wife and mistress of John York. Additional hospital personnel include the security team, rapid response team, pastoral care and physicians, all of whom are called into the scenario as the students need them.

Bill's mother has a strategic role in the scenario. She becomes very aggressie if the students ignore her son's symptoms, starts crying, and calls the supervisor to report the unit. If blood is ordered, she really turns on the aggressive behavior. The wife and mistress of John York visit at the same time. The mistress is obviously pregnant. A conflict emerges between the two females which causes John to start coughing violently when attempting to intervene ultimately leading to the dehiscence of the wound.

The dehisced bowel is made by filling a condom with cranberry oatmeal and placing plastic rings at intervals to replicate segments of the bowel. Fake skin is made from Vaseline and cornstarch tinted to match the simulator's skin tone. Fake skin is used to cover the bowel with a portion left open. Sutures are inserted into the skin, but where the dehiscence is, the ties are broken. Blood is applied to the bowel and an abdominal dressing is applied. The normal incision was made by a seamstress using material matching the simulator's skin tone and thick black thread to mimic sutures. The ends have Velcro to hold the material in place.

If primary health care providers are unavailable, a volunteer from the affiliate hospital could be used to portray all three primary health care providers using different accents. The health care provider makes rounds on the patients and seeks out the charge nurse as well as the nurse assigned to each patient thereby providing an opportunity for the nursing students to communicate directly with a primary health care provider to either obtain orders or give a report on the patients (practice SBAR).

The use of oxygen in the room forces the student to think about safety and education, especially related to the finding of the cigarettes. A different sound for each patient call bell allows staff to distinguish which patient requires assistance. Videotaped recordings can be used for debriefing, peer evaluations, self-evaluations, remediation, and review for unavoidable nursing student absences. Planning and collaboration among faculty, interdisciplinary team, and the simulation coordinator are critical for successful completion of the scenario. To facilitate setup, each patient should have a designated container to store essential supplies. Reflective journaling was instituted to provide an opportunity for students to discuss the fidelity of the scenario and to assess their readiness for practice. Use of affiliate hospital personnel helped to ensure currency and accuracy of the treatment regimens. Recommended allowed a time frame for the scenario would be 2 hours, 1 hour for the scenario and 1 hour for debriefing.

I. RECOMMENDATIONS FOR FURTHER USE

This scenario is quite complex, therefore it requires placement in upper level nursing courses, a leadership course, or as part of a capstone course. Although the current use is in an ASN program, it could be used for undergraduate baccalaureate nursing students and/or BSN completion program as well. In addition, the scenario could be adapted for use as part of an orientation for new graduates or competency assessment in the acute care setting.

J. HOW SIMULATION-BASED PEDAGOGY HAS CONTRIBUTED TO IMPROVED STUDENT OUTCOMES

This scenario was developed to assess the students' readiness for practice both from an individual and a program viewpoint. The scenario fosters the evaluation of self and peers, which will be required in practice. Students often verbalize a more accurate evaluation of their peers' performance, but are reluctant to score their peers accordingly on the graded rubric. This provided an opportunity to discuss the implications of substandard performance on safe patient care.

K. EXPERT RECOMMENDATIONS AND WORDS OF WISDOM

Additional patients could be added, or more crisis situations developed to increase the complexity or add variety to the scenario. Also, the setting could be adapted to be in a clinic, physician's office, or an intensive care unit. Dressing the human simulators in street clothes would better mimic the different settings. The scenario can be run using mid-fidelity or static simulators. Originally, we used static simulators with labels applied to indicate vital signs and other assessment data.

You can be very creative and use things that have happened in the clinical setting such as having a visitor go into an asthma attack because there were flowers in the room, smuggling a cat into the hospital for a patient, and transporting a visitor to the emergency department when labor started.

Our recommendation would be to allow a minimum of 2 hours for this simulation, so the scenario and debriefing are not rushed. Our class time now is only 1 hour, allowing 30 minutes for the scenario and 30 minutes for debriefing. This shortened time frame is not conducive for successful completion of objectives.

L. EVALUATION OF BEST PRACTICE STANDARDS AND USE OF CREDENTIALED SIMULATION FACULTY

Components of International Nursing Association for Clinical Simulation in Learning Standard VIII: Simulation Enhanced Interprofessional Education (Decker et al., 2015) are evident through the involvement of interprofessional team members from the affiliated hospital. The students have verbalized an appreciation of this interprofessional approach as they did not know the roles and responsibilities of the security officer, pastoral care, and the rapid response (advanced practice nurses) team. This has increased their knowledge of the roles of other members of the health care team and improved their understanding of nursing's role in an interprofessional approach to care.

Components of Standard IX: Simulation Design (Lioce et al., 2015) are apparent through the use of content experts to ensure the validity of treatment regimens, prebriefing activities designed to prepare students, and the use of the certified health care simulation educator (CHSE) simulation lab coordinator to ensure fidelity of the scenario. The CHSE has assisted faculty in their role of facilitating and debriefing scenarios through role modeling and providing educational opportunities on the topics. Elements of Standard VI: Debriefing Process (Decker et al., 2013) are applied throughout the debriefing session, which is completed immediately following the simulation includes the interprofessional personnel.

REFERENCES

American Association of Colleges of Nursing. (2008). *The essentials of baccalaureate education for professional nursing practice.* Washington, DC: Author. Retrieved from http://www.aacnnursing.org/Portals/42/Publications/BaccEssentials08.pdf

Decker, S., Fey, M., Sideras, S., Caballero, S., Rockstraw, L., Boese, T., ... Borum, J. C. (2013). Standards of best practice: Simulation standard VI: The debriefing process. *Clinical Simulation in Nursing, 9*(S6), S26–S29. doi:10.1016/j.ecns.2013.04.008

Decker, S. I., Anderson, M., Boese, T., Epps, C., McCarthy, J., Motola, I., ... Lioce, L. (2015). Standards of best practice: Simulation standard VIII: Simulation-enhanced interprofessional education (Sim-IPE). *Clinical Simulation in Nursing, 11*(6), 293–297.

Dreifuerst, K. L. (2015). Getting started with debriefing for meaningful learning. *Clinical Simulation in Nursing, 11*(5), 268–275. doi:10.1016/j.ecns.2015.01.005

Dusai, T. K. (2014). Five fast fixes: Debriefing. *Clinical Simulation in Nursing, 10*(9), 485–486. doi:10.1016/j.ecns.2014.06.002

Eberhardt, S. (2014). Improve handoff communication with SBAR. *Nursing, 44*(11), 17–20.

Lasater, K. (2007). Clinical judgment development: Using simulation to create an assessment rubric. *Journal of Nursing Education, 46*(11), 496–503.

Lioce, L., Meakim, C. H., Fey, M. K., Chmil, J. V., Mariani, B., & Alinier, G. (2015). Standards of best practice: Simulation standard IX: Simulation design. *Clinical Simulation in Nursing, 11*(6), 309–315.

National Council of State Boards of Nursing. (2015). NCLEX-RN examination: Test plan for the National Council Licensure Examination for Registered Nurses. Retrieved from https://www.ncsbn.org/2016_NCLEX_RN_Test_Plan.pdf

CHAPTER 42

SIMCamp: Trauma Simulation, Rapid-Cycle Deliberate Practice Team Training

Kimberly Bilskey and Leslie Catron

Trauma is the known leading cause of death and acquired disability in children and adolescents (Curtis et al., 2016; McKenzie, 2016). Initial intervention in the emergency department (ED) makes a tremendous impact on patient outcomes and adhering to developed protocols, activating adequate appropriate resources, and ensuring competent use of equipment is necessary to mitigate severity of injury (Curtis et al., 2016; McKenzie, 2016). Interprofessional teamwork is vital for patient safety. Valley Children's Healthcare, Madera, California children's hospital with 356 beds developed a task force to achieve its transition to a pediatric trauma center competent in safely resuscitating pediatric trauma patients. Challenged with training a large trauma staff to meet accreditation requirements for level II trauma designation required a new programmatic approach. Literature demonstrated that the curriculum was in the early stages of development (Zimmermann et al., 2015), so the burgeoning interprofessional simulation program was charged with building a formidable simulation training program and curricula for trauma team training.

A. IMPLEMENTATION OF SIMULATION-BASED PEDAGOGY IN YOUR INDIVIDUALIZED TEACHING AREA

Transitioning from academic simulation to hospital simulation requires a change in mindset. There are three inherent differences: time for simulation, knowledge of the learners, and payment to the learner for education time. In the college setting, there is more running time for a scenario to unfold and debrief the learners; students are novice learners and *they* pay for their education.

A fourth difference is shared by both simulation locations, adult learners have an innate fear of appearing not to know something. Whereas on my (Leslie) return to the children's hospital as the interprofessional simulation coordinator, it was astonishingly apparent that there was less time for in situ teaching; in the lab and in the classroom, learners ranged from competent to expert, and only *mandatory* education was paid for by the departments, meaning elective participation required high learner motivation to come in on a day off. The fear of appearing less than competent is magnified when knowledge, experience, and confidence have developed beyond school, so stress and defenses become barriers for the learners to overcome.

Presented early on with a request for this crucial team training, overcoming barriers quickly became important. Teaming up with the ED clinical educator (Kim), who had recently trained in simulation theory, fidelity, and debriefing, and the medical simulation director, a pediatric intensive care internist with extensive background in simulation (trauma and ICU) from her residency and employment at a large medical center, the 6 weeks of curriculum preparation began.

A focus on the Advanced Trauma Life Support (ATLS) protocol (Acosta et al., 2010) was primary. Multiple decisions needed to be made:

1. Interprofessional objectives were based on the *Core Competencies for Interprofessional Collaborative Practice* (Interprofessional Education Collaborative Expert Panel, 2011).
2. Trauma core objectives focused on the Pediatric Trauma Resuscitation Checklist developed and shared by Children's National Hospital (Kelleher, Jagadeesh Chandra Bose, Waterhouse, Carter, & Burd, 2014).
3. What scenarios would be used and what will the measurable focused objectives be using the International Nursing Association for Clinical Simulation in Learning Standards of Best Practice: Simulation[SM] Simulation Design (2016)?
4. What location will be used (in situ was chosen due to the realistic environment and access to equipment)?
5. Early scenario development will be done with subject matter experts (emergency physicians, trauma surgeons, trauma educator, and staff) to ensure accuracy and standard of practice.
6. Supplies and equipment necessary for scenario realism will be needed.
7. What is the best time for staff participation (early morning was chosen because of low patient census at that time)?
8. Identify stakeholders and schedule meetings (emergency unit director, trauma medical director, emergency physicians, emergency trauma coordinator, charge nurses, and multiple supervisors and managers will be needed later for whole-system activation).
9. Will training be mandatory or elective for staff (the department director elected to ensure on-shift staff time and later paid for participants' mandatory time to attend the SIMCamp)?

With the first three in situ trainings each held monthly, it was immediately apparent not enough staff would be able to participate to meet the Level II Pediatric Trauma designation survey deadline. Plus, in the first simulation, 27 process gaps were identified that required changes for staff to better function in their roles.

Drawing from academic experience with multiple students, the simulation team regrouped and the concept of SIMCamp (Simulation Intensive Mastery Course) was born. This model was based on rapid-cycle deliberate practice simulation (Doughty, 2015). With 2 and a half months of planning, the first SIMCamp was launched for 39 participants; each paid to attend a 2-hour session. In teams of five to seven, learners cared for three pediatric trauma patients, scaffolding simple to complex care. Time and number of scenarios can be adjusted as can the number of learners; training can be done with one to seven learners at a time. Debriefings were held after each session and focused on the interprofessional team and scenario objectives to embed learning. Realism and fidelity were imperative to learning. An emergency medical services (EMS) report was given in the prebriefing, and the human patient simulator (HPS) was moulaged appropriately for the patient situation. Results were remarkable, with participants engaging and visibly gaining knowledge, skills, and actions between the first to the third scenarios. Chaos became controlled flow of care and this was observed later in real patient cases as this staff not only performed better, but also mentored each other.

An unexpected educational outcome was the ability to use the SIMCamp model in other multiple staff training sessions requiring learning situations, as demonstrated with extracorporeal life support (ECLS) training, hospitalist emergency medical response team (EMRT) training, and hospitalists training.

B. EDUCATIONAL MATERIALS AVAILABLE IN YOUR TEACHING AREA AND RELATED TO YOUR SPECIALTY

It was helpful to work in a hospital committed to ongoing staff development. Each unit had a clinical educator who was resourceful in collecting and reusing supplies for "education use only."

The ED educator accumulated these, so simulation supplies were plentiful. The interprofessional simulation program was in the beginning stages of development and was part of the clinical education budget. Combined with the trauma and ED department funds, further supplies needed were able to be purchased. Doing the training in the ED trauma resuscitation room provided the equipment necessary for patient care. Plus, there was a supply room in immediate proximity. It was agreed that any supplies taken from stock would be charged to the ED and saved, if possible, for future trauma simulation. In planning, an exhaustive list of supplies and equipment was developed ensuring everything was available for the staff with quick turn-around for the next scenario.

Materials were placed in plastic covered boxes labeled for each scenario and each session (three scenarios, four sessions). After running the first session, it was discovered that most of the supplies could be reused and only liquids (blood, vomit, urine, etc.) and consumables (bandages, syringes, etc.) needed replacement. So those were stocked in quantity ahead of time. The session boxes were abandoned and only the scenario boxes remained and were restocked as needed in between simulations.

C. SPECIFIC OBJECTIVES FOR SIMULATION USAGE WITHIN A SPECIFIC COURSE AND THE OVERALL PROGRAM

The interprofessional simulation program team in collaboration with the trauma team was to develop curricula that would assess:

1. Competency of trauma team members in the care of a pediatric trauma patient, including the use of a trauma resuscitation checklist
2. System processes for the care of a pediatric trauma patient
3. Latent safety threats in caring for a pediatric trauma patient and the function of the trauma team

D. INTRODUCTION OF SCENARIO

Setting the Scene

Each patient simulation experience takes place in the local pediatric acute care hospital ED, preferably in the trauma resuscitation room. It can be in any medical–surgical hospital ED or in an academic setting made to resemble an ED patient room (see recommendations for further use).

Technology Used

A high-fidelity 6-year-old HPS and monitor with Wi-Fi capability is used. The technology of Wi-Fi enables transporting the patient into the trauma room with EMS personnel transferring the patient from the gurney to the table. This transfer contributes to the trauma process and realism of the scenario. This technology ensures the simulation technician running the manikin will not be in the way of patient care and will be able to visualize and hear the care interventions.

A high-fidelity 2-month-old infant HPS and monitor is also used, ours was tethered to the compressor and computer, which requires a wheeled cart in order to be transported and setup in the patient room.

Description of Participants

No scripts were developed. Each participant was expected to function in the role assigned by the lead nurse when the participant entered the trauma resuscitation room. A sticker was provided for each role identifying who each individual was to help new team members coming into the situation. The sticker is placed on the individual's personal protective equipment (PPE).

E. RUNNING OF THE SCENARIO

1 Month to 2 Weeks Before Training

In advance of the simulation, we communicated with the ED, trauma coordinator, physicians to provide in advance dates, time, and responsibilities and to answer all questions to be sure everything is clarified.

1 Week Before Training

Volunteers from the ED staff were requested to help with SIMCamp. It took two extra volunteer staff to help with setup and breakdown the day of SIMCamp. Supplies were gathered, prepared, and inventoried so that needed items could be ordered. The HPS is checked for any technology challenges.

Day Before Training

Equipment, supplies, and HPS are packed and ready to be moved to the trauma resuscitation room.

Day of Training

Usual setup time is 1.5 hours if moulage is to be applied. The goal is to have the trauma resuscitation room ready and the patient on the EMS gurney before staff arrives.

Note: A prebrief should be done with every simulation to follow the International Nursing Association for Clinical Simulation and Learning INACSL Standards of Best Practice: Simulation^SM Facilitation (2016) to acquaint the participants with the HPS. If moulaged, then cover the HPS with towels or sheets so as not to give away the scenario before proceeding.

Note: If there are patients and parents in the proximity of the training, it is extremely important to take the time to connect with them to explain what is taking place (usually done by the simulation coordinator) as follows:

1. Introduce yourself.
2. Provide a brief explanation indicating that you are doing a staff training for patient care in an emergency. It is NOT real although it may appear like it is. Do not worry; the patient is a computerized doll and is not really a patient. This is strictly a training device.
3. Ask whether you may shut the curtain/door so you do not upset their child.
4. Reassure them that the staff will be checking on them frequently and they can call for staff at any time if they have a concern about their child.

We are in the process of also putting this information on a small, laminated card in English and Spanish to further provide a safe and comfortable environment for patients and families.

The HPS patient is then placed on an EMS gurney and removed from the emergency trauma resuscitation room, located somewhere out of sight of the trauma staff. The dispatcher takes the EMS report from the radio call and gives this to lead nurse, who provides a report to the team. This is done near the room where the simulation will take place so as not to disrupt patient care in the ED.

The simulation technician uses the scenario template or "road map." (We have developed our own template after much revision.) This is the key to staying the course in reaching the objectives of the simulation. The scenario is moved forward based on the participant actions as outlined on the template. But, of course, participant actions do not follow a specific sequence as they occur simultaneously in a trauma. It becomes important that a trauma educator and/or physician (often in our case the medical simulation director) stay with the technician to guide the running of the scenario. By doing this, changes can be made off the "road map" to either move the participants back on track, challenge them, and/or complicate the patient condition. Adding complications to the experience can be done for participants who are doing well and will end the scenario sooner than expected, which happens with highly experienced staff.

F. PRESENTATION OF A COMPLETED TEMPLATE

Titles

Three scenarios are presented: (a) Motor Vehicle Collision With Blunt Abdominal Injury, (b) Respiratory Distress With Blunt Chest Injury, and (c) Motor Vehicle Collision With Penetrating Abdominal and Head Injuries

Scenario Level

Novice to expert

Focus Area

Pediatrics, prehospital emergency trauma, emergency trauma level I/level II, academic simulation

Participant Objectives

Interprofessional Objectives

1. Communicate one's roles and responsibilities clearly to team members (roles and responsibilities)
2. Demonstrate ethical conduct and quality care in one's contributions to team-based care (values and ethics)
3. Express one's knowledge and opinions to team members involved in patient care with confidence, clarity, and respect, working to ensure common understanding of information, treatment, and care decisions (communication)
4. Perform effectively on teams and in different team roles that support collaborative practice and team effectiveness (team and teamwork)

Scenario Objectives

At the end of the course the participant will be able to:

1. Verbalize the roles of the trauma team and use effective closed-loop team communication
2. Identify and gather appropriate supplies and resources based on patient information before EMS arrival
3. Initiate EMS time-out for report to the trauma team before moving the patient to ED gurney
4. Upon patient arrival, prioritize and implement the Primary Survey–ABCDE (airway, breathing, circulation, disability, exposure) survey (American College of Surgeons Committee on Trauma, 2012) based on a trauma resuscitation checklist
5. Provide and demonstrate the ability to appropriately resuscitate and manage care for the trauma patient
6. Recognize and intervene to maintain the patient's airway and prevent aspiration
7. Use correct intubation equipment and technique

8. Recognize and intervene to maintain the patient's ventilation and respiratory status
9. Provide the appropriate equipment and assist with chest tube placement
10. Initiate and administer massive transfusion protocol
11. Recognize the need for communication with the operating room (OR) team and expedite transport to the OR

Setting the Scene

Equipment and Supplies

Equipment needed: Standard set up of an ED trauma resuscitation room: trauma resuscitation checklist, emergency drug sheet and medication resource binder, nonrebreather mask, endotracheal tube, bag valve mask (BVM), cervical collar (c-collar), backboard, chest tube drainage chamber, chest tube, thoracostomy tray, 20-gauge intravenous (IV) cannulas, intraosseous needle and gun, 1 L normal saline (NS), IV tubing, rapid infuser tubing, orogastric tube (OG), bedside blood analysis equipment, lab tubes, clothing, blanket, backpack, toy, and pacifier

Roles for All Scenarios

Lead RN: Focus on staff and physician needs, global view of patient care, delegation
Right-hand RN: Medications
Left-hand RN: Fluids, IVs, blood products, procedures
Recorder RN: Documentation
Respiratory care practitioner (RCP): Airway management; two practitioners may be used
Unlicensed assistive personnel: Vital signs, monitor, labs, runner
Emergency room physician: Accepts patient, provides initial care
Trauma surgeon: Arrives following level I trauma activation by the lead RN and assumes care
EMS personnel (simulation facilitators fill this role): Brings the patient to room, gives the mechanism of injury, injuries, vital signs, and treatments, or mechanism, injury, vital signs, treatment (MIVT).

Scenario Implementation

Scenarios take place in situ in the ED trauma resuscitation room. See Exhibit 42.1 for details.

G. DEBRIEFING GUIDELINES

Several models of debriefing have been used over time in the hospital, but in developing the interprofessional simulation program and receiving training from the Harvard Institute Center for Medical Simulation, specifically, the Debriefing Assessment for Simulation in Healthcare (DASH) rater training workshop, a decision was made to utilize the "debriefing with good judgment" approach (Rudolph, Simon, Dufresne, & Reamer, 2006, p. 49). Trauma simulations can be highly stressful and emotionally charged as trauma staff not only strive for perfection while the situation can conjure memories from real trauma patient experiences that ended in less than perfect team dynamics or outcomes. A framework for debriefing is therefore important. Using INACSL Standard V (Decker et al., 2013) and validating debriefers with the DASH tool provided a structure for quality debriefing. The advocacy and inquiry model (Rudolph et al., 2006) for participant reflection gives the debriefer a look into the learner's frame of reference and critical thinking while keeping the focus on the goal to change behavior and take that new behavior to the clinical setting.

Exhibit 42.1	Three SIMCamp Trauma Simulations		

Scenario 1 Title

Motor Vehicle Collision With Blunt Abdominal Injury

Scenario 2 Title

Respiratory Distress With Blunt Chest Injury

Scenario 3 Title

Motor Vehicle Collision With Penetrating Abdominal and Head Injuries

Simulator level:

High-fidelity 6-year-old HPS with cardiac monitor and Wi-Fi capability. Abdominal bruising for seat belt injury was created by using blue eye shadow and dark-pink blush placed over a thin layer of petroleum jelly (helps prevent staining and easier cleanup). The bruising was placed to the abdomen where the seat belt rested. Use pictures off the internet to help guide you.

Simulator level:

A high-fidelity 2-month-old infant HPS with cardiac monitor and laptop. Fingertip bruising to the anterior and posterior bilateral ribcage was created by using blue eye shadow and dark-pink blush. Makeup was placed on the fingertips of an adult and then transferred to the HPS over a thin layer of petroleum jelly using the thumbs on the anterior chest and the rest of the fingers on the posterior chest. Pat out to smudge just a little for realism.

Simulator level:

High-fidelity 6-year-old HPS with cardiac monitor and Wi-Fi capability. Abdominal bruising was created by using blue eye shadow and dark-pink blush placed over a thin layer of petroleum jelly. The bruising was placed to the abdomen where the seat belt rested. Penetrating abdominal injury was created with ink from a pen placed through the lower left abdomen skin. Latex tubing* was placed at open entry site and run under the torso skin up the side of the chest and out the neck of the HPS. The tubing was filled with simulated blood and clamped at the end. During the scenario, three 60-mL syringes were used to create active abdominal bleeding. The head laceration was created with a premade wound, a piece of a plastic cup to simulate glass, and simulated blood.

*Latex tubing was ¼ inch × 3/32 inch × 60 inches. CAUTION: Be sure to wear gloves if allergic to latex or have another person prepare this part of the moulage.

(continued)

Exhibit 42.1	Three SIMCamp Trauma Simulations *(continued)*	
Scenario 1 Title	**Scenario 2 Title**	**Scenario 3 Title**
Motor Vehicle Collision With Blunt Abdominal Injury	Respiratory Distress With Blunt Chest Injury	Motor Vehicle Collision With Penetrating Abdominal and Head Injuries
Scene 1	**Scene 1**	**Scene 1**
EMS radio call	Mother presents to triage with her 9-month-old baby girl. She states she found her blue and having trouble breathing. Triage nurse notes patient to be pale and lethargic with subcostal retractions. The triage nurse contacts the charge nurse to notify her that she is bringing the patient to the resuscitation room. The charge nurse pages resuscitation team.	**EMS radio call**
STAT trauma standard call in Unit 41, Paramedic Jones		Stat trauma standard call in
		Unit 41, Paramedic Jones
ETA: 5 minutes		ETA: 5 minutes
6-year-old, male, 22.5 kg		6-year-old, male, 22.5 kg
Stat trauma, rollover MVC, back seat passenger side, lap seat belt only	**Learner actions**	Stat trauma, rollover MVC, back seat passenger side, + seat belt
Cervical spine precautions and backboard in place	Team members respond to page and state role as they enter the room.	C-spine and backboard in place
Initially disoriented on scene and now Glasgow	Don PPE.	GCS = 7 before intubation
Coma Scale = 9		HR: 180 beats/minute, BP: 70/30 mmHg, RR: 18 breaths/minute assisted
HR: 140 beats/minute, BP: 90/40 mmHg,		
RR: 32 breaths/minute		Forehead laceration with embedded glass actively bleeding; firm abdomen with bruising, abrasions, and penetrating injury actively bleeding; capillary refill 4 sec; distal pulses weak × 4
Firm abdomen with bruising and abrasions, capillary refill 4 sec, distal pulses weak × 4		
1 L NS infusing through 20-gauge IV to right AC		1 L NS infusing through 20-gauge IV to right AC
Unknown medical history, medications, and allergies		Unknown medical history, medications, and allergies
Learner actions		**Learner actions**
Page ED trauma team to the room.		Page ED trauma team to the room.
Page out appropriate trauma team activation.		Page out appropriate trauma team activation.
Prepare the trauma resuscitation room for patient arrival gathering anticipated supplies based on EMS report.		Prepare the trauma resuscitation room for patient arrival by gathering anticipated supplies based on EMS report.
Don PPE.		Don PPE.

Scene 2

EMS time-out

Mechanism: Rollover MVC, back seat passenger side, lap seat belt only

Injuries: Abdominal bruising and abrasions, possible head injury due to declining GCS and emesis ×1

Vital signs: HR: 135 beats/minute, BP: 91/43 mmHg, RR: 30 breaths/minute

Treatment: C-spine, backboard, 20-gauge IV right AC, 1 L NS, oxygen

Learner actions

Trauma team pauses to listen to EMS report before moving patient to ED gurney.

Scene 2

Vital signs: HR: 185 beats/minute, RR: 44 breaths/minute, BP: 80/48 mmHg, SpO_2: 94%, Temp: 98.6°F

Primary assessment findings:

Airway: clear

Breathing: Lung sounds clear, decreased on right side

Circulation: Capillary refill 4 sec, pulses 3+, dusky

Disability: GCS = 12

Exposure/environment: Bruising noted to anterior and posterior chest

Verbal sounds: Cries when touched

Mother (a confederate) remains in the room and is anxious but appropriate. May ask occasional questions but is not an obstacle to care.

Learner actions

Place on the monitor.

Complete primary survey.

Put nonrebreather on the patient.

Place PIV.

Page appropriate trauma team activation.

Scene 2

EMS time-out

Mechanism: Rollover MVC, back seat passenger side, + seat belt

Injuries: Forehead laceration with embedded glass actively bleeding, firm abdomen with bruising, abrasions and penetrating injury actively bleeding

Vital signs: HR: 180 beats/minute, BP: 70/30 mmHg, RR: 16 breaths/minute assisted

Treatment: C-spine, backboard, 20-gauge IV right AC, 1 L NS, intubated

Learner actions

Trauma team pauses to listen to EMS report before moving patient to ED gurney.

(continued)

Exhibit 42.1 Three SIMCamp Trauma Simulations *(continued)*

Scenario 1 Title	Scenario 2 Title	Scenario 3 Title
Motor Vehicle Collision With Blunt Abdominal Injury	Respiratory Distress With Blunt Chest Injury	Motor Vehicle Collision With Penetrating Abdominal and Head Injuries
Scene 3	**Scene 3**	**Scene 3**
Vital signs: HR: 135 beats/minute, RR: 30 breaths/minute, BP: 91/43 mmHg, SpO$_2$: 97%, Temp: 97°F	**Vital signs:** HR: 198 beats/minute, RR: 18 breaths/minute, BP: 80/48 mmHg, SpO$_2$: 84%, Temp: 98.6°F	**Vital signs:** HR: 180 beats/minute, RR: 16 breaths/minute, assisted, BP: 70/30 mmHg, SpO$_2$: 99%, Temp: 96°F
Primary assessment findings:	Assessment: Capillary refill 4 sec, pulses 3+, dusky, breath sounds absent on right side	Primary assessment findings:
Airway: Large emesis, gurgling respirations	PIV attempts unsuccessful	Airway: clear, endotracheal tube
Breathing: Lung sounds clear	**Learner actions**	Breathing: lung sounds clear, assisted ventilation
Circulation: Capillary refill 4 sec, pulses 1+, pallor, cool skin	Recognize patient is deteriorating due to pneumothorax.	Circulation: capillary refill 4 sec, pulses 1+, pallor, cool skin
Disability: GCS = 9, PERRL	Prepare for needle decompression, gather supplies.	Disability: GCS = 7, PERRL
Exposure/environment: Abdominal distension, bruising and abrasions noted, cool skin	Decompress right lung.	Exposure/environment: Forehead laceration with embedded glass actively bleeding, firm abdomen with bruising, abrasions and penetrating injury actively bleeding, cool skin
Verbal sounds: Moaning, gurgling respirations	Prepare for chest tube placement, gather supplies.	**Learner actions**
Learner actions	Place chest tube in right pleural space.	Apply pressure to actively bleeding wounds.
Suction airway.	Reassess airway, breathing, perfusion and vital signs.	Place on the monitor.
Place on the monitor.	Place intraosseous needle for fluid replacement therapy.	Complete primary survey.
Complete primary survey.	Administer NS bolus via rapid infusion technique.	Place second large bore IV.
Place the second IV.	Reassess patient after interventions.	Administer NS bolus via rapid infusion technique.
		Place OG to decompress abdomen and protect the airway.
		Initiate massive transfusion protocol.

Scene 4

Vital signs: HR: 145 beats/minute, RR: 6 breaths/minute, BP: 80/35 mmHg, SpO$_2$: 90%, Temp: 97°F

Assessment: capillary refill 4 sec, pulses 1+, GCS 7

Patient is nonresponsive.

Learner actions

Recognize deteriorating patient.

Perform assisted ventilation with bag and mask.

Prepare for intubation using RSI medications, gather supplies.

Insert OG tube to decompress abdomen and protect airway.

Scene 4

Vital signs: HR: 132 beats/minute, RR: 30 breaths/minute, BP: 88/52 mmHg, SpO$_2$: 94%, Temp: 98°F

Assessment:

Airway: Clear

Breathing: Lung sounds clear, equal, chest tube in place

Circulation: Capillary refill 3 sec, pulses 2+, skin warm and pale, IO to right tibia infusing NS bolus

Disability: GCS = 14, PERRL

Exposure/environment: Bruising noted to anterior and posterior chest

Learner actions

Order portable chest x-ray.

Recognize patient's response to interventions.

Prepare for transport to PICU/OR.

Initiate social worker and CPS referral.

Scene 4

Vital signs: HR: 210 beats/minute, RR: 16 breaths/minute assisted, BP: 58/26 mmHg, SpO$_2$: 94%, Temp: 95.8°F

Assessment: Capillary refill 6 sec, pulses 1+

Learner actions

Recognize deteriorating patient.

Rapidly infuse blood products immediately on arrival.

Continue to hold pressure to actively bleeding wounds.

Reassess patient after interventions.

(continued)

505

Exhibit 42.1 Three SIMCamp Trauma Simulations *(continued)*

Scenario 1 Title	Scenario 2 Title	Scenario 3 Title
Motor Vehicle Collision With Blunt Abdominal Injury	Respiratory Distress With Blunt Chest Injury	Motor Vehicle Collision With Penetrating Abdominal and Head Injuries
Scene 5		**Scene 5**
Vital signs: HR: 120 beats/minute, RR: 24 breaths/minute, assisted, BP: 90/50 mmHg, SpO$_2$: 99%, Temp: 98°F		**Vital signs:** HR: 170 beats/minute, RR: 16 breaths/minute assisted, BP: 75/48 mmHg, SpO$_2$: 98%, Temp: 97.5°F
Assessment: Capillary refill 3 sec, pulses 2+		Assessment: Capillary refill 4 sec, pulses 1+
Learner actions		**Learner actions**
Check ETT placement, capnography, place on a ventilator.		Recognize patient's response to interventions.
Order portable chest x-ray.		Continue infusing blood products per massive transfusion protocol.
Recognize patient's response to interventions.		Prepare for immediate transport to the OR.
Prepare for transport to PICU/OR.		

AC, antecubital; BP, blood pressure; CPS, child protective services; ED, emergency department; EMS, emergency medical services; ETA, estimated time of arrival; ETT, endotracheal tube; HPS, human patient simulator; HR, heart rate; IO, intraosseous; IV, intravenous; MVC, motor vehicle collision; NS, normal saline; OG, orogastric tube; PEERL, pupils are equal, round, and reactive to light; PICU, pediatric intensive care unit; PIV, peripheral intravenous; PPE, personal protective equipment; RR, respiratory rate; RSI, rapid sequence intubation.

Because of the short debriefing time between scenarios (15–20 minutes), the debriefer needs to listen carefully for thoughts, concerns, questions that bring focus to the scenario's primary objectives. Team dynamics are always the focus, not a single individual. A stop–start scenario debrief rapid cycle model was chosen later and proven to work best with this type of curriculum. It proved successful with participants, allowing for real-time critical thinking.

Upon entering the debriefing room, the facilitator notes to the group that they have a lot to talk about and guides them in beginning to unpack their thoughts about what they just experienced.

Note: An attempt has been made to avoid the expression of feelings or emotions; the intent is to bring the learners to collectively examine their experience. In doing so they will express their stress and frustration, but there will be less focus on not liking something or being angry.

As this dialogue unravels, learners will state how they were forgetful in doing something, slow to respond, and/or did not communicate to an individual. It is important to always acknowledge this but not dwell on the individual's missed step. Many concerns are embedded in the interprofessional objectives, so reassure the learner these will be covered in a team discussion. It is interesting to note that in a relatively short period of time, a comment is made that *directly* hits an objective. Quickly acknowledge and begin with, "Let's talk about that."

As a facilitator, it is imperative to keep the simulation and debriefing environment nonpunitive. Understanding the art of advocacy and inquiry, one can bring the team to know the correct way of doing things, but the facilitator must remain curious about the individual's critical thinking process. In this way, the action no longer requires defense, but rather clinical reasoning. Instead of the facilitator teaching, ask the team how they could have helped in the situation. This brings the group into a collaborative effort to teach, support each other, and problem solve.

Example

Staff member: "I didn't get the OG tube down before the intubation."

Facilitator: "I did notice that didn't happen after the doctor asked twice, but I'm curious about what you were thinking at the time, can you fill me in?"

There could be one of several answers that provide a frame of reference:

#1 "I heard it but didn't know where they were kept."

This is a process issue. Ask the team how they could have helped find the OG tube.

Someone who knows should step up and provide the answer, showing the way.

#2 "I've not done this yet on a child"

This is a skill issue (novice nurse). Ask the team how they could have helped. Most respond that they should speak up and not be afraid to say they didn't know how.

The educator or facilitator should speak up then and offer time to practice.

#3 "I didn't hear the doctor say he wanted an OG tube passed."

This is a communication issue. Ask the team whether anybody heard the doctor. If someone did, then ask how this could be solved in the future. It's a close-the-loop communication problem. Was there too much noise in the room? Should the lead nurse have asked the team to bring it down a little so the doctor could be heard?

Focus back on team communication, support, and the mental models they share. This creates cohesiveness, builds trust, and has proven to be extremely positive for this hospital's trauma staff.

Usually, there is time to focus on two to three objectives in the short period of time allowed for the debriefing. The facilitators cannot be afraid to keep the group on track and tactfully shutdown sidebar conversations. This is where learning happens and behavior changes. Remember, if the facilitator is talking during the debrief, then the participant is not learning. Good debriefing is about asking open ended questions, reflection, and dialogue.

H. SUGGESTIONS/KEY FEATURES TO REPLICATE OR IMPROVE

The planning of SIMCamp was thorough, so during the follow-up planning debrief only the process gaps or team challenges needed to be addressed. Knowing that the simulation would be repeated the following year, the trauma and simulation team did decide on the following changes:

1. Decide the dates earlier in the year with the ED director and begin earlier coordination with the medical simulation director's work schedule to ensure availability.

2. SIMCamp dates must ideally be put out for staff to sign-up at least 3 months in advance so they can fit this education class into their work schedules.

3. Communicate early with the trauma surgeons (allow 3 months once dates are decided) to ensure surgeons' availability. Their presence was requested in evaluations by the staff as they felt this would be helpful for team dynamics and cohesiveness.

4. Often high patient census within the hospital requires staff to be called in on their day off. This happened during the first SIMCamp. Some staff had volunteered to help with the setup and break-down of the simulation on their day off. Since they were in the hospital, ED leadership requested they come, clock-in, and assume patient care. For future SIMCamps, it was agreed that an algorithm needs to be created to stipulate when volunteers can be pulled to work as staff. This will eliminate miscommunication and frustration that erodes teamwork.

5. During set up between simulations, it is important to reapply petroleum jelly to the HPS when doing touch-up moulage using makeup, so as not to stain the skin.

6. We did not videotape the SIMCamps as part of setting up psychological safety for the participants, but also because the debriefing time is too short to play back even a segment that has been marked. This will be considered for the future.

7. Using the true form of the rapid cycle, the stop–start style of 10-second debriefing while in the scenario was considered and is now implemented in other SIMCamps. The challenge with longer scenarios is they might not be able to finish, so flexibility is key in letting go of the ending. But using this method would give participants the opportunity to have immediate formative feedback with self-correction thereby embedding learning.

I. RECOMMENDATIONS FOR FURTHER USE

Adaptations

Originally this curriculum was specifically designed for pediatric hospital trauma team development. But after running the scenarios multiple times, debriefing, revising, and validating the content, it became readily apparent that the SIMCamp model could be applied in varying forms in multiple settings. Timing for SIMCamp could be reduced or expanded, hospital departments could adapt for focused education, clinics the same, and colleges and universities most of all, could use the multiple scenario SIMCamp model with few or many students as a Campus Clinical Day.

1. Colleges and universities can collaborate and/or partner with local hospital EDs to replicate a trauma resuscitation room. The simulation lab could be set up to have similar equipment, supplies, and arranged to replicate the trauma resuscitation room the students will encounter. Clinical staff from the hospital can volunteer time to come for the day and run or be in the scenario to help the learners grasp the concepts of pediatric trauma. Strong relationships between academia and service can be strengthened.

2. The hospital could provide clinical simulation days for clinical academic partners. Student lab fees could cover costs of supplies used at the hospital. The SIMCamp staff would collaborate with the instructors and apply theory to hands-on learning.

3. The SIMCamp model can be used extensively in the college/university setting as a way to teach multiple students. The model can fit into all curricula. Using three or more scenarios over a day, week, or even month, from simple to complex, allows the students to scaffold their learning of patient care. Coordinating with the theory provides the base for learning in the clinical simulation. Rotation of students allows for four to six participants to be in the simulation while others are in skills training.

Outcome From Trauma SIMCamp

This SIMCamp curriculum is completely adaptable to any department and curriculum needing interprofessional collaborative practice and learning. Although this scenario is pediatric trauma, it can be modified for adult trauma. Session time, scenario length, debriefing period, and a number of simulations can all be adjusted easily to fit the situation. This curriculum model has been adapted to extracorporeal life support (ECLS) pump specialist training, which happens for 2 days once a month and 3 days twice a year. Further, a new training program for hospitalists was developed following the SIMCamp format. Physicians trained with the medical simulation director in four simulation experiences focused on rapid response and code blue team leadership. Nursing and respiratory clinical educators acted in bedside staff roles but were instructed not to initiate patient care interventions, except at the direction of the physician. The first three scenarios were conducted using stop–start to quickly identify a variation from algorithms. This provided immediate correction and starting again with new behavior. The last scenario provided a complete patient case and debriefing at the end of the day's learning. This format could be used in academia with a specific course or module to embed learning.

Recommendations for Variation in the Scenarios

More time for each session would allow for:

1. Simulation scenarios to unfold
2. Debriefing time with participate reflection
3. Start–stop during the scenario itself in which a 10-second debrief and course correction is made
4. The addition of an electronic health record (EHR); at present all documentation is on paper but in the future, with new software, there is the opportunity to complete trauma resuscitation on an EHR
5. Increased complexity based on team experience; by knowing the audience the scenario can be individualized

Evaluation

Formative feedback during debriefing was used with the advocacy and inquiring model. An interprofessional team simulation evaluation was designed with questions to provide as little subjective opinion as possible but still using a qualitative Likert scale. This provided excellent feedback indicating that the objectives were met and participants felt SIMCamp was valuable to their personal clinical development.

K. EXPERT RECOMMENDATIONS AND WORDS OF WISDOM

1. What you have used in one place can be used in another
2. Debrief, regroup, reconsider, revise
3. After doing a simulation one way you may need to regroup and realized that not all the staff can be trained this way in a timely manner

4. Build on a "germ" of an idea
5. Gather the troops and create from a thought. SIMCamp was born this way.
6. Plan, plan, plan
7. You cannot overthink a project but you can underthink it
8. Creativity counts from ALL stakeholders. Know who they are, talk to them face-to-face
9. In running a scenario, you need to ebb and flow (be flexible) while keeping the objectives in your sights. This is done ONLY if you KNOW the patient case inside and out
10. Always say, "THERE IS A WAY"
11. Faced with obstacles, unknowns, cynics, "we don't know how, we never done it before," the answer is: "Of course we can!" Then go find your resources and work it out.

L. EVALUATION OF BEST PRACTICE STANDARDS AND USE OF CREDENTIALED SIMULATION FACULTY

This simulation program applies the INACSL Standards of Best Practice in Simulation[SM] (INACSL, 2016) with all simulation activities and education development. This interprofessional simulation education model is based on these standards and on the Interprofessional Education Collaborative Expert Panel (2011) *Core Competencies for Interprofessional Collaborative Practice.* Particular to this SIMCamp, the protocols for ATLS, trauma nursing core course, and the trauma resuscitation checklist were used.

The INACSL Standards of Best Practice in Simulation (2016) as referenced by the editors in Chapter 1, were used in the development of the trauma curricula and scenario development.

The simulation coordinator is a Certified Healthcare Simulation Educator (CHSE) through the Society for Simulation in Healthcare (SSIH), received DASH Rater Training from the Harvard Center for Medical Simulation, and obtained a Certificate in Simulation Education from Bryan LGH College of Health Sciences. Furthermore, the coordinator has a master's degree.

The value of professional development through simulation cannot be stressed enough. The field of simulation education and research is expanding rapidly and keeping up with the educational and technological changes is vital to an innovative, cutting-edge program. Creativity comes from networking and collaboration. Attending conferences and connecting with expert colleagues through listservs may provide resources and solutions to problems encountered or just great ideas for improvement. The educational background and experience of this simulation coordinator and medical simulation director provided a foundation for SIMCamp, but it took a team to bring the idea to fruition and see it through. The experience of both these individuals was imperative during the challenging moments in creating SIMCamp. There is always a way to learn from an experience, it just takes thinking beyond the status quo.

ACKNOWLEDGMENT

Sincere appreciation to Valley Children's Healthcare for their enthusiastic support in the development of this program. Special thanks to Dr. Tara Lemoine, DO, Pediatric Intensivist and Medical Simulation Director for her overwhelming creativity, collaboration, and passion for seeing interprofessional simulation grow at Valley Children's.

REFERENCES

Acosta, C. D., Kit Delgado, M., Gisondi, M. A., Raghunathan, A., D'Souza, P. A., Gilbert, G.,...Wang, N. E. (2010). Characteristics of pediatric trauma transfers to a level I trauma center: Implications for developing a regionalized pediatric trauma system in California. *Academic Emergency Medicine,* *17*(12), 1364–1373.

American College of Surgeons Committee on Trauma. (2012). *Advanced trauma life support: Student course manual.* Chicago, IL: Author.

Curtis, K., McCarthy, A., Mitchell, R., Black, D., Foster, K., Jan, S.,…Holland, A. J. (2016). Paediatric trauma systems and their impact on the health outcomes of severely injured children: Protocol for a mixed methods cohort study. *Scandinavian Journal of Trauma, Resuscitation and Emergency Medicine,* *24,* 69.

Decker, S., Fey, F., Sideras, S., Caballero, S., Rockstraw, L., Boese, T.,…Borum, J. C. (2013). Standard of best practice: Simulation standard VI: The debriefing process. *Clinical Simulation in Nursing, 9*(9), S26–S29.

Doughty, C. (2015). Rapid cycle deliberate practice pediatric simulation scenarios. *MedEdPORTAL Publications, 11,* 10134. doi:10.15766/mep_2374-8265.10134

International Nursing Association for Clinical Simulation and Learning Standard Committee. (2016, December). Standards of best practice: Simulation: Simulation Design. *Clinical Simulation in Nursing, 12*(6S), S5–S12.

Interprofessional Education Collaborative Expert Panel. (2011). *Core competencies for interprofessional collaborative practice: Report of an expert panel.* Washington, DC: Author.

Kelleher, D. C., Jagadeesh Chandra Bose, R. P., Waterhouse, L. J., Carter, E. A., & Burd, R. S. (2014). Effect of a checklist on advanced trauma life support workflow deviations during trauma resuscitations without pre-arrival notification. *Journal of the American College of Surgeons, 218*(3), 459–466.

McKenzie, L. (2016). Nationwide Children's Center for Injury Research and Policy: Safety innovation. Retrieved from http://www.nationwidechildrens.org/safety-innovation

Rudolph, J. W., Simon, R., Dufresne, R. L., & Raemer, D. B. (2006). There's no such thing as "non-judgmental" debriefing: A theory and method for debriefing with good judgment. *Simulation in Healthcare, 1*(1), 49–55.

Zimmermann, K., Holzinger, I. B., Ganassi, L., Esslinger, P., Pilgrim, S., Allen, M.,…Stocker, M. (2015). Inter-professional in-situ simulated team and resuscitation training for patient safety: Description and impact of a programmatic approach. *BMC Medical Education, 15,* 189.

CHAPTER 43

Teaching Quality, Safety, and Process Improvement Through Root Cause Analysis Simulation

Jared M. Kutzin

A. IMPLEMENTATION OF SIMULATION-BASED PEDAGOGY IN YOUR INDIVIDUALIZED TEACHING AREA

There is robust literature examining the use of both low- and high-technology simulation for learning in undergraduate and graduate nursing education. Most reports focus on the outcomes of simulation learning for increasing knowledge and improving clinical skills. However, there is a dearth of studies examining the use of simulation learning for graduate nurses preparing for nonclinical roles, such as nursing administration.

The use of multiple simulation modalities for clinical skills acquisition has increased in nursing education. This is due in part to increased student enrollment, faculty shortages, and limited clinical sites, as well as the understanding of the role of deliberate practice in education to ensure high-quality, safe care for patients. Sources contain frequent discussion of the advantages and disadvantages of the use of simulation in nursing education. Advantages include limited or no risk to actual patients, assurance of more opportunities to practice a variety of skills, enhanced knowledge, and immediate feedback by faculty. Disadvantages frequently noted are the high cost of time and equipment and the need for the technical knowledge and support inherent in this method (Hravnak, Tuite, & Baldisseri, 2005).

Many sources report on the efficacy of simulation use for student performance or confidence, both at a graduate and undergraduate level. Bremner, Aduddell, Bennett, and VanGeest (2006) reported on 615 undergraduate students and found improved performance and confidence in the assessment skills learned using simulation. Moule, Wilford, Sales, and Lockyer (2008) reported greater confidence in students exposed to simulation before starting their clinical experience. Other studies have found benefits to student-reported confidence or skills with the use of simulation, particularly when the learning is highly technical (Alinier, Hunt, Gordon, & Harwood, 2006; Brannan, White, & Bezanson, 2008; Feingold, Calaluce, & Kallen, 2004).

For graduate nurses and advanced practice nurses (APNs; nurse practitioners, clinical nurse specialists, nurse-midwives, and nurse anesthetists), the use of simulation is generally limited to acquiring various clinical skills or clinical management scenarios. Examples include advanced cardiac life support (ACLS) training, crisis management training, and clinical assessment skills acquisition (using standardized patients) in graduate APN education.

Hravnak, Tuite, and Baldisseri (2005) described teaching critical care technical skills to acute care nurse practitioners and clinical nurse specialists using high-fidelity patient simulators and reported positive student responses. Tiffen, Graf, and Corbridge (2009) evaluated low-fidelity simulation as compared with lecture and case study to teach cardiac and respiratory assessment to APN students. They found that the group using simulation achieved greater confidence in these skills than the group taught using a more traditional educational approach. Corbridge and colleagues (2008) and Haskvitz and Koop (2004) also found more self-reported confidence among graduate nursing students learning to manage complicated patient scenarios. Corbridge, Robinson, Tiffen, and Cobridge (2010) also reported a preference for simulation over a more traditional learning method for teaching mechanical ventilation to a group of nurse practitioner students. Two other reports described the use of simulated patient scenarios for teaching end-of-life and palliative care (Gillan, Jeong, & van der Riet, 2014) and may show promise for high-fidelity simulation scenarios (Shawler, 2011; Wakefield, Cooke, & Boggis, 2003).

Simulation is also being used in the health care field to promote team training (Murphy, Curtis, & McCloughen, 2016) and nontechnical skills such as teamwork, communication (Härgestam, Lindkvist, Brulin, Jacobsson, & Hultin, 2013; Tofil et al., 2014), collaboration, and leadership (Jankouskas et al., 2007). The use of simulation in nursing education continues to broaden. Decker, Sportsman, Puetz, and Billings (2008), among others, call for a continued assessment of simulation as a valid and reliable method for the acquisition and long-term retention of knowledge and skills. Recognizing the preference for simulation training by students and the reported increased learning and confidence in clinical skills, we attempt to expand the use of simulation beyond clinical and teamwork skills into the management and administrative courses of graduate nursing education. Although incorporating simulation into the root cause analysis (RCA) process and error identification is increasing, its use in undergraduate and graduate nursing education is still limited (Lambton & Mahlmeister, 2010; Simms, Slakey, Garstka, Tersigni, & Korndorffer, 2012).

In addition to schools that use simulation for students, hospitals use simulation to train and educate clinical staff. The current, common focus of many simulation programs, especially hospital-based simulation programs, is on teaching clinical or interpersonal (teamwork and communication) skills. Such topics include shoulder dystocia skills and team training, cardiac arrest team training, and the breaking of bad news.

In addition, graduate faculty often advise simulation facilities that they cannot find ways of implementing simulation into their curricula or they do not see the utility in trying to bring this technique into their classes. However, some graduate faculty have long embraced standardized patients, a form of simulation, in the education of advanced clinical providers for specific skills training. This chapter discusses the implementation of a hybrid simulation program for nonclinical skills, which was implemented in a graduate nursing class focused on quality, safety, and process improvement.

B. EDUCATIONAL MATERIALS AVAILABLE IN YOUR TEACHING AREA AND RELATED TO YOUR SPECIALTY

The program was initially implemented at the New York Simulation Center for Health Sciences (NYSIM), a New York University Langone Medical Center–City University of New York joint simulation center, located at Bellevue Hospital. The faculty initially involved with this program were associated with Hunter–Bellevue School of Nursing in New York City, which had access to the facility. Since the initial implementation, this program has been hosted at various hospital-based simulation facilities and national and regional conferences to demonstrate how simulation can be used to teach about quality, safety, and process improvement.

C. SPECIFIC OBJECTIVES FOR SIMULATION USE WITHIN A SPECIFIC COURSE AND THE OVERALL PROGRAM

Initially, the simulation was included in a course that focused on how nurse leaders and other health care professionals work in integrated networks and apply leadership and management theories to patient safety and quality-of-care topics.

Simulation was added to this course, which allowed the graduate nursing students to have an experiential learning opportunity focusing on the hazards that may lead to medical errors, how to identify the root causes of the error using specific analytic methods, and how to develop an action plan using process-improvement strategies that would permanently solve the root causes. Since the initial implementation, this course has been taught as a continuing-education program for licensed health care providers (nurses, physician assistants, physicians, etc.).

The scenario is designed for learners to interact with standardized participants (SPs) who play the role of health care providers involved with a medical error. When used as part of a graduate student curriculum, this activity takes place at the end of the semester after students have discussed the role of nursing management, oversight of regulatory agencies, and patient safety and quality.

D. INTRODUCTION OF SCENARIO

Setting the Scene

Before attending the simulation experience, learners should be familiar with the process of performing an RCA, including tools, such as fishbone diagrams and process mapping. Students typically spend about 2.5 hours learning and discussing the differences between RCA and failure mode effects analysis (FMEA), as well as specific tools used to improve health care quality, such as:

1. Pareto charts (Tagues, 2005)
2. Ishikawa diagrams (fishbone; Tagues, 2005)
3. Flow charts (National Patient Safety Foundation [NPSF], 2016)
4. The five-why's method of reaching the root cause (Tagues, 2005)
5. Cause-and-effect diagrams (NPSF, 2016)

Through a variety of classroom exercises and discussions, students are taught why errors occur, how systems fail, the levels of harm that result from medical errors, and how health care attempts to identify and reconcile medical mistakes. Although originally taught in a traditional bricks-and-mortar classroom environment, using online educational modules (either homemade or publicly available), such as the Institute for Healthcare Improvement (IHI) open courses, can be substituted for traditional instructor-led training. Online education can be used to provide knowledge in preparation for an in-person simulation session focusing on conducting an RCA. In addition, both learners and faculty should review the NPSF's (2016), *RCA²: Improving Root Cause Analyses and Actions to Prevent Harm* as a reference for how to conduct an RCA.

To begin the session, learners are positioned in small groups of five to seven, either in one large classroom or in separate small rooms. These teams are meant to simulate the teams that would conduct an RCA after a medical mistake has been identified. Each team is presented with a simulated incident report that gives high-level information regarding the case, such as the patient's name, where the incident occurred, and what the reporting individual thinks happened. This can be tailored so that it accurately reflects the local institution's format.

The incident report for this specific case states that the patient, Jane Dolan, was an inpatient, currently on hospital day 4 for the treatment of pneumonia, who suffered a cardiac arrest. The cardiac arrest team responded and provided treatment, including chest compressions and defibrillation. The patient was then found to be wearing a bracelet that indicated the patient had an active do not resuscitate (DNR) order. The resuscitation was stopped. However, the primary nurse indicated to the code team that she did not think the patient had a DNR. The team monetarily paused their efforts until clarification of the DNR status was obtained. The incident report was filed because of the treatment (possible delay or wrong care) provided to the patient. The teams are now tasked with identifying what occurred, why it occurred, and how to prevent such situations in the future.

Technology Used

To facilitate the scenario, a high-fidelity manikin should be in a patient bed. A saline lock should be placed in the patient's arm. Vitals signs are heart rate (HR): 90 beats/minute, blood pressure (BP): 110/70 mmHg, respiration rate (RR): 20 breaths/minute, oxygen saturation (SpO_2): 94% on 2 L oxygen via nasal cannula). The patient wristband identifies the patient as Jane Dolan. Standard telemetry monitors are in place, including a bedside electrocardiography (EKG) monitor, BP monitor, and pulse oximeter. A code cart stocked with standard medications and a defibrillator are available in the hallway as is a stool for chest compressions. Other equipment needed "off stage" include a patient chart and color-coded medical wristbands.

The learners can watch the scenario from a remotely located room via closed-circuit television, through a one-way mirror, or can even be in the simulation room watching as observers.

Objectives

At the conclusion of this program, learners should be able to:

1. Discuss the differences between RCA and FMEA
2. Conduct an RCA to identify the causes of the error
3. Develop an improvement strategy that will alter the outcome of the case

Description of Participants

Standardized participants (SPs) play the roles of a primary nurse, code team nurse (ICU nurse), code team doctor (team leader), code team medical student, and respiratory therapist (or anesthesiologist).

E. RUNNING OF THE SCENARIO

SPs play the role of the primary nurse and the code team and have rehearsed the scenario before the course. Rehearsing before the scenario not only allows the SPs to be familiar with how to run the scenario, but also allows them to accurately give responses and portray their characters during the interview process previously described. The SPs have been given a script of their respective roles and understand the frame of mind of their character. The complete scenario, including SP frames of mind, is available in Exhibit 43.1.

In summary, the scenario begins with the primary nurse entering the patient's room to perform an initial assessment. The nurse recognizes that the patient is missing the appropriate identification bands to signify she has an allergy to a medication. The nurse retrieves what they believe to be the correct wristband (blue) and applies it to the patient. After administering an antibiotic and leaving the patient room, the patient suffers a cardiac arrest. The responding team sees the blue wristband and recognizes this as a DNR wristband. A conversation ensues during the cardiac arrest regarding the patient's code status. It is subsequently found that the patient does NOT have a DNR and the nurse applied the wrong wristband. An incident report is filed, which leads to the present day and the teams of learners needing to complete an RCA.

Once all of the learner groups have had the opportunity to interview the SPs, they are provided with 20 minutes to complete their RCA and develop a root cause statement and complete their flowcharts, Ishikawa diagrams, or other tools they used to reach the root causes. While the groups are completing this, faculty advisors circulate and ensure that students are on track in reaching a plausible root

Exhibit 43.1	Human Patient Simulation: Mrs. Jane Dolan	
Time	**Vital Signs**	**Participant Cues**
Time 0: 0 min	HR: 90 beats/minute sinus rhythm BP: 110/70 mmHg RR: 20 breaths/minute SpO_2 94% 2 L	The patient has just been admitted and is resting comfortably in bed. At this time the patient has no specific complaints. The patient states her breathing is better after being treated in the emergency department. A nurse is in the room completing an admission assessment and implementing the plan of care, including making sure the patient identification bands (ID, allergy, and no blood draw) are placed on the patient, and then hangs the antibiotics (ceftriaxone). The nurse places a blue wristband, which he or she believes signals an allergy to penicillin, and a red wristband, signaling no blood draw, on the patient. The nurse completes the tasks, double-checks that the patient is comfortable, and exits the room.
Time 1: 2 min	HR: 130 beats/minute sinus tachycardia BP: 90/50 mmHg RR: 28 breaths/minute, wheezing SpO_2 92% RA	The nurse is summoned back into the room via patient monitor alarm and the patient calling out for the nurse. The patient complains of dizziness, lightheadedness, and a general feeling of "not feeling well." The nurse calls out for help—looking for "local assistance," but no one is available and no one responds to the request. The nurse reassures the patient and asks questions such as: "What are you feeling? When did it start? Describe it in more detail." The patient answers with: "Trouble swallowing, difficulty breathing, can't catch my breath. Started a few minutes ago with a funny feeling in my mouth and throat." The nurse looks around the room, checks the medications, and stops the infusion (realizing this may be anaphylaxis). The nurse begins providing oxygen via nonrebreather mask for the patient's difficulty breathing.
Time 2: 2.5 min	HR: Ventricular tachycardia BP: 0/0 mmHg RR: 0 breaths/minute SpO_2 88%	The patient becomes unresponsive. Nurse again calls for help, this time by calling a code—pushing the code button, speaking with a unit coordinator, calling on a phone, and so on. The nurse puts the head of the bed down and begins prompt CPR.
Time 3: 3.5 min	HR: Ventricular tachycardia BP: 0/0 mmHg RR: 0 breaths/minute SpO_2 88%	The code team arrives with the code cart and defibrillator from the hallway and begins caring for the patient. The primary nurse turns over care to the code team by giving a verbal report. The primary nurse provides the code team with the situation (S), background (B), and assessment (A): S—Patient is in cardiac arrest. B—Patient was admitted for IV antibiotic for pneumonia. Patient has a history of CABG × 2, diabetes, HTN. A—IV antibiotics were infusing when patient became tachycardic, tachypneic, and then developed a pulseless ventricular tachycardia arrest.

(continued)

Exhibit 43.1	Human Patient Simulation: Mrs. Jane Dolan *(continued)*

Time	Vital Signs	Participant Cues
		Code team begins to provide resuscitation.
		Junior MD begins compressions.
		ICU RN places defibrillation pads on the patient and turns defibrillator on (on direction from code leader).
		RRT or other member begins using BVM and securing an airway with appropriate devices (oral airways, intubation).
		Code team leader says to make sure the IV medication infusion is stopped, defibrillator pads are attached quickly, and asks that epinephrine 1 mg IV be made ready. The code leader has an intense focus on making sure the defibrillator is used quickly. He or she continually states, "Get the defibrillator on. Is it ready? Make sure the defibrillator is hooked up."
Time 4: 5 min		Two cycles of CPR are completed—code team nurse prepares to administer epinephrine and, before administration, notices a blue wristband signifying "DNR" on the patient's wrist. The ICU nurse calls everyone's attention to this by asking, "Is this patient DNR?"
		The code team asks the primary nurse for confirmation and the primary nurse, who is standing in the corner of the room, hesitantly states, "I … I don't believe the patient to is DNR…. I don't think so."
		The code team asks the nurse to get the chart to confirm the code status while they debate whether they should continue resuscitation (compressions can be continued, but defibrillation is delayed, and medications are held while the patient status is confirmed).
Time 5: 6 min	HR: Asystole BP: 0/0 mmHg RR : 0 breaths/ minute SpO$_2$ as indicated by actions of code team	While the code team debates whether they should continue and while the primary nurse is out looking for the chart, the patient deteriorates to asystole.
		The nurse returns a few moments later with the chart, which identifies the patient as a full code—the nurse is flipping through the chart and does not find DNR paperwork and states as such.
		The code team double-checks with the nurse by asking, "Are you sure the patient is a full code?"
		The primary nurse confirms the patient's status and the resuscitation is continued after the delay.
		The code team can no longer provide defibrillation because the rhythm has changed to asystole.
		The resuscitation continues for two additional rounds of CPR (2–3 minutes) before being stopped and the patient is pronounced dead.
		An alternative to this ending, for those organizations not wanting to have the patient die, is to have a delay in defibrillation, but the heart rhythm remains in ventricular tachycardia (a shockable rhythm). The conclusion of the case can have the patient be successfully resuscitated with the patient being transferred to the ICU, however, because of the delay in defibrillation, the patient experiences irreversible brain damage (harm).

BP, blood pressure; BVM, bag–valve–mask; CABG, coronary artery bypass graft; CPR, cardiopulmonary resuscitation; DNR, do not resuscitate; HR, heart rate; HTN, hypertension; ICU, intensive care unit; IV, intravenous; RA, room air; RR, respiratory rate; RRT, rapid response team.

cause. On reaching a root cause(s), they then work as a group to identify a solution to the root cause(s) they determined. Potential solutions include, but are not limited to:

1. Education
2. Change in wristband design (including words on the wristband or different shapes)
3. Standardizing wristband colors
4. Relocating wristbands into separate cabinets
5. Policy of posting a DNR in the patient room via a sign

After finalizing their RCA and solution, student groups share their findings with their classmates.

The scenario takes approximately 3 hours to complete, although up to 4 hours may be necessary for novice learners. Large groups can be accommodated with this program. Up to 35 learners (five groups of seven learners) have participated at one time.

F. PRESENTATION OF COMPLETED TEMPLATE

Title

Leadership and Managment

Focus Area

Patient safety, health care quality, process improvement

Scenario Description

The students arrive and are placed into small groups that are meant to simulate the teams that conduct an RCA. The teams review an incident report that describes the misidentification of a patient's DNR status. At this time, the teams should organize themselves in preparation for conducting an RCA. A team leader as well as a facilitator, time keeper, and recorder should be identified. The remaining individuals can self-select into other roles, such as "process experts" in which they are responsible for asking questions of the SPs related to specific areas of concern. The organization of the team is a process that the facilitator should observe and be prepared to debrief at the conclusion of the event. Similar to many clinical scenarios in which teamwork and communication make up a majority of the objectives, here, too, teamwork and communication have an impact on the success of the team conducting the RCA.

After organizing themselves as a team, SPs are introduced to the groups. The SPs introduce themselves by name and role and spend approximately 10 minutes with each group being interviewed. At this point, the facilitator should be listening and observing each of the groups. Debriefing points from this stage of the exercise include nonverbal communication techniques (how the teams arranged themselves in relation to the SP), verbal communication skills (types and order of questions asked), and how the individual team members functioned as an ad-hoc team.

After interviewing each of the SPs, the teams spend up to 30 minutes working to create a flowchart and identifying opportunities to improve the system to prevent such an error from occurring in the future. Following the team's discussion of their findings and system improvements, the simulation is demonstrated, and the learners witness the case in real time.

The scenario includes a primary nurse (SP) assessing and treating a patient who then goes into cardiac arrest. The primary nurse activates the code team, who respond and treat the patient until they identify a DNR wristband. The resuscitation is stopped, but discussion about the legitimacy of the wristband ensues. This delay in care affects the patient outcome. The initial patient data form is shown in Exhibit 43.2. The full scenario is detailed in Exhibit 43.1.

Depending on the level of the learner and the comfort of the facilitator, the level of harm presented in the scenario can span from no harm to death. Slightly modifying the incident report, the SPs' responses, as well as the objectives of the program can lead to a vastly different experience for the learners. Simple modifications can include stopping compressions in addition to defibrillation and having the delay result in loss of brain function or patient death. Although the process for conducting an RCA should not change as it relates to the level of harm caused, the opportunity for the facilitator to introduce an array of other topics for discussion is available when the scenario is modified. For example, the facilitator can discuss with the learners how to manage the reactions of the individuals involved (caring for the caregiver), the incorporation of a "just culture" into the process, or the role of settling claims with the family after a serious adverse event.

An additional customization of this program is to rerun the scenario with some or all of the fixes the teams have identified. The facilitator can preplan with the SPs to either make mistakes or not make mistakes the second time based on the interventions suggested. A list of suggested improvements and their relative strength is available in Appendix A.

Setting the Scene

Equipment needed (part 1): Standardized participants (at least five), flip chart (one per group), incident report (paper copy, one per group), diagrams used as part of an RCA (fishbone, flow chart, etc.).

Equipment needed (part 2): Simulator (with patient monitor), medical equipment (code cart [intubation equipment and bag-valve-mask, BVM], defibrillator, resuscitation medications [simulated—epinephrine, atropine, bicarb]), oxygen hookup, pulse oximeter, BP cuff, stethoscope, stool (for compressions), medical record (electronic or paper), patient ID band—white, red wristband indicating "no blood draw" placed on the wrist by the admitting nurse, and blue wristband indicating "allergy" placed on wrist by admitting nurse. Plastic patient wristbands can be used; however, we used 1 inch of ribbon cut to length with double-sided tape on one end to simulate the wristbands without words.

Simulator level: Part 1—SP Part 2—high-fidelity

Participant roles: The five standardized participants should not be class participants; rather, they should be professional medical or nursing staff or others practiced and briefed on their roles.

Exhibit 43.2	Data Form for Patient Jane Dolan

Patient Data Form

Name: Jane Dolan

Demographics:

Age: 74 years old

Occupation: Retired librarian

Pertinent past medical history: CABG × 2 (5 years earlier), diabetes, HTN, breast cancer, appendectomy (40 years earlier), lumpectomy with lymph node removal (left side)

Presenting symptoms, illnesses, injuries, and recent surgeries:

Current medications: Plavix, aspirin, glucophage, hydrochlorothiazide

Allergies: Penicillin

Visit history: Recent admit for 4 days of continually worsening cough, chest discomfort, and fever. Admitted through the ED to the medical telemetry floor. The patient has had the initial admission paperwork completed and is getting settled on the floor. The patient is admitted for IV antibiotics and is being monitored because of her past medical history.

CABG, coronary artery bypass graft; ED, emergency department; HTN, hypertension; IV, intravenous.

The SPs should not hide the aforementioned information from the learners, but should not prompt them either. The SPs do not have to give each group the same information if the questions from the students do not allow for it.

An example of the conversation the primary nurse may have is:

Group interviewing: "Why do you think this error occurred?"
Actor: "There's probably a few reasons."
Group interviewing: "Can you explain what you mean?"
Actor: "Well, to be honest, I was a bit tired."
Group interviewing: "Why were you tired?"
Actor: "Well this is my second job, and I had already worked 3, 12-hour days (or shifts) when they asked me to stay late."

The aforementioned comments from each standardized participant describe numerous reasons the error occurred:

Primary nurse: Fatigue, patient overload, lack of standardization of wristbands between jobs and across the health care community, environment (bands stored all together), work overload (too much going on during the admission process)

Code team junior clinician: Role on the code team (focus on compressions), no training in looking for bracelets or knowing what they mean, culture (did not think they could speak up)

ICU nurse: Environment (bands do not have writing on them), need a work-around in the ICU (not a standardized process)

Code team senior clinician: Focused on one or two tasks and did not take a global view (did not see the bracelet)

Respiratory therapist/anesthesia: Focused on the airway, should probably look for the patient's status (is not located near the wrist to see the wristband); it is unclear as to why some conditions get wristbands and others do not

Scenario Implementation

Exhibit 43.1 described the full scenario, and Exhibit 43.3 provides pre/post course survey for the learners.

G. DEBRIEFING GUIDELINES

Debriefing of this program is multifaceted. Debriefings should be conducted throughout the course at natural break points, such as after the teams interview the SPs but before they begin working on potential solutions, after the potential solutions have been presented by each team of learners, after the scenario is demonstrated without the suggested fixes, and again after the scenario is rerun with the suggested fixes. The facilitator can focus on a variety of topics in each debrief, including but not limited to:

1. What roles did the team assign to each member and how did the team assign roles during the initial team formation?
2. Who was the team leader? Why is it important to have a team leader in the boardroom, just like at the bedside?
3. What could have been done differently to make the team work more effectively? How did it feel interviewing the staff?
4. What did the teams discover during the interviews?

Exhibit 43.3	Pre/Post Survey of Students				
Criterion	**Strongly Disagree**				**Strongly Agree**
I feel confident in explaining the difference between a root cause analysis and a failure modes effect analysis.	1	2	3	4	5
I have witnessed an error (real or simulated) that has led to patient harm.	1	2	3	4	5
I can identify major causes of errors in health care.	1	2	3	4	5
I can list the levels of patient harm that may occur.	1	2	3	4	5
I am familiar with the tools to conduct a root cause analysis.	1	2	3	4	5
I can describe how to create and use a fishbone diagram (Ishikawa diagram).	1	2	3	4	5
I can describe the Plan-Do-Check-Act (PDCA) cycle of process improvement.	1	2	3	4	5
I know how to ask questions to get to the underlying cause of an error.	1	2	3	4	5

5. What causes did the teams come up with?
6. What could the teams do differently to uncover additional root causes?
7. What interventions could the teams implement to prevent this type of error from happening in the future?
8. What other solutions could the teams use to prevent the root cause in the future?

In addition to debriefing the learners, the opportunity exists to have the SPs take part in the debrief so that the learners can hear from the perspective of the SPs and how they felt being interviewed. Variations in team dynamics, nonverbal communication (i.e., positioning of chairs), and how they conducted the interviews can be discussed.

H. SUGGESTIONS/KEY FEATURES TO REPLICATE OR IMPROVE

The scenario has been implemented with a variety of audiences, including graduate nursing students and expert simulation users and has received positive feedback from all participants. The scenario requires significant preparation by the faculty member and the simulation team and the SPs. Skilled SPs are required to successfully run this scenario, and it is recommended that they be clinicians skilled in simulation, as accurately responding to the learner's questions may require improvisational responses.

We dedicated 2 hours to a review of RCA tools in a session before the simulation so that learners understood the basic concepts of the tools they were expected to use during the simulation and subsequent encounter with the actors. Using a case study that demonstrates the RCA tools may add value to the lecture-style review so that students have an example from which to draw from when they begin putting the tools into practice.

We also found it helpful to provide the students with a diagram demonstrating the effectiveness of various interventions in health care once the teams have brainstormed their own ideas. This "take home" allows them to recall which interventions are most likely to prevent the incident from occurring in the future. An "action hierarchy" can be found in the RCA^2 document produced by the NPSF (2016, p. 17).

I. RECOMMENDATIONS FOR FURTHER USE

In addition to using the clinical scenario to discuss and use the tools of an RCA, the clinical scenario presented earlier can be used to have discussions about ethics as well as the policy and procedure for how to handle a situation in which a patient is mistakenly identified as a DNR. The format described can be used with alternate clinical scenarios, such as attaching the patient to the wrong oxygen source (connecting the patient to an air regulator [yellow] instead of an oxygen regulator [green]) or other identified patient safety issue. This would lead to the discovery of different root causes and potential system solutions to prevent these errors.

J. HOW SIMULATION-BASED PEDAGOGY HAS CONTRIBUTED TO IMPROVED STUDENT OUTCOMES

We have found that using role play and simulation in the manner described earlier has improved learners ability to conduct an RCA. Learners have reported feeling more confident with the interview process, diagramming the statements of participants, and identifying opportunities to fix system concerns.

K. EXPERT RECOMMENDATIONS AND WORDS OF WISDOM

The importance of interdisciplinary team training for health care professionals has been established. Many organizations are now beginning to also recognize the need for education of front-line clinical staff about systems and how they impact the quality and safety of care. Although topics, such as RCA and FMEA, are often discussed in a lecture-style setting during the postbaccalaureate academic education of health professionals, the firsthand experience is often lacking. The true introduction to these topics typically only occurs once students become licensed and are unfortunately involved in an adverse event requiring investigation. Although newly licensed health professionals are not typically involved in the process of investigating or responding to errors, they often hear about the "investigation" that takes place following an "occurrence" and may be unfairly biased by colleagues' perceptions of the response to the error by the organization and other staff.

The role of simulation in training health care providers in patient safety and health care quality topics is still in its infancy. Encouraging interprofessional teams of learners to participate in a training program such as the one described earlier has value not only in academic institutions but also in practice sites as well. Many clinicians do not understand how systems impact their daily work. Nor, do they understand the process that quality-and-safety professionals go through to identify and prevent errors. Learners who have taken part in this program often focus on the clinical topics, such as the quality of CPR or the team dynamics of the staff, rather than on the myriad other factors that converged to result in the error. Refocusing their attention to the patient safety issues expands their knowledge base beyond clinical treatments to better understand how the system they are working in impacts patient care.

L. EVALUATION OF BEST PRACTICE STANDARDS
AND USE OF CREDENTIALED SIMULATION FACULTY

The aforementioned scenario is in line with the International Nursing Association for Clinical Simulation and Learning (INACSL) Standards of Best Practice (INACSL, 2013/2016) and the American Association of Colleges of Nursing (AACN) *Essentials of Master's Education in Nursing*. As per the INACSL Standards of Best Practice, the facilitation methods describe using a low-technology simulation in an educationally appropriate manner and then incorporates high-technology simulation as necessary to further the understanding of the learners (INACSL, 2013/2016). The debriefing process is paramount in the aforementioned curriculum and the debriefing involves talking with the learners about their feelings regarding interviewing the SPs and what worked well and what could be improved on.

Essentials I, II, III, IV, VI, and VII of the AACN *Essentials of Master's Education in Nursing* (2011) are met through the completion of this program. Essential I (Background for Practice from Sciences and Humanities), Essential II (Organizational and Systems Leadership), Essential III (Quality Improvement and Safety), Essential IV (Translating and Integrating Scholarship into Practice), Essential VI (Health Policy and Advocacy), and Essential VII (Interprofessional Collaboration for Improving Patient and Population Health Outcomes) all address the integration of quality, safety, process improvement, and leadership skills into the curriculum (AACN, 2011).

REFERENCES

Alinier, G., Hunt, B., Gordon, R., & Harwood, C. (2006). Effectiveness of intermediate-fidelity simulation training technology in undergraduate nursing education. *Journal of Advanced Nursing, 54*(3), 359–369.

American Association of Colleges of Nursing. (2011). *The essentials of master's education in nursing*. Washington, DC: Author.

Brannan, J. D., White, A., & Bezanson, J. L. (2008). Simulator effects on cognitive skills and confidence levels. *Journal of Nursing Education, 47*(11), 495–500.

Bremner, M. N., Aduddell, K., Bennett, D. N., & VanGeest, J. B. (2006). The use of human patient simulators: Best practices with novice nursing students. *Nurse Educator, 31*(4), 170–174.

Corbridge, S. J., McLaughlin, R., Tiffen, J., Wade, L., Templin, R., & Corbridge, T. C. (2008). Using simulation to enhance knowledge and confidence. *Nurse Practitioner, 33*(6), 12–13.

Corbridge, S. J., Robinson, F. P., Tiffen, J., & Corbridge, T. C. (2010). Online learning versus simulation for teaching principles of mechanical ventilation to nurse practitioner students. *International Journal of Nursing Education Scholarship, 7*, Article 12.

Decker, S., Sportsman, S., Puetz, L., & Billings, L. (2008). The evolution of simulation and its contribution to competency. *Journal of Continuing Education in Nursing, 39*(2), 74–80.

Feingold, C. E., Calaluce, M., & Kallen, M. A. (2004). Computerized patient model and simulated clinical experiences: Evaluation with baccalaureate nursing students. *Journal of Nursing Education, 43*(4), 156–163.

Gillan, P. C., Jeong, S., & van der Riet, P. J. (2014). End of life care simulation: A review of the literature. *Nurse Education Today, 34*(5), 766–774. doi:10.1016/j.nedt.2013.10.005

Härgestam, M., Lindkvist, M., Brulin, C., Jacobsson, M., & Hultin, M. (2013). Communication in interdisciplinary teams: Exploring closed-loop communication during in situ trauma team training. *British Medical Journal Open, 21*(10), e003525. doi:10.1136/bmjopen-2013-003525

Haskvitz, L. M., & Koop, E. C. (2004). Students struggling in clinical? A new role for the patient simulator. *Journal of Nursing Education, 43*(4), 181–184.

Hravnak, M., Tuite, P., & Baldisseri, M. (2005). Expanding acute care nurse practitioner and clinical nurse specialist education: Invasive procedure training and human simulation in critical care. *AACN Clinical Issues, 16*(1), 89–104.

International Nursing Association for Clinical Simulation and Learning. (2013, updated 2016). INACSL standards of best practice: Simulation. Retrieved from https://www.inacsl.org/i4a/pages/index.cfm?pageID=3407

Jankouskas, T., Bush, M. C., Murray, B., Rudy, S., Henry, J., Dyer, A. M., . . . Sinz, E. (2007). Crisis resource management: Evaluating outcomes of a multidisciplinary team. *Simulation in Healthcare, 2*(2), 96–101.

Lambton, J., & Mahlmeister, L. (2010). Conducting root cause analysis with nursing students: Best practice in nursing education. *Journal of Nursing Education, 49*(8), 444–448.

Moule, P., Wilford, A., Sales, R., & Lockyer, L. (2008). Student experiences and mentor views of the use of simulation for learning. *Nurse Education Today, 28*(7), 790–797.

Murphy, M., Curtis, K., McCloughen, A. (2016). What is the impact of multidisciplinary team simulation training on team performance and efficiency of patient care? An integrative review. *Australasian Emergency Nursing Journal, 19*(1), 44–53. doi:10.1016/j.aenj.2015.10.001

National Patient Safety Foundation. (2016). *RCA²: Improving root cause analyses and actions to prevent harm.* Boston, MA: Author.

Shawler, C. (2011). Palliative and end-of-life care: Using a standardized patient family for gerontological nurse practitioner students. *Nursing Education Perspectives, 32*(3), 168–172.

Simms, E. R., Slakey, D. P., Garstka, M. E., Tersigni, S. A., & Korndorffer, J. R. (2012). Can simulation improve the traditional method of root cause analysis: A preliminary investigation. *Surgery, 152*(3), 489–497.

Tagues, N. (2005). *The quality toolbox* (2nd ed.). Milwaukee, WI: ASQ Quality Press.

Tiffen, J., Graf, N., & Corbridge, S. (2009). Effectiveness of a low-fidelity experience in building confidence among advanced practice nursing graduate students. *Clinical Simulation in Nursing, 5*(3), 113–117.

Tofil, N. M., Morris, J. L., Peterson, D. T., Watts, P., Epps, C., Harrington, K. F., . . . White, M. L. (2014). Interprofessional simulation training improves knowledge and teamwork in nursing and medical students during internal medicine clerkship. *Journal of Hospital Medicine, 9*(3), 189–192. doi:10.1002/jhm.2126

Wakefield, A., Cooke, S., & Boggis, C. (2003). Learning together: Use of simulated patients with nursing and medical students for breaking bad news. *International Journal of Palliative Nursing, 9*(1), 32–38.

APPENDIX A

Standardized Participant Responses to Team Interview Questions and Frames of Reference

	Primary Nurse	Code Team Nurse (ICU Nurse)	Code Team Leader	Code Team Provider (Jr. MD/Medical Student/PA)	Respiratory Therapist
Patient responsibility (workload)	Responsible for seven patients during this shift	Has a patient assignment in the ICU (currently two patients)	Responsible for managing all the ICU patients (12)	Is on the medical service, responsible for up to 25 patients at a time	Covers a few units but all therapists respond to "code calls"—the respiratory therapist happened to be the first one there
Duty hours	Works 12-hours shifts. Was asked to stay an extra 4 due to a sick call. Has already worked 36 hours in previous 3 days. The incident occurred toward the end of the shift.	Works 12-hour shifts.	Works 12-hour shifts. Seven days on and then 7 days off. The incident occurred on the third day of work.	If resident—limited to 80 hours per week on average over a 2-week period; if medical student—no real limits, students shadow the residents so basically it amounts to about 75 hours per week.	8-hour shifts
Other commitments	Works two jobs (one is at another hospital) and has a family.	Family	Family, children	Schoolwork	Family
Frame of reference regarding wristband	Thinks a blue band indicates allergy (in actuality blue band signifies DNR at this hospital. At the "other" hospital it signifies allergy)	Blue band = DNR—the hospital standard. Nurse put a sign above the patient's bed for easy reference, with big letters: DNR.	Thinks that the blue band = DNR. Isn't sure because it's a nursing task and leader doesn't get involved.	Thinks that the blue band = DNR. Isn't sure because it's a nursing task and code team doesn't get involved.	Is pretty sure the blue band = DNR. Hospital does a yearly competency about all the wristband colors.
Location of wristbands	All of the patient bands (ID, DNR, allergy, no blood draw, fall alert, etc.) are kept at the nurse's station in the same cabinet.	They keep the wristbands separated in bins in the ICU. But they also put a sign in the patient's room.	In the ICU there's a BIG sign above a patient's bed which indicates a DNR. Assumes this is normal practice throughout the hospital.	Doesn't know.	Doesn't know.

(continued)

(continued)

	Primary Nurse	Code Team Nurse (ICU Nurse)	Code Team Leader	Code Team Provider (Jr. MD/Medical Student/PA)	Respiratory Therapist
Application of wristbands	Believes the emergency department should have put the wristbands on the patient. The floor nurse cannot be responsible for that task, especially since the admissions process is cumbersome and takes a long time.	Thinks the emergency department should identify the patient with the wristbands, but knows that sometimes they do not. Besides, the wristband is just a way of getting information quickly; the document MUST be in the chart. They keep the document on the cover of the chart so they do not have to look for it.	N/A	N/A	N/A
Responsibility during code	Responsible for recognizing and activating the code team.	Responds to code to assist the floor nurse with medications and defibrillation.	Team leader at the event who provides medical management. Big focus is on early defibrillation. If the rhythm is V tach or V fib, then the earlier the shock the better. In addition, do NOT interrupt check compressions. Push hard and push fast.	Compressions: Major focus is on pushing hard and fast as per the ACLS and BLS guidelines. The guidelines state to push at a rate of at least 100 compressions per minute and to a depth of at least 2 inches deep.	Airway: Maintain a patent airway either through a BVM or intubation. CPR should NOT be stopped to intubate.

Recognition of wristband	Thinks the blue wristband = allergy alert.	Noticed the wristband on the patient and said something to the team leader, but did not recognize it right away as medications were not given for a few minutes as per protocol. Only when nurse went to give the medication did he or she see the wristband. It's not on the nurse's "to-do list" when responding. If the primary nurse calls, then this nurse believes the primary nurse knows the patient's wishes.	The responsibility isn't this person's job. His or her job is to respond and lead the code. The primary nurse needs to know when to call the team.	Noticed the wristband on the patient but didn't really know exactly what it meant. Thought it may mean DNR, but since there are no words on the wristband, wasn't sure. The overhead page colors are listed on the back of the ID (code gray, code red, etc.), but not the wristband colors.	Did not really see the wristband since he or she was at the head of the bed, but doesn't understand how the blue wristband can mean anything other than DNR. Blue = airway = DNR. However, there is not wristband for "do not intubate," maybe there should be?
Ability to speak up	Felt comfortable in the room until the mistake was recognized. Did not know what was going on. Is not involved in a lot of code responses. His or her role is to provide information, not really to get involved.	Spoke up right away. Noticed the wristband and said something.	Believes it's everybody's job to work together.	Did not feel comfortable speaking up as provider was not 100% sure about the colors.	The team leader did a good job asking about the airway patency.

(continued)

(continued)

	Primary Nurse	Code Team Nurse (ICU Nurse)	Code Team Leader	Code Team Provider (Jr. MD/Medical Student/PA)	Respiratory Therapist
Medical management	Knows about CPR and pushing hard and pushing fast. Knows to get a stepstool and lower the bed. Is certified in BLS every 2 years.	Is certified in ACLS every 2 years.	Is certified in ACLS. Knows that getting the defibrillator pads on the patient is the most important things and was really focused on that. A 1-minute delay in defibrillation decreases the chance of survival by 10%. Since the code committee reviews the data each month the leader was really focused on getting the pads on early for an in-hospital cardiac arrest.	Took ACLS once.	Has not taken ACLS in a while, but is very proficient with airway skills.
Years in practice/length of service	In practice for 4 years; worked at this hospital for 3	In practice fo 8 years; worked at this hospital for 5	Attending physician in critical care for 14 years	Depends on role (med student vs. resident vs. PA)	In practice for 12 years, at this hospital for 9
Other information	Attends hospital in-service as required. Wristbands are not covered on an annual basis.	Attends hospital in-service as required. Has a workaround in the ICU (described previously). This is necessary because the wristbands do not have words on them.	Thinks the nurse should be sure of the code status before calling the team.	Isn't really concerned with wristband colors because it's not really relevant to them on a daily basis.	Isn't sure why there is a DNR bracelet but not a DNI bracelet. What if a patient does not want to be intubated but his or her heart is still beating?

ACLS, advanced cardiac life support; BLS, basic life support; BVM, bag-valve–mask; CPR, cardiopulmonary resuscitation; DNI, do not intubate; DNR, do not resuscitate; ICU, intensive care unit; V fib, ventricular fibrillation; V tach, ventricular tachycardia.

CHAPTER 44

Student-Generated Scenarios
for Senior Simulation Day

Karen M. Daley and Robin S. Goodrich

A. IMPLEMENTATION OF SIMULATION-BASED
PEDAGOGY IN YOUR INDIVIDUALIZED TEACHING AREA

Implementation of simulation-based pedagogy progressed rapidly at Western Connecticut State University over the initial 5 years of the simulation program. At the time, all simulations were done on static manikins and were primarily skill based. As the lead instructors in the capstone course in the spring semester of 2008, we felt it very important to expose senior students to high-fidelity simulation. High-fidelity simulation allows the student to link theory, use the nursing process, and apply curricular content using a multidisciplinary approach. Additional advantages of high-fidelity simulation include enhancement of psychomotor skills and collaboration with peers and faculty in a nonthreatening environment.

Obtaining our first human patient simulator (HPS) took several tries and much effort over a 2-year period. Once obtained, we made it an immediate priority to introduce high-fidelity simulations at the senior level. This effort turned out to be extremely timely. That year, one of the regional hospitals began competency testing using the HPS. Our graduates, it was reported, were some of the only new graduates who excelled in the testing.

As time went by, simulation was introduced at all levels of the program. By the time the seniors arrive in the capstone course, the students have become accustomed to interacting with the HPS and have developed their own "simulation personalities." For instance, some came hungry for as much simulation as possible. Others arrived and announced that they had done so much simulation, they were "sick and tired of it!" The year this scenario was introduced, the students arrived and stated they had not done enough simulation and were asking for dedicated time in a nontesting situation to reacquaint themselves with the HPS. As with all capstone courses, our job as faculty is to assess each group's final learning needs and meet them as the best way we see fit. However, this year it was apparent that the capstone course itself was so anxiety producing that testing on the simulators did not seem feasible. In fact, once the students had completed their intensive capstone course clinical practicum, assessing competencies was not an issue.

Encouraging and supporting critical thinking is, however, a continuous challenge, and simulations serve as a fun yet challenging way to work to synthesize all that has been learned throughout the program as well as within the capstone course. Larew, Lessans, Spunt, Foster, and Covington (2006) suggest that groups of students be asked to develop scenarios as an experiential learning exercise. As a result a "Senior Simulation Day" was created as a substitution for a clinical day to meet the needs of this group of seniors, in which seniors were asked to create student-generated scenarios. Since the introduction of this scenario, other authors have expressed the value of having students teach each other during simulations (Dumas, Hollerbach, Stuart, & Duffy, 2015) and encouraging peer-led simulations as a "valuable educational approach" (Valler-Jones, 2014).

B. EDUCATIONAL MATERIALS AVAILABLE IN YOUR TEACHING AREA AND RELATED TO YOUR SPECIALTY

In 5 years, simulation facilities tripled in the nursing department. In the academic year 2002–2003, when the university held a centennial celebration, nursing graduates from 30 years ago returned and stated that the nursing labs had remained "much the same" as when they were students. Since then, the nursing department has worked tirelessly to upgrade and renovate the original nursing lab and expand the facilities to now include three nursing labs, with a fourth ICU lab. Each of these labs houses an HPS with a designated area and equipment for use with that HPS. In addition, we have found that a student resource center with textbooks, a seminar table, and references are essential for debriefing, processing, and redoing scenario plans. Students have access to online resources and drug references as well as the entire lab. Initially without the space or facilities for using a control room for simulations, the lab was upgraded to remote access for instructors who would like to run the scenarios remotely from the HPS. Often, these scenarios are run by only one instructor, and having a scenario control person is often not possible.

C. SPECIFIC OBJECTIVES OF SIMULATION USE WITHIN A SPECIFIC COURSE AND THE OVERALL PROGRAM

The objective of this simulation experience is to test senior nursing students' basic program outcome competencies and knowledge synthesis through creation of one simulated scenario of an advanced medical–surgical disease/condition, integrating the nursing process, communication skills, nursing skills, and critical thinking. Students then try to "stump" their classmates by testing the observing group's knowledge of the medical–surgical problem.

D. INTRODUCTION OF SCENARIO

Setting the Scene and Technology Used

Students are instructed to "mock up" a high-fidelity HPS to make the scenario as real as possible. They are given full access to the medical–surgical lab and are allowed to use any equipment they need from the lab supplies, including intravenous (IV) machines, IVs, and Foley catheters.

Objectives

Students will be able to identify a common medical–surgical problem from their recent clinical experiences and create a scenario that allows the following:

1. Portrays assessment factors and vital statistics common to that problem
2. Uses a chart and medication record with the appropriate drugs and dosages for that disease
3. Shows common psychosocial issues and concerns through communication with the patients, health care providers, and significant others
4. Requires interventions and evaluations appropriate to the standard of care for the medical–surgical problem being covered, which result, through the playing out of the scenario, in an improvement in the patient's condition

The National Council of State Boards of Nursing's (NCSB) National Council Licensure Examination for Registered Nurses (NCLEX-RN®) test plan categories and subcategories (NCSBN, 2015) addressed within this scenario include the following:

Safe and effective care environment category: *Management of care* (collaboration with interdisciplinary team, delegation, establishing priorities, ethical practice, informed consent, legal rights and responsibilities, and resource management), *Safety and infection control* (standard/transmission-based/other precautions/surgical asepsis and safe use of equipment); **Health promotion and maintenance:** *Techniques of physical assessment*; **Psychosocial integrity:** *Coping mechanisms, Therapeutic communication*; **Physiological integrity:** *Basic care and comfort* (elimination, nonpharmacological comfort interventions, personal hygiene, rest, and sleep), *Pharmacological and parenteral therapy* (dosage calculation, expected effects/outcomes, medication administration, parenteral/IV therapies, pharmacological agents/actions, pharmacological pain management), *Reduction of risk potential* (diagnostic tests, laboratory values, potential for complications of diagnostic tests/treatments/procedures, system-specific assessments, therapeutic procedures), *Physiological adaptation* (hemodynamics, illness management, medical emergencies)

Description of Participants

We encouraged all students in the group who created each scenario to become involved in the scenario. One student is the scenario controller and runs the computer as the scenario progresses. The HPS is the patient, and the other students may become the wife, doctor, nurse, or other participants at the discretion of the student creators.

E. RUNNING OF THE SCENARIO

Students are instructed to access the following simulation assignment from the course website 1 week before the simulation day.

NUR 375 Nursing Practicum

Senior Simulation Day
    This day is designed to refamiliarize you with the HPS SimMan. Many hospitals now test basic nursing competencies of new graduates in orientation with the SimMan. Today, we will be creating scenarios from your experience or your imagination. We will split the group in two, and one group will test the other on an advanced medical–surgical scenario.

Objective

To test senior nursing students on one advanced medical–surgical disease/condition, integrating the nursing process, communication skills, nursing skills, and critical thinking.

Instructions

Please access the NURSIM site.

1. Print out the Laerdal Scenario Planning Worksheet (Laerdal Medical, 2008a), first two pages only, and the Scenario Validation Sheet (Laerdal Medical, 2008b) and bring them to clinical on Simulation Day.
2. View the SimMan Introduction PowerPoint presentation about simulation and SimMan.
3. Feel free to browse other documents or links. If you want to know more about the computers hiding in SimMan and the setup, you can look at the SimMan/SimBaby PowerPoint presentation (we do not have SimBaby yet).

Assignment

- Design a medical–surgical scenario based on a real patient or a simulated patient to run for another group of students as if you are the instructor.
- You will need to mock up SimMan to look as "real" as possible. You can use any equipment in the White Hall Nursing Lab, for example, IVs, the IV machine, medication, carts, Foleys, and so on.
- You may decide to use other students as actors, for example, the distraught wife, the rude doctor, the inattentive nurse.
- Write out how the scenario will progress on the second page of the planning sheet. Include dialog, SimMan settings (respiratory rate [RR], pressure [P], blood pressure [BP], temperature [T], pulse oximeter, etc.), and equipment needed. Include all the knowledge you want to test on the crucial aspects of the disease/condition and medications. List all nursing assessments and interventions needed in order for the patient to improve.
- Just like a play, all scenarios have a beginning, middle, and end, so do not forget to plan for an ending (e.g., the patient with difficulty breathing is breathing better). But scenarios often take on a life of their own, so limit it to 15 minutes.
- Good luck and have fun.

Before arriving for the simulation day, students should download and print the scenario template and evaluation criteria. Students are also instructed to brainstorm on their own about comprehensive scenarios that test in-depth knowledge about common problems they encountered in the capstone clinical. Students are instructed to produce a chart, medication sheet, and history for their simulated patient, keeping in mind that they will need to construct the scenario much like they would write a play. On Senior Simulation Day, faculty introduce each group to the simulation technology from the instructor's side. Faculty demonstrate simulation technology and the features of the HPS to the student groups. Students are expected to run the scenario in its entirety themselves. Faculty support is available, although independence of the group is encouraged.

F. PRESENTATION OF COMPLETED TEMPLATE

A total of 37 students in five clinical groups were given this assignment. The capstone course coordinator, who is the resident expert on simulation, attended all simulation events along with the clinical instructors. A total of six scenarios were created by the students. Three are presented here. In the end, only four clinical groups participated due to timing issues and scheduling (maternity leave, family emergencies, and illness). Those not participating were given an alternate assignment.

SAMPLE STUDENT-GENERATED SENIOR SCENARIOS 1 TO 3

Scenario 1

Title

Joe Money

Scenario Level

Senior scenario

Focus Area

Nursing 375 nursing practicum

Scenario Description

Joe Money is a 59-year-old man found on the scene unresponsive with a BP of 180/90 mmHg, weak thready pulses, no reflexes, flaccid extremities, fixed pinpoint pupils, and a history of drug and alcohol (ETOH) abuse. Transported to the emergency room, where his BP is now 230/108 mmHg, with severe respiratory depression progressing to apnea. Patient may also have a head trauma and increased intracranial pressure. When his clothes are removed, $800, a switchblade, and a syringe are found in his jean pockets.

Scenario Objectives

1. Demonstrates proper assessment for drug overdose and trauma with appropriate interventions, including assessment of airway, breathing, and circulation (ABCs).
2. Performs assessment and interventions for increased intracranial pressure.
3. Staff uses proper safety precautions for potential drug-abuse patients.

Setting the Scene

Equipment Needed

HPS, patient monitor, O$_2$ hookup, pulse oximeter, BP cuff, stethoscope, paper chart for documentation, syringe, money, fake switchblade, two large-bore IVs, IV machine, Foley catheter, several vials of mock IV push drugs, and IV access syringes

Resources Needed

Textbooks, drug books, and computer access

Simulator Level

High-fidelity

Participant Roles

Student to run the computer for the HPS.
> *Scene 1:* Student to play a drug user and a student to play Joe Money, two students to play emergency medical technicians (EMTs) who transport the patient.
> *Scene 2:* HPS plays Joe Money and two students play emergency room nurses.

Scenario Implementation

Initial scene takes place in an apartment as Joe Money sells drugs to a customer and then sits down to drink alcohol and smoke crack cocaine. Joe Money passes out, and emergency medical technicians (EMTs) are called.

Scenario resumes in the emergency department (ED), where the patient is now played by the HPS. Two emergency room nurses are assessing the patient and reporting the results to the observing students, who are making suggestions and recommendations for care. Students use the nursing process as a guiding framework for moving through the scenario.

Initial Settings for HPS

BP: 180/90 mmHg at the scene then 230/108 mmHg in the ED. Variable bradycardia with irregular beat, shallow and slow respirations of 5 to 10 progressing to Cheyne–Stokes and then apnea.

Electrocardiogram (EKG) shows a bundle branch block typical of cocaine abuse. ED nurse (played by student) reports weak thready pulse; toxicology screen positive for cocaine and high blood alcohols levels; blood gasses of P_{CO_2}: 32, pH: 7.54, O_2: 47, Na: 147, and glucose: 181. Results of CT scan show multiple bilateral deep and superficial cerebral hematomas.

Required Student Assessments and Actions

___Identify symptoms of respiratory depression and cardiac abnormality
___Initiate two large-bore IVs
___Suggest C-spine (cervical spine) x-ray, CT scan, and arterial blood gases (ABGs) based on assessment findings and history
___Raise head of the bed secondary to increasing intracranial pressure
___Assess blood tests, toxicology screen, and urinalysis
___Insert Foley and assess drainage of 3,000 mL over 1 hour as a sign of diabetes insipidus/increasing intracranial pressure
___Obtain EKG and recognize bundle branch block as a sign of cocaine abuse
___Administer medications prescribed. Check dosages and five rights
___Assess results of x-rays and ABGs and recommend actions
___Suggest airlift transport to a level 1 trauma hospital once stabilized

Evaluation Criteria

___Students who have created the scenario use the nursing process to cue the observing students to make recommendations about patient care. Cues are adequate for recognition by the observing students.
___Students observing were able to recognize signs and symptoms as drug and alcohol overdose and proceed with appropriate interventions and safety precautions.
___Students observing were able to recognize the signs and symptoms of possible trauma and follow diagnostic protocol to assess and begin interventions for trauma and increasing intracranial pressure.
___Students observing were able to connect the cardiac arrhythmia with the patient's drug abuse.
___Students observing were able to accurately assess abnormal blood gases and suggest treatment.
___Students observing were able to suggest correct medication and dosages to treat patient's condition.
___Patient stabilizes enough for transport, but students watch for signs of impending herniation and possible negative outcome.

Scenario 2

Title

Addison Jane

Scenario Level

Senior scenario

Focus Area

Nursing 375 nursing practicum

Scenario Description

Addison Jane is a 62-year-old White female with a history of hypertension and hyperlipidemia who was found by a bystander in her driveway near gardening tools, clutching her chest and appearing pale. In addition, she has blood on her right earlobe. Patient weighs 165 pounds and is allergic to aspirin and penicillin. Her medications are unknown. Pregnant daughter is called and is nearby in the ED.

Scenario Objectives

1. Uses initial assessment/focused history when evaluating patient
2. Prioritizes and initiates emergency patient care with stabilization of the cervical spine
3. Performs automated external defibrillation
4. Understands how to clear patient during the delivery of shocks in defibrillation
5. Demonstrates assessment of patient's response to resuscitation
6. Properly documents events during the emergency care

Setting the Scene

Equipment Needed

HPS, patient monitor, O₂ hookup, bandages, pulse oximeter, BP cuff, stethoscope, and paper chart

Resources Needed

Textbooks and computer access for database search and evidence-based practice

Simulator Level

High-fidelity

Participant Roles

Two nurses, doctor who yells incorrect orders, pregnant family member whose water breaks in the middle of the code, and a student to run the computer for the HPS

Scenario Implementation

Initial settings for the HPS

HR: 62 beats/minute, BP: 106/72 mmHg, RR: 12 breaths/minute, pulse oximeter: 94%

Required Student Assessments and Actions

___Performs initial assessment and cervical spine immobilization
___Performs EKG and recognizes deterioration to ventricular fibrillation with no BP and HR of less than 140 beats/minute
___Correctly performs cardiopulmonary resuscitation (CPR) with the use of a bag-valve mask
___Applies automated electronic defibrillator (AED)
___Administers three shocks at the correct setting, despite physician giving incorrect orders
___Performs CPR
___Establishes IV access
___Gives medications as appropriate: Epinephrine q (every) 3 to 5 minutes; atropine q 3 to 5 minutes
___Patient response to interventions: Return to bradycardic sinus rhythm with vital signs (VS) of BP: 85/52 mmHg, P (pulse): 34 beats/minute, O₂ 88%, with weak thready pulse and normal heart sounds
___Interventions continue with remedication of atropine and the addition of amiodarone with improvement of VS to BP: 104/68 mmHg, P: 65 beats/minute, and O₂: 94%
___Once stabilized, patient is recommended to be sent for head and neck evaluation and MRI

Evaluation Criteria

___Correct interventions result in the stabilization of the patient.

___Students who have created the scenario use the nursing process to cue the observing students to make recommendations about patient care. Cues are adequate for recognition by the observing students.

___Students observing are able to recognize signs and symptoms of possible trauma and severe hypovolemia.

___Students observing are able to follow proper protocol in directing the sequence of CPR.

___Students take proper safety precautions.

Scenario 3

Title

Dolly

Scenario Level

Senior scenario

Focus Area

Nursing 375 nursing practicum

Scenario Description

Dolly is a 45-year-old woman admitted with a methicillin-resistant *Staphylococcus aureus* (MRSA) infection of a wound. Her temperature at home was 102°F, with complaints of overall achiness, loss of appetite, and diaphoresis. She has a past medical history of type II diabetes, hypertension, increased cholesterol blood levels, and depression. Wound is currently a stage 3 in the lumbar sacral area. She weighs 325 pounds and is 5 feet, 4 inches tall.

Scenario Objectives

1. Students will be able to state some orders a doctor would write for the signs and symptoms observed.
2. Students will be able to state five continuous orders for a patients with a suspected pulmonary embolism (PE).
3. Students will be able to state five discharge orders for someone recovering from a PE.

Setting the Scene

Equipment Needed

HPS, patient monitor, O_2 hookup, bandages, pulse oximeter, BP cuff, stethoscope, paper chart, thermometer, nasal cannula (NC), IV machine, and IV bag with vancomycin and IV bag with heparin and secondary line, primary line

Resources Needed

Textbooks and computer access for database search and evidence-based practice

Simulator Level

High-fidelity

Participant Roles

Uninterested RN, patient technician, and medical doctor (MD)

Scenario Implementation

Initial settings for HPS BP: 130/70 mmHg, P: 72 beats/minute, RR: 12 breaths/minute, temperature(T): 102°F

Day 1 in the emergency room

Dolly is complaining of decreased appetite and not feeling well. She is found to have a fever of 102°F and a stage 3 lumbar sacral ulcer. After culture, the wound is found to be infected with MRSA. Patient is admitted to the floor with an IV infusion of vancomycin.

Day 3 on the patient floor

8 a.m.: White blood count (WBC) 541 cells/mm^3, no complaint of (c/o) of pain, BP: 130/72 mmHg, P: 85 beats/minute, T: 99.2°F, O$_2$: 98% on room air (RA). Patient refuses to get out of bed since admission. Only uses bedpan.

12 p.m.: Patient care technician comes in for VS and reports them to the RN: BP: 130/79 mmHg, RR: 26 breaths/minute, P: 120 beats/minute, T: 100.2°F, O$_2$ 94% on RA. Patient states, "My chest hurts, and I can't breathe." RN seems uninterested in patient and says she is going on break and will check on patient after her break. Tells patient care technician to keep an eye on the patient.

13 p.m.: RN finally gets around to assessing patient and finds wheezing, 7/10 substernal chest pain on a 0-to-10 scale. Nonproductive cough and increased anxiety. O$_2$ has dropped to 86%, and pulse is 130. RN puts oxygen on patient 2 L NC, and O$_2$ comes up to 90%.

RN proceeds to call MD, who orders EKG, cardiac enzymes, chest x-ray (CXR), and 1 mg morphine IV.

14 p.m.: Results

EKG: Sinus tachycardia

Cardiac enzymes: Negative

CXR: Infiltrates, elevated diaphragm on right side. Doctor suspects PE and orders baseline coagulation studies: prothrombin time (PT), partial thromboplastin tine (PTT), and international normalized ration (INR); spiral CT to verify PE; heparin bolus 10,000 U and maintenance 1,600 U per hour.

15 p.m.: VS as follows: BP: 120/70 mmHg; RR: 20 breaths/minute, P: 100 beats/minute, T: 99.0°F; O$_2$, 97% on 2 L NC; pain level 5/10 on a 0-to-10 scale and given 1 mg morphine IV

MD continuous orders: High Fowler, incentive spirometer every 2 hours, out of bed as soon as possible with the assistance of physical therapy; Thromboguards, monitor blood values especially PT, INR

Day 7: discharge:

MD discharge instructions: Decrease weight, take Coumadin as prescribed, Thromboembolic-deterrent (TED) stockings, initiate visiting nurses, active range of motion exercise to all extremities, get out of bed as much as tolerated, do not dangle or cross legs

Required Student Assessments and Actions

___Students in scenario assess and intervene in the emergency room based on the recommendations of observing students

___Assess VS, wound, and do a focused assessment/history of patient

___Obtain IV access and begin antibiotic therapy
___Transfer to floor with orders
___Assessment of VS on day 3 by RN
___Evaluation of assessment data by RN and interventions at the bedside by administering O_2
___Use of situation, background, assessment, recommendation (SBAR) format in communication with the MD
___Order and obtain required blood and diagnostic tests
___Evaluate blood tests and communicate with the MD
___Set up and administer heparin as ordered
___Interact appropriately with the patient to explain new orders
___Delegate appropriate interventions to patient care technician. Communicate clearly
___Discuss discharge follow-up with patient

Evaluation Criteria

___Students who have created the scenario use the nursing process to cue the observing students to make recommendations about patient care. Cues are adequate for recognition by the observing students. Students observing were able to recognize signs and symptoms as wound infection and PE.
___Students observing were able to recommend scenario students follow diagnostic protocol to assess and begin interventions for wound infection and PE.
___Students observing were able to connect the immobility related to a wound infection with the consequence of PE. Students observing were able to accurately assess abnormal lab test and diagnostic test and suggest treatment.
___Students observing were able to suggest correct medication and dosages to treat patient's condition.
___Patient stabilizes for discharge, and students recommend proper home care follow-up.
___Students observing and participating recognize communication issues and discuss how effective communication and teamwork would improve outcomes in this scenario.

G. DEBRIEFING GUIDELINES

Instructors worked with the student scenario creators to create objectives and outcomes for each scenario. General questions reviewed in the debriefing were as follows:

1. What disease process was being portrayed in the scenario?
2. What were the key assessment factors and VS parameters important in the scenario?
3. Did the scenario follow the known standard of care for the medical–surgical problem?
4. Was there anything new that you learned as a result of the scenario?
5. What were the crucial nursing interventions and evaluation points necessary for the patient's condition to improve?
6. Was the scenario realistic and engaging?

H. SUGGESTIONS/KEY FEATURES TO REPLICATE OR IMPROVE

These student-generated scenarios are an excellent synthesis exercise in which students are required to access all knowledge and skills learned in order to evaluate their peers with regard to their knowledge and skills. Posting the assignment gave students time to review and ask questions of their individual instructors. In addition, the use of, and access to the entire lab and all equipment was important to promote the "realness" of the simulation. Students were encouraged to be as creative as possible throughout the scenario generation, which seemed to be a very enjoyable part of the exercise. Students showed enthusiasm for all roles, including running the computer program, which we believed might have been a hindrance. The students demonstrated how quickly they are able to learn and adapt to new technology as active participants in a nonthreatening and collaborative setting.

I. RECOMMENDATIONS FOR FURTHER USE

Student-generated scenarios should be used as a creative and exciting alternative to testing. We have all found that even in the best faculty-developed scenarios, students have ideas and suggestions that change the running of scenarios written by instructors. This format, although not appropriate at the lower levels, allows students to show what they know in who were safe, supportive environment while testing knowledge, skills, and critical thinking of the graduating senior. The instructor role became one of support, encouragement, and resource person. At least one instructor was recruited into the scenario to play a role. Instructors commented they were "amazed" at how well the students did and how comprehensive the student-generated scenarios were.

J. HOW SIMULATION-BASED PEDAGOGY HAS CONTRIBUTED TO IMPROVED STUDENT OUTCOMES

Simulation-based pedagogy has contributed to improved student outcomes in two significant ways: improved demonstration of critical thinking abilities and knowledge-based application of principles of safety, communication, and team collaboration.

In student-generated scenarios, each group of students found that there was a need to outline the case being presented from a critical thinking perspective. Each scenario needed to be complete and accurate, but also able to anticipate the critical thinking of the other students through cueing the students observing to help them move along in the scenario. Once all the pertinent facts of the case were checked and verified, the chart was set up and the students had to ask, "Will they recognize this as abnormal and know what to do?" Using their own knowledge and checking references available, the students then were able to piece together the scenario using the nursing process as a template for how the other students would process information and come to conclusions. Senior students found that the use of the nursing process facilitated the learning of the other students during the scenario and in debriefing.

Safety, communication, and team collaboration were essential in the successful development and implementation of the scenario. Safety issues were addressed repeatedly without guidance of the instructors and in fact were often used as a part of the scenario in need of recognition and correction during the scenarios. Communication among nurses, patients, families, and other health care providers was also an essential element of each scenario. Effective communication resulted in improved patient outcomes during the simulations. Teamwork and collaboration with members of the health care team were emphasized in each simulation. As the simulations evolved, the observing students made recommendations, and each team member worked together to carry out nursing interventions. Included as part of the team were family members who were used to clarify and explain the circumstances surrounding the scenario.

Students commented that this type of scenario made them realize how much more they knew than previously thought. Most students commented how much more confident they felt in their abilities after doing these simulations. In addition, students suggested that more simulation within the curriculum would be beneficial at all levels of the program.

In summary, we thought student-generated scenarios contributed not only to increased application of critical thinking, safety, communication, and teamwork, but also to increased levels of confidence of graduating seniors. In this way, student-generated scenarios, as an endpoint learning exercise for graduating seniors, affirm the use of simulation-based pedagogy not only as a test of competency, but also as a demonstration of the skill and knowledge level required at the end of an undergraduate nursing program.

K. EXPERT RECOMMENDATIONS AND WORDS OF WISDOM

Many years have passed since the inception of this scenario. Both authors have moved on from actively creating and implementing scenarios for nursing students to overseeing nursing programs as administrators. Both continue to be champions of simulation-based pedagogy as an essential tool in maintaining the highest standards of quality delivery of nursing education at all levels. Although not implemented as written in some time, we believe this scenario has stood the test of time and is still as relevant as when it was written. In the beginning, when this book was originally written, there was not a plethora of well-designed simulations. There was one reference on "how to do" simulation; we were novices filled with passion and drive common among our peers—to do the best thing to help nursing students succeed. What was uncommon at the time was this newfangled "high-fidelity simulation" and educators who believed this new educational tool could revolutionize nursing education and improve educational outcomes. This revolution has become an evolution of practice and thought in which simulation-based pedagogy, instead of being a add-on, has become fully integrated throughout the nursing curriculum. It is not something we should do, simulation-based pedagogy is what we all do and is now common in nursing education.

Our recommendations and words of wisdom are to follow your passion even if those around you are unsure of your ideas. Simply said, in doing the right thing as a nursing educator, innovative and yes, new-fangled ideas may propel you and your colleagues into innovative change.

L. EVALUATION OF BEST PRACTICE STANDARDS AND USE OF CREDENTIALED SIMULATION FACULTY

At the time of the writing of this scenario, no standards existed. In comparing this scenario with the The International Nursing Association for Clinical and Simulation Learning (INACSL, 2013/2016) standards, it appears even at this early stage of development, we were using the same framework of best practice although it was in its infancy. In reviewing the standards, each of the standards appear in some form throughout the scenarios proposed in this chapter.

At the time of the writing of this scenario, there were no credentialed simulation faculty and no process for gaining certification or obtaining a credential; just two enthusiastic faculty who believed these scenarios would make a difference. We continue to assert that senior nursing students are capable of constructing peer-to-peer scenarios to test program outcomes as a summative teaching and learning experience.

REFERENCES

Dumas, B. P., Hollerbach, A. D., Stuart, G. W., & Duffy, N. D. (2015). Expanding simulation capacity: Senior-level students as teachers. *Journal of Nursing Education, 54*(9), 516–519.

International Nursing Association for Clinical Simulation and Learning. (2013, updated 2016). INACSL standards of best practice: Simulation. Retrieved from https://www.inacsl.org/i4a/pages/index.cfm?pageID=3407

Laerdal Medical. (2008a). Scenario planning worksheet. Retrieved from http://simulation.laerdal.com/forum/files/folders/checklists worksheets/entry8.aspx

Laerdal Medical. (2008b). Scenario validation checklist. Retrieved from http://simulation.laerdal.com/forum/files/folders/checklists worksheets/entry9.aspx

Larew, C., Lessans, S., Spunt, D., Foster, D., & Covington, B. G. (2006). Innovations in clinical simulation: Application of Benner's theory in an interactive patient care simulation. *Nursing Education Perspectives, 27*(1), 16–21.

National Council of State Boards of Nursing. (2015). NCLEX-RN examination: Test plan for the National Council Licensure Examination for Registered Nurses. Retrieved from https://www.ncsbn.org/RN_Test_Plan_2016_Final.pdf

Valler-Jones, T. (2014). The impact of peer-led simulations on student nurses. *British Journal of Nursing, 23*(6), 321–326.

CHAPTER 45

Assessing for Elder Abuse: The Importance of Interprofessional Collaboration

Lee-Anne Stephen, Dawna Williams, and Pamela Causton

A. IMPLEMENTATION OF SIMULATION-BASED PEDAGOGY IN YOUR INDIVIDUALIZED TEACHING AREA

The influence of interprofessional collaboration on patient outcomes is well supported by the literature. As a result, interprofessional education (IPE) is becoming a key focus in nursing education. Providing interprofessional content to a student aids in the development of teamwork, collaboration, and cooperation skills (Zhang, Thompson, & Miller, 2011). IPE improves health outcomes for patients and strengthens health care systems (World Health Organization, 2010).

Interprofessional simulation (IPS), through experiential learning, can aid in the development of knowledge and skill required for collaborative practice (Murdoch, Bottorff, & McCullough, 2013). IPS can also have a positive influence on students' attitudes and perceptions of their own and others' unique contribution to the health care team (Murdoch et al., 2013). Thus, IPS scenarios are an excellent way to support the development of interprofessional collaboration, role clarification, and leadership skills of health care students.

A needs assessment should be completed before the development of a simulation scenario (Lioce et al., 2015). When creating this scenario, the authors reviewed current trends in nursing education, feedback from clinical partners, and our health studies programs' curricula.

B. EDUCATIONAL MATERIALS AVAILABLE IN YOUR TEACHING AREA AND RELATED TO YOUR SPECIALTY

The educational materials available at the University of the Fraser Valley (UFV) are discussed in Chapter 23.

C. SPECIFIC OBJECTIVES FOR SIMULATION USAGE WITHIN A SPECIFIC COURSE AND THE OVERALL PROGRAM

Learning Objectives

The scenario was designed to help students recognize scopes of practice and develop interprofessional skills. These skills include communication, collaboration, and shared leadership. Through interprofessional collaboration and communication, the team (bachelor of science in nursing [BSN], practical nursing [PN], and health care assistant [HCA] students) should determine that their patient has experienced elder abuse. Each student is required to complete an assessment and identify a unique piece of information about the patient. If students share this information with their team members, the outcome will be the successful identification of elder abuse. If collaboration among the students does not occur, this may be missed. The level of student for each program will depend on when elder abuse and interprofessional practice is taught. It is our suggestion that the scenario is most applicable at the latter end of their training.

Student Learning Activities

Review patient scenario, including social history, medical history (past/current).
Review principles of teamwork and collaboration.
Review scope of practice for disciplines involved in the simulation experience.
Review gerontology theory, including dementia/delirium and pharmacology.

The key elements in the scenario that relate to the National Council of State Boards of Nursing (NCSBN; 2015)—National Council Licensure Examination for Registered Nurses (NCLEX-RN®) test plan include:

Safe and effective care environment: *Management of care* (assignment, delegation and supervision, collaboration with interdisciplinary team, referrals); **Health promotion and maintenance:** (aging process); **Psychosocial integrity:** (abuse/neglect, family dynamics, therapeutic communication); **Physiological integrity:** *Pharmacological and parenteral therapies* (pharmacological pain management)

The College of Registered Nurses of British Columbia (CRNBC; 2015) entry-level RN practice competencies that this scenario supports include:

Standard I: Professional responsibility and accountability
Self-regulation competencies 1, 2, and 6
Standard II: Knowledge-based practice
Specialized body of knowledge competency 27
Ongoing comprehensive assessment competencies 39 and 42
Health care planning competency 55
Standard III: Client-focused provision of service
Client-focused provision of service competencies 83 and 84

D. INTRODUCTION OF SCENARIO

Setting the Scene

This scenario is set in a private room on a subacute hospital unit. The patient should be on a stretcher alone in the room.

Technology Used

The HPS used in this scenario could be a Sim Essential or Nursing Anne and should look like an elderly male. Ideally, there will be live-feed software so that students can observe the scenario in a debriefing room.

Objectives

1. Demonstrate an understanding of own scope of practice within the health care setting.
2. Recognize and respect diversity of another health care provider's scope of practice.
3. Demonstrate effective communication with members of a professional health care team.

4. Collaborate with members of the health care team to provide safe patient care.
5. Act on leadership opportunities within one's own scope of practice.

Description of Participants

Mr. Morgan, a widowed, 81-year-old male, was brought into the emergency room (ER) by his son and daughter-in-law because of increased confusion over the last few days. His son states that Mr. Morgan fell and hit his head 5 days ago. Since that time he has been confused and agitated, the family is not able to cope in the home setting, and they are requesting admission. The son gave a brief health history and then left without providing further contact information or notifying the nursing staff.

E. RUNNING OF THE SCENARIO

Students are required to have read the patient history and completed all preassigned activities prior to coming to the simulated setting.

During prebriefing, it is the faculty member's responsibility to ensure that the students feel psychologically safe. This is significant because this could be the first time that these students have worked together and there could be power dynamics at play among the students. The prebriefing should also include a review of the student confidentiality agreement, realism challenges of the simulated environment, participant roles, student expectations, and the simulation suite. The students will be reminded that the focus of this simulation is communication, collaboration, and leadership; they are informed that they can call a time-out when they have information to share with the other team members; and they will have time to discuss roles, plan patient care, and ask questions.

Questions the facilitator could ask during prebriefing might include: Do you know what your scope of practice is in this situation? What is the role of the BSN, PN, and HCA in the clinical setting? What are the similarities among these roles? Who are your resources in relationship to your scope of practice? What are leadership characteristics for bedside health care providers? Once roles have been assigned, students enter the room at predetermined intervals to allow time for the development of therapeutic relationships and the completion of assessments/care as outlined in the scenario objectives. The scenario ends when a student recognizes that the patient has experienced elder abuse and verbalizes the need to intervene. Students do not necessarily need to provide interventions based on physical assessment findings but should identify verbal statements of neglect and assess physical findings of abuse and neglect.

Small student groups are important when implementing this scenario so that students feel comfortable sharing their thoughts within the group. Each discipline should be represented as it would be clinically. The observers will have a worksheet that focuses on collaboration and communication. The timeframe should be 30 minutes for briefing, 20 minutes for hands-on-care, and a 1 to 1.5 hour debriefing.

F. PRESENTATION OF A COMPLETED TEMPLATE

Title

Enhancing Interprofessional Collaboration

Scenario Level

Students enrolled in the later phase of the nursing program

Focus Area

Interprofessional collaboration and geriatric assessment

Scenario Description

Shift Report

Mr. Morgan was admitted to the subacute unit for overnight observation. An HCA was assigned 1:1 for patient safety. The patient slept well and was orientated × 3 throughout the night. Assessment and diagnostic findings were all normal. He woke up at 6 a.m. and was hungry, so breakfast was ordered and his morning medications given. He has been complaining of pain to his right side on movement.

Patient History

Patient information: Samuel Morgan; date of birth (DOB) April 8, 1936; Allergies—sulfa (hives)

Social background: Married to Beatrice for 33 years/widowed for 2 years. Born in England, immigrated with his parents to Canada as a young boy. Lives with his son and daughter-in-law and two twin grandsons since his transient ischemic attack (TIA). Retired site supervisor for the Department of Highways. Religion: Roman Catholic. Languages: English, French, and Italian.

Medical history: TIA 1 year ago cholecystectomy in 1992; fractured rt. radius 8 months ago. Smoked for 40 years. Peripheral vascular disease (PVD), hypertension, non-insulin-dependent diabetes.

Health Assessment Results

Labs: All normal—urinalysis, complete blood count (CBC), electroytes, glucose

X-ray: Evidence of old fracture, but no current breaks

Vitals: Weight 85 kg (187 pounds); height: 5 feet, 11 inches, blood pressure (BP): 159/78 mmHg, heart rate (HR): 72 beats/minute and regular, respiratory rate (RR): 18 breaths/minute, O_2 saturation 95%.

Medication Record: (See Exhibit 45.1)

Scenario Objectives

The HCA student enters the room and has the first 5 minutes of the simulation scenario to develop a therapeutic relationship with the patient and keep the patient safe. The PN student and BSN student review their plan of care outside the patient room.

The BSN student then enters the room and introduces self to Mr. Morgan. This student then leaves the room and enters the medication preparation area/zone of silence in the simulation suite. The zone of silence is a simulated space where team members can communicate freely. In this space, the BSN student will look through Mr. Morgan's chart.

The PN student then enters the room and performs an assessment. If the BP cuff is removed the student should find a hand-shaped bruise under cuff and various old and new bruises on Mr. Morgan's body. The focus will most likely be on the patient's pain as he is complaining of excruciating pain to the arm the BP cuff is not attached to (the site of the old fracture). The PN student then goes into the medication room/zone of silence to look up pain medications that Mr. Morgan can receive.

Exhibit 45.1	Medication Record—Metoprolol

Metoprolol, 10 mg PO

Glyburide, 10 mg BID

Hydromorphone, 0.25–0.5 mg IV q 4 h PRN

Metformin, 200 mg BID

Tylenol, 1,000 mg QID

Ketorolac, 15–30 mg IV q 8 h PRN

BID, twice a day; IV, intravenous; OD, once a day; PRN, as needed; QID, four times a day.

When information is being transferred between the team members in the zone of silence, the other team member should stay in role, and sit quietly at the bedside.

Setting the Scene

Equipment needed

Stethoscope, thermometer, O$_2$ sat monitor, BP cuff,

human patient simulator, name band, allergy band, hospital gown, saline lock, dressing on left arm, bedside table, sputum cup, denture cup, urinal, tissues, food tray,

medication administration record (MAR). On the MAR morning medications have been signed for; variety of pain medication options; old chart; current chart; lab and x-ray results; alcohol swabs; sharps container.

physician orders indicating diabetic diet, activity as tolerated (AAT), routine vitals, blood sugars assessed four times a day (QID), maintain saline lock

Participant Roles

Patient: The most important aspect of the patient role is to provide the verbal cues/set the stage regarding the abuses he has experienced. He should divulge more to the least educated of the team to empower this member and enhance communication/collaboration among all team members. He is alert and oriented. Through the course of the simulation, the patient will disclose that living with his son is a benefit to his son as he helps pay the rent and bills at his son's house. He states that he is sometimes in the way of the busy family, and is often left alone. His adaptive equipment (glasses, dentures, hearing aids) are worn and malfunctioning. He will complain of pain when the BP cuff is inflated over the hand-print bruise as well as severe pain to his alternate wrist/arm.

When discussing possible analgesia options with the care team, the patient should disclose that his daughter-in-law sometimes gives him medication during the afternoon to help him sleep if she is going out.

His son seems angry all the time and his daughter-in-law is often short with him. With the appropriate questioning, the patient will divulge that sometimes he is hit or pushed by his son, but he will provide the excuse that this son has a very stressful job and does not mean anything by it.

BSN student: You are the assigned team leader and will be participating in a supportive leadership role. After the report is provided for the team, allow the HCA student 5 minutes with Mr. Morgan. Knock on the door, go in and introduce yourself as the student nurse and team leader. Let Mr. Morgan know that you will be checking in on him throughout the shift. Proceed into the medication room/zone of silence and review the medical history and health assessment. Be mindful that this is the PN student's assigned patient and he or she is responsible for this patient. Both the HCA and PN student roles will defer to you for direction for anything beyond their scope of practice.

PN student: Mr. Morgan is your *assigned* patient for the shift. He has an HCA student assigned to him 1:1. You are responsible for the assessment, direction, and evaluation of care for Mr. Morgan throughout the simulation exercise. Communicate any significant findings with your team leader and work within your scope of practice.

HCA student: You have been assigned to Mr. Morgan 1:1 to observe and care for him today. After receiving the report, go into the room and introduce yourself to Mr. Morgan. Engage him in a conversation and try to make him feel comfortable. Talk to him about his home life and family for 5 minutes. Your goal is to ensure patient safety and establish a therapeutic relationship. The PN student is the primary nurse and will be responsible for this patient. You should report any assessment or significant findings to the PN student. When the BSN and PN students are collaborating in the medication room, sit quietly at the bedside.

Scenario Implementation

Initial Settings for the HPS/Equipment

The patient should have old and new bruises on his legs, a hand impression on the arm where the BP cuff will be applied, an abrasion on the side of his right eye (one steri-strip in place, slightly bruised eye),

Mepore on his right lower forearm, saline lock in situ, and a wristband and allergy band. Vital signs: BP: 159/78 mmHg, HR: 72 beats/minute and regular, RR: 18 breaths/minute, and O_2 saturation 95%.

Expected/Required Student Assessments and Actions

HCA: Wash hands upon entering the room. Introduce self and explain role to Mr. Morgan. Assess room. Communicate with Mr. Morgan about his family and home environment. Recognize cues of elder abuse when communicating with Mr. Morgan. Communicate assessment findings with PN student. Collaborate as part of the health care team.

BSN: Wash hands on entering the room. Introduce self and explain role to Mr. Morgan. Administer medications if PN student needs assistance. Recognize signs and symptoms of abuse from the chart and when conversing with the patient. Collaborate with team members regarding assessment findings and nursing care.

PN: Wash hands on entering the room. Introduce self and explain role to Mr. Morgan. Complete a comprehensive physical assessment—including pain. Recognize signs and symptoms of elder abuse. Collaborate with team members regarding assessment findings and nursing care.

Instructor Interventions

The instructor supplies the patient voice to cue students to abuse unless a standardized patient is used.

Facilitate briefing and debriefing.

Evaluation Criteria

Use the list in the section titled expected/required student assessment and actions to develop a checklist for evaluation of student actions during the hands-on-care portion of the simulation experience. Students should complete an evaluation of the simulation experience, so that they can identify areas of strength and improvement for clinical practice. A reflective evaluation of facilitation skills should be completed by the facilitator.

G. DEBRIEFING GUIDELINES

Issues to Consider

Debriefing should focus on the following concepts: leadership, collaboration, scope of practice (roles and responsibilities), communication, and diversity. In addition during debriefing, ensure that students understand their own and others' roles and responsibilities as well as shared scope of practice in relation to the provision of safe patient care in the hospital setting.

Student Questions

Reaction

1. What successes did the team achieve?
2. What challenges did the team experience?

Analysis

1. Provide examples of informal leadership characteristics that you saw portrayed by your BSN, PN, and HCA peers.
2. Describe shared roles/overlapping roles.
3. Discuss the diversity of the roles of the health care team and how they influence patient safety.
4. Describe differences in roles when you needed to ask for assistance/support from a member of the team.
5. Describe the collaboration that was evident. What were its strengths and what did you feel could have been done differently?
6. Identify the communication strategies that you noticed. What were the strengths and what did you feel could have been done differently?
7. How did the collaboration among team members contribute to safe patient outcomes?

Summary

1. Have you ever witnessed or participated in an interprofessional event in the clinical setting?
2. How will this simulated learning event assist you when interacting with different professionals in the clinical setting?

H. SUGGESTIONS/KEY FEATURES TO REPLICATE OR IMPROVE

This simulation scenario has been pilot tested. During the pilot test, we found that the interaction between Mr. Morgan and the team members was the key to effective student learning. Using an experienced faculty member as the voice of the patient enhances students' learning in this scenario.

I. RECOMMENDATIONS FOR FURTHER USE

This scenario could be expanded to include a variety of other health care professionals. For example, social work students, physiotherapy students, or medical students could be incorporated into this learning activity. The number of students actively involved in the scenario will dictate the length of the simulation experience. Incorporating an extended briefing with an interprofessional class would allow students to engage in icebreaking activities and increase the feeling of safety among the different team members.

Changing the ethnicity of the patient could add a cultural safety component to this simulation. This would encourage students to consider cultural aspects when caring for an individual.

J. HOW SIMULATION-BASED PEDAGOGY HAS CONTRIBUTED TO IMPROVED STUDENT OUTCOMES

The literature supports the use of simulation learning when providing IPE. This learning experience will increase students' awareness of one another's scope of practice, unique contributions to the health care team, ability to collaborate, and understanding of leadership.

K. EXPERT RECOMMENDATIONS AND WORDS OF WISDOM

Similarities among the different nursing roles should be a focus of this experience. Often, differences are highlighted and this can strengthen power dynamics in the clinical setting. If students focus on similarities and their unique roles in the health care setting, this may minimize some of the negative interactions that occur among the RN, LPN, and HCA in clinical settings.

Ensuring there is adequate time during briefing and debriefing is fundamental to the learning that will occur during this experience. Helping students unpack the importance of knowing and respecting one another's unique roles and knowledge base as well as the importance of communication and collaboration is essential. This may not always occur quickly. During debriefing, focus on how shared responsibility of patient care facilitated the discovery of elder abuse.

L. EVALUATION OF BEST PRACTICE STANDARDS AND USE OF CREDENTIALED SIMULATION FACULTY

As mentioned in Chapter 23, the UFV Health Studies Simulation committee has developed a simulation scenario template based on the International Nursing Association for Clinical Simulation and Learning (INACSL, 2013/2016) Simulation Standards of Best Practice, to help ensure consistency in simulation design. Simulation professional development is offered annually to all faculty in the School of Health Studies.

REFERENCES

College of Registered Nurses of British Columbia. (2015). *Competencies in the context of entry level registered nurse practice in British Columbia.* Vancouver, BC: Author.

International Nursing Association for Clinical Simulation and Learning. (2013, updated 2016). INACSL standards of best practice: Simulation. Retrieved from https://www.inacsl.org/i4a/pages/index.cfm?pageID=3407

Lioce, L., Meakim, C. H., Fey, M. K., Chmil, J. V., Mariani, B., & Alinier, G. (2015). Standards of best practice: Simulation standard IX: Simulation design. *Clinical Simulation in Nursing, 11*(6), 309–315. doi:10.1016/j.ecos.2015.03.005

Murdoch, N. L., Bottorff, J. L., & McCullough, D. (2013) Simulation education approaches to enhance collaborative healthcare: A best practices review. *International Journal of Nursing Education Scholarship, 10*(1), 307–321. doi:10.1515/ijnes-2013-0027

National Council of State Boards of Nursing. (2015). NCLEX-RN examination: Test plan for the National Council Licensure Examination for Registered Nurses. Retrieved from https://www.ncsbn.org/RN_Test_Plan_2016_final.pdf

World Health Organization. (2010). Framework for action on interprofessional education and collaborative care. Retrieved from http://apps.who.int/iris/bitstream/10665/70185/1/WHO_HRH_HPN_10.3_eng.pdf?ua=1

Zhang, C., Thompson, S., & Miller, C. (2011). A review of simulation-based interprofessional education. *Clinical Simulation in Nursing, 7*(4), e117–e126. doi:10.1016/j.ecns.2010.02.008

CHAPTER 46

Post-Concussion Syndrome

*Doris French, Andrew Booth, Michael J. Shoemaker, Jeanine Beasley,
Geraldine Jacobus Terry, Margaret Devoest, Samantha Scanlon, and Philip Van Lente*

A. IMPLEMENTATION OF SIMULATION-BASED
PEDAGOGY IN YOUR INDIVIDUALIZED TEACHING AREA

The Midwest Interprofessional Practice and Research Center (MIPERC) is a consortium of universities and health care institutions working together to support interprofessional practice and education. The center was developed out of the Office of the Vice Provost for Health at Grand Valley State University (GVSU) and is a multi institutional organization comprising more than 25 organizational and more than 150 individual members. Within MIPERC there are six champion workgroups that help to carry out its mission, which is to identify ways that the members can develop collaborative, innovative, and interprofessional initiatives across disciplines, learning institutions, and health care systems. Also residing within MIPERC is the student organization, Promoting Interprofessional Education for Students (PIPES). This group meets six times per academic year and is supported by the Simulation Champion workgroup. This workgroup consists of faculty members from several health disciplines lead by coleads Andrew Booth, DHEd, PA-C, and Michael J. Shoemaker, DPT, PhD. The rest of the workgroup is made up of Jeanine Beasley, EdD, OTR/L, CHT, FAOTA; Margaret de Voest, PharmD; Phil Van Lente, MD; Samantha Scanlon, BSN RN; Geraldine Jacobus Terry, MD, MSN, RN; and facilitator Doris French, MSN, RN, CNOR, NE-BC. The workgroup facilitates two interprofessional simulations per year that serve as a culminating event during which students can experience interacting with students from other health disciplines, to learn from, with, and about other the professions. The PIPES meetings and simulations also count as activities for an interprofessional certificate available through MIPERC.

B. EDUCATIONAL MATERIALS AVAILABLE IN
YOUR TEACHING AREA AND RELATED TO YOUR SPECIALTY

GVSU's Simulation Center consists of three areas. Two areas are adjacent to two large clinical skills labs, and one smaller simulation lab is located on the fourth floor. Each of the areas is equipped with cameras and microphones that are a part of a recording, streaming software package, Simulation iQ Enterprise, from Educational Management Solutions (EMS) in Exton, Pennsylvania.

One of the areas is a hospital suite, which is a large room with one ICU hospital room and four medical–surgical hospital rooms contained within it. This area also has a two-bed ward area and control room for both recording purposes and manikin operation. The hospital suite contains many high-fidelity, newborn and adult manikins. Medium- and low-fidelity manikins are available and used for appropriate skills development or scenarios. This area also comes equipped with functioning headwalls, beds, crash cart, medication dispensing unit, and other equipment needed to set the appropriate environment for the scenarios being done.

Adjacent to the hospital suite is the standardized patient suite, which has eight outpatient examination rooms located within it. These rooms are complete with patient assessment tables, functioning headwalls, and is stocked with various assessment supplies. This suite also contains space for training or small-group meetings.

A smaller simulation room is located on the fourth floor. This is a two-bed hospital room divided by curtains. It contains the same equipment located in the hospital suite, but has an attached conference or small classroom divided from the simulation area with a wall containing two one-way windows and a door. The classroom has projection capabilities as well as two computer workstations for controlling manikins.

The simulation center also has three debriefing rooms, one observation room with 16 computer stations, and a standardized patient reception area. Two of the debriefing rooms and the observation room are equipped with cameras and microphones, making them flexible space for simulated care conferences.

C. SPECIFIC OBJECTIVES FOR SIMULATION USAGE WITHIN A SPECIFIC COURSE AND THE OVERALL PROGRAM

Interprofessional simulation experiences provide students with the opportunity to interact directly with other health-discipline students to practice interprofessional collaboration so they can effectively be ready to practice teamwork and team-based care (Interprofessional Education Collaborative [IPEC], 2016). Objectives for interprofessional education [IPE] simulations include gaining competence in the following four areas (IPEC, 2016).

1. Values and ethics for interprofessional practice
2. Roles and responsibilities for collaborative practice
3. Interprofessional communication competencies
4. Interprofessional team and teamwork competencies

The IPE simulations are available to both undergraduate and graduate students from any university who wish to attend.

D. INTRODUCTION OF SCENARIO

Setting the Scene

This scene takes place in an interprofessional post-concussion clinic. Patients coming to this clinic are those patients who have been seen in an emergency department (ED) or physician office that were diagnosed with a concussion 1 to 2 weeks before follow-up neuro assessment. This is an office setting with examination tables, functional assessment equipment, including ophthalmoscope, otoscope, and sphygmomanometer.

Technology Used

Standardized patients (the same number as the number of groups)
Family members or confederates (the same number as the number of groups)
Examination tables

Otoscopes
Ophthalmoscopes
Sphygmomanometers
Stethoscope
Assessment tools, including reflex hammer, tongue depressors, paper clip
Foam squares for balance assessment
Post-Concussion Symptom Scale (2015)
Mini-Mental State Examination (Folstein, Folstein, & McHugh, 1975)
The Balance Error Scoring System (2011) https://theconcussionblog.files.wordpress.com/2011/02/bessprotocolnata09.pdf developed by researchers and clinicians at the University of North Carolina's Sports Medicine Research Laboratory, Chapel Hill, NC.
King–Devick Eye Tracking Test (Galetta et al., 2011)
Long Division Math Problem

Objectives

The learning objectives for the simulation were based on the following four IPEC competencies (IPEC, 2016):

RR1. Communicate one's roles and responsibilities clearly to patients, community members, and other professionals.
RR2. Recognize one's limitations in skills, knowledge, and abilities.
RR6. Communicate with team members to clarify each member's responsibility in executing components of a treatment plan or public health intervention.
RR9. Use unique and complementary abilities of all members of the team to optimize health and patient care.
CC2. Communicate information with patients, community members, and health care team members in a form that is understandable, avoiding discipline-specific terminology when possible.
CC3. Express one's knowledge and opinions to team members involved in patient care and population health improvements with confidence, clarity, and respect, working to ensure common understanding of information, treatment, care decisions, and population health programs and policies.
CC4. Listen actively, and encourage ideas and opinions of other team members.

Participants

Students: The students participating in this simulation were both undergraduate students and graduate students in health-related programs from GVSU's Kirkoff's College of Nursing both prelicensure and doctor of nursing professional (DNP) students, athletic training (AT) students, and students studying allied health sciences, physical therapy (PT), occupational therapy (OT), as well as physician assistant (PA) students.

Patients: Because PIPES is a voluntary, independent student group we did not know the number of students or the discipline well in advance of the event date. The RSVP deadline was 2 weeks before the simulation to allow us to determine group size and distribution of disciplines. We found we had a greater number of undergraduate nursing students sign up so we recruited from that group of students to play the patient roles.

Parent (either mother or father): Again because of the greater number of nursing students, we also recruited from that group of students to play the parent roles.

Care team: Each team had an undergraduate nurse, OT, PT, and an AT student. There were limited numbers of PA and nurse practitioner (NP) students. We distributed them among the teams, but some teams did not have an advanced practice provider.

Observers: We did not have any observers for this event as everyone participated.

Faculty: The PT, OT, nursing, medical, and PA faculty provided input for training the nursing students portraying patients. A training video was made of the training by the PT faculty member, and sent as to all of the student actors 1 week before the simulation event. The simulation workgroup as a whole provided input as to how the parent role needed to be portrayed and trained the family members 30 minutes before the event. The nursing faculty member briefed the students participating in the event. All faculty circulated among the groups during the event with one faculty member responsible for timing the scenario. All faculty participated in debriefing.

E. RUNNING OF THE SCENARIO

All clinical testing materials and documents were provided to students before the simulation and were also printed and available at each simulation station. Students were preassigned from the RSVP list to interprofessional groups according to their discipline. Name tags, which included group designation, were made in advance and given to the students as they signed in. Door signs with the group name were posted on all of the simulation rooms so the students could determine where to go after the briefing. During sign-up any student who came to the event and who had not previously RSVP'd was assigned to a group making sure to match the student with his or her specific discipline. Because the event was well attended, students and faculty met in the auditorium for briefing. While the large group was being briefed final training was taking place with the students portraying the patients and family members. Briefing/training was planned for 30 minutes, the simulation for 30 minutes, and the debriefing for 30 minutes.

F. PRESENTATION OF COMPLETED TEMPLATE

Title

Interprofessional Post-Concussion Simulation

Scenario Level

Novice

Focus Area

Interprofessional competencies

Scenario Description

The scenario takes place in an examination room of a post-concussion clinic. The patient is seen by an interprofessional care team for a patient assessment to determine whether it is physically safe for the patient to return to team competition. The typical patient is between 14 and 18 years of age and is a member of a sports team. A parent is required to accompany his or her child. The care team consists of a PT, OT, RN, AT, and a midlevel health care provider, such as an NP or PA.

The patient being seen is a 16-year-old Olympic-level gymnast presenting to the interprofessional post-concussion clinic for follow-up evaluation as directed by the ED physician. Ten days earlier, she sustained a head injury during vaulting practice. Her medial left wrist had previously been hurting with pronation/supination and hyperextension (Bernstein, 2016), and had "given out" during initial contact on a vaulting attempt. This resulted in a head-on collision with the vault. There was no loss of consciousness (LOC) but she was apparently "dazed" afterward. Later that night she vomited and her parents brought her to the ED for further evaluation. Head CT and cervical spine plain films for right-sided neck pain were negative. She was instructed to rest and not return to sports until after a follow-up assessment at the post-concussion clinic. She did not go to school last week, and started back yesterday.

She now presents with continued neck pain and headache, along with a left wrist pain. She and her mother/father are eager for her to return to training because of an upcoming important regional meet next week.

The mother/father answers all questions that are asked of the patient. The parent is also defensive and anxious about the patient not being able to continue with her training.

A medication history reveals that the daughter is taking Vicodin 1 to 2 tabs every 6 hours for head/neck pain with good relief. During questioning the mother/father confesses to giving the daughter Valium (one tablet, unsure whether it was 5 or 10 mg) 36 hours ago to help with her anxiety about returning to school and to help with her social withdrawal and depression. The mother/father assumes this depression is the result of not being able to continue with her training.

Scenario Objectives

1. To participate in an interprofessional simulation
2. To communicate one's roles and responsibilities clearly to "patient," a "family member," and other students in the group
3. To recognize one's skills, knowledge, and abilities
4. To communicate with team members to clarify each member's responsibility in executing components of the patient assessment
5. To use unique and complementary abilities of all members of the team to plan patient care
6. To organize and communicate information from the assessment to the "patient" and "family member" in language that is understandable, avoiding discipline-specific terminology when possible
7. To express one's knowledge and opinions to other members of the team involved in assessing the post-concussion patient with confidence, clarity, and respect, working to ensure common understanding of information and treatment and care decisions
8. To listen actively and encourage ideas and opinions of other team members

Accomplishing the objectives of this interprofessional simulation provides the students with a beginning competency in communication when working on an interprofessional team, which is Essential VI of the *Essentials of Baccalaureate Education for Professional Nursing Practice* as described by the American Association of Colleges of Nursing (AACN; 2008). It also provides the opportunity for students to "learn about, from and with each other to enable effective collaboration and improve health outcomes" as defined by the World Health Organization in 2010 and referred to in the "Standards of Best Practice: Simulation Standard VIII: Simulation-Enhanced Interprofessional Education" (Decker et al., 2015). Interprofessional communication is also incorporated into the National Council Licensure Examination for Registered Nurses (NCLEX-RN®) test plan as one of the integrated processes that are distributed throughout the examination (National Council of State Boards of Nursing [NCSBN], 2015).

Setting the Scene

The Simulation Champion workgroup supporting the PIPES group started meeting 4 months before the post-concussion simulation event. We discussed the idea of designing a simulation tailored to the disciplines that signed up to participate in the event. The workgroup discussed possible conditions that could be adapted to a broad range of disciplines.

The decision for announcing the simulation event and RSVP dates were made, keeping in mind the length of time for design, determining logistics, and busy schedules. We decided to make the announcement before the January PIPES meeting and then established the RSVP link. The RSVP deadline was set for January 31, 2016.

The workgroup had designed a small tabletop simulation for the PIPES group in November 2015, which was well received by students. This simulation required the students to compile a handover report for another group after reading a small case study. The feedback given demonstrated the student's discomfort with the simulation environment and fears he or she would not be able to contribute due to his or her level of knowledge, which was unfounded. With this feedback the group felt the students would be successful with a more robust scenario. As concussions have been a hot topic for student and professional athletes the Simulation Champion workgroup decided to develop a simulation around post-concussion assessment. This subject could also be tailored to multiple disciplines.

A large number of nursing students signed up for the event. In order to have care groups without multiple nurse members the work group decided to ask these students whether they would participate in the simulation by playing the role of the patient and parent. Once we received confirmation that those students were willing to participate in that capacity, we could then distribute the rest of the nursing students among the care groups. A total of 67 students RSVP'd from seven disciplines, including OT, PT, graduate and undergraduate nursing, PA, AT, and allied health sciences.

We had a discussion about which student materials to give for the needed foundational knowledge regarding concussions; a decision was also made about the assessment tools that would be used to determine return to play after a concussion. State guidelines were also reviewed. The decision was made to send links to two articles: "Update: Evaluation and Management of Concussion in Sports" written by the American Academy of Neurology (2013) and "Diagnosis and Management of Sport-Related Concussion Best Practices" (National Collegiate Athletic Association [NCAA], 2016), and a YouTube video of a vault accident. These links would be emailed to all students who had submitted an RSVP.

Students who agreed to portray a patient or parent were sent a recording made by Michael Shoemaker, PhD, DPT, the PT faculty member, instructing them on how they should act and what movements to make. The "patients" were also instructed on how to respond to the various assessment tests. The various assessment tools were also sent out to all students for review. The Post-Concussion Symptom Scale (2015) was prescored to help save time during the event (Lovell et al., 2006).

Scenario Implementation

The students were divided into 12 care groups with each group having at least one nurse, PA, or NP and OT, PT, and AT student as available. The allied health students assisted with information management as needed according to their focus area. Name tags were made for each student with a medical symbol added to the name tag that matched a room number. These symbols helped the students identify which group they were in and where they would complete the scenario. Two students had not RSVP'd so they were assigned a group on arrival.

All students reported to a large auditorium for prebriefing. While the nursing faculty member was providing the prebrief information, students playing the patients and parents were being trained by the PT and OT faculty members in the simulation area. Other members of the team were distributing testing material and other equipment necessary for the completion of the scenario.

Once prebriefing was completed, the students divided into their groups and reported to the simulation area to find their room assignments. Once all students were just outside their rooms, the faculty members gave the signal to start the simulation. Each group was given 50 minutes to complete its assessments and offer their recommendations to the patient and family. When all the groups had completed the scenario, they all returned to the auditorium for a large group debriefing.

Evaluative Criteria

1. Were the students playing the patient and family member effective in engaging the care team? In other words, were they realistic?
2. How did the students interact with each other? Was their communication clear?
3. Did the students recognize overlap or role blurring?
4. Was the scenario too complicated, having too many tasks to complete in the time frame that was allotted?
5. Was the scenario robust enough so all of the disciplines were able to participate and use their skills?

G. DEBRIEFING GUIDELINES

1. How did the team work together?
2. Did the team communicate its role with the patient and did the team communicate in a way the patient could understand?
3. Was the scenario realistic?
4. Were the objectives of the simulation met?
5. Did everyone feel he or she was able to participate?

H. SUGGESTIONS/KEY FEATURES
TO REPLICATE OR IMPROVE

Negative outcomes from this simulation event included:

- We did not advertise this simulation well enough.
- All of the information needed from the students to design the simulation was not asked for during the sign-up process. This resulted in time spent reconnecting with students to obtain all the necessary information, resulting in inefficient time management.
- The groups could have used more help, so faculty recruitment should have been done as well.
- The students indicated that there were not enough midlevel providers to make referrals for further evaluation of the wrist injury that contributed to the accident causing the concussion.

Positive features of this simulation were the use of students as simulated patients and parents. Other positive outcomes were:

- Students appreciated the experience of interacting with other disciplines while still a student.
- The assessment tools made the scenario more realistic
- This simulation experience reconfirmed that the student had chosen the proper profession.
- Students enjoyed and learned new perspectives from playing the patient and parent.
- The students knew that some of the professions overlapped, but it was interesting for them to see how each discipline differed beyond the overlap.
- Assessment tools differed among professions.
- Communication with patients and family was handled differently among disciplines and students liked seeing these different approaches.
- Students who were concerned they were not at a high enough level in their studies remarked they were still able to participate and felt comfortable doing so.

I. RECOMMENDATIONS FOR FURTHER USE

Most of the planning was adequate for this simulation. The RSVP deadline was set far enough in advance so the simulation event could be planned, the students could be grouped according to discipline, and the training material could be sent out. However, this event could have been better advertised to recruit medical, nurse practitioner (NP), and pharmacy students.

Comments from the debriefing session were noted, but a formal survey would have been helpful to identify improvements. Overall, the students spoke up during debriefing, but there may have been some smaller issues that could have arisen from a survey that did not surface because students felt uncomfortable sharing in a large group.

The overall subject captured interest from all of the various disciplines and helped students engage in the scenario. Complications from concussions have received more awareness through the media recently and the enactment of legislation surrounding these injuries has seen families seeking out help for student athletes. Multidisciplinary care is recognized as a key element of success of these patients (Hugentobler, Vegh, Janiszewski, & Quatman-Yates, 2015). The simulation workgroup viewed this simulation as a success and, with slight modifications, it could be used with a variety of disciplines.

J. HOW SIMULATION-BASED PEDAGOGY HAS CONTRIBUTED TO IMPROVED STUDENT OUTCOMES

Group communication was monitored by walking around from group to group during this interprofessional simulation. The students explained what they were doing, encouraged other members of the group to participate, and, in some circumstances, taught a different profession an assessment skill that they approached just a little differently, which made the skill easier to accomplish. The students were focused and engaged in the scenario. The groups communicated in a relaxed manner. No one reported worrying whether something was a "PA" job or a "PT" job. The focus was on making a good assessment.

Listening to the debriefing discussion after this event, one of the students brought up how the professions overlap and how interesting it was to see the differences beyond the overlap. Experiencing the roles firsthand and learning new perspectives may help each of these students provide improved patient care. They may be better prepared to know who to ask when their scope of practice is exceeded or how to prepare the patient for the next step of care. The students reported an improved ability to work as a team member.

K. EXPERT RECOMMENDATIONS AND WORDS OF WISDOM

1. Always leave plenty of time between the RSVP deadline and the simulation for assigning groups and distributing necessary learning materials.
2. Design a realistic setting to allow student immersion in the scenario.
3. Have supplies and equipment organized so everything is set up and ready to go.
4. Have enough knowledgeable staff to provide help with logistics during the event. The less confusion there is, the more confident the students may feel.

L. EVALUATION OF BEST PRACTICE STANDARDS AND USE OF CREDENTIALED SIMULATION FACULTY

All of the MIPERC workgroups are tasked with helping students achieve interprofessional competence. These competencies were created by experts from six different professions who came together to create the IPEC. The goal of the IPEC is to help prepare future health professionals for enhanced team-based care of patients and improved population health outcomes (IPEC, 2016). The workgroups refer to these competencies when creating activities or learning situations for our students. The individual learning opportunities created by the workgroups use the basics in gaining interprofessional competence that is integrated with guidelines for learning methodologies for simulation. Our simulation practices are based on standards set forth by Society for Simulation in Healthcare (SSIH; Committee for Accreditation of Healthcare Simulation Programs, 2016) and International Nursing Association for Clinical Simulation and Learning (Decker et al.,

2015). Individual program curriculum standards are also in place for the health care professions involved in this simulation.

REFERENCES

American Academy of Neurology. (2013). Update: Evaluation and management of concussion in sports. Retrieved from https://www.aan.com/uploadedFiles/Website_Library_Assets/Documents/3Practice_Management/5Patient_Resources/1For_your_Patient/6_Sports_Concussion_Toolkit/evaluation.pdf

American Association of Colleges of Nursing. (2008). *The essentials of baccalaureate education for professional nursing practice.* Washington, DC: Author. Retrieved from http://www.aacn.nche.edu/education-resources/BaccEssentials08.pdf

Balance Error Scoring System. (2011). Retrieved from http://knowconcussion.org/wp-content/uploads/2011/06/BESS.pdf

Bernstein, J. (2016). TFCC injury. In J. Bernstein (Ed.), *Musculoskeletal medicine for medical students* (11th ed.). Rosemont, IL: American Academy of Orthopaedic Surgeons. Retrieved from http://orthopaedicsone.com/display/MSKMed/TFCC+injury

Committee for Accreditation of Healthcare Simulation Programs. (2016). Core standards and measurement criteria. *Society for Simulation in Healthcare Accreditation.* Retrieved from http://www.ssih.org/Portals/48/Accreditation/2016%20Standards%20and%20Docs/Core%20Standards%20and%20Criteria.pdf

Decker, S. I., Anderson, M., Boese, T., Epps, C, McCarthy, J, Motola, I.,...Scolaro, K. (2015). Standards of best practice: Simulation standard VIII: Simulation-enhanced interprofessional education (Sim-IPE). *Clinical Simulation in Nursing, 11*(6), 293–297. doi:10.1016/j.ecns.2015.03.010

Folstein MF, Folstein SE, & McHugh PR. (1975). "Mini-mental state". A practical method for grading the cognitive state of patients for the clinician. *Journal of Psychiatric Research, 12*(3), 189–198.

Galetta, K. M., Barrett, J., Allen, M., Madda, F., Delicata, D., Tennant, A. T.,...Balcer, L. J. (2011). The King-Devick test as a determinant of head trauma and concussion in boxers and MMA fighters. *Neurology, 76*(17), 1456–1462.

Hugentobler, J. A., Vegh, M., Janiszewski, B., & Quatman-Yates, C. (2015). Physical therapy intervention strategies for patients with prolonged mild traumatic brain injury symptoms: A case series. *International Journal of Sports Physical Therapy, 10*(5), 676–689.

Interprofessional Education Collaborative. (2016). *Core competencies for interprofessional collaborative practice: 2016 update.* Washington, DC: Author.

Lovell, M. R., Iverson, G. L., Collins, M. W., Podell, K., Johnston, K. M., Pardini, D., ... Maroon, J. C. (2006). Measurement of symptoms following sports-related concussion: Reliability and normative data for the post-concussion scale. *Applied Neuropsychology Adult, 13*, 166–174. Retrieved from http://www.hawaiiconcussion.com/PDF/Post-Concussion-Symptom-Scale.aspx

National Collegiate Athletic Association. (2016). Diagnosis and management of sport-related concussion best practices. Retrieved from http://www.ncaa.org/health-and-safety/concussion-guidelines

National Council of State Boards of Nursing. (2015). *NCLEX-RN examination: Test plan for the National Council Licensure Examination for Registered Nurses.* Retrieved from https://www.ncsbn.org/RN_Test_Plan_2016_Final.pdf

CHAPTER 47

Integrating Telehealth in a Simulated Multidisciplinary Rural Health Simulation

Rebecca J. Ventura

A. IMPLEMENTATION OF SIMULATION-BASED PEDAGOGY IN YOUR INDIVIDUALIZED TEACHING AREA

Health care consists of health care professionals in both clinical and nonclinical roles, working side by side or perhaps, unseen. Education and research are focusing on multidisciplinary and interdisciplinary cooperation, as health care strives for better and more efficient patient care. The participants in this scenario are students who are enrolled in five different College of Health programs: health services administration (HSA), health information management (HIM), health information technology (HIT), registered nursing (RN), and medical assistant (MA). Health care professionals work closely with other ancillary persons, professionals, and practitioners; however, many do not understand the important role that others play. These participants represent a small sample of health care's nonclinical and clinical professionals.

As health care faculty, we are constantly looking for innovative ways to *reach* our students and technology seems to be one answer. High-fidelity simulation laboratories can create a supervised and "safe" environment for students to practice their skills. Instructors have the ability to build case scenarios ranging from simple to complex that can meet any learning objective. Anything is a possibility as long as it is designed to meet objectives (Lioce et al., 2015).

Now add telehealth: According to the American Telemedicine Association, "Over half of all U.S. hospitals now use some form of telemedicine" (2016, "How Typical Is Telemedicine," para. 1). Telehealth is ever increasingly becoming the norm for the health care industry. As a university, we are privileged to have purchased four telemedicine carts that use telehealth technology. In September 2013, Davenport University's Veteran Bachelor of Science (VBSN) program received a grant from the Health Resources and Services Administration (HRSA). This initiative began with the VBSN program because of the military's high regard for cutting-edge technology in the medical field. By purchasing and piloting telehealth equipment, our students are able to use this technology to help leverage the experiences of service members who are familiar with the equipment from their military experience. Telehealth has brought about a new age of medicine for all medical professionals.

B. EDUCATIONAL MATERIALS AVAILABLE IN YOUR TEACHING AREA AND RELATED TO YOUR SPECIALTY

The university has four bachelor of science in nursing (BSN) programs located at four different campuses. Each campus boasts a fundamentals laboratory, a simulation laboratory (SimMan® 3G, SimMom® with baby and Neonate) as well as a telemedicine cart.

C. SPECIFIC OBJECTIVES FOR SIMULATION USAGE WITHIN A SPECIFIC COURSE AND THE OVERALL PROGRAM

The incorporation of multidisciplinary students and the use of simulation and telehealth are part of the goals for the College of Health Professions (CoHP). The dean of the CoHP has encouraged collaboration among different health programs to share simulation scenarios and equipment and to foster camaraderie among faculty members. Her foresight is founded in research and best practices. According to Dillon, Nobel, and Kaplan (2009), patient and health care professional's job satisfaction were increased and patient outcomes improved, when interdisciplinary workers collaborated on patient care. Communication between interdisciplinary and multidisciplinary professionals is paramount for effective patient care. Understanding and appreciating each role that health care professionals provide help communication and can foster mutual respect.

With telemedicine increasing in health care, the university made it a priority to educate its current students. The purchase of four telehealth carts with telehealth-compatible electronic (E) stethoscopes provides real-world and practical learning for all CoHP students. Our population is aging and technology is advancing. Sometimes there is a disconnect among patients, family members, and even health care professionals. Technology can be a barrier, but with training and familiarity at the college level, future health care professionals can become more comfortable using this technology (Benhuri, 2010). These students will graduate and it is to be hoped that they will embrace as well as advocate the use of technology in their patient care.

D. INTRODUCTION OF SCENARIO

Prescenario #1: 25 Minutes

The majority of the students were active participants in a voluntary simulation scenario 1 year before the combination telehealth and simulation event. The previous simulation event was requested by students to learn more about the simulation laboratory and its capabilities. One of the goals of the students was to be introduced to the simulation laboratory in a nontesting manner. The simulation laboratory was strictly used for second-year nursing students; this appeared to be an intimidating factor for many of the students.

The simulation laboratory coordinator introduced herself and gave a brief overview of the capabilities of the SimMan 3G. The students were encouraged to explore and to interact with the simulator. The coordinator explained SimMan 3G's bedside monitor information and his capabilities. Although some of the students were initially timid, they joined in with the other students, discovering SimMan's many moving parts, tubes, and wounds. All of the students had current cardiopulmonary resuscitation (CPR) cards, so the coordinator asked whether the students would like to practice CPR. Every student performed chest compressions on SimMan 3G.

The students' learning outcome was to become familiar with the simulation lab. The author's learning outcomes were that the students became familiar with simulation lab and that they would want to come back and learn more. Although these learning outcomes seemed simple, they were an important first step in introducing simulation as a learning tool. After the simulation scenario, the students asked for more simulation scenarios. They wanted more, and they seemed excited to learn!

Prescenario #2: 15 Minutes

The same group of students wanted to learn about telehealth. The telemedicine cart was brought to the classroom so that the students could see and interact with the technology. They turned it on, practiced moving the camera, and plugged in the e-stethoscope. The students received an overview of the benefits and challenges facing telehealth. The manufacturer provided a brief video that showed the potential clientele and applications that were available. This presentation led to the discussion of incorporating a simulated event that required the use of telehealth.

Pre scenario #3: 30 Minutes

Each student was given an assignment to research how telehealth could affect them as professionals and as potential patients. Each student was to reflect about his or her future role in health care and how telehealth would fit into their chosen profession.

Setting the Scene and Implementation

This simulation used inclement weather in a rural setting as the scene. Owing to heavy snowfall, a young pregnant female arrives at a rural health care clinic. She states that she is having contractions and is not able to make it to the hospital. She is alert and able to answer questions. The students are not given any patient history, but are encouraged to ask the patient questions. The patient states that she has had minimal prenatal care at another facility.

A call for help to all available personnel to assist was initiated by the RN working in the facility. The students are brought to the patient's bedside, where the RN assists the students in obtaining a set of vital signs and positioning the patient for delivery. The first baby is delivered and placed into the infant warmer. However, the patient is still experiencing pain and states she feels the need to continue to push. The fetal heart tone monitor is placed on her abdomen and indicates there is a fetal heart rate. The patient is carrying another baby, but with each contraction, the heart rate drops.

The decision to contact the physician on call using telehealth is made. The faculty member calls the physician and allows the conversation to progress. Students report what they are seeing and answer the physician's questions. A medication for pain is ordered and an HIT student asks the patient whether she is allergic to any medications. An MA student asks her pain level and a nursing student yells out the adverse reactions. Our telehealth physician asks for updated vital signs on both the patient and baby #1. The telehealth monitor camera focuses in and out on the patient. The students can see the camera viewing the entire room. They assist the patient with the second delivery as well as get supplies, read vital signs, examine the babies, and reposition the patient.

The student roles were not assigned to allow student-led delegation as well as student role autonomy. Students are led to believe that the patient is having one baby, but two babies are delivered while consulting the on-call physician via telehealth.

Equipment and Technology Used

This simulation used:

1. High-fidelity SimMom with baby and neonate
2. Hospital bed
3. Bedside patient monitor—blood pressure, heart rate, respiratory rate, and pulse oxygenation reading
4. Fetal heart tone monitor
5. Infant warmer
6. Gloves
7. E-stethoscopes
8. Two telemedicine carts (one cart was in simulation laboratory and one cart was at a different location)

Objectives

1. Introduce simulation and telehealth to multidisciplinary students in a nontesting format.
2. Participate in a multidisciplinary collaborative simulation scenario using telehealth technology.
3. Implement appropriate communication techniques using telehealth technology within an emergent childbirth simulation scenario.

Participant Roles

The patient was portrayed by SimMom with a faculty member (simulation coordinator) supervising students, who wanted to deliver or "push out" baby #1 or baby #2. This faculty member was the only RN in the scenario. The second faculty member stood by the telemedicine cart and facilitated the scenario by asking questions and stopping the simulation to move students or redirect students. The students were not placed into specific roles. If a nonclinical student wanted to help deliver a baby or read a vital sign, this was allowed and encouraged. The students answered questions from both faculty members, other students, and the telehealth on-call physician. If the student did not know the answer, another student could answer, or the faculty provided the answer. The remote on-call physician (telehealth) was played by a faculty member who was located 100 miles away.

E. RUNNING OF THE SCENARIO

The simulation coordinator and the author discussed the learning objectives as well as the students' preassignment. It was decided to use the SimMom and baby for our "emergency" scenario. Many of the students had some experience with childbirth, and it was felt that this scenario would lend itself to the objectives. We discussed that no fatalities or near fatalities would occur to continue with our theme.

The patient was a healthy, full-term pregnant female who was unable to make it to the hospital because of inclement weather. The patient was put into a gown and had a full set of vital signs performed. She was placed in the lithotomy position on the bed. The students were encouraged to ask the patient questions. The simulation coordinator answered their questions and directed students to use telehealth to call the "on-call physician." Students answered questions from the physician and followed his orders. Although the orders were appropriate for the patient, it was important to remember the students' different skill levels. The exercise was focused on the learning outcomes.

The students helped deliver the first baby with assistance from the faculty and physician. As they placed the first baby in the incubator, the simulation coordinator stated that another baby was imminent. The students worked together to deliver the second baby, take care of the patient and first baby, call the father and family (as directed by the patient), gather supplies, take vital signs, read the monitor, and communicate with the telehealth physician.

F. PRESENTATION OF COMPLETED TEMPLATE

Title

Integrating Telehealth in a Simulated Multidisciplinary Rural Health Simulation

Scenario Level

This simulated event uses telehealth as an educational tool to engage and integrate multidisciplinary participant roles in a simulated rural emergency scenario. The use of telehealth in this scenario met the learning outcomes as well as an increased participants' knowledge of their future roles as health care providers.

Focus Area

This scenario was geared toward multidisciplinary students with different skill sets.

Scenario Description and Setting the Scene

This simulation used inclement weather in a rural setting as the scene. Owing to heavy snowfall, a young pregnant female arrives at a rural health care clinic. She states that she is having contractions and is not able to make it to the hospital. The students, with the help of faculty and the on-call physician via telehealth, assist the patient in delivering two healthy babies.

Scenario Objectives

1. Introduce simulation and telehealth to multidisciplinary students.
2. Participate in a multidisciplinary collaborative simulation scenario using telehealth technology.
3. Implement appropriate communication techniques, using telehealth technology, within an emergent childbirth simulation scenario.

G. DEBRIEFING GUIDELINES

This scenario lasted 45 minutes. This did not give adequate time to debrief before students had to leave for class. Again, the collaboration was extended to fit everyone's busy schedule, and this was a volunteer event. Students were asked to email the author the following qualitative reply: What were your thoughts about the scenario and the use of simulation and telehealth?

There was an approximately 75% return on requested feedback to the simulation event. The students were descriptive and pointed out positive aspects as well as some areas to improve for better flow and believability. All the students stated that they wanted to participate in another combination scenario.

It was interesting that the nonclinical students seem to appreciate the event as much as the clinical students. One of the HIM student's replied, "I really enjoyed seeing how the telehealth works. As an HIT/HIM student, it was nice to see because it would be easier to explain how it works and to know how to bill or code for this new technology." A quote from an HSA student stated, "As a future administrator, knowing Davenport University students are receiving this training with this type of technology builds my confidence in the abilities of new graduates. Combining the telemedicine and Sim lab demonstrations clearly showed everyone how telemedicine can be used by each of us and be applied to an endless variety of situations." Overall, the students' feedback was positive and indicated that they felt the scenario was educational as well as nonstressful.

H. SUGGESTIONS/KEY FEATURES TO REPLICATE OR IMPROVE

It was challenging and took a great amount of collaboration to have all of the students (who were volunteering to do this scenario) attend the simulation before any scheduled classes, work with the simulation coordinator and the remote faculty member, reserve the simulation laboratory, and have the telemedicine cart available. It is suggested that a date for simulations be designated well in advance to allow for busy schedules. As this was a volunteer event, the date and time were chosen by the participating students. The majority of the students had a class following the event, which was convenient for the students but not ideal for running this event and providing debriefing time. The time should be closely monitored, as the simulation was very interactive and face paced. There was not enough time to debrief the students and faculty in this event; therefore, the formal feedback was delayed.

There should be a limited amount of people in the simulation laboratory. The scenario brought several faculty members, advisors, and other students who wanted to watch the scenario. Although 12 participants (including faculty) had registered for the simulation and telehealth scenario, the simulation laboratory's observers grew. There was no person delegated to address observers or visitors. The noise level seemed to grow as the scenario progressed and the students became more engaged. This seemed to stimulate conversation from visitors, which was positive and encouraging, but not conducive to communication. It would be advisable to have someone limit the access to the area or have a designated person to monitor visitors.

A suggestion was made that next time this telehealth scenario was run, the nonclinical students might have greater input and participation. Spending more time in prescenario conference and providing more detail about the scenario would help the nonclinical students prepare for their roles. The HIT/ HIM students could research billing codes for telehealth services, patient privacy practices, as well as current and pending laws regarding provider reimbursement. The HSA students would be able to address the availability of services, training, budget, and how telehealth could benefit their organization. Including different CoHP program faculty and leadership may benefit the student scenario by adding program-specific content.

I. RECOMMENDATIONS FOR FURTHER USE

The scenario stimulated conversation about the roles of the other students and met the learning objectives. It was suggested that one of the preconferences be focused on the different roles of health care providers as well as include program-specific faculty in both the preconference and simulation event.

J. HOW SIMULATION-BASED PEDAGOGY HAS CONTRIBUTED TO IMPROVED STUDENT OUTCOMES

As a CoHP faculty member, I had the privilege of mentoring an incredible group of health care students. I was able to find common ground by using simulation and telehealth. This chapter discusses how a multidisciplinary group of students with different skill levels were able to effectively use simulation and telehealth to meet the learning objectives, but more important, connect with health care professionals.

K. EXPERT RECOMMENDATIONS AND WORDS OF WISDOM

This simulation event's first learning outcome was to introduce simulation and new technology to students. This group of students had stated that they were nervous about the simulation laboratory technology and telehealth, but were interested in using both of them. They were nervous that they would make a mistake or that they would not know the answer to a question. I have found that students want to perform well in a simulation scenario, but seem to be afraid of making mistakes when the simulation is the best place to make mistakes. This event encouraged and allowed students to experience simulation and telehealth in a nontesting format. Although student feedback reflected that the scenario was educational, the participating students stated that the event was a lot of fun and they wanted more.

L. EVALUATION OF BEST PRACTICE STANDARDS AND USE OF CREDENTIALED SIMULATION FACULTY

This simulation and telehealth exercise was conducted under the supervision and direction of the simulation laboratory and clinical coordinator for the BSN program, who is an RN with more than 10 years of ICU experience and holds a Simulation Certificate from Drexel University, and an Army Nurse Corps registered nurse veteran with more than 20 years of emergency department/ critical care experience. The on-call physician was portrayed by a combat-medic-trained veteran with telehealth experience. For this exercise, the video conferencing or real-time telehealth application was used (Center for Connected Health Policy, 2016). The following International Nursing Association for Clinical Simulation in Learning (INASCL) standards were referenced: Standard VII: Participant Assessment and Evaluation (Sando et al., 2013), Standard VIII: Interprofessional Education (Decker et al., 2015), and Standard IX: Simulation Design (Lioce et al., 2015).

ACKNOWLEDGMENT

Health Resources and Services Administration (HRSA) of the U.S. Department of Health and HumanServices (HHS) under grant number UF1HP26488 and title "Veterans to BSN Program" for $1,217,446, with 0% financed with nongovernmental sources.

REFERENCES

American Telemedicine Association. (2016). How typical is telemedicine? Retrieved from http://www .americantelemed.org/main/about/telehealth-faqs-

Benhuri, G. (2010). Teaching community telenursing with simulation. *Clinical Simulation in Nursing, 6*(4), e161–e163. Retrieved from http://www2.eerp.usp.br/Nepien/DisponibilizarArquivos/ Telenursing_and_simulation.pdf

Center for Connected Health Policy. (2016). Video conferencing. Retrieved from http://www.cchpca .org/what-is-telehealth/video-conferencing

Decker, S. I., Anderson, M., Boese, T., Epps, C., McCarthy, J., Motola, I., . . . Lioce, L. (2015). Standards of best practice: Simulation standard VIII: Simulation-enhanced interprofessional education (Sim-IPE). *Clinical Simulation in Nursing, 11*(6), 293–297.

Dillon, P. M., Noble, K. A., & Kaplan, L. (2009, March/ April). Simulation as a means to foster collaborative interdisciplinary education. *Nursing Education Perspectives, 30*(2), 87–90. Retrieved from http:// search.proquest.com

Lioce, L., Meakim, C. H., Fey, M. K., Chmil, J. V., Mariani, B., & Alinier, G. (2015). Standards of best practice: Simulation standard IX: Simulation design. *Clinical Simulation in Nursing, 11*(6), 309–315.

Sando, C. R., Coggins, R. M., Meakim, C., Franklin, A. E., Gloe, D., Boese, T., . . . Borum, J. C. (2013). Standards of best practice: Simulation standard VII: Participant assessment and evaluation. *Clinical Simulation in Nursing, 9*(6S), S30–S32.

CHAPTER 48

Interprofessional Team Simulation: Pediatric Rapid Sequence Intubation in Respiratory Failure Due to Severe Bronchiolitis

Jeff Bishop, Maureen M. Ryan, Melissa Holland, and Emma Carrick

A. IMPLEMENTATION OF SIMULATION-BASED PEDAGOGY IN YOUR INDIVIDUALIZED TEACHING AREA

Life-threatening presentations and critical events do not occur with high frequency in pediatric hospital units. One such high-stake event is emergency intubation of children. To develop individual competence, it is estimated that learners need to participate in 20 to 30 of these procedures to obtain competence (Bernhard, Mohr, Weigand, Martin, & Walther, 2012; Kusel, Farina, & Aldous, 2014). Victoria General Hospital (VGH) serves as the regional referral site for pediatrics and 11,000 pediatric patients come through the emergency department, 2,000 of whom are admitted to our pediatric ward and intensive care unit per year (ChildHealth BC, 2014). Within this patient population, we perform pediatric intubation an estimated 25 to 30 times per year outside of the operating room. This mirrors the low rate of pediatric intubation across pediatric units in North America (Nishisaki et al., 2011). VGH is also a regional training center for physicians, nurses, and respiratory therapists. Many of the graduates complete their training and then work in smaller rural centers where the frequency of pediatric intubations is even lower than in the urban hospitals. Thus, the expectation that health professional practitioners obtain and maintain competence during prelicensure training in this critical procedure through clinical exposure is not reasonable. However, simulation-learning events provide a venue by which prelicensure and licensed health care practitioners can learn and practice pediatric intubation without compromising patient safety. Indeed, simulating this necessary clinical learning has been shown to be equivalent to the intensive patient-based learning when measuring individual skill acquisition (Hall et al., 2005).

Here at the Island Medical Program of the University of British Columbia, we have opted to use a scenario of respiratory failure due to bronchiolitis as the basis for leveled simulation learning. Our prelicensure learners encounter the scenario during their preclinical and clinical training in the simulation lab and during postgraduate training, either in the simulation lab or during an in situ simulation on the pediatric ward.

This chapter focuses on the experience of undergraduate nurses, physicians, and respiratory therapy students who are seeing the scenario for the first time in a team environment: interprofessional education (IPE).

B. EDUCATIONAL MATERIALS AVAILABLE IN YOUR TEACHING AREA AND RELATED TO YOUR SPECIALTY

In advance of the simulation, learners are provided with the detailed case outline, medication lists, and evaluation checklists that preceptors use when teaching. We use a flipped learning model (Betihavas, Bridgman, Kornhaber, & Cross, 2016) and Table 48.1 outlines the required and optional resources to be reviewed before attending the simulation session.

Learner Preparation

Presimulation learning material:

1. OpenPediatrics module on recognizing respiratory distress (16-minute duration): www.openpediatrics.org/assets/video/recognizing-respiratory-distress (Kleinman, 2013)
2. OpenPediatrics scenario of a patient with bronchiolitis requiring intubation (12-minute duration): www.openpediatrics.org/assets/video/common-intubation-scenarios-bronchiolitis (Wolbrink, 2015). Note that the choice of induction agents (propofol) is different from our suggested agent (ketamine).

C. SPECIFIC OBJECTIVES FOR SIMULATION USAGE WITHIN A SPECIFIC COURSE AND THE OVERALL PROGRAM

Interprofessional team simulation provides a safe and effective context to practice prelicensure health professional student collaborative teamwork around a patient care event that they will encounter in future as a health care professional. Experiential learning theory guides clinical practice coursework across curricula. Each health professional student licensure competencies cite competency in interprofessional patient care and teamwork. For example, nursing students must meet the standards of practice of interdisciplinary competency outlined by the College of Registered of Nurses British Columbia (CRNBC) Standard 3: Client-Focused Provision of Service (CRNBC, 2013) during clinical courses before their licensure examination (NCLEX). Similarly, medical students must meet competencies as described by the Medical Council of Canada to meet their professional licensing objectives (Licentiate of the Medical Council of Canada Exam [LMCC] part I).

We have learned that students who wish to engage in the interprofessional patient simulations must be able to clearly articulate their roles and have the psychomotor skills requisite to perform their role during the simulation as indicated by the International Nursing Association for Clinical Simulation and Learning (INACSL) Standard VIII: Simulation-Enhanced Interprofessional Education (Sim-IPE; Decker et al., 2015) of the INACSL Standards of Best Practice.

The scenario may be our students' first exposure to a child in respiratory failure and/or is the first time they have been involved in a simulated intubation of a child. We know that one of the major contributors to errors during rapid sequence induction (RSI) is a result of problematic communication or team functioning (Nishisaki et al., 2011). Thus we remove the cognitive load associated with diagnosis and management planning for our novice teams by providing the full case scenario details to them before the simulation session. Formally structuring the simulation and providing learners with the foreknowledge of the required steps helps ensure that the simulation proceeds with a systematic interprofessional team working toward the expected goals.

D. INTRODUCTION OF SCENARIO

Setting the Scene and Technology Used

Learners arrive in the simulation space and are introduced to each other and the preceptors present. Sessions take place in a simulation lab or in situ using a high- or moderate-fidelity human patient

Table 48.1	Medication Chart	
Medication	**Dose**	**Considerations**
Acetaminophen	15 mg/kg	May be given orally or rectally.
Antibiotics		
Ampicillin	100–200 mg/kg/24 hr divided q 6 hr	Antibiotics are not effective in this case of bronchiolitis but would be used for pneumonia.
Ceftriaxone	50–100 mg/kg im/IV once daily	
Gentamicin	7.5 mg/kg/24 hr div. q 8 hr	
Vancomycin	60 mg/kg/24 hr div. q 6 hr	
Bronchodilators		
Epinephrine (nebulized)	2.5 mL of 1:1,000 neb.	Efficacy of bronchodilators in bronchiolitis is debated. Not effective for respiratory failure because of apnea.
Ventolin (nebulized)	1.25 or 2.5 mL neb.	
Steroids		
Dexamethasone	0.15–0.6 mg/kg	Steroids are not effective in this case of bronchiolitis, but would be used for asthma.
Prednisone	1 mg/kg	
Intubation medications		
Premedication		
Atropine	0.01 mg/kg	Not given routinely in intubation but for patient of this age, may be helpful to prevent or treat bradycardia during laryngoscopy.
Sedation		
Ketamine	2 mg/kg	Suggested agent for our hospital
Midazolam	0.1 mg/kg (max 8 mg)	
Fentanyl	2 mcg/kg	
Etomidate	0.3 mg/kg	Not available in our hospital.
Propofol	1–4 mg/kg IV	Cardiac depression is likely with large doses.
Paralysis		
Succinylcholine	2 mg/kg	
Roccuronium	1 mg/kg	

(continued)

Table 48.1	Medication Chart *(continued)*	
Medication	**Dose**	**Considerations**
Maintenance of sedation post intubation		
Morphine infusion	10–40 mcg/kg/hr	
Midazolam infusion	1–4 mcg/kg/min	
Other medications		
3% Hypertonic saline	5 mL	Not effective as an emergency treatment

IV, intravenous; q every.

simulator (HPS) and large video screen for displaying laboratory results, radiology images, and other supplemental materials, including a video of, pediatric patients with respiratory distress. All equipment required for the scenario is laid out in advance with the appropriate sizes preselected for the learners.

Prebriefing

We begin with introductions of team members and the roles and expectations of all participants. We review the setting, resources available, and the objectives of the session and emphasize the safe nature of the learning environment as a place where mistakes are welcomed as learning opportunities.

Objectives

The Canadian Interprofessional Health Collaborative (CIHC) National Interprofessional Competency Framework outlines competencies required for effective interprofessional collaboration within six domains: (a) role clarification; (b) team functioning; (c) patient-/ client-/ family-/ community-centered care; (d) collaborative leadership; (e) interprofessional communication; and (f) interprofessional conflict resolution (CIHC, 2010). For our novice learners, we focus on role clarification, team functioning, collaborative leadership, and interprofessional communication domains as an introductory first level during the simulation and debriefing. Mutually beneficial learning objectives across prelicensure curricula include a practice opportunity to:

1. Gain knowledge and practice about their role and other health team members when responding to respiratory distress and implementing RSI.
2. Understand the principles of teamwork dynamics and group/team processes to enable effective interprofessional collaboration and shared decision making.
3. Share decision making and leadership and accountability for actions, responsibilities, and roles as defined within the professional scope of practice.
4. Communicate with each other in a collaborative, responsive, and responsible manner.

Description of Participants

We limit the care team to a maximum of five learners, including at least one nursing learner, one physician learner, and, when available, a respiratory therapy learner in his or her senior year of training at the undergraduate level. Roles are assigned as team leader, recorder, medication preparer, airway support person, and miscellaneous support person (depends on training pathway of the learner). We assign one facilitator to alter HPS parameters and provide supplemental material, such as labs or imaging, as requested by the team. The other facilitator is tasked with carefully observing team behavior and leading the debriefing process afterward.

One key point that we have identified is the importance of not asking learners to pretend to be a different professional. We emphasize that as professionals we train for very different jobs and that pretending to be a member of a different profession is not appropriate. When medical students are asked to prepare medications, they are not pretending to be nurses; they are physicians preparing medications. Similarly, if nursing students perform the physical tasks associated with managing an airway, they are not respiratory therapists but rather nurses whose scope of practice may include tasks associated with airway management. We have found that this distinction of task performance versus role play as a member of a different profession removes what can be a barrier to the suspension of disbelief necessary to run the simulation. It also helps prepare learners for the real-life clinical situation of having to perform tasks normally done by another professional because of lack of resources, as may occur in small centers with limited staffing.

E. RUNNING OF THE SCENARIO

After the orientation to space and equipment is completed, learners are presented with a video of a child in severe respiratory distress. They are asked as a group to identify the clinical features observed, including increased work of breathing, as demonstrated by tachypnea, indrawing, tracheal tug, nasal flaring, grunting, and see-saw breathing. The Pediatric Assessment Triangle is used to highlight that the child is in severe respiratory distress with a moderately altered mental status and prolonged capillary refill (Dieckmann, Brownstein, & Gausche-Hill, 2010) The absence of stridor is noted as a learning point that this is more likely a case of lower respiratory tract illness than upper tract pathology. Once the video has been reviewed, learners are assigned their specific roles and are provided a few minutes to meet as a team to discuss their strategy and approach to the patient. The scenario then begins as the team begins to interact with the HPS.

F. PRESENTATION OF COMPLETED TEMPLATE

Title

Pediatric RSI in Respiratory Failure Due to Severe Bronchiolitis

Scenario Level

Prelicensure health professional students

Focus Area

Pediatric acute care hospital setting: Emergency admission of a 4-month-old in respiratory distress

Scenario Objectives

All Learners

- Describe and identify clinical signs of respiratory distress.
- Describe and identify clinical and laboratory signs of respiratory failure.
- Identify and treat oxygenation difficulties.
- Identify and treat ventilation difficulties.
- Describe features of lower respiratory tract illness versus upper respiratory tract illness.
- Administer oxygen therapy.
- Identify apnea and intervene with one's scope of practice.

- Perform as a team the steps of a modified pediatric RSI *(modified RSI includes bag-valve mask ventilation [BVM], whereas in a classic RSI no BVM ventilation occurs;* Morrow et al., 2015).

Physician Learners

- Identify and treat the complications of severe bronchiolitis with respiratory failure.
- Act as team leader for pediatric RSI, including the performance of endotracheal tube placement and tube securement.

Nursing Learners

- Administer bronchodilators (salbutamol and epinephrine).
- Participate in pediatric RSI, including preparing and administering RSI medications.

Respiratory Therapy Learners

- Administer bronchodilators (salbutamol and epinephrine).
- Prepare for and participate in pediatric RSI, including the performance of equipment preparation, endotracheal tube placement, and tube securement.

Setting the Scene

Equipment Needed

HPS:

Laerdal SimBaby, Laerdal SimPad, and monitor

Multimedia:

Video of respiratory distress (not included as consent only given for use at our center); chest x-ray: preintubation; laboratory investigations: complete blood count (CBC), capillary blood gas, electrolytes, blood urea nitrogen (BUN), creatinine, glucose; chest x-ray: postintubation

Airway equipment:

Simple oxygen mask, nasal prongs, nonrebreather mask, nebulization mask, self-inflating bag and mask, oral airway/nasal trumpet, laryngeal mask airway, laryngoscope and blade, endotracheal tube, stylet, end tidal carbon dioxide device (in line and Pedicab colour change), Yankauer suction, tape to secure tube, Nicobar to secure tube, pediatric video laryngoscope

Other equipment:

Nasogastric tube, intravenous (IV) tubing and extensions, two IV bags set up for injection (i.e., one bag on the floor serves as the "patient" end and allows for the appropriate volume of simulated medications to be injected via and injection port), medication pump, Broselow tape, medication resources (see Table 48.1) plus access to BC Children's Hospital online resource (Esau, 2013), mock medication vials for all medications listed, drug monographs, intubation checklist.

Participant Roles

Participants play themselves and work within their scope of practice through the phases outlined in Exhibit 48.1, where we describe the infant status, goals of care, and a timeline of completion.

Exhibit 48.1	Scenario Phases		
Phase	**Status**	**Goals of Care**	**Time**
1	**History:** A previously healthy 4-month-old boy (Liam) has returned to the ED after being seen 2 days ago. He was unwell with URTI symptoms 3 days ago and was found to be positive for RSV. When initially seen in the ED, Liam only had a mildly increased work of breathing, was feeding well, and was not desaturated. Today he has progressively worsened with an increased work of breathing, inability to feed, and no urine output for several hours. Liam has a 3-year-old sibling who has been unwell for almost a week with URTI symptoms. He has NOT had a fever. **Past history:** Liam was born at term with no pregnancy or delivery complications. He has been well before this illness. **Meds:** Vitamin D 400 units daily **Immunizations:** Has received his routine 2-month and 4-month vaccines. **Allergies:** No known allergies **Development:** No concerns; he is meeting appropriate age milestones. **Family history:** No chronic respiratory illness (no asthma, cystic fibrosis, etc.) **Social:** Lives with parents, both of whom have mild cold symptoms. Liam has a 3-year-old sibling who has been unwell for almost a week with URTI symptoms. No pets. No travel. No ingestions. No foreign body exposures. **On examination: 6 kg** Cries to painful stimulation. Minimal response to touch/voice. Increased WOB: In-drawing, tracheal tug, nasal flare, grunting, see-saw breathing Capillary refill 3 seconds peripheral; less than 2 central Temp: 37°C HR: 170 beats/minute (normal sinus rhythm) BP: 75/38 mmHg O_2 sat: 83% room air (improves to 90% with mask or nasal prongs)	Recognize moderate/severe respiratory distress. Recognize lower respiratory tract illness (wheeze, crackles). Apply oxygen therapy. Establish IV access (successful first time). Investigations: Labs, CXR Consider trial of bronchodilators (not effective).	10 min

(continued)

Exhibit 48.1	Scenario Phases (*continued*)		
Phase	**Status**	**Goals of Care**	**Time**
2	Minimal improvement with oxygen therapy and bronchodilators	Identify apnea/respiratory failure.	5 min
	HR: Increases to 185 beats/minute over 2 minutes followed by episodes of apnea and desaturation,	Initiate PPV.	
		Set up for intubation.	
	BP: 78/40 mmHg		
	O_2 sat: 88% with increasing desaturation, events during apnea; sats increase to 94% with PPV via bag valve mask.		
	The patient begins to have apneic spells and desaturations.		
3	Intubation via RSI	Follow intubation checklist.	10–15 min
	Island Health intubation checklist is available on the intranet of Island Health as a policy and practice statement and is printed out and attached to the intubation cart for practitioners' reference.		

BP, blood pressure; CXR, chest x-ray; ED, emergency department; HR, heart rate; IV, intravenous; PPV, positive pressure ventilation; RSV, respiratory synctial virus; URTO, upper respiratory tract infection; WOB , work of breathing.

Scenario Implementation

Exhibit 48.1 details phases of the simulation scenarios. The team members place appropriate monitoring equipment—EKG, saturation probe, blood pressure cuff—and turn on the patient monitor. A team member may be delegated or identify his or her role to collect an initial set of vital signs and perform a primary assessment. A medical student gives an order to another student to start an IV, which is placed without difficulty. The team lead may order or consult with team members to order laboratory investigations.

Initial laboratory investigations and radiographic investigation results demonstrate hypoventilation though an increased CO_2 on a capillary blood gas and a lack of laboratory markers of bacterial pneumonia (normal white blood cell count, normal C-reactive protein, and normal procalcitonin). The chest radiograph demonstrates mild bilateral increased opacification hyperinflation and peribronchial cuffing without focal infiltrate. Learners who do not read the radiograph are expected to consult with a radiologist who can be reached by phone and who helps to interpret it as likely representing bronchiolitis without evidence of pneumonia.

These initial steps take 10 to 15 minutes. Once they have been completed, the facilitator lowers the respiratory rate of the HPS, and the O_2 saturations are decreased. If deterioration is not quickly recognized by any team member, the facilitator turns to the cues offered in Exhibit 48.2. The team transitions at this point to setting up for and completing RSI.

For novice learners, we have found that the logistics of completing RSI can be quite overwhelming. We provide facilitators with the Exhibit 48.2 cue sheet outlining times when it may be useful to have a confederate step in.

The confederate plays the role of a senior-level physician or nurse who can then take over the team leader role in the RSI and helps assign experience-appropriate roles to each of the learners. As has been shown by Long, Fitzpatrick, Cincotta, Grindlay, and Barrett (2016), the use of a checklist can be helpful for high cognitive load tasks, such as intubation, and Exhibit 48.3 provides an example of the one we use in clinical practice at our hospital.

Exhibit 48.2	Teaching Cues for Facilitators

Learners may have reviewed the Canadian Pediatric Society position statement on bronchiolitis describing how minimal investigations and treatments are needed. This case, however, demonstrates severe lower respiratory tract disease and respiratory failure.

If team members do not reassess and notice the baby's respiratory rate decreasing and oxygen saturation levels decreasing, the facilitator can prompt: "The baby appears to be tiring. The baby is having apnea episodes with the color change."

Consideration for noninvasive respiratory support (high-flow oxygen, CPAP, BiPAP may occur. These interventions would not be appropriate in the presence of apnea.

Learners may require prompting to identify a lack of response to bronchodilators. Consider a confederate for this role, who indicates:

"You do not see any difference with that Ventolin."

"The baby is still working very hard to breathe."

Similarly, prompting may be required if apnea is not quickly identified:

"He has stopped breathing."

"Should we bag him?"

The time required for RSI may exceed the allotted simulation duration and/or some learners may be so uncomfortable with performing the RSI that they choose to not proceed with this step.

If the team is struggling to complete the process, consider having a senior physician and/or nurse arrive (confederate) and assume the role of team leader. Learners can then perform the tasks required under the direction of an experienced practitioner.

BiPaP, bi-level positive airway pressure; CPAP, continuous positive airway pressure; RSI, rapid sequence induction.

Exhibit 48.3	Checklist of Care Goals

Time	Goal	Achieved? Y or N	Notes (Observed Behaviors by Care Team)
10 min	Identify severe respiratory distress. *Tachypnea, tachycardia, indrawing, tracheal tug, nasal flare, grunting, see-saw breathing*		
	Identify lower respiratory tract illness. If needed, prompt learners (during debrief) regarding findings of LRTI (wheeze, crackles) versus URTI (stridor).		
	Apply monitors.		
	Assess ABCs and provide airway support. *Application of oxygen, suction of nasal and oropharynx, place patient in sniffing position, possible chin lift or jaw thrust*		

(continued)

Exhibit 48.3	Checklist of Care Goals *(continued)*		
Time	**Goal**	**Achieved?** **Y or N**	**Notes (Observed Behaviors by Care Team)**
	Establish IV access.		
	Initiate IV fluid. *Crystalloid with or without dextrose*		
	Trial of bronchodilators (optional)		
	Order CXR.		
	Order other investigations.		
5 min	Identify respiratory failure. *Apneic periods, increasing somnolence, desaturation*		
	Escalate provision of oxygen and airway management. *Repeat previous steps with airway opening via jaw thrust or chin lift as a must-see component.*		
	Review investigations ordered and identify failure to ventilate. *(Elevated CO_2, clinical inadequacy of respiratory effort)* Review clinical status and identify failure to oxygenate. *(Desaturation despite provision of oxygen)*		
	Identify apnea (nonresolving).		
	Provide assisted ventilation and oxygenation via positive pressure, bag-valve mask ventilation.		
	Identify need for definitive airway via RSI.		
10–15 min	Review intubation checklist and set up for RSI (see checklist for details of each step). • *Patient preparation* • *Equipment preparation* • *Team preparation* • *Outcomes preparation*		
	Complete RSI. • *Medication administration* • *Placement of ETT* • *Maintain saturations >88% during procedure* • *RSI steps performed efficiently and effectively*		

(continued)

Exhibit 48.3	Checklist of Care Goals (*continued*)		
Time	**Goal**	**Achieved?** **Y or N**	**Notes (Observed** **Behaviors by** **Care Team)**
	Post-RSI confirmation of tube placement *(Clinical examination and qualitative or* *quantitative EtCO$_2$)* • *EtCO$_2$ present* • *Adequate bilateral chest rise* • *Mist in the ETT* • *Auscultation of bilateral axilla and epigastric region* • *Improvement in patient saturations*		
	Post-RSI care • *Placement of gastric decompression tube* • *X-ray confirmation of location* • *Ongoing sedation and analgesia* • *Initial ventilator settings or ongoing hand ventilation* • *Transfer of patient to intensive care setting*		

ABCs, airway, breathing, circulation; CXR, chest x-ray; ETT, endotracheal tube; IV, intravenous; LRTI, lower respiratory tract infection; RSI, rapid sequence intubation; URTI, upper respiratory tract infection.

The same checklist that is provided during the simulation is followed during the RSI procedure. The scenario ended with the successful placement of the endotracheal tube as confirmed by clinical status and presence of end-tidal CO$_2$. Further steps, such as the placement of a nasogastric tube, ongoing sedation and paralysis, and patient monitoring, are discussed with the team as we transition to the debriefing phase.

G. DEBRIEFING GUIDELINES

We allocate 30 minutes for the scenario and 30 minutes for the postscenario debriefing. Our facilitators use a combination of our scenario's task-specific checklist and an advocacy inquiry approach (Rudolph, Simon, Rivard, Dufresne, & Raemer, 2007) to review observed behaviors and facilitate the team discussion. In the advocacy-inquiry debriefing, an observation statement is followed by an inquiry into what the student was thinking and what the student was responding to to facilitate learning in a psychologically safe environment. For example, "I noticed that when the baby started to go quiet and was apneic and team member X asked whether you wanted to start bagging you did not respond and focused on the medication order" (advocacy) followed by "I am wondering what was important for you at that moment? How you were assessing the patient responses?" (inquiry). By inquiring into the student thinking, the facilitator allows the student to reflect on his or her decisions and consider ways to respond to similar, future situations as an individual and a team member.

H. SUGGESTIONS/KEY FEATURES
TO REPLICATE OR IMPROVE

In the ideal setting, we have at least two faculty members present with representation from different professions to observe and debrief on individual and team performance. When this is not possible, we have learners who are not participating in the scenario closely observe the actions of the members of their profession using the objectives checklist as a guide. Observers might also be provided with a copy of a standardized data-collection tool, such as the Mayo High Performance Teamwork Scale, and identify examples of the dimensions of teamwork described in the tool (Malec et al., 2007) during the postscenario debrief.

I. RECOMMENDATIONS FOR FURTHER USE

The learners referred to in this chapter are novice teams in contrast to teams composed of fully qualified professionals already employed and working with VGH. We also use the scenario for the improvement of team dynamics and crisis resource management when performed by staff-level practitioners in the emergency department trauma bay and the pediatric ICU. For teams of expert practitioners, identification of where equipment is stored in the trauma bay and selection of appropriate sizes adds task to the scenario.

When the scenario is run in situ for expert teams, we add the presence of a parent who is quite upset who requires support throughout the scenario. The parental support is usually provided by our unit social worker and/or a registered nurse and helps us to meet a further interprofessional competency: family-centered care (CIHC, 2010). When available, we also include our clinical pharmacist in the medication preparation process.

J. HOW SIMULATION-BASED PEDAGOGY HAS CONTRIBUTED TO IMPROVED STUDENT OUTCOMES

We have completed this simulation scenario numerous times with prelicensure and post-licensure learners across care areas, including the simulation lab, the emergency department, pediatric ward, and pediatric ICU. One somewhat surprising observation has been that learners who have completed the scenario state that they appreciate the opportunity to improve their own performance through repetition and find the in situ experience especially helpful once they are practicing as unrestricted graduate professionals. Although we have not measured the effect objectively, we do feel that frequent practice and simulation of pediatric RSI has made our novice- and expert-level team more comfortable and proficient when faced with actual patients requiring intubation.

We have designed a good stepwise introduction to the clinical practices on the unit. Leveling the scenarios to the learner keeps them engaged in learning and prepares them to practice. Students who are prepared for unit practices instill confidence in their mentors.

Motivating and engaging experienced practitioners into simulation events can be difficult. From our experience thus far, having students in situ helps to remove this barrier of discomfort. The students are fully engaged in the simulation sessions and debrief thereby making it an environment of interactive learning. They take on roles and procedures in simulation events that they may normally shy away from because of lack of experience and confidence at the bedside. The students offer questions to the group, thereby opening up a conversation that perhaps may not have been started by a more experienced nurse for fear of being judged for something the nurse did not know.

As in situ simulation becomes a more accepted routine activity, we hear requests for more simulation and positive comments on the benefits of simulation. Students and practitioners tell us over and over that they encounter similar patient care experiences in their practice as encountered in the simulated patient scenarios...and they know how to respond safely and effectively.

K. EXPERT RECOMMENDATIONS
AND WORDS OF WISDOM

Having representatives from the three key professions as well as an adequate number of trained facilitators present for the sessions requires considerable coordination and collaboration. We believe our collaborative efforts in IPE providing safe and effective teaching and learning contributes to creating safe and effective practitioners. Promoting simulation as a tool for quality improvement has helped us to promote in situ simulation as a routine and valuable part of our practice.

L. EVALUATION OF BEST PRACTICE STANDARDS
AND USE OF CREDENTIALED SIMULATION FACULTY

We have noted throughout this chapter the frameworks and standards of practice that inform our work. Our clinical faculty members are content experts in pediatric care, experienced teachers, and recipients of the trainer approach in simulation facilitation.

REFERENCES

Bernhard, M., Mohr, S., Weigand, M. A., Martin, E., & Walther, A. (2012). Developing the skill of endotracheal intubation: Implication for emergency medicine. *Acta Anaesthesiologica Scandinavica, 56*(2), 164–171.

Betihavas, V., Bridgman, H., Kornhaber, R., & Cross, M. (2016). The evidence for "flipping out": A systematic review of the flipped classroom in nursing education. *Nurse Education Today, 38,* 15–21.

Canadian Interprofessional Health Collaborative. (2010). A national interprofessional competency framework. Retrieved from http://www.cihc.ca/files/CIHC_IPCompetencies_Feb1210.pdf

ChildHealth BC. (2014). Children's emergency department tiers of service. Retrieved from http://childhealthbc.ca/?drawer=Tiers%20of%20Service

College of Registered of Nurses British Columbia. (2013). *Professional standards for registered nurses and nurse practitioners.* Vancouver, BC, Canada: Author. Retrieved from https://crnbc.ca/Standards/Lists/StandardResources/128ProfessionalStandards.pdf

Decker, S., Anderson, M., Boese, T., Epps, C., McCarthy, J., Motola, I.,...Scolaro, K. (2015). Standards of best practice: Simulation standard VIII: Simulation enhanced interprofessional education (Sim-IPE). *Clinical Simulation in Nursing, 11,* 293–297.

Dieckmann, R. A., Brownstein, D., & Gausche-Hill, M. (2010). The pediatric assessment triangle: A novel approach for the rapid evaluation of children. *Pediatric Emergency Care, 26*(4), 312–315.

Esau, R. (2013). *Pediatric drug dose guidelines.* British Columbia Children's and Women's Hospital Pharmacy, Therapeutics and Nutrition Committee. Retrieved from http://pedmed.org

Hall, R. E., Plant, J. R., Bands, C. J., Wall, A. R., Kang, J., & Hall, C. A. (2005). Human patient simulation is effective for teaching paramedic students endotracheal intubation. *Academic Emergency Medicine, 12*(9), 850–855.

Kleinman, M. (2013). Recognizing respiratory distress [Video broadcast and written material]. Retrieved from https://www.openpediatrics.org/assets/video/recognizing-respiratory-distress

Kusel, B., Farina, Z., & Aldous, C. (2014). Anaesthesia training for interns at a metropolitan training complex: Does it make the grade? *South African Family Practice, 56*(3), 201–205.

Long, E., Fitzpatrick, P., Cincotta, D. R., Grindlay, J., & Barrett, M. J. (2016). A randomised controlled trial of cognitive aids for emergency airway equipment preparation in a paediatric emergency department. *Scandinavian Journal of Trauma, Resuscitation and Emergency Medicine, 24,* 8.

Malec, J. F., Torsher, L. C., Dunn, W. F., Wiegmann, D. A., Arnold, J. J., Brown, D. A., & Phatak, V. (2007). The Mayo High Performance Teamwork Scale: Reliability and validity for evaluating key crew resource management skills. *Simulation in Healthcare, 2*(1), 4–10.

Morrow, D., Pascucci, R., Wolbrink, J., Smallwood, C., Manning, M., Craig, N.,...Bullock, K. (2015). Respiratory care curriculum: Invasive mechanical ventilation. Retrieved from https://www.open pediatrics.org/curriculum/respiratory-care-curriculum-invasive-mechanical-ventilation

Nishisaki, A., Nguyen, J., Colborn, S., Watson, C., Niles, D., Hales, R.,...Nadkarni, V. M. (2011). Evaluation of multidisciplinary simulation training on clinical performance and team behavior during tracheal intubation procedures in a pediatric intensive care unit. *Pediatric Critical Care Medicine, 12*(4), 406–414.

Rudolph, J. W., Simon, R., Rivard, P., Dufresne, R. L., & Raemer, D. B. (2007). Debriefing with good judgment: Combining rigorous feedback with genuine inquiry. *Anesthesiology Clinics, 25*(2), 361–376.

Wolbrink, T. (2015). Common intubation scenarios: Bronchiolitis [video broadcast and written material]. Retrieved from https://www.openpediatrics.org/assets/video/common-intubation-scenarios -bronchiolitis

CHAPTER 49

Prevention and Management
of Operating Room Fires

Nancy A. Moriber

A. IMPLEMENTATION OF SIMULATION-BASED
PEDAGOGY IN YOUR INDIVIDUALIZED TEACHING AREA

The use of simulation technology in health care education, certification, and recertification is becoming commonplace. In fact, students and practitioners alike are expecting to come in contact with simulation as part of the continuing-education process. Up to now, the focus of simulation in education has been on formative evaluation, where participants use simulation to reflect on their individual strengths and limitations, so that they can develop the skills necessary to integrate knowledge into practice (Glavin & Gaba, 2008). Increasingly, however, simulation as a summative assessment tool is becoming more popular in order to evaluate participants' readiness for practice. Simulation as a summative assessment tool allows for assessment of the critical thinking, prioritization, and interprofessional skills necessary for the provision of safe patient care in a highly complex patient-care environment (Glavin & Gaba, 2008).

The Fairfield University Egan School of Nursing and Health Studies (SON) has integrated simulation-based pedagogy across programs. The ultimate goal is to use simulation for both educational enrichment and assessment of student performance so that students can develop and demonstrate the attainment of the highly complex critical decision-making and communication skills necessary for nurse anesthesia practice. The following scenario can be used for both formative and summative assessment, and is applicable to senior-level undergraduate and entry-level advanced practice students (master's and doctoral preparation). It can also be used for continuing education with licensed practitioners who are involved in perioperative care.

This chapter focuses on the prevention and management of operating room (OR) fires. The students participating are required to identify high-risk situations, institute preventative measures, and appropriately manage an OR fire that occurs. The scenario is based on recommendations set forth by the American Society of Anesthesiologists Task Force on Operating Room Fires (2013).

B. EDUCATIONAL MATERIALS AVAILABLE IN YOUR
TEACHING AREA AND RELATED TO YOUR SPECIALTY

As stated in Chapter 32, the SON is moving into a new building and state-of-the-art simulation center on the Fairfield University campus in the fall of 2017. This facility embraces the simulation-based pedagogy adopted by the SON and has been designed to foster the development of psychomotor, cognitive, and affective clinical skills in the students enrolled in all programs. It is equipped with two fully functional ORs, as well as critical care, acute care, and primary care facilities to facilitate simulation across programs. Control rooms are adjacent to the simulation rooms and are designed to allow separation of the facilitators from the students participating in the scenarios to increase fidelity. The control rooms are equipped with the capability of recording and transmitting to adjacent classrooms in real time in order to facilitate effective debriefing.

In addition to the high-fidelity simulation rooms, independent skills labs have been incorporated to house the low-fidelity simulators and static trainers, which can also be used to supplement learning within the high-fidelity simulation environment. A stand-alone 20-bed graduate health assessment lab with integrated audiovisual capabilities for recording and debriefing will also be available for use. Faculty will have the ability to use recorded sessions for formative and summative evaluation of student performance within the health care setting.

The proposed scenario is run in the anesthesia room, which is fully equipped to simulate the operative environment. The scenario can be modified to other health care settings, where oxygen-enriched environments and fuel or ignition sources exist.

C. SPECIFIC OBJECTIVES FOR SIMULATION USAGE WITHIN A SPECIFIC COURSE AND THE OVERALL PROGRAM

The overarching objectives for this simulation focus on the development and implementation of crisis management, critical thinking, and interprofessional communication skills. They are consistent with the program essentials for undergraduate- and graduate-level education as set forth by the American Association of Colleges of Nursing (AACN; 2006, 2008, 2011). At the completion of the simulation the student is able to:

1. Implement crisis resource management skills in the perioperative setting.
2. Use critical thinking skills and current practice guidelines in the management of crisis situations.
3. Assume leadership roles in crisis situations.
4. Collaborate effectively with members of the perioperative care team and other health professionals during critical situations.
5. Communicate with peers and other health care professionals in the provision of patient-centered care.

This scenario is designed for undergraduate nursing students who have completed their medical–surgical training and have spent some time in the perioperative setting (from admission to the postanesthesia care unit). It can also be implemented at the graduate level in advanced-practice specialty courses for students whose primary area of practice is in the critical care or operative setting. This can include students enrolled in nurse anesthesia, clinical nurse specialist, or acute care nurse practitioner programs at either the master's or doctoral level.

This scenario addresses the following Baccalaureate Essentials (AACN, 2008):

Essential II: Basic Organizational and Systems Leadership for Quality Care and Patient Safety, Objectives 1, 2, 5 to 8
Essential VI: Interprofessional Communication and Collaboration for Improving Patient Health Outcomes, Objectives 2 to 6
Essential VII: Clinical Prevention and Population Health, Objective 9
Essential VIII: Professionalism and Professional Values, Objectives 1, 2
Essential IX: Baccalaureate Generalist Nursing Practice, Objectives 4, 12, 14

This scenario addresses the following Master's Essentials (AACN, 2011):

Essential II: Organizational and Systems Leadership, Objectives 1, 2
Essential III; Quality Improvement and Safety, Objectives 5 to 7
Essential V: Informatics and Healthcare Technologies, Objectives 1 to 5
Essential VII: Interprofessional Collaboration for Improving Patient and Population Outcomes, Objectives 3, 4, 6
Essential IX: Master's-Level Nursing Practice, Objectives 3, 11

This scenario addresses the following Doctoral Essentials (AACN, 2006):

Essential I: Scientific Underpinnings for Practice, Objectives 1, 2
Essential II: Organizational and Systems Leadership for Quality Improvement and Systems Thinking, Objective 2
Essential VI: Interprofessional Collaboration for Improving Patient and Population Health Outcomes, Objectives 1 to 3
Essential VIII: Advanced Nursing Practice, Objectives 2 to 4

D. INTRODUCTION OF SCENARIO

Setting the Scene

This scenario takes place in the OR. A 27-year-old, otherwise healthy male has just been taken into the OR where he is scheduled to undergo an excisional biopsy of an enlarged submandibular lymph node under general anesthesia with a laryngeal mask airway (LMA). The patient is placed on the OR table and attached to standard monitoring equipment, including EKG, blood pressure (BP) cuff, pulse oximeter, and end-tidal carbon dioxide monitoring. It is up to the OR team to determine the level of fire risk and implement appropriate precautionary measures, and manage the crisis situation as it develops. This scenario begins when the patient enters the operating suite.

Technology Used

In order to run this scenario, it is necessary to have a high-fidelity human patient simulator (HFHPS) so that the students involved in the simulation can visualize and respond to the hemodynamic changes that are implemented as part of the scenario. In addition, they are able to take the appropriate steps in the management of a compromised airway. If an HFHPS is not available, an actor can be substituted, but the instructors need to get more creative with displaying hemodynamic changes. If simulated patients are used it will also be necessary to provide adequate training to ensure that required behaviors are displayed during the scenario.

Access to patient records, either in electronic or paper format, is also necessary. As many hospitals use electronic records in the OR, access to electronic records would offer greater scenario realism and allow participants (anesthesia and nurses) to chart as would be appropriate in an actual surgical case. Audiotaped recordings of common OR sounds should be incorporated into the scenario to simulate the authenticity of noisy and hectic operative environment. Finally, video-recording equipment will be necessary so that the scenario can be taped for playback for evaluation and discussion purposes during debriefing sessions. If recording is planned, written permission should be obtained at the start of any simulation session or, ideally, on entrance into the training program. A blanket release form can be obtained and used to cover all simulation sessions in which a student participates during his or her educational experience.

Objectives

At the completion of this scenario, the student is able to:

1. Identify the three components of the "fire triad."
2. Identify procedures at high-risk for the development of OR fires
3. Implement preventative measures for OR fires
4. Discuss the early-warning signs of fire in the OR
5. Appropriately manage OR fires
6. Develop skills as a team leader, patient advocate, and effective communicator

The National Council Licensure Examination for a Registered Nurse (NCLEX-RN®) test plan categories and subcategories (National Council of State Boards of Nursing [NCSBN], 2015) addressed in this scenario include the following:

Safe and effective care environment: *Management of care* (advocacy, case management, collaboration with interdisciplinary team, establishing priorities, ethical practice, performance improvement [quality improvement], resource management), *Safety and infection control* (accident/injury prevention, emergency response plan, handling hazardous and infectious equipment, reporting of incident/event/irregular occurrence/variance, safe use of equipment); **Psychosocial integrity:** *Crisis intervention therapeutic communication*; **Physiological integrity:** *Reduction of risk potential* (potential for alterations in body systems, potential for complications from surgical procedures and health alterations), *Physiologic adaptation* (medical emergencies, pathophysiology).

Description of Participants

A total of five participants are required to run this scenario properly. Students involved take on the role of surgeon, anesthesia care provider, surgical scrub technician (certified surgical technologist [CST]), circulating nurse, and OR assistant or this can be run as an interprofessional simulation with students/practitioner from each of these specialties. In some situations, a second circulating nurse can be substituted for the anesthesia care provider because some surgical procedures are done under local anesthesia and sedation is not required. In these circumstances, a second circulating nurse is responsible for monitoring the patient and providing supplemental oxygen. Assessment can be conducted on one or all of the participants as it is essential that all members of the operative team work together to assure patient safety because the management of an OR fire requires a coordinated effort on the part of all participants. Therefore, the entire team should be evaluated with respect to its ability to function as part of the emergency response. The students must have completed a fire safety module, and ideally had exposure to medical–surgical nursing and the OR environment. If the simulation is run with graduate students it could be modified to include advanced airway management skills, especially if working with students in nurse anesthesia or critical care tracks.

The student taking on the role of circulating nurse is given the role of team leader and would be required to identify a high-risk operative procedure and to designate team roles for the prevention and management of an OR fire. The student assuming the role of the surgeon is responsible for controlling the ignition source in the form of the electrocautery and for placing surgical drapes, which can serve as a source of fuel for the OR fire. The surgeon is also required to *announce* the intent to use the ignition source during the surgical procedure. The student assuming the role of the CST is responsible for assisting the surgeon in the surgical procedure and participating in the management of the OR fire. The student taking on the role of anesthesia care provider is responsible for monitoring the patient's hemodynamic status, providing supplemental oxygen, and sedation as required. Finally, the student assuming the role of the OR assistant carries out tasks as directed by the circulating nurse such as obtaining equipment, activating the fire alarm, or assisting with the transport of the patient. All individuals participating in the scenario should have completed a fire safety module before the simulation is conducted.

Finally, two faculty members are required to run the simulation. One faculty member operates the patient simulator and acts as the voice of the patient. The other faculty member is embedded in the scenario so that someone is available to help facilitate movement and guide the students should it become necessary. If five students are not available for the simulation, the faculty member can serve as the surgeon and actively participate in the scenario. If a second faculty member is not available, it will still be possible to run the simulation but no one will be available to help guide the students if they require prompting at any point in time.

Controlling the Fuel Triad

As prevention of OR fires require manipulation of the "fire triad" by minimizing or avoiding an oxidizer-enriched atmosphere near the surgical site, managing ignition sources, and managing fuel sources, each member of the OR team has a specific role in the prevention of a fire. As surgical prep solutions serve as one of the primary fuel sources, it is the responsibility of the circulating nurse to ensure that prep solutions have dried and alcohol has dissipated before draping the patient. The surgeon is responsible for announcing that he is planning on using an ignition source before activating it, and the anesthesia care provider is responsible for minimizing the flow of oxygen into the surgical field. The fraction of inspired oxygen (FiO_2) delivered to the patient should be guided by the patient's oxygen saturation and pockets of oxygen under the drapes should be avoided. This requires effective closed-loop communication to verify steps before proceeding.

E. RUNNING OF THE SCENARIO

Before running the scenario, it is essential that all students have completed the didactic and clinical components necessary to effectively manage the scenario. Students should complete a fire safety module covering the "fire triad," identification of high-risk procedures, and prevention and management procedures. In addition, students should ideally have had some exposure to the OR in their clinical rotations, as this is a highly specialized environment in which there is significant interaction among many members of the health care team. It is difficult for students to take on these roles if they have not been given the opportunity to observe practitioners in the work environment. Students should also be made aware of the general purpose of the scenario—management of an OR fire—and provided with specific guidelines before attending the simulation session so that they can prepare appropriately.

All equipment necessary for running the scenario is available in the simulation room, including materials for the "fire triad" such as surgical prep solutions, surgical drapes, an electrocautery unit (can be simulated), and oxygen delivery systems. In order to simulate a fire, a smoke machine or dry ice is necessary. Participants need easy access to the materials required to extinguish a fire, including saline solution and a fire extinguisher.

F. PRESENTATION OF THE COMPLETED TEMPLATE

Title

Prevention and Management of Operating Room Fires

Scenario Level

This scenario can be modified to run with students at the baccalaureate, master's, and doctoral levels. All members of the perioperative team, regardless of their background, have a role in the prevention and management of these emergencies.

Focus Area

Emergency response, medical–surgical nursing, and operating room nursing

Scenario Description

Mr. Burnes is a 27-year-old male who comes to the OR for surgical excision of an enlarged left submandibular lymph node under monitored anesthesia care (MAC). He was in his usual state of health until 1 week before admission when he noticed a painless, hard mass under his jaw. He has had no other symptoms except for a 10-pound weight loss over the past 3 months. He is extremely anxious and tells the anesthetist that he does not want to hear or see anything.

He has no significant past medical history and is on no medication. He had a tonsillectomy at age 4 without complications. He is allergic to iodine. The scenario begins after the patient is brought to the operating suite by the anesthesia care provider and is placed on the monitors. Oxygen is placed at 3 L/min via nasal cannula. The surgeon, circulating nurse, and CST are already in the OR.

Scenario Objectives

At the completion of the simulation the students will be able to:

1. Identify the three components of the "fire triad"
2. Identify procedures at high-risk for the development of OR fires
3. Implement preventative measures for OR fires
4. Discuss the early-warning signs of fire in the OR
5. Appropriately manage OR fires
6. Develop skills as a team leader, patient advocate, and effective communicator

Setting the Scene

Equipment Needed

High-fidelity simulator; video-recording device; patient monitor; blood pressure (BP) cuff; EKG; pulse oximeter; oxygen flow meter; nasal cannula and face mask; intravenous line; intravenous pole; surgical prep solution; surgical drapes; sterile gowns; basic surgical set, including clamps, scissors, retractors, scalpels without blades, forceps; electrocautery devise, surgical sponges; irrigation solution and container; fire extinguisher; smoke machine; patient record (mock anesthesia and OR record); mock oxygen shut off valve

Resources Needed

Fire safety manual, phone to activate fire alarm

Simulator Level

High-fidelity simulation

Participants Roles

Five participants: circulating nurse (student role), CST (student role), anesthesia care provider (student role), surgeon (faculty facilitator or student), OR assistant (student), and faculty member to operate simulator

Scenario Implementation

Initial Settings for the High-Fidelity Simulator

BP: 128/80 mmHg, heart rate (HR): 98 beats/minute, respiratory rate (RR): 18 breaths/minute, arterial oxygen saturation (SpO_2): 99%

Required Student Assessments and Actions

___ Identifies procedure as high risk for fire.
___ Notifies OR team of the presence of an oxygen enriched environment.
___ Collaborates with team and articulates each practitioner's role in prevention:
   ___ Anesthesia care provider: Minimizes oxygen concentration to 21% before using the ignition source.
   ___ Surgeon: Announces intent to use ignition source and waits 1 to 3 minutes before use.
   ___ Circulating nurse: Allows prep solutions to dry.
   ___ CST: Moisten sponges and gauze on surgical field.
___ Preps patient and allows solution to dry before draping.
___ Drapes patient and conducts fire prevention time-out before incision.
___ Identifies early-warning signs of fire on the drapes such as unexpected flash or flame, presence of smoke or heat, unusual sounds (pop, snap) or odors, discoloration of the drapes or unexplained patient movement or complaint.
___ Halts procedure and calls for evaluation of situation.
___ If fire is present immediately ensures that:
   ___ All flow of oxygen is stopped by anesthesia care provider.
   ___ All drapes and burning materials are removed by surgeon and CST.
   ___ Burning materials are extinguished by pouring saline or suffocating.
   ___ OR assistant obtains fire extinguisher.
___ If fire persists in the OR (student performs or delegates): activates fire alarm, evacuates patient, closes OR door, and turns gas supply off to room.
   ___ Performs a head-to-toe focused assessment in collaboration with surgeon and anesthetist to determine extent of injury and airway involvement.
   ___ Reports OR fire to appropriate hospital and risk management personnel.

Instructor Interventions

The instructor running the simulator acts as the voice of the patient and is required to make appropriate changes to the patient's status in response to student behaviors. If the early-warning signs of fire go undetected, the faculty member embedded should provide verbal cues to the participants, facilitate student performance, and provide guidance in accordance with the terminal objectives.

Evaluation Criteria

Student performance in this scenario is evaluated using the rubric presented in Table 49.1 based on the degree to which he or she performs in appropriate order, with or without coaching, the actions outlined earlier. The effectiveness of this simulation as a learning tool can be assessed using a program's existing simulation assessments or course evaluation tools. It is essential to make sure that information regarding the students' overall impression of the simulation, including what worked well, what did not, and where improvement/change might be beneficial, is obtained so that improvements can be made to the simulation experiences.

Table 49.1	Evaluation Criteria for "Prevention and Management of an Operating Room Fire" Scenario		
Student Behavior	**Independent**	**Prompting**	**Appropriate Order**
Identifies procedure as high risk.			
Notifies OR team of the presence of an oxygen-enriched environment.			
Collaborates with team and articulates each practitioner's role in fire prevention:			
a. Anesthesia care provider: Minimizes oxygen concentration to 21% before using the ignition source.			
b. Surgeon: Announces the intent to use ignition source and waits 1–3 minutes before use.			
c. Circulating nurse: Allows prep solution to dry.			
d. CST: Moistens sponges and gauze on surgical field.			
Preps patient and allows solution to dry before draping.			
Drapes patient and conducts time-out reinforcing fire prevention before incision.			
Identifies early-warning sign of an operating room fire.			
Initial assessment is carried out in less than 10 minutes.			
Halts procedure and calls for evaluation of the situation.			
If the fire is present immediately ensures that:			
a. All flow of oxygen is stopped by anesthesia care provider.			
b. All drapes and burning materials are removed by surgeon and CST.			
c. Burning materials are extinguished by pouring saline or suffocating the fire.			
If fire persists in OR (performs or delegates):			
a. Activates fire alarm.			
b. Evacuates patient.			
c. Closes OR door.			
d. Turns off gas supply to room.			

(continued)

Table 49.1	Evaluation Criteria for "Prevention and Management of an Operating Room Fire" Scenario *(continued)*

Student Behavior	Independent	Prompting	Appropriate Order
Performs a head-to-toe focused assessment in collaboration with surgeon and anesthesia care provider to determine extent of injury and airway involvement.			
Reports OR fire to appropriate hospital and risk management personnel.			

CST, certified surgical technologist; OR, operating room.

G. DEBRIEFING GUIDELINES

Debriefing is essential if effective learning is to occur during a simulation experience because it encourages reflection, critical thinking, and group discussion. Video-taping capabilities would enhance the overall experience as well because it would give all students (participants and observers) the opportunity to reflect back on specific components of the simulation and constructively discuss individual and group performance. Students should be provided with the evaluation criteria before viewing the taped simulation so that they can compare and contrast actual performance with expected behaviors. Questions used to facilitate discussion should be open ended but focused enough so that they encourage student participation in the debriefing session. Some specific questions include:

1. Overall, how do you think the management of the OR fire went? What do you think you could have done differently? What would you do the same?
2. How can you manipulate the "fire triad"?
3. What would you have changed in your plan of care if the patient was sick or elderly and required high oxygen concentrations to prevent hypoxia?
4. What are some of the barriers to fire prevention/management in the OR?
5. How can you facilitate communication/collaboration among team members?
6. How would your management have differed if this were an airway fire?

H. SUGGESTIONS/KEY FEATURES TO REPLICATE OR IMPROVE AND RECOMMENDATIONS FOR FURTHER USE

OR fires are rare but when they occur can have devastating and permanently disfiguring consequences for the patient. *OR fires* are defined as fires that occur on or near patients who are under anesthesia (Caplan et al., 2008). These include surgical fires, which occur on or in a patient cavity, and airway fires, which occur within a patient's airway or within the anesthesia breathing circuit. Airway fires are uniquely challenging because they involve some degree of direct tissue injury and can impair a patient's ability to oxygenate effectively. Therefore, understanding the etiology, prevention, and management of all types of OR fires is essential for any provider working in or around the operative suite. As the management of an OR fire is a team effort, it would be ideal for participants in this scenario to rotate through the roles to gain experience in addressing all aspects of the fire triad. At any given time, any member of the surgical team may be called on to perform any of these tasks. They are not practitioner specific in any way.

As there are many types of OR fires that practitioners need to be able to manage, this scenario can be modified to target all types and incorporate advanced clinical skills such as those required in advanced practice nursing specialties. For example, this scenario could be modified for use in nurse anesthesia educational programs by changing the surgical procedure that the patient is undergoing to a tonsillectomy. This would require the usage of advanced airway management skills and would lend itself to the development of an airway fire in the scenario. Obviously, the terminal behavior objectives and evaluation criteria would need to be revised to address the additional requirements of the scenario, but the basic template would remain unchanged. In addition, the scenario could be built on and the focus changed to the address the postburn management by perhaps the acute care nurse practitioner. The possibilities are truly endless.

J. HOW SIMULATION-BASED PEDAGOGY CONTRIBUTES TO IMPROVED STUDENT OUTCOMES

Students enjoy using simulation as a learning tool because it provides them with the opportunity to develop psychomotor, cognitive, and affective skills in a less-threatening and safe environment. Students are able to take their management of patients down different pathways and see both the positive and negative consequences of their actions. As a result, they tend to not only have a better understanding of the physiologic and pharmacologic principles underlying patient management, but rate their overall educational experiences more positively.

Educators embrace simulation because it allows them to expose students to complex and rare clinical situations that may not be encountered during training. Using simulation, students can incorporate their didactic knowledge into their clinical acumen so that they are better prepared to handle these situations in actual practice. Simulation also helps educators in the remediation of students struggling in the clinical setting, especially if video-taping capabilities are available. Students can visualize their patient-care management and work with their instructors to develop mutually agreed on action plans. This is essential for "buy in" from students in these situations.

K. EXPERT RECOMMENDATIONS AND WORDS OF WISDOM

Crises occur in all practice settings and a coordinated, rapid response is essential to ensure the best possible outcomes for patients. However, not all practitioners possess the fundamental knowledge or skill to manage them appropriately. Fire-safety training is a key component of any institution's safety program and high-fidelity simulation is an ideal tool to use to reinforce these principles as thankfully, perioperative fires are rare. It is therefore recommended that nurses at all levels of clinical training and expertise participate in simulations that target these specific crisis situations.

L. EVALUATION OF BEST PRACTICE STANDARDS AND USE OF CREDENTIALED SIMULATION FACULTY

As discussed in Chapter 32, SON is in the process of becoming a Society for Simulation Healthcare (SSH) Accredited Program. The school is currently using the International Nursing Association for Clinical Simulation and Learning (INACSL) standards across programs and disciplines as a framework to confirm that faculty have the knowledge, skills, and abilities to facilitate quality health care simulation activities. The director of simulation is a graduated INACSL Fellow for year 2016 and is completing the Sim Lead fellowship for the National League for Nursing (NLN), which concluded in January 2017. She is also cochair of the state-wide sim consortium, the Health Care Simulation Network of Connecticut (CT), a subgroup of CT League for Nursing. The SON sees simulation as an integral component of the educational pedagogy linking the classroom to the clinical practice arena.

REFERENCES

American Association of Colleges of Nursing. (2006). *Essentials of doctoral education for advanced nursing practice.* Washington, DC: Author. Retrieved from http://www.aacnnursing.org/Portals/42/Publications/DNPEssentials.pdf

American Association of Colleges of Nursing. (2008). *Essentials of baccalaureate education for professional nursing practice.* Washington, DC: Author. Retrieved from http://www.aacnnursing.org/Portals/42/Publications/BaccEssentials08.pdf

American Association of Colleges of Nursing. (2011). *Essentials of master's education for advanced practice nursing.* Washington, DC: Author. Retrieved from http://www.aacnnursing.org/Portals/42/Publications/MastersEssentials11.pdf

American Society of Anesthesiologists Task Force on Operating Room Fires. (2013). Practice advisory for the prevention and management of operating room fires: An updated report by the American Society of Anesthesiologists Task Force on operating room fires. *Anesthesiology, 118*(2), 1–20.

Caplan, R. A., Barker, S. J., Connis, R. T., Cowles, C., de Richemond, A. L., Ehrenwerth, J., . . . Wolf, G. L. (2008). Practice advisory for the prevention and management of operating room fires. *Anesthesiology 108*(5), 786–801. doi:10.1097/01.anes.0000299343.87119.a9

Glavin, R. J., & Gaba, D. M. (2008). Challenges and opportunities in simulation and assessment. *Simulation in Healthcare: Journal of the Society for Simulation in Healthcare, 3*(2), 69–71.

National Council of State Boards of Nursing. (2015). *NCLEX-RN examination for the National Council Licensure Examination for Registered Nurses.* Chicago, IL: Author.

CHAPTER 50

Teaching and Learning Experiences on Safe Patient Transfers by Occupational Therapy and Nursing Students

Sharon R. Flinn and Julie L. Polanic

A. IMPLEMENTATION OF SIMULATION-BASED PEDAGOGY IN YOUR INDIVIDUALIZED TEACHING AREA

Early mobility of seriously ill patients results in fewer falls, lower ventilator-associated events, fewer pressure ulcers, and fewer catheter-associated urinary tract infections, as well as reducing hospital costs and improving functional independence in routine care (Fraser, Spiva, Forman, & Hallen, 2015). The ability of a patient to perform safe bed-to-chair transfers is considered one of the three gatekeeper tasks for establishing the destination of a patient at discharge, either the potential of independent living versus care in a skilled nursing facility or nursing home setting (Mokler, Sandstrom, Griffin, Farris, & Jones, 2000). Although this intervention benefits a majority of patients, potentially 29% of this group can be harmed during an assisted transfer (Guillaume, Crawford, & Quigley, 2016). In addition, 21% to 69% health care professionals report work-related musculoskeletal symptoms because of strenuous patient handling (Lee, Lee, & Gershon, 2015; Olkowski & Stolfi, 2014). In spite of the academic training that occurs for health care professionals in patient handling techniques, 40% report unsafe practices and injuries related to unanticipated actions, which can take place during patient transfers (Dyrkacz, Mak, & Heck, 2012). Therefore, a teaching and learning approach was selected to maximize self-efficacy and to improve patient handling skills for nursing and occupational therapy (OT) students.

B. EDUCATIONAL MATERIALS AVAILABLE IN YOUR TEACHING AREA AND RELATED TO YOUR SPECIALTY

Davenport University's Department of Nursing simulation laboratory currently houses six adjustable hospital beds; two examination tables; four high-fidelity human patient simulators, including SimMom, SimJunior, SimMan, and SimNewB; and three low-fidelity human patient simulators. The control center is capable of transmitting in real time and there is space available for debriefing. Additional equipment available includes armless chairs, intravenous (IV) supplies, urinary catheters, blood pressure (BP) equipment, and gait belts, all of which allow students to participate in this scenario. This scenario can be set up using minimal equipment to simulate the patient bedside.

C. SPECIFIC OBJECTIVES FOR SIMULATION USAGE WITHIN A SPECIFIC COURSE AND THE OVERALL PROGRAM

This scenario is intended for those enrolled in OCTH 636: Analysis of Environment, Task, and Activity for a graduate occupational therapy (OT) program and NURS 317: Health Assessment in Nursing, a second-year class in a 4-year baccalaureate program. Demographic data are provided for each group in Table 50.1.

The overall learning objective of the simulation is to safely transfer patients using proper body mechanics and preventing injury or harm to self or patient. Specific student activities are based on each discipline's learning objectives, including:

Occupational Therapy

1. Learn best practices for sit-stand transfers.
2. Facilitate higher levels of Bloom's taxonomy: comprehension, analysis, and evaluation.
3. Improve self-efficacy that assures one's perceived ability to safely perform patient transfers.
4. Reinforce interprofessional collaboration and common knowledge in proper patient-handling techniques between nursing and OT.

Nursing

1. Identify and develop nursing assessment skills.
2. Provide holistic, culturally sensitive, safe, and effective therapeutic nursing interventions in collaboration with individuals and families in multiple settings.
3. Identify the principles of the teaching–learning process to educate individuals and peers.
4. Identify and evaluate patient outcomes.
5. Identify and revise the plan of care based on individual patient outcomes.
6. Identify research and evidence-based information for application to nursing.

D. INTRODUCTION OF SCENARIO

Setting the Scene

The simulation takes place in a mock patient room. The patient lies flat in bed in a supine position. The OT student introduces the session to the nursing students, reviews a list of competencies for safe patient handling, and administers self-efficacy and learning-style inventories. The nursing student transfers an OT student, acting as the patient with an IV, from the bed to a chair on the side of the bed using a stand-pivot technique.

Table 50.1	Demographic Data	
Characteristics	**OT Students**	**Nursing Students**
Age	Mean: 26 years old *SD*: 5.01 years, range: 23–45 years	Mean: 26 years old *SD*: 7.7 years, range: 19–51 years
Gender	3 male, 23 female	3 male, 34 female
Ethnicity	23 White, 1 African American, 2 Asian	36 White, 1 African American

OT, occupational therapy; *SD*, standard deviation.

Technology Used

None

Objectives

Facilitate a teaching and learning style of interaction between OT and nursing students that results in the safest demonstration of a safe stand-pivot transfer for patients needing minimal to moderate assistance.

Description of Participants

The OT students play the role of the instructor, the patient, and the assessor. The nursing student plays the role of the health care professional transferring a patient.

E. RUNNING OF THE SCENARIO

The simulation experience and roles of each student are introduced as a formative assignment in a class in each discipline. A teaching and learning style of education is selected to facilitate inter-professional collaboration in acquiring the skills of safe patient handling techniques and proper body mechanics. This approach demonstrates the recall of tasks in previous courses, supports trial-and-error learning, and develops in-class strategies to be successful. The expectation is that students' preparation is crucial to the simulation and that active participation and "thinking on your feet" problem-solving skills are essential to completing the experience successfully. Despite the role assigned to the student, personal life experiences in working with patients is valued and encouraged in the process of learning.

F. PRESENTATION OF COMPLETED TEMPLATE

Title

Safe Patient Transfers by OT and Nursing Students

Scenario Level

Second-semester master's of occupational therapy students and first-semester BSN students

Focus Area

Inpatient care

Scenario Description

Patient History

An 84-year-old male patient, oriented, was admitted 24 hours ago with pneumonia, a past history of cardiovascular disease, atrial fibrillation, a blood disorder, and a history of falls.

Health Assessment Results

Nursing students complete a focused assessment of the patient, including vital signs, cardiac and respiratory systems, to identify any changes in patient condition before proceeding through the scenario.

Medication Record

Nursing students conduct a brief interview, including documentation of medications the patient takes on a routine basis, to identify potential interactions before proceeding through the simulation.

Scenario Objectives

For the scenario, National Council of State Boards of Nursing (NCSBN, 2015) National Council Licensure Examination for Registered Nurses (NCLEX-RN®) test plan categories address the following areas:

Safe and effective care environment: (collaboration with interdisciplinary team, continuity of care, establishing priorities); **Physiological integrity:** (basic care and comfort, safety and infection control); **Health promotion and maintenance; Psychosocial integrity**

    For student nurses, the American Association of Colleges of Nursing (AACN) *Essentials of Baccalaureate Education for Professional Nursing Practice* (AACN, 2008) addressed by scenario objectives include:

    Essential II: Basic Organizational and Systems Leadership for Quality Care
    Essential VI: Interprofessional Communication and Collaboration for Improving Health Care Outcomes
    Essential VIII: Professionalism and Professional Values

Setting the Scene

Environment

Medical–surgical, intensive care unit, acute, inpatient rehabilitation

Equipment needed

Working hospital bed with adjustable side rails and electronic controls for raising the head of the bed and height of the mattress, a bedside table to store props, a chair with arms for each hospital bed

Resources needed

Props include hand sanitizer, gait belt, blood pressure (BP) cuff, and stethoscope, intravenous (IV) tubing, and tape

Participants needed

One nursing student, three occupational therapy students, and one occupational therapy faculty observer/ adviser

Scenario Implementation

Expected/Required Student Assessments/Action

Presimulation (OT Students)

1. Complete terminology quiz on patient handling
2. Discuss unique roles in a teaching and learning environment
3. Review and practice criteria for transfer training in simulation lab as required by the participation style of teaching assigned to the group (Pendleton & Schultz-Krohn, 2013)

Patient Safety

1. Introduce self and wash hands
2. Assess patient ability preactivity; take BP
3. Share with patient the rationale for bed-to-chair transfer

Prepare Environment

1. Position chair at a 30° angle to bed
2. Position IV pole on transfer side
3. Use proper body mechanics; first practice

Pretransfer Positioning

1. Raise bed to sitting position
2. Bring feet off the edge of the bed
3. Shift patient body to sitting position
4. Adjust bed height so feet are flat on floor
5. Scoot patient buttocks to edge of the bed
6. Stabilize lower body of the patient with your knees
7. Provide clear directions to the patient on his or her role in the transfer
8. Use proper body mechanics; second practice

Stand-Pivot Transfer

1. Check patient response for pulse, dizziness, any other observations
2. Apply gait belt and grab it in the back of the patient
3. Stand, turn buttocks with smooth, controlled movements to chair
4. Ensure patient leg is against chair and hands on armrest
5. Lower patient smoothly
6. Use proper body mechanics; third practice

Review and Practice Criteria for Body Mechanics

1. Stay close to the patient
2. Position your body to face the patient
3. Keep a neutral spine
4. Keep wide base of support; heels down
5. Bend knees; use legs, not your back
6. Walk with the patient; avoid rotating when bending

Day of Simulation

1. Instructors set up environment and equipment to specifications
2. BSN students are assigned to one of three teaching groups:
   Observation dominant (OD): two peer observations, one hands-on demo
   Participation dominant (PD): one peer observation, two hands-on demos
   Participation only (PO): No peer observations, three hands-on demos
3. OT instructor reviews simulation, answers questions from OT students
4. OT student assumes roles, greets nursing students, and requests presimulation self-efficacy and learning-style inventory forms completed by the nursing students

5. OT student introduces simulation, verbally reviews posted competencies for stand-pivot transfer and proper body mechanics, provides 0 to 2 demonstrations based on BSN student assignment

6. BSN student demonstrates competencies for stand-pivot transfers and proper body mechanics without posted form, immediately prompted by OT students on performance except for final BSN student hands-on demonstration

7. All students discuss competencies and personal experiences with real patients that may improve the quality of the demonstration

8. OT student confirms satisfactory completion of competencies for each BSN student

9. OT student requests postsimulation self-efficacy and learning-style inventory forms from the nursing student

10. Expected activity run time: 30 minutes/BSN student

Instructor Interventions

The OT instructor is present during the simulations and provides direct prompts to the OT student instructors if errors occur in the performance of the stand-pivot transfer and/or body mechanics. However, students are encouraged to answer their questions within the group.

Evaluation Criteria

The written competencies for stand-pivot transfers and proper body mechanics are used.

G. DEBRIEFING GUIDELINES

During the simulation, there is an immediate student-to-student feedback, from an occupational therapy student to a nursing student. Following the completion of the simulation, every student was asked to contribute personal challenges, outlining strengths and areas of growth, the perception of the other discipline as a student and a professional, and opportunities for future collaboration as health care professionals. Twenty minutes were provided for guided reflection and debriefing time. Student and instructor dialogue for each discipline is important to clarify the simulation scenario and to identify any recommendations for change. Instructor-to-instructor debriefing provides an opportunity to further develop the simulation experience.

H. SUGGESTIONS/KEY FEATURES TO REPLICATE

This simulation built on the knowledge obtained in regular classroom activities by challenging students to be active participants who are invested in preventing a frequently occurring clinical concern. It provided BSN students the ability to refresh mobility skills learned in the first 7 weeks of their second academic year and 6-week clinical experience within the nursing program. OT students were presented with the responsibility of setting up a competency-based, safe experience for the nursing students. This scenario combined the techniques of safely transferring patients with the application of proper body mechanics. Students from both disciplines were able to meet and collaborate in a nonthreatening environment with a shared purpose to provide safe patient care. Positive reports were received from cohorts.

I. RECOMMENDATIONS FOR FURTHER USE

Several changes would be useful based on student and instructor feedback. They include:

1. This simulation can occur in the first 7 weeks of the BSN student's second academic year, before their first clinical experience. This could prevent serious injury to students or patients and reinforces safe transfer practices before their acute inpatient encounter.
2. A second simulation can replace this scenario and explore the use of standardized patients instead of classmates. Varying ages, medications, and conditions would be applied to provide a more realistic approach to basic patient care. Increased levels of difficulty would be introduced with common scenarios involving patients from postoperative, cardiac, pulmonary, chronic medical, respiratory, urinary, and orthopedic settings (Baird, Raina, Rogers, O'Donnell, & Holm, 2015).
3. Simulation can include other health care professionals, such as physical therapy graduate students, to maximize self-efficacy and improve patient-handling skills.

J. HOW SIMULATION-BASED PEDAGOGY HAS CONTRIBUTED TO IMPROVED STUDENT OUTCOMES

Simulation-based pedagogy has contributed to improved student outcomes by increasing self-efficacy (individual's belief that he or she can succeed in executing a task) and expanding critical thinking skills. A simulation scenario can be modified to include a disease or skill that the student has been unable to observe in the clinical environment or include a variable such as a combative patient. Practicing in a controlled, safe environment allows the students to accrue knowledge and competency necessary for successful completion of the nursing and occupational therapy curriculum.

K. EXPERT RECOMMENDATIONS AND WORDS OF WISDOM

Collaborating with another discipline in providing a simulation experience indicates to the students how valuable the interdisciplinary team is in providing safe patient care. Although not always easy to insert into an already full nursing and occupational therapy curriculum, it is worth the time to use this simulation scenario to improve patient-handling skills with your students.

L. EVALUATION OF BEST PRACTICE STANDARDS AND USE OF CREDENTIALED SIMULATION FACULTY

Collaboration between occupational therapy and nursing requires the ability to maintain professional integrity of the participants. In this scenario, mutual respect for various disciplines is expected and supported. To achieve the desired outcome of the scenario, each teaching and learning experience between the occupational therapy and nursing students must be received in a safe learning environment. Constructive feedback is encouraged but must be delivered in a respectful manner (Gloe et al., 2013). Simulation experiences provide increased knowledge and improved clinical thinking in the BSN prelicensure student. Therefore, the use of credentialed simulation faculty is encouraged to ensure evidence-based practices in the simulation experience. Currently, our campus does not employ a certified simulation educator, but we do follow evidence-based guidelines in our simulation scenarios. Two current faculty members have completed a certificate in the simulation from Drexel University.

Occupational therapy students were required to analyze data from this experience for another course. Posters were created by the occupational therapy students, and a formal session was scheduled to present findings and to encourage discussion with occupational therapy and nursing faculty and students.

REFERENCES

American Association of Colleges of Nursing. (2008). *The essentials of baccalaureate education for professional nursing practice*. Washington, DC: Author. Retrieved from http://www.aacnnursing.org/Portals/42/Publications/BaccEssentials08.pdf

Baird, J. M., Raina, K. D., Rogers, J. C., O'Donnell, J., & Holm, M. B. (2015). Wheelchair transfer simulations to enhance procedural skills and clinical reasoning. *American Journal of Occupational Therapy*, 69(Suppl. 2), 1–8. doi:10.5014/ ajot.2015.018697

Dyrkacz, A. P., Mak, L. Y., & Heck, C. S. (2012). Work-related injuries in Canadian occupational therapy practice. *Canadian Journal of Occupational Therapy [Revue Canadienne D'ergotherapie]*, 79(4), 237–247.

Fraser, D., Spiva, L., Forman, W., & Hallen, C. (2015). Original research: Implementation of an early mobility program in an ICU. *American Journal of Nursing*, 115(12), 49–58.

Gloe, D., Sando, C. R., Franklin, A. E., Boese, T., Decker, S., Lioce, L., . . . Borum, J. C. (2013). Standards of best practice: Simulation standard II: Professional integrity of participant(s). *Clinical Simulation in Nursing*, 9(6S), S12–S14.

Guillaume, D., Crawford, S., & Quigley, P. (2016). Characteristics of the middle-age adult inpatient fall. *Applied Nursing Research*, 31, 65–71.

Lee, S. J., Lee, J. H., & Gershon, R. R. (2015). Musculoskeletal symptoms in nurses in the early implementation phase of California's safe patient handling legislation. *Research in Nursing & Health*, 38(3), 183–193.

Mokler, P. J., Sandstrom, R., Griffin, M., Farris, L., & Jones, C. (2000). Predicting discharge destination for patients with severe motor stroke: Important functional tasks. *Neurorehabilitation and Neural Repair*, 14(3), 181–185.

National Council of State Boards of Nursing. (2015). NCLEX-RN examination: Test plan for the National Council Licensure Examination for Registered Nurses. Retrieved from https://www.ncsbn.org/RN_Test_Plan_2016_Final.pdf

Olkowski, B. F., & Stolfi, A. M. (2014). Safe patient handling perceptions and practices: A survey of acute care physical therapists. *Physical Therapy*, 94(5), 682–695. doi:10.2522/ptj.20120539

Pendleton, H. M., & Schultz-Krohn, W. (2013). *Mobility in Pedretti's occupational therapy practice skills for physical dysfunction* (7th ed.). St. Louis, MO: Elsevier Mosby.

CHAPTER 51

Professional Integrity in Interdisciplinary Simulation: Creating Workforce Relationships in Occupational Therapy and Nursing

Theresa L. Leto

A. IMPLEMENTATION OF SIMULATION-BASED PEDAGOGY IN YOUR INDIVIDUALIZED TEACHING AREA

The Master of Science in Occupational Therapy program at Davenport University in Grand Rapids, Michigan, is a new graduate program for the university. The occupational therapy program achieved initial accreditation from the Accreditation Council for Occupational Therapy Education (ACOTE) in April 2016. The curriculum consists of seven semesters that progress student learning from the basic tenets and theoretical perspectives of occupational therapy to the knowledge, skills, and critical thinking required for managing the complex care of a diverse client base.

The Institute of Medicine (IOM; 2003) identifies five core competencies for the delivery of quality health care that is required of all health care providers. These core competencies serve as an overarching aim for quality health services. Interdisciplinary simulation exercises occur in the first semester of the program involving occupational therapy and nursing students, and were based on two of these competencies.

The first competency is the ability to provide patient centered care. This competency targets specific skills for meeting the needs of patients, including respect for patients' individual values and preferences, as well as the communication skills required to maintain a therapeutic relationship with patients. The second of the competencies, the ability to work in interdisciplinary teams, requires skills in collaboration as well as effective communication. When stated another way, quality health care is dependent on strong professional relationships. Occupational therapy practitioners connect with nurses in every clinical setting. These professional relationships then, should be forged early in the educational curriculum and fostered throughout a professional program regardless of the discipline. To this end, interdisciplinary simulations with occupational therapy and nursing students begin in the first semester of the Davenport University occupational therapy program.

In the first semester, two courses involve simulations. One course, OCTH 616: Fundamentals and Scope of Occupational Therapy Practice, as the title implies, introduces the fundamentals and scope of occupational therapy practice. In this course, the emphasis is placed on communication with both clients and professional colleagues throughout a person-centered health care relationship. Communication strategies learned in this course include but are not limited to active listening, clear delivery of information, ethical communication, respecting the values and differences of others, and collaborative goal setting for occupational therapy interventions. Interdisciplinary simulations were created to apply specific concepts and skills from classroom learning.

The second course in the first semester linked to the simulations was OCTH 621: Acute and Chronic Conditions: Effect on Occupational Performance. This course includes the study of body systems and pathology, and explores the effects of illness and disease on a person's ability to engage in daily occupations. The student learning outcomes of this course assist the occupational therapy student in anticipating and predicting the effect of disease, illness, and injury on an individual's functional abilities. The content of this course also assists the student in developing an understanding of the medical environment as well as skills in monitoring and measuring clinical signs of activity intolerance. During the first semester, there are three interdisciplinary simulation exercises. The interdisciplinary simulation that follows focuses on professional communication and is seated within these two courses.

B. EDUCATIONAL MATERIALS AVAILABLE IN YOUR TEACHING AREA AND RELATED TO YOUR SPECIALTY

The simulation met the design concepts established by the International Nursing Association for Clinical Simulation and Learning (INACSL) as outlined in *INACSL Standards of Best Practice: Simulation*[SM] (INACSL, 2013/2016). The simulation was directly related to concepts taken from classroom learning activities. Spaces used for the simulation included classroom areas used by the occupational therapy program and modified to best replicate the health care environment in which the scenario might occur that established physical fidelity. The simulation occurred in a large classroom with desks and chairs arranged much like a therapy gym or outpatient setting located in a hospital or rehabilitation facility. Traditionally, in these settings, there are multiple therapists and clients involved in the rehabilitation process at the same time, which can create a high-level of activity and a lack of privacy. In this sense, the simulation environment created high psychological fidelity. At the start of the semester, occupational therapy and nursing faculty collaborated for scheduling, as well as reviewing and modifying the procedures for the simulation. Planning included consideration of the number of students from each discipline, scheduling of the simulation within the semester, timing protocols, use of the physical environment, the equipment needed and faculty supervision needed for each simulation planned for the semester.

C. SPECIFIC OBJECTIVES FOR SIMULATION USAGE WITHIN A SPECIFIC COURSE AND THE OVERALL PROGRAM

The overall objective of the simulation exercise was to meet the 2013 educational standards established by ACOTE (American Occupational Therapy Association [AOTA], 2011). Table 51.1 shows the ACOTE standards addressed by the OCTH 616 and OCTH 621 courses in contrast to the American Association of Colleges of Nursing (AACN) *Essentials of Baccalaureate Education for Professional Nursing Practice* (AACN, 2008). Specific objectives for the simulation were based on these standards.

D. INTRODUCTION OF SCENARIO

Setting the Scene

The scenario included a list of equipment and supplies needed to replicate the simulation. The supplies and equipment were available in both the occupational therapy and nursing programs.

Table 51.1	Comparison of Professional Program Educational Standards	
Accreditation Standards for a Master's-Degree-Level Educational Program for the Occupational Therapist (AOTA, 2011)	*The Essentials of Baccalaureate Education for Professional Nursing Practice* (AACN, 2008)
Effectively communicate and work interprofessionally with those who provide services to individuals, organizations, and/or populations in order to clarify each member's responsibility in executing an intervention plan.	Demonstrate appropriate team building and collaborative strategies when working with interprofessional teams.
Explain the role of occupation in the promotion of health and the prevention of disease and disability for the individual family and society.	Contribute the unique nursing perspective to interprofessional teams to optimize patient outcomes.
Demonstrate knowledge and understanding of the AOTA code of ethics, ethics standards, and standards of practice and use them as a guide for ethical decision making in professional interactions, client interventions, and employment settings.	Demonstrate the professional standards of moral, ethical, and legal conduct. Access interprofessional and intraprofessional resources to resolve ethical and other practice dilemmas.
Use standardized and nonstandardized screening and assessment tools to determine the need for occupational therapy intervention. Evaluate client's occupational performance in ADL, IADL, education. Work, play, rest, sleep, leisure, and social participation using standardized and nonstandardized assessment tools.	Conduct comprehensive and focused physical, behavioral, and psychological–spiritual, socioeconomic, and environmental assessment of health and illness parameters in patient using developmentally and culturally appropriate approaches.
Demonstrate therapeutic use of self, including one's personality, insights, perceptions and judgments, as part of the therapeutic process in both individual and group interaction. Provide therapeutic use of occupation, exercises and activities.	Engage in caring and healing techniques that promote a therapeutic nurse–patient relationship.

Source: 2011 Accreditation Council for Occupational Therapy Education (ACOTE®) Standards. Originally published in 2012 in *American Journal of Occupational Therapy, 66*, S6–S74. http://dx.doi.org/10.5014/ajot.2012.66S6. Copyright© 2012 by the American Occupational Therapy Associated. Used with permission.

ADL, activities of daily living; AOTA, American Occupational Therapy Association; IADL, instrumental activities of daily living.

Technology Used

There is no technology required beyond the physical environment replicating the clinical setting.

Objectives

The student will:

1. Demonstrate therapeutic communication through completion of an occupational profile
2. Demonstrate competency in a selected skill in screening, evaluation, and referral within a scenario
3. Demonstrate understanding of the code of ethics and standards of practice and its use in decision making

Description of Participants

Participants in the simulation included the occupational therapy students, nursing students, and faculty from both disciplines. Nursing students portrayed a standardized patient in the scenarios. Faculty were present from both disciplines and acted as facilitators. The facilitators were seasoned clinicians with deep knowledge of content and the skill base to be addressed by the simulation.

E. RUNNING OF THE SCENARIO

The scenarios were developed to reinforce the knowledge and skills acquired in classroom learning activities. This simulation exercise lasted approximately 2 hours in length and was strategically positioned in the semester to best match the course content. For example, occupational therapy students learned about therapeutic communication and specific pathologies before the simulation. In additional, occupational therapy students learned standards of practice and the occupational therapy code of ethics. Nursing students had progressed through the nursing program whereby they possessed a good understanding of the diagnoses and conditions portrayed in the standardized patient scenarios.

The path of the session was directed by the occupational therapy student and the responses from the standardized patients during the simulation. Students were provided with performance expectations verbally and in writing 1 week in advance of the simulation. Students were permitted to orient themselves to the simulation environment at their own convenience any time before the day of the simulation if they chose to do so. Students were encouraged to review relevant readings and practice skills that applied to the scenario. Before the start of the simulation, students were reassured that the results of the experience were confidential. However, as the students were in an open space during the simulation, they may have been observed by their peers. They were oriented to the physical space and the location of the equipment likely needed during the simulation verbally and through a visit to the simulation environment at their discretion. Student expectations were stated again immediately before the start of the simulation. The simulation included the element of time pressure and the student was responsible for the flow and pacing of the simulation. Once the simulation had begun, it was allowed to progress without interruption unless a safety concern developed. Otherwise, the facilitator observed the simulated interventions as they unfolded (INACSL, 2013/2016). At the end of the simulation, nursing students stepped out of their role as the standardized patient and provided direct feedback to the occupational therapy students about the effectiveness of communication strategies employed during the session.

F. PRESENTATION OF COMPLETED TEMPLATE

Title

Simulation #1—Occupational Profile

Scenario Level

The level of this scenario is intended for an advanced beginner

Focus Area

Occupational therapy, general practice

Scenario Description

The occupational therapy scenario replicates an outpatient therapy setting. The patient arrives in the occupational therapy department with a physician referral and is evaluated by the occupational therapist. Occupational therapy and nursing students arrive in the occupational therapy classroom and separate into to their respective roles. Occupational therapy students function as therapists while nursing students function as standardized patients referred to occupational therapy for intervention. The nursing student randomly chooses a patient identity that includes a brief history and specific behavioral characteristics that are portrayed during the interaction. The gender of the standardized patients modified to reflect the gender of the nursing student playing the role of the patient. The patient's identity and history are withheld from the occupational therapy student. The identities for the standardized patients include:

- A 27-year-old with a history of a traumatic brain injury; the injury is a result of a ride on the back of a four-wheeler that was driven by the spouse
- A 30-year-old single parent with a flexor tendon injury to the dominant hand
- A 65-year-old with the diagnosis of left cerebral vascular accident affecting the dominant upper limb; this patient is new to a long-term care facility and is hoping to be a temporary resident
- A 50-year-old who works in a factory that assembles small parts with electrical wiring and now has an upper limb injury sustained on the job
- A 70-year-old divorced person newly released from the hospital after right-knee replacement with complications; this patient currently lives with his daughter but wants to return to an apartment located on the upper level of an apartment building

Scenario Objectives

1. The occupational therapy student obtains information from the patient through an occupational profile to include the patient'soccupational history and experiences, daily habits and routines, interests, values and current concerns.
2. The occupational therapy student implements therapeutic communication strategies, including interview techniques, to elicit information from the patient necessary to complete the evaluation process.

The scenario reflects the following AOTA (2011) standards:

Standard B.4.0: Screening, Evaluation and Referral
Standard B.5.7: Demonstrate Therapeutic Use of Self

The AACN *Essentials of Baccalaureate Education for Professional Nursing Practice* (AACN, 2008) reflected in the scenario:

Essential IX: Baccalaureate Generalist Nursing Practice

The National Council of State Boards of Nursing (NCSBN, 2015) test plan for the National Council Licensure Examination for Registered Nurses (NCLEX-RN°) addressed in the simulation include the following:

Psychosocial integrity (therapeutic communication, therapeutic environment)

Setting the Scene

Equipment Needed

___ Large open area to replicate clinical space
___ Tables and chairs
___ Occupational therapy referrals reflecting each patient scenario
___ Timing implement such as a timer
___ Optional props simulating documentation
___ Optional props simulating characteristics of the standardized patient

Participant Roles

Patient

The patient is ambulatory and enters the clinic area. The patient presents the referral to a faculty member who acts as the office receptionist. The patient is seated in the clinical waiting area until the therapist is ready to begin the session. The patient is assigned to a therapist by the receptionist. The patient displays the behavioral characteristics consistent with the assigned diagnosis and contextual elements described to the patient in each scenario, which is unknown to the therapist at the start of the evaluation session. For example, the single parent with the flexor tendon injury is unable to complete some parenting responsibilities because of the injury. This patient is also unable to work and has financial concerns that would impact full participation in occupational therapy that would improve his or her functional capacity.

Therapist

The therapist is professionally dressed. The therapist greets the patient and introduces him-or herself by name and asks the patient how he or she prefers to be addressed. The therapist confirms the information presented on the referral sheet presented by the patient. The therapist describes the evaluation process and provides an approximate length of the therapy session. He or she asks about the patient's comfort and pain level and moves forward with the occupational profile using therapeutic communication techniques. These techniques could include strategic questions that are open ended in nature, pacing questions as indicated by the patient's responses, and active listening. The therapist responds to the patient's behavior and responses to interview questions according to occupational therapy standards of practice. He or she terminates the session based on standards of practice, including scheduling of subsequent therapy appointment and distribution of a business card.

Scenario Implementation

The simulation is implemented within the time frame of scheduled course hours. Students are expected to pace the session such that it is initiated and terminated in a 15-minute time frame. Students are expected to arrive prepared for the simulation knowledgeable about characteristics typically associated with the diagnosis.

Instructor Interventions

The facilitator only intervenes if the safety of patient or therapist is compromised.

Evaluation Criteria

Exhibit 51.1 shows the assessment completed by the nursing students as feedback to the occupational therapy students from the standardized patient perspective.

Exhibit 51.1			

OT Student Name _____   Nursing Student Name _____

Start time: End time:

Nursing student feedback to OT student

Therapeutic interaction	Yes	No	Comments
OT student introduced himself/herself.			
OT student explained occupational therapy.			
OT student made eye contact.			
OT student established rapport.			
OT student's affect matched the affect of the client.			
OT student facilitated conversation through strategic questioning.			
OT student responded to behaviors of client appropriately/therapeutically.			
OT student was able to elicit client's perspective on current concerns, goals, and desired outcome of intervention.			
OT student used active listening strategies, including but not limited to: ☐ Sharing observations ☐ Acknowledging feelings ☐ Clarifying and validating ☐ Reflecting and paraphrasing			
Other comments:			

OT, occupational therapy.

G. DEBRIEFING GUIDELINES

Issues to Consider

Time

Allow enough time for debriefing so that meaningful reflection and summary can take place. Initial debriefing occurred directly following the simulation. Time constraints limited the depth of reflection that helps the student connect the experience with the objectives of the simulation. Debriefing occurred the following time the class met together, however, since a full week had elapsed, active student engagement in the conversation was limited. Students were invited to make an appointment with faculty for further analysis and reflection of their session. As faculty was present during the simulation, additional information and analysis of performance could be shared. Additional debriefing may be considered balanced with the amount of class time needed, room reservations, schedules among the disciplines, and other technical considerations.

Confidentiality

As multiple simulations occurred simultaneously and in a shared space, students were in full view of one another and could see and hear peer performances. Students received immediate feedback from the nursing students so confidentiality of the session and the feedback received may have been inadvertently compromised.

Feedback Bias

Nursing students were familiarized with the feedback tool. However, assessment of student performance by another student is subjective. Some nursing students were uncomfortable providing feedback that might appear negative to occupational therapy students, especially if they were of the opposite sex.

H. SUGGESTIONS/KEY FEATURES TO REPLICATE OR IMPROVE

There are many advantages in using high-fidelity simulation. Through the use of standardized patients, occupational therapy students build on specific skills in a safe environment with a minimal safety risk. The occupational profile simulation can be modified for any occupational therapy practice setting such as hospital, rehabilitation, home health or long-term care settings. In the future, the simulated patient scenarios can increase in complexity with heightened expectations of student performance as the students move through the occupational therapy program. Allowing more time for debriefing immediately following the simulation would be more meaningful to the students in terms of content, but also in relieving anxiety about their own performance. There may be a way to structure debriefing such that faculty could thoroughly document observations on an electronic tool, such as a computer or tablet, and deliver this level of feedback directly to the student's electronic account for private viewing. In this way, the student would receive feedback from the standardized patient as well as a skilled observer directly after the simulation.

I. RECOMMENDATIONS FOR FURTHER USE

When replicating this simulation, a structured format, such as a template, to help the standardized patients prepare for their roles should be included. For this experience, in an attempt to make written instructions clear and brief, in some cases, the description and background story of the standardized patients and their identified concerns were a bit sparse. As the nursing students were familiar with typical characteristics of specific diagnoses in the scenarios, they were able to accurately portray the patient. Pilot testing the simulation may have acknowledged this gap (INACSL, 2013/2016).

The scenarios can be further developed to require the use of the Department of Nursing simulation lab. A portion of the simulation lab at Davenport University is designed to reproduce a traditional medical–surgical unit in a hospital. Including content in the scenario that demonstrates more complex patient behaviors, adding a caregiver, assessing for activity intolerance, and monitoring vital signs would be practical modifications to the scenario that would allow students of both disciplines to meet their respective educational standards. In the more complex standard patient scenario, the pressures of clinical reasoning, rapid problem solving, and decision making that is part of practice in a hospital setting can be recreated. The students could demonstrate proficiency in any number of procedural and caring skills required in general practice.

J. HOW SIMULATION-BASED PEDAGOGY HAS CONTRIBUTED TO IMPROVED STUDENT OUTCOMES

To assess the impact of simulation on student outcomes, analysis of student performance was based on skilled observation by faculty, classroom discussions, and course evaluations. Student commentary indicates that students highly value all experiential learning opportunities, however, students report that high-fidelity simulation helps them gain confidence in their existing skills and prompts "feeling like a therapist." It also helps them identify areas for individual improvement.

The high-fidelity simulation seems to move the students closer to professional practice as they prepare for direct patient care. Students also highly valued the interdisciplinary nature of this simulation. Students of different disciplines were required to work together during the simulation to achieve an outcome, much like professional practice.

K. EXPERT RECOMMENDATIONS AND WORDS OF WISDOM

This simulation exercise presents an opportunity for the student to gain insight into his or her personal communication style. Students can confuse therapeutic communication with conversational communication where skills in redirection, limit setting, or crisis management are not required. This experience prompts deeper reflection and provides concepts for discussion throughout the semester. The challenges in planning this simulation surrounded coordinating space, student groups, establishing clear objectives, and time. For example, occupational therapy students may be available but students from another discipline may not be. Institutions may require room reservations be made a year in advance. The recommendation is to begin planning, at minimum, one semester before the simulation is scheduled to occur. When collaborating with another discipline, objectives need to be clearly articulated so that all participants understand that the objectives drive the simulation.

The design of future simulations allows time to fully pilot the simulation scenarios before implementation. For example, the amount of time needed for debriefing and resetting the simulation space was unanticipated. Piloting may also have eliminated the pressure associated with completing the simulation with all students in the time frame allotted. Enough time for deep reflection on the experience is added so that students can integrate new learning with existing knowledge.

L. EVALUATION OF BEST PRACTICE STANDARDS AND USE OF CREDENTIALED SIMULATION FACULTY

Currently, ACOTE or other official documents of the American Occupational Therapy Association (AOTA) provides no standards for the use of simulation or credentialing in occupational therapy education. Occupational Therapy Council (2013) has guidelines for simulation used in occupational therapy education but no standards and these guidelines are based on published evidence in other disciplines (Harris, 2016). Faculty involved in this simulation were advanced practice clinicians and educators. Previous teaching experience in curriculum development and educational strategies supported the development of the simulation. In addition to this experience, INACSL best practice standards (INACSL, 2013/2016) provided detailed information for the design as well as a glossary of terms that facilitated understanding of the standards. This is particularly helpful as literature shows that some terms about simulation in education can be used erroneously (Beaubien & Baker, 2004). Simulation in occupational therapy education is gaining momentum and the INACSL standards provide guidance until the time that discipline-specific standards or expectations are established. INACSL best practice standards (2013/2016) can offer design guidance to educators of many health care disciplines, particularly if they are new to simulation or curriculum design. These standards can provide a common language furthering the development of workforce relationships.

REFERENCES

American Association of Colleges of Nursing. (2008). *Essentials of baccalaureate education for professional nursing practice.* Washington, DC: Author. Retrieved from http://www.aacnnursing.org/ Portals/42/Publications/BaccEssentials08.pdf

American Occupational Therapy Association. (2011). Accreditation Council for Occupational Therapy Education standards and interpretive guide. Retrieved from http://www.aota.org/Education -Careers/Accreditation/StandardsReview.aspx

Beaubien, J. M., & Baker, D. P. (2004). The use of simulation for training teamwork skills in health care: How low can you go. *Quality and Safety in Healthcare, 13*(Suppl. 1), i51–i56. doi:10.1136/ qshc.2004.009845

Harris, J. (2016). Simulation in occupational therapy education. *Occupational Therapy Now, 18*, 18–19.

Institute of Medicine. (2003). *Health professions education: A bridge to quality.* Washington, DC: National Academies Press.

International Nursing Association for Clinical Simulation and Learning. (2013, updated 2016). INACSL standards of best practice: Simulation. Retrieved from http://www.inacsl.org/i4a/pages/index .cfm?pageid=3407

National Council of State Boards of Nursing. (2015). *NCLEX-RN examination: Test plan for the National Council Licensure Examination for Registered Nurses.* Retrieved from https://www.ncsbn.org/ RN_Test_Plan_2016_Final.pdf

FURTHER READING

Bethea, D. P., Castillo, D. C., & Harvison, N. (2014). Use of simulation in occupational therapy education: Way of the future? *American Journal of Occupational Therapy, 68*, S32–S39. doi:10.5014/ ajot.2014.012716

Greidanus, E., King, S., LoVerso, T., & Ansell, L. D. (2013). Interprofessional learning objectives for health team simulations. *Journal of Nursing Education, 52*(6), 311–316.

Herge, E. A., Lorch, A., Deangelis, T., Vause-Earland, T., Mollo, K., & Zapletal, A. (2013). The standardized patient encounter: A dynamic educational approach to enhance students' clinical healthcare skills. *Journal of Allied Health, 42*(4), 229–235.

Occupational Therapy Council (2013). Occupational therapy council accreditation standards explanatory guide: The use of simulation in practice education/fieldwork. Retrieved from http://otcouncil.com .au/wp-content/uploads/2012/09/Explanatory-notes-for-simulation-in-practice-education-July -2013.pdf

Yeung, E., Dubrowski, A., & Carnahan, H. (2013). Simulation-augmented education in the rehabilitation professions: A scoping review. *International Journal of Therapy & Rehabilitation, 20*(5), 228–236.

CHAPTER 52

Interprofessional Disaster Simulation

Doris French, Andrew Booth, Michael J. Shoemaker, Margaret Devoest, Jeanine Beasley, and Julie A. Bulson

A. IMPLEMENTATION OF SIMULATION-BASED PEDAGOGY IN YOUR INDIVIDUALIZED TEACHING AREA

The Midwest Interprofessional Practice and Research Center (MIPERC) is a consortium of universities and health care institutions working together to support interprofessional practice and education. The center was developed out of the office of the vice provost for health at Grand Valley State University (GVSU) and is a multi-institutional organization comprised of over 25 organizational and over 150 individual members. Within MIPERC there are six champion workgroups that help to carry out its mission, which is to identify ways that the members can develop collaborative, innovative, and interprofessional initiatives across disciplines, learning institutions, and health care systems. In addition, residing within MIPERC is the student organization, PIPES (Promoting Interprofessional Education for Students). This group meets six times per academic year and is supported by the Simulation Champion Workgroup. This workgroup consists of faculty members from several health disciplines lead by coleads Andrew Booth, DHEd, PA-C, and Michael J. Shoemaker, DPT, PhD. The rest of the workgroup members are Jeanine Beasley, EdD, OTRL, CHT, FAOTA; Julie Bulson, MPA, BSN RN, NEA-BC; Margaret Devoest, PharmD; Vicki Swendroski, MSN RN, CPAN, CHSE; Phil Van Lente, MD; Cathy Harro, MS PT, NCS; Barb Boomstra, BSN RN; and facilitator Doris French, MSN RN, CNOR, NE-BC. The workgroup facilitates two interprofessional simulations per year that serve as a culminating event in which students can experience interacting with students from other health disciplines, learning from, with, and about other the professions. The PIPES meetings and simulations also count as activities for an interprofessional certificate available through MIPERC.

B. EDUCATIONAL MATERIALS AVAILABLE IN YOUR TEACHING AREA AND RELATED TO YOUR SPECIALTY

GVSU's simulation center consists of three areas. Two areas are located on the third floor adjacent to two large clinical skills labs, and one smaller area is located on the fourth floor. Each of the areas is equipped with cameras and microphones that are a part of a recording/streaming software package (Simulation iQ Enterprise from Education Management Solutions, Exton, PA), used to manage educational videos.

One of the areas located on the third floor is a hospital suite, which is a large room with five smaller hospital rooms and a two-bed ward contained within it. One of the rooms is representative of an intensive care unit and the remaining four are medical–surgical hospital rooms. This area also has a control room for both recording purposes and manikin operation. The hospital suite contains many high-fidelity manikins from newborn to adult. Medium- and low-fidelity manikins are available and used for appropriate skills development or scenarios. This area also comes equipped with functioning headwalls, hospital beds, a crash cart, medication-dispensing unit, and other equipment needed to set the appropriate environment for the scenarios.

Adjacent to the hospital suite is the standardized patient suite, which has eight outpatient examination rooms located within it. These rooms are complete with patient assessment tables, functioning headwalls, and stocked with various assessment equipment and supplies. This suite also contains space for training standardized patients or small-group meetings.

A smaller simulation room is located on the fourth floor. This is a two-bed hospital room divided by curtains. It contains the same equipment located in the hospital suite but has an attached conference or small classroom divided from the simulation area with a wall containing two one-way windows for observation and a door. The classroom has projection capabilities as well as two computer workstations for controlling manikins.

The simulation center also has three debriefing rooms, one observation room set up with 16 computer stations configured for live streaming, and a standardized patient reception area. Two of the debriefing rooms and the observation room are equipped with cameras and microphones making them flexible space for simulated care conferences.

C. SPECIFIC OBJECTIVES FOR SIMULATION USAGE WITHIN A SPECIFIC COURSE AND THE OVERALL PROGRAM

Interprofessional simulation experiences provide students with the opportunity to directly interact with other health discipline students to practice interprofessional collaboration so they can effectively be ready to practice teamwork and team-based care (Interprofessional Education Collaborative [IPEC], 2016).

Objectives for interprofessional education (IPE) simulations include gaining competence in the following four areas:

1. Values and ethics for interprofessional practice
2. Roles and responsibilities for collaborative practice
3. Interprofessional communication competencies
4. Interprofessional team and teamwork competencies (IPEC, 2016)

D. INTRODUCTION OF SCENARIO

Setting the Scene

This scene takes place in a rehabilitation hospital. It is late afternoon at the end of March, and the hospital has just been struck by a tornado. There is significant damage to one side of the third floor, which requires that seven rehab inpatients be relocated to the second floor of the hospital. There are many staff members still available, including several social workers who had been conducting care conferences earlier in the afternoon.

Technology Used

13 standardized patients
1 low-fidelity human simulator, with a cuffed tracheostomy tube attached to a ventilator, an Ambu bag, and a cervical collar in place

1 Hoyer lift
1 stair chair
1 evacuation sled
1 wheelchair
1 walker
1 portable oxygen tank
7 hospital beds with standard hospital furniture such as night stands and overbed tables

Objectives

The learning objectives for the simulation were based on the following four IPEC competencies (IPEC, 2016):

RR3: Engage diverse health care professionals who complement one's professional expertise, as well as associated resources, to develop strategies to meet specific patient care needs.

RR5: Use the full scope of knowledge, skills, and abilities of available health professionals and health care workers to provide care that is safe, timely, efficient, effective, and equitable.

CC4: Listen actively, and encourage ideas and opinions of other team members.

CC8: Communicate the importance of teamwork in patient-centered care and population health programs and policies consistently.

Description of Participants

Students: The students participating in the simulation were both graduate and undergraduate students in health or health-related programs. Students were invited from three different universities to participate; two medical residents from the Grand Rapids Medical Education Partners were asked to help facilitate the scenario. The programs represented were undergraduate nursing social work, physician assistant sudies (PA), public health, pharmacy, medicine, and physical therapy (PT).

Patients: Six of the seven patients were played by PT students and one was a low-fidelity human simulator.

Family members: The family members of the patient with a C2 fracture, portrayed by the low-fidelity human simulator, and the patient who was aphasic because of a cerebral vascular accident (CVA) were portrayed by PT students. The rest of the family members were assigned randomly from the student RSVP list.

Caregivers: The students who were not assigned to a patient or family member were divided into seven groups composed of two providers (either a medical student or PA or two PA students), a nursing student, and one or two PT students. There were four pharmacy students who served as a pharmacist assigned to the second floor, a night shift second-floor pharmacist, and a third-floor pharmacist. The fourth pharmacy student played the part of the third-floor sender, whose duty was to record the patient name, the time leaving the unit, and where the patient was going. A master's in public health (MPH) student served as the receiver of the second-floor unit and recorded the patient name, time received, and bed assignment. The four social work students, who were having a care conference at the rehab facility, were divided among the seven groups to offer help where needed. Finally, the two medical residents played physicians who were completing rounds of their patients when the tornado struck.

Observers: There were seven extra students who attended the simulation who had not signed up in advance. They were provided with the simulation objectives and were assigned to observe and record their impressions to share during debriefing. There was one observer for each group.

Faculty: The PT faculty, Michael J. Shoemaker, DPT, PhD, and Cathy Harro, MS, PT, NCS, instructed the PT students to portray the individual patient conditions and provided dressings and other props to help set the stage. One faculty member served as the on-site incident commander along with the director of disaster preparedness from one of the local hospitals, Julie Bulson, MPA, BSN RN,

NEA-BC. The remaining faculty from the various disciplines provided logistical help with tasks such as sign in, name tags, photo consents, and so forth. All faculty helped with briefing and debriefing.

E. RUNNING OF THE SCENARIO

Students were assigned to specific groups in an attempt to divide the disciplines as evenly represented as possible. Other students were given roles that fell outside the seven disciplines represented such as sender or receiver. The students then gathered in a large classroom adjacent to the simulation area to receive their briefing. At the end of the briefing, a faculty member opened the door and announced that a tornado just hit the building and the patients need to be moved. We need everyone's help now! The students then were dispersed to the simulation area and helped to find their patient, then told to start planning their patient's evacuation. As there was only one stair chair and one evacuation sled, the groups had to communicate with each other to determine which patient should be evacuated first using these scarce resources.

Faculty members circulated throughout the simulation areas and gave encouragement or helped with finding supplies or equipment that the students needed. The students were given 45 minutes to complete the scenario. All patients were successfully evacuated in 36 minutes.

F. PRESENTATION OF COMPLETED TEMPLATE

Title

Interprofessional Disaster Simulation

Scenario Level

Novice

Focus Area

Interprofessional competencies

Scenario Description

There are seven inpatients located on the third floor of a Midwest rehab hospital. The seven patient cases were as follows:

1. Total knee arthroplasty who has just been weaned from intravenous (IV) pain control to oral pain medication before admission to the rehab hospital who has weight-bearing restrictions and needs help transferring
2. Total hip arthroplasty with a history of atrial fibrillation, oral pain medications, weight-bearing restrictions, special needs for transferring, international normalized ratio (INR) is 6
3. Cerebrovascular accident (CVA) with aphasia, agitation, balance issues, and an agitated family member
4. Neuropathic foot ulcer, negative pressure wound therapy dressing, weight-bearing restrictions
5. Traumatic brain injury, agitation
6. C2 fracture (ventilated), mechanical ventilator, specific transfer needs, agitated family member.
7. A patient who is recovering from extensive chemotherapy in hospital for muscle strengthening, balance issues, and neutropenic precautions

It is March and a tornado has touched down, destroying one end of the third-floor corridor, which necessitates all the patients be moved to the second floor. The students need to determine who should be transferred first and which method of transfer would be the best. Then they must evacuate their patients safely down the stairway.

Scenario Objectives

1. Participate in an interprofessional simulation
2. Engage with diverse health care professionals who complement one's professional expertise as well as associated resources to develop strategies to meet specific patient care needs
3. Use the full scope of knowledge, skills, and abilities of available health professionals and health care workers to provide care that is safe, timely, efficient, effective, and equitable
4. Listen actively and encourage ideas and opinions of other team members
5. Communicate the importance of consistent teamwork in patient-centered and community-focused care

The accomplishment of the objectives for this interprofessional simulation provide the students with a beginning competency for communication when working on an interprofessional team, which is one of *The Essentials of Baccalaureate Education for Professional Nursing Practice* as described by the American Association of Colleges of Nursing (AACN; 2008). It also provides the opportunity for students to "learn about, from and with each other to enable effective collaboration and improve health outcomes" as defined by the World Health Organization in 2010 and referred to in the "Standards of Best Practice: Simulation Standard VIII: Simulation-Enhanced Interprofessional Education" (Decker et al., 2015, p. 294). Interprofessional communication is also incorporated into the NCLEX-RN® (National Council Licensure Examination) for Registered Nurses test plan as one of the integrated processes that are distributed throughout the examination (National Council of State Boards of Nursing [NCSBN], 2015).

Setting the Scene

The MIPERC simulation workgroup supports the PIPES student group. The workgroup met in early September to determine the topic of the simulation. At the time GVSU was conducting a university-wide read of *Five Days at Memorial* (Fink, 2013). This book told of the care patients received at a New Orleans hospital post Hurricane Katrina. The group thought that a disaster scenario would include roles by many different disciplines making it an ideal topic for our-end-of-year IPE simulation event (Mendenhall, 2006).

The PIPES group meets once a month during the fall and winter semesters. Speakers from various disciplines are asked to speak about their perspectives on interprofessional care for patients and its importance to patient safety and outcomes. Since the simulation topic was chosen in September, we were able to schedule speakers that would give students the requisite knowledge and insight into a disaster. One speaker talked about medical ethics in a disaster situation referring to *Five Days at Memorial* (Fink, 2013), for example. The speaker scheduled just before the simulation is the director for emergency preparedness at one of the local medical institutions, Julie Bulson, MPA, BSN RN, NEA-BC. She talked with the students about disaster preparedness and the various provider roles needed during a disaster. She also provided videos of the proper use of a stair chair and evacuation sled. The link to these videos was sent out to all students who RSVP'd for the simulation event.

Before the simulation the PT students were given instruction on their portrayal of the various medical conditions and were bandaged or given an application of moulage according to the condition they were portraying. A cuffed tracheostomy tube was inserted into a low-fidelity manikin representing the patient with the C2 fracture and then attached to a ventilator. An Ambu bag was stored in a nearby bedside cabinet, and a Hoyer lift and portable oxygen tank were located nearby. Other ambulatory aids for patients, such as walkers, crutches, and wheelchairs, were brought to a nearby storage area. The stair chair and evacuation sled were available in the simulation suite for the students to use.

Signage was made to help direct the students to the briefing/debriefing rooms. Other signs were made to designate the second-floor receiving area. Case report sheets were created before the event and given to the individual groups, and station signs were displayed by each patient bed.

Scenario Implementation

Immediately after briefing a faculty member entered the room and announced, "A tornado has hit the hospital. We need to evacuate the second floor. I need everyone to help with this situation." Other faculty members then urged the students out of the classroom and took them to the simulation area. There they were instructed to find their group and begin planning their patient's evacuation.

The "third-floor rehab unit" was chaos for the first few minutes, but faculty members facilitated the organization of the student groups, and soon they were interacting and carrying out all the duties needed to evacuate the patients. As many of the students were not familiar with our simulation center, we needed enough faculty to assist students in finding equipment, medications, and so forth.

Evaluative Criteria

1. Were students interacting with other roles?
2. Did the students portray knowledge of the situation?
3. Were they able to complete the scenario?
4. Could the students immerse themselves in the scenario?
5. Were there enough resources?

G. DEBRIEFING GUIDELINES

Our debriefing questions are based on the Core Competencies for Interprofessional Collaborative Practice (IPEC, 2016). As we based the objectives on those competencies, the debriefing questions were used to determine whether we had met those objectives.

The following were the initial questions for debriefing:

1. What were the key items noted by the observers?
2. Did everyone feel he or she had a place or was needed?
3. How were communications among the team members?
4. Did all the patients know the roles of the care team?
5. Did the team work well together?

H. SUGGESTIONS/KEY FEATURES TO REPLICATE OR IMPROVE

Improvements

Overall, there was good feedback about the simulation. Some suggestions from the students were:

1. Some students who were not familiar with our simulation center thought it would have been nice to have more knowledge of the facility before the simulation.

2. Instead of announcing the hospital had been hit by a tornado and everyone's help is needed now, have someone come in and shout out in a panic to let everyone know the urgency of the situation.

3. There were no patient charts just a sheet with patient information. Next time an actual chart for the students would be helpful.

Keep the Same

The things the students felt were good about the simulation were:

1. The students liked being able to participate in the simulation. They were able to have a hands-on experience with a stair chair and evacuation sled, which they felt they would not get as a student.

2. Roles in an IPE situation sometimes get lost because one is so focused on the task. This scenario allowed team leaders to emerge and participants felt safe to speak up about their expertise.

3. Good support is given to the patient and family.

4. Good explanations and support were given by faculty.

I. RECOMMENDATIONS FOR FURTHER USE

This simulation took many meetings and hours to develop and plan. The workgroup did not include our facilities department in the planning to set the stage, so the scene could have been more real if the facilities department was involved in the planning process, including more visual and auditory cues such as sirens and plastic hung to simulate structural damage.

Another issue was assigning groups so that all disciplines were distributed appropriately. The RSVP process began 2 weeks before the event. RSVPs should have been completed 2 weeks before the event and made clear that if the student did not RSVP he or she would be an observer. This way there would have been time to offer tours of the facility to students who came from the other two universities.

A formal evaluation tool was not developed for this event. Outcomes could be measured more specifically had a tool been developed. Some students spoke up during the debriefing about possible improvements, but there may have been other suggestions that the students were not willing to verbalize to the group as a whole.

The students were well prepared with the materials that were sent to them and the lectures preceding the event were beneficial. Many of the students attended all of the lectures and reviewed the video of the evacuation equipment, as well as the slide show presentation from our guest lecturer, Julie Bulson, MPA, BSN RN, NEA-BC, who is a local director of emergency preparedness.

Suggestions made by the participants during the debriefing were good and will be incorporated into future simulations. It was felt that students gained confidence in their roles as caregivers and team members. During the debriefing, the students verbalized that the physicians did not know everything about emergency evacuation and that the PTs needed to help with transfers, especially with the use of the Hoyer lift. Although the roles blurred at times, each participant still retained his or her expertise, contributing to the overall care of the patient. The literature suggests that students do not always have the opportunity to participate as a caregiver in a disaster situation before graduating (Jennings-Sanders, Frisch, & Wing, 2005) so this experience was very valuable to those who participated.

J. HOW SIMULATION-BASED PEDAGOGY HAS CONTRIBUTED TO IMPROVED STUDENT OUTCOMES

An alumnus of the PA program returned to participate in an open house for the simulation center. She described how, during her first physical assessment as a student, she listened to lung sounds through the patient's gown. She explained to open-house visitors that she made many mistakes during her simulations, but each event helped her. She credits the simulations for allowing her to establish rapport with her patients and build her self–confidence to become a successful clinician. Simulating events in which multiple roles need to work together to provide care for a patient helps students communicate more effectively and clarifies their scope of practice. They also learn different perspectives and new techniques for communicating with patients.

K. EXPERT RECOMMENDATIONS AND WORDS OF WISDOM

- Have the students RSVP no less than 2 weeks before the event.
- Preplan student groups and color code to help organize the students during the sign-in procedure.
- Work with the facilities department to plan for additional props for better realism in the environment.
- Make sure there is enough personnel to help with the sign-in the process so it is organized and efficient.

L. EVALUATION OF BEST PRACTICE STANDARDS AND USE OF CREDENTIALED SIMULATION FACULTY

All of the MIPERC workgroups are tasked with helping students achieve interprofessional competence. These competencies were created by experts from six different professions that came together to create the IPEC. The goal of IPEC is to help prepare future health professionals for enhanced team-based care of patients and improved population health outcomes (IPEC, 2016). The workgroups refer to these competencies when creating activities or learning situations for our students. The learning opportunities created by workgroups are based on gaining interprofessional competence but must integrate this with best practices for simulation as a learning modality. The simulation practices, used by MIPERC, are based on standards set forth by Society for Simulation in Healthcare (SSIH; Committee for Accreditation of Healthcare Simulation Programs, 2016a, 2016b) and the International Nursing Association for Clinical Simulation and Learning (Decker et al., 2015). Individual program curriculum standards are also in place for the health care professions involved in this simulation.

REFERENCES

American Association of Colleges of Nursing. (2008). *The essentials of baccalaureate education for professional nursing practice.* Washington, DC: Author. Retrieved from http://www.aacnnursing.org/Portals/42/Publications/BaccEssentials08.pdf

Committee for Accreditation of Healthcare Simulation Programs. (2016a). Core standards and measurement criteria. *Society for Simulation in Healthcare Accreditation.* Retrieved from http://www.ssih.org/Portals/48/Accreditation/2016%20Standards%20and%20Docs/Core%20Standards%20and%20Criteria.pdf

Committee for Accreditation of Healthcare Simulation Programs. (2016b). Teaching/education standards and measurement criteria. *Society for Simulation in Healthcare Accreditation.* Retrieved from http://www.ssih.org/Portals/48/Accreditation/2016%20Standards%20and%20Docs/Teaching-Education%20Standards%20and%20Criteria.pdf

Decker, S. I., Anderson, M., Boese, T., Epps, C., McCarthy, J., Motola, I., . . . Scolaro, K. (2015). Standards of best practice: Simulation standard VIII: Simulation-enhanced interprofessional education (Sim-IPE). *Clinical Simulation in Nursing, 11*(6), 293–297. doi:10.1016/j.ecns.2015.03.010

Fink, S. (2013). *Five days at memorial*. New York, NY: Crown Publishers.

Interprofessional Education Collaborative. (2016). *Core competencies for interprofessional collaborative practice: 2016 update*. Washington, DC: Author.

Jennings-Sanders, A., Frisch, N., & Wing, S. (2005). Nursing students' perceptions about disaster nursing. *Disaster Management & Response, 3*(3), 80–85.

Mendenhall, T. J. (2006). Trauma-response teams: Inherent challenges and practical strategies in interdisciplinary fieldwork. *Families, Systems, & Health, 24*(3), 357–362. doi:10.1037/1091-7527.24.3.357

National Council of State Boards of Nursing. (2015). NCLEX-RN examination: Test plan for the national council licensure examination for registered nurses. Retrieved from https://www.ncsbn.org/RN_Test_Plan_2016_Final.pdf

The Simulation Journey Continues

CHAPTER 53

Learning to Write Like a Nurse in Clinical Simulations

Lillian Campbell

DO NURSES WRITE?

Often, nurses do not identify the written communication that they use in clinical contexts as "writing." The essays that they write for nursing courses? The articles that they publish in scholarly journals? Sure, those are writing. But the to-do lists that help them to organize patient care? The extensive notes in a patient's chart? Nope, not writing. As a writing scholar and teacher, I have always found this distinction puzzling. However, as my research has increasingly brought me into conversation with nursing students about how they learn to "write" in the field, I have also come to see it as detrimental. It keeps both nursing students and instructors from recognizing connections between the assignments they write in nursing classes—from nursing philosophy statements to patient care plans—and their future writing as professional nurses.

Of course, this challenge is not unique to the field of nursing. Students in many professional educational tracks struggle to recognize how classroom-based writing prepares them for writing in their future fields. However, nursing education is unique in its incorporation of clinical simulations, which exists in a space between the traditional nursing classroom and the clinical context. As such, clinical simulations offer a rich opportunity for students to notice and discuss the different kinds of writing they encounter in clinical contexts, to practice designing texts that help them to coordinate care, and to reflect critically on the effectiveness of their simulated writing experiences.

In this chapter, I briefly introduce genre theory from writing studies to help nursing instructors understand the challenges of teaching professional writing in classroom contexts. Subsequently, I specifically discuss what makes learning to "write like a nurse" so challenging and how the simulation context can address these limitations. Finally, I offer several suggestions for how instructors can leverage different aspects of clinical simulations to help students practice writing and reading a range of nursing documents.

GENRE THEORY AND CLASSROOM-BASED WRITING

Writing scholars believe that learning to communicate in a discipline or a professional context entails much more than learning standards for grammatical or technical correctness and much more than acquiring a repertoire of texts to reproduce on command. As nursing students negotiate the interpretation of a physician's orders or prepare assessment information to begin a conversation with the physician, they are also being initiated into value systems, tacit ways of thinking and behaving, and a hierarchy of clinical power relationships. And just as they have the capacity to act flexibly within these modes of communication, its texts are also acting on them—shaping their worldview and their interactions with people and things in powerful ways. Thus, learning disciplinary and professional communication is also a way of learning how to be and act within a community.

Rhetorical genre theory is one framework used for writing studies that attempts to capture the complexity of this interrelationship between texts and individual identities (Bawarshi & Reiff, 2010). Here, the term *genre* describes formalized modes of communication, like business memos or patient medical history forms. Writers often think about genres as a set of rules on how information should be organized and communicated, but this does not account for the way that genres are tied to their social contexts. Instead, genre theorists argue that we should think about how a genre's features emerge because of its particular situation, audience, and purpose. For example, the categories of a patient medical history form are not arbitrary but instead reflect the medical field's prioritization of physical symptoms over psychosocial patient information (Bawarshi, 2003).

Rhetorical genre theory also highlights how genres play a complex part in shaping individual worldviews and relationships to one another. For example, Paré's (2000) study of social work students' transitions into hospital writing found that they had to learn to adapt their identities as students who emphasized social relationships into the more technical, scientific writing forms that were expected by a medical audience. Thus, Paré demonstrated how genres are one means by which individuals come to inhabit and embody a field or institution's dispositions. He was particularly struck by the discourse of loss that accompanied this genre learning.

Fundamentally, writing scholars have argued that genres function quite differently in classrooms than in the "real world." In professional and public contexts, genres always participate in complex systems that include other genres, people, practices, and materials to make action possible. In classrooms, however, genres are typically produced for evaluation by the instructor rather than for the coordination of action. Russell (1997) draws on activity theory to address this distinction, arguing that while professionals in a workplace setting acquire genres as tools that support them in achieving the larger objects of their organization, genres are often treated as the object in classroom contexts. Similarly, Wardle (2009) describes how many of the assignments that students produce in writing classrooms are "mutt genres" that "mimic genres that mediate activities in other activity systems, but within the (classroom) their purposes and audiences are vague or even contradictory" (p. 774). Even when students are specifically asked to write for an imagined audience outside of the classroom, their writing is still being evaluated as the object by an instructor, which creates what Russell describes as double binds.

At the same time, students do not just have trouble connecting the types of writing they do for their classes into the workplace, their writing processes and approaches to learning new genres rarely transfer either. In "Learning to Write Professionally," Freedman and Adam (1996) describe very different genre-acquisition processes in school and workplace settings. In school, guidance tends to come before writing, projects are completed once handed in, feedback is evaluative, and no revision is expected. In the workplace, guidance often comes after completing a draft, the project is never fully complete (past projects keep living even after completion as they are referenced for future writing), feedback is intended to be incorporated into revision, writing is often done collaboratively, and writing experiences, which are rarely scaffolded, emerge organically from the organization's needs. This litany of differences raises the question of how classroom assignments and activities can better prepare students for genre learning in their public and professional lives.

In response, recent research in writing studies calls for classroom-based genre teaching that emphasizes rhetorical awareness and flexibility and moves students away from merely reproducing certain types of texts with technical accuracy. Devitt (2004) describes this as the difference between teaching for genre awareness instead of genre acquisition. Teaching for genre awareness entails focusing on form and context as constantly intertwined and calling student attention to the importance of cultural and situational influences on genre choices. Devitt emphasizes the need to teach genres as flexible, varied, and open to creativity by showing students multiple examples of a genre, some that push the limits of the genre conventions and exemplify creativity.

Overall, as writing scholars have come to recognize the immense complexity of genres and, therefore, classroom-based genre teaching, reactions have varied from radical calls for the abolition of writing courses (Crowley, 1998; Smit, 2004) to more measured discussions of ways to create classrooms that are more authentic rhetorical contexts in and of themselves (Bawarshi, 2003; Feldman, 2008). Clinical simulations offer one possibility for "teach(ing) a genre explicitly in the process of performing a rhetorical action" (Russell & Fisher, 2009, p. 165). This chapter offers suggestions for how simulation-based genres have the potential to support a practice-based understanding of professional genres that can translate into clinical contexts. In conversation with the many perspectives on genre learning offered here, I emphasize throughout how classroom-based simulations can position students as communicators with agency in their future fields, oriented toward nursing genres as both flexible and potentially fallible.

LEARNING TO WRITE LIKE A NURSE

Many of the limitations discussed earlier regarding classroom-based genre teaching broadly apply to the teaching of nursing genres as well. However, as with any discipline, nursing genres come with their unique set of challenges tied to the community's values and practices. Specifically, given the necessity of technical correctness within the nursing profession, there is a tendency for instructors to focus on lower order concerns like formatting, citation, and grammar that would be associated with a genre-acquisition framework rather than a genre-awareness framework (Devitt, 2004). This section briefly overviews some of the distinct qualities of nursing writing assignments as discussed in the relevant literature. I have demonstrated how the assignments that nursing students produce for their classes can lack intertextual connections and purpose about their profession. Students then have trouble both understanding where there might be room for flexibility within their writing and imagining the role writing plays in their future careers. This provides context for the rest of the chapter and my discussion of how simulation genres can position students quite differently by fostering rhetorical responsiveness and creativity.

As Gimenez (2008) points out in his survey of nursing and midwifery students at the United Kingdom University, research on writing in nursing tends to focus on the experiences of post-registration nurses, with a particular emphasis on supporting graduate and professional nurses in publishing. This research is part of the burgeoning field of the workplace or professional/technical writing scholarship, but results in limited documentation of the writing experiences of baccalaureate nurses. Meanwhile, baccalaureate nursing students are expected to produce a lot of writing, in a wide range of different genres, throughout their undergraduate years: "Beginning in their first undergraduate semester, nurses are asked to compose a gamut of texts: from descriptions of patients they encounter during their first experience on a hospital floor to descriptions of competing nursing theories" (Ariail & Smith, 2008, p. 248).

Both students and instructors can struggle to understand the relationship between this range of assignments and the work of professional nurses. The nursing student in Ariail and Smith's (2008) study identified one of the biggest challenges of writing assignments for students as "[not] understanding the purpose of the assignments" (p. 259), which they attribute to "nursing's theory–practice divide as experienced by students in many professional programs whose curricula demand writing but whose day-to-day practices do not, at least in academic forms" (p. 259). Meanwhile, the nursing field heavily emphasizes the use of writing for "documentation." This focus on documentation along with the valuing of precision and brevity in the field can lead to a heightened focus on the technical aspects of structure, grammar, and citation in writing assignments as opposed to more conceptual concerns like context, audience awareness, organization, argument, and integration of sources. Ariail and Smith (2008) discuss this trend as it connects to the field's worldview, more broadly:

> Nursing faculty outline structure and criteria for grading. In standardizing the genres their students produce, these health care professionals treat writing as they treat insertion of a Foley catheter. Sure, it may have a certain unpleasantness associated with it, but there is a procedure that can be

followed to make it as painless as possible, for nurse and patient, for nurse writer and nurse grader. The guidelines are indeed "helpful," in that they provide basic structures and expectations. However, they fall short in that they do not recognize that the microcosmic guidance they give may, in fact, undercut more macrocosmic and subjective criteria like clarity, significance, or quality. . . . In classical rhetorical terms, they sacrifice invention at the altar of arrangement and style. (p. 258)

Here, in drawing the analogy between assignment criteria and procedures for Foley catheter insertion, the authors highlight how nurses' professional values can shape their approach to teaching writing assignments. They also observe how this can occur at the expense of understanding the relationship between conventions and the nurse's rhetorical situation.

Meanwhile, in their research, Ariail and Smith (2008) found that faculty expressed a sense of loss regarding more creative or open-ended writing. In trying to help students learn the genres of the field with explicit assignments and writing guidelines that focus on form or structure, instructors "wonder if they are sacrificing the more humanistic, creative attributes for which the profession is valorized" (p. 245). Of course, this is a larger tension for the genres of the field. Nursing genres exist in comprehensive genre systems and are a source of information for medical professionals from a range of different backgrounds and with a wide variety of priorities. In *Writing in the Health Professions*, Heifferon (2005) advises students, "Emotion in charts is unadvisable; if you have particular difficulties with patients, it's best to air those in your team meetings with other staff members" (p. 294). The fact-based, list-oriented genres of nursing documentation then exist in part because of their role in interdisciplinary communication. However, this means, "the texts that grow out of nurse–patient interactions might not be accurate depictions of the core helping relationship" (Ariail & Smith, 2008, p. 262). Ultimately, the tension between teaching students the writing strategies they need to communicate efficiently and effectively with other health care professionals and teaching them what it means to interact compassionately with patients and family "like a nurse" undergirds the range of assignments that nursing students encounter in their baccalaureate courses.

There is also a way, however, that both nursing instructors and students may not be recognizing and valuing the opportunities for supporting genre learning that exists in less creative or open-ended assignments. For example, even an assignment that asks students to summarize an academic article necessitates that they make strategic choices about which information to foreground based on their assessment of what is valued within a community. Summary assignments are thus deeply situated, relying on students' burgeoning understanding of the discipline. As a field, nursing has tended to prioritize technical and content-based correctness in assessing writing, but there are certainly ways to approach assignments to emphasize the development of disciplinary identity and possibilities for rhetorical flexibility. As I will show, simulated contexts create additional opportunities for leveraging flexible teaching of nursing genres.

STRATEGIES FOR TEACHING WRITING IN CLINICAL SIMULATIONS

In a clinical simulation setting, much like other professional contexts, students are learning about the possible subject positions available to nurses. One mode of this learning is the wide range of genres that circulate in a given situation. In simulations, students consult patient records, prioritize physician's orders, interpret lab results, and document their interventions. These texts are not just derivative, designed to look like their clinical counterparts merely for show. Instead, they operate to authentically regulate activity, support interactions, and contribute to the nursing students' care and treatment of their patient within the simulation context. This means that they also avoid some of the pitfalls that scholars have identified for the classroom-based writing assignments. They operate as "tools" for coordinating activity and not simply "objects" for evaluation by the instructor. In this section, I discuss some of the different strategies that instructors can use to leverage the unique positioning of simulated genres and best support student learning.

Facilitate Backward- and Forward-Reaching Reflection

One of the best ways to help students benefit from their writing experiences in simulations is to explicitly ask them to connect those experiences to their writing in the classroom and clinical placements. Recent educational research on knowledge transfer has found that to help students take learning from one context and apply it in a different context, instructors should ask them to be reflective about possible connections across contexts. Strategies for fostering these reflections include asking students to think about similarities and differences between writing tasks (Bawarshi & Reiff, 2010) and creating opportunities for backward reaching (making connections to previous writing experiences) and forward reaching (reflecting on how they might mobilize this knowledge in the future; Fraizer, 2010; Perkins & Salomon, 1988).

Using a few minutes of debriefing to reflect on how the genres that students encountered during simulations were similar or different from those in the classroom and clinical would likely yield interesting results. For example, students might notice that physicians' orders in simulations are rarely prioritized or organized in the same way they might be in a hospital. This could lead to a fruitful conversation about how the goals of the simulation are different because it is designed to support collaborative problem solving among students to prioritize tasks. Or instructors could ask students to think about how the information that they documented about their patient during the simulation compared to a patient care plan they wrote for their clinical course. Here, students might be able to recognize how both were governed by the nursing process but the care plan allowed for them to delve much more deeply into the epidemiology of patient conditions, although documentation in simulations focused more on interventions. These kinds of conversations will likely have the added benefit that students will be able to understand the purpose of classroom writing better and value its role by tying it to writing experiences in simulations and clinical practicums. Table 53.1 lists some different genres in each context that instructors could refer to prompt connection making and reflection.

Overall, by making connections among genres across contexts and tying the characteristics of different genres to the larger goals of the situation, instructors can help students to think critically about why hospital genres look the way they do. Rather than thinking about the electronic health record as just a form to be filled out, then students can start to consider why particular categories are there and the efficacy of a record's organization. This encourages a flexible orientation to hospital genres that also recognizes the potential for modification or revision if the situation demands different modes for communicating information.

Table 53.1	Written Genres Across Contexts

Clinical experiences
- – Medication database
- – Physician's orders
- – Electronic health records
- – Nurse's notes

Simulation context
- – Medication database
- – Physician's orders
- – Patient chart
- – Other students' notes

Class experiences
- – Textbook readings
- – Writing assignments
- – Reading notes
- – Written exam questions

Support Student-Designed Texts

Some of the genres that nursing students encounter in simulations are predesigned for the simulation context. The preparation sheet and physician's orders, for example, are likely provided to you and your students in a particular form. With these prewritten genres, students have less of an opportunity to think strategically about a text's content and design. This is why it is also important to call their attention to the student-designed texts that play a role in coordinating their simulated care.

As students begin a simulation, they may be taking with them notes that they took during their preparation work. Throughout the scenario, they may use these nurse's notes to help them prepare for a call to the physician, report to other nurses on their team the information they are gathering about a patient, or organizing their handoff to the subsequent nursing team. A group of students may be making use of whiteboards in the simulation room to write down notes about the patient or create a "to-do" list for themselves as a team. If you do not have an electronic charting system, these whiteboards may even be a place where students document patient care.

Again, it would be easy for both students and instructors to overlook these brief and intermediary writing experiences in the simulation, but research in writing studies suggests these are particularly rich moments for student writers. As they design texts to coordinate patient care, students are drawing on their previous knowledge about different modes of communication in the hospital and making strategic choices about how to best organize and prioritize information. In fact, writing researchers are calling for instructors to create opportunities for students to design genres just like this that coordinate classroom activities. For example, Roundtree (2014) proposes "an instructor might construct a memo assignment by which students must relay data to one another for completing the next major assignment or another course in the degree plan. In this way, the memo serves another end—namely helping finish another assignment" (p. 114). Thus, one of the things that nursing instructors can do to support learning about writing in simulation contexts is simply to encourage students to be aware of and make use of these makeshift written genres that coordinate the activities of the simulation.

In addition, student-designed texts can further support learning when they are collaboratively designed and thus, genre knowledge is shared across a group of students. For example, a group may create a shared "to-do" list at the beginning of the shift to help them prioritize and assign tasks, or members might gather at the end of their shift to create notes for their patient handoffs. As collaborative learning scholar Bruffee (1999) argues, for novice writers who are finding their way into new professional communities, there is real value in negotiating these writing experiences together. Bruffee also highlights the importance of creating space for an intermediary, makeshift genre within those contexts:

> In collaborative learning, the route to fluency in the language of a new community is paved with ad hoc intermediary languages that students devise themselves to serve their own purposes as they work through the assigned task... non-foundational teaching will almost certainly teach students to quack. But on the way they will also learn to gobble, honk, peep, and squawk. (p. 77)

What is visibly lacking in many of the writing assignments we bring into our classrooms is this capacity to "gobble, honk, peep, and squawk." However, when a group of students comes together during a simulation to decide how to take notes on a patient's progress, for example, each member brings a range of earlier genre knowledge, creativity, and possibilities to the conversation. Then, when they use their text to share information, they experience first hand how it supports them or deters them from translating their findings to other students, the physician, or the patient. At the same time, instructors can support students in critically reflecting on their genre design by using debriefs to leverage peers as a source of audience response and feedback.

Create Opportunities for Constructive Feedback

One of the biggest advantages for genre learning in simulation contexts is that students are given the opportunity to experience firsthand how effective both predesigned and self-designed genres are in supporting the simulation's activities. However, this opportunity can only really be leveraged if instructors can facilitate conversations that prompt active reflection on what it was like to use these genres in context. Students likely feel most comfortable critiquing a genre based on its deviation from a set structure. For example, if you provided them with a template to help chart patient care on the whiteboard, peers readily identify where groups deviated from this given structure. To best support learning, however, these conversations should focus less on the technical specifics of the genre and more on the genre's effectiveness about its purpose, audience, and situation.

One of the questions that instructors often ask during debriefing to prompt student reflection is, "How did that feel?" A similar question targeted specifically at genres in the simulation could be quite effective. For example, "How did using the electronic health record feel? How did it support or interrupt your care?" Debriefs can also leverage peers as a source of audience feedback, asking, for example, an incoming group of nurses how the handoff felt and what information might have needed more attention or discussion. The peers' responses could then be tied back to the student-designed notes to think about modifications that would have helped to better capture the needed information. Ideally, this reflective questioning enables students to recognize different modes of communication as potentially fallible, capable of causing them to overemphasize tasks rather than responding to patient needs, for example, or leave out the key problem in a conversation with the physician. Overall, providing students with space to critically reflect on how their writing both supports and detracts from their care has rich potential for making them more thoughtful and responsive communicators in the future.

CONCLUSIONS

Without instructor guidance, students are unlikely to identify the writing in clinical simulations as "writing" at all. The simulation scenario presents such an exciting challenge that the many texts that students are interacting with and using to document care could easily go unnoticed. This would be a shame because the simulation context presents a unique opportunity for genre acquisition. Unlike in a classroom, the writing students are doing in simulations is goal oriented and has an authentic audience that relies on its success. Meanwhile, unlike in a clinical context, students still have the reflective space of the debrief to think critically about how their writing helped to coordinate their care and to talk through possible strengths and limitations of nursing genres. Thus, with a little instructor guidance, writing in simulations can bridge students' classroom and clinical writing experiences and help them to value their classroom writing while also better understanding the challenges of writing like a nurse.

REFERENCES

Ariail, J., & Smith, T. G. (2008). Concept analysis: Using an academic nursing genre for writing instruction in nursing. In B. Heifferon & S. C. Brown (Eds.), *Rhetoric of healthcare: Essays toward a new disciplinary inquiry* (pp. 243–263). Cresskill, NJ: Hampton.

Bawarshi, A. (2003). *Genre and the invention of the writer: Reconsidering the place of invention in composition.* Logan: Utah State University Press.

Bawarshi, A., & Reiff, M. J. (2010). *Genre: An introduction to history, theory, research, and pedagogy.* West Lafayette, IA: Parlour Press.

Bruffee, K. (1999). *Collaborative learning: Higher education, interdependence, and the authority of knowledge* (2nd ed.) Baltimore, MD: Johns Hopkins University Press.

Crowley, S. (1998). *Composition in the university: Historical and polemical essays. Pittsburgh series in composition, literacy, and culture.* Pittsburgh, PA: University of Pittsburgh Press.

Devitt, A. (2004). *Writing genres.* Carbondale: Southern Illinois University Press.

Feldman, A. (2008). *Making writing matter: Composition in the engaged university.* Albany: State University of New York Press.

Fraizer, D. (2010). First steps beyond first year: Coaching transfer after FYC. *WPA Writing Program Administration, 33*(3), 34–57.

Freedman, A., & Adam, C. (1996). Learning to write professionally: "Situated learning" and the transition from university to professional discourse. *Journal of Business and Technical Communication, 10*(4), 395–427.

Gimenez, J. (2008). Beyond the academic essay: Discipline-specific writing in nursing and midwifery. *Journal of English for Academic Purposes, 7*(3), 151–164.

Heifferon, B. (2005). *Writing in the health professions. Allyn and Bacon series in technical communication.* New York, NY: Pearson Longman.

Paré, A. (2000). Writing as a way into social work: Genre sets, genre systems, and distributed cognition. In P. Dias & A. Paré (Eds.), *Transitions: Writing in academic and workplace settings* (pp. 145–166). Cresskill, NJ: Hampton.

Perkins, D. N., & Salomon, G. (1988). Teaching for transfer. *Educational Leadership, 46*1), 22–32.

Roundtree, A. K. (2014). *Computer simulation, rhetoric, and the scientific imagination: How virtual evidence shapes science in the making and in the news.* Lanham, MD: Lexington Books.

Russell, D. (1997). Rethinking genre in school and society: An activity theory analysis. *Written Communication, 14*(4), 504–554.

Russell, D. R., & Fisher, D. (2009). Online, multimedia case studies for professional education: Revisioning concepts of genre recognition. In J. Giltrow & D. Stein (Eds.), *Genres in the internet: Issues in the theory of genre* (pp. 163–191). Amsterdam, the Netherlands: John Benjamins.

Smit, D. (2004). *The end of composition studies.* Carbondale: Southern Illinois University Press.

Wardle, E. (2009). "Mutt genres" and the goal of FYC: Can we help students write the genres of the university? *College Composition and Communication, 60*(4), 765–789.

CHAPTER 54

How to Assess Our Own Expertise: Certification and Accreditation

Leland J. Rockstraw, Rita M. Coggins,
Carol R. Sando, and Jared M. Kutzin

DEFINITIONS

For purposes of this chapter, the authors present the following definitions of terms:

1. *Certificate of attendance*—Certificates of attendance or participation are provided to participants who have attended or participated in classes, courses, or other educational or training programs. The certificate awarded at the completion of the program signifies that the participant was present and, in some cases, that the participant actively participated in the program. Demonstration of accomplishment of the intended learning outcomes by participants is not a requirement for receiving the certificate. Therefore, possession of a certificate of attendance or participation does not indicate that the intended learning outcomes have been accomplished by the participant. Examples include certificates of attendance provided at many conferences (Institute for Credentialing Excellence [ICE], 2010).

2. *Certification*—Professional or personnel certification is a voluntary process by which individuals (participants) are evaluated against predetermined standards for knowledge, skills, or competencies. Participants who demonstrate that they meet these competency standards, by successfully completing the assessment process, are granted a time-limited credential. To retain the credential, individuals must demonstrate continued competence. The credential awarded by the certification program provider denotes that the participant possesses particular knowledge, skills, or competencies. The assessment is independent of any specific class, course, or other education or training program (ICE, 2010).

   CHSE—certified health care simulation educator

   CHSE-A—certified health care simulation educator—advanced

   CHSOS—certified health care simulation operations specialist

3. *Accreditation*—The process by which a credentialing or educational program is evaluated against standards defined by a third party. When in compliance with these standards, the program is awarded recognition. Accreditation is valuable because it enables organizations to demonstrate to the profession it represents and to the general public it serves, that their program has met the stringent standards set by the credentialing community. Accreditation also enhances a program's credibility and legitimacy by providing impartial, third-party oversight of a conformity assessment system (ICE, 2010).

BACKGROUND

History

Since the time of Florence Nightingale, nursing has based its practice on scientific principles that guide decisions based on research findings. The branch of knowledge we know as the art of nursing has arranged these truths or facts as best practices for clinical application, education, and future research endeavors. The use of simulation has entered the mainstream in health care education and practice. As simulation research evolves, the science of simulation contributes substantively to healthcare education and evidence-based practice.

Certification standardizes beliefs and practices that constitute high-quality simulation experiences. The process of certification has evolved through intentional deliberations that resulted in policy decisions. Certification in simulation is the logical next step, following recognition of simulation as a viable means of health care instruction, the increase in simulation centers, and the development of the simulation standards by the International Association for Clinical Simulation and Learning (INACSL).

The positive consequences of certification on simulation curriculum design and outcomes has been demonstrated in the literature. More than 160 studies, reports, and articles suggest that certified teachers in classrooms profoundly impact student learning. Similar results have been documented in the simulation literature. The connection between professional certification and the organization of instruction is evident in improved participant learning (National Board for Professional Teaching Standards, 2017). The notion of health care simulation certification has developed only recently. "Certification" may take many forms. There are intensive weeklong seminars that provide training to novice and experienced simulation educators and culminate with certificates of completion awarded to attendees. Basic core competencies in simulation learning methods, scenario building, and integration into health care curricula, specifically in nursing, are some of the topics presented (Monash University, 2012; National League for Nursing [NLN], n.d.). Postgraduate coursework in simulation is also available, along with academic degrees focused on simulation-based education. Although knowledgeable and experienced simulation experts offer these seminars, there is no central certifying agency for these academic-based courses, which would provide a reliable, best practice simulation program for individuals or institutions.

Historically, the National League for Nursing Accrediting Commission (NLNAC) and the Commission on Collegiate Nursing Education (CCNE) provide accreditation for nursing education programs by performing a systematic review of practices, outcomes, and operations that demonstrate adherence to standards associated with the nursing services provided. The Society for Simulation in Healthcare (SSH) began accrediting health care simulation programs in four key areas: assessment, research, teaching and education, and systems integration (SSH, 2012), but this accreditation is focused on simulation programs, not academic programs. The creation of the simulation standards by the INACSL as well as the certification and accreditation programs by SSH have initiated the process of requiring scientifically sound and consistent simulation practice founded on research-based principles.

From Societal Values to Professional Certification

Certification and accreditation offer assurances to the public that an individual or institution provides accurate and reliable simulation instruction and evaluation. Achieving certification suggests that the individual is able to perform at a predetermined level of expertise, in order to provide simulation experiences or services in a consistent and accurate manner within the scope of simulation knowledge and competencies. As stated earlier, certification in simulation can be earned by meeting the eligibility requirements for the certification test, applying for certification, and ultimately taking and passing the international certification examination.

Certification, Fellowships, and Certificates of Attendance

The determination to obtain new knowledge may be daunting. Understanding the myriad options available to novice simulation users is important. Clarifying the differences among certification, fellowship, and certificate of attendance especially aids understanding.

As presented in this chapter's definition of terms: certification evaluates against predetermined standards for knowledge, skills, or competencies. The method of evaluation can be examinations (knowledge), demonstration (skills), or a mixture of testing and demonstration (competencies). It is also a common practice to maintain certification, requiring the individual to continually demonstrate competence by attending education sessions specific to the field of certification. Some examples of health care certifications are critical care registered nurse (CCRN) and certified emergency nurse (CEN) credentials. One of the first health care simulation certifications offered was the SSH's certification program. It offers certification as a health care simulation educator (CHSE), an advanced credential, the CHSE-A, and certification in health care simulation operations (CHSOS).

The SSH's development of a simulation certification process began with an analysis of practice, developing an examination blueprint and piloting the examination. The CHSE blueprint was completed in 2011 and includes five domains: professional values and capabilities; knowledge of simulation principles, practice, and methodology; educating and assessing learners using simulation; managing overall simulation resources and environments; and engaging in scholarly activities. The CHSOS certification launched in 2014 and also includes five domains: concepts in health care and simulation; simulation modalities and technologies; health care simulation program practices, processes, and procedures; professional role development; and instructional design and theory. Although the CHSE and CHSOS credential are examination based, the CHSE-A credential requires a portfolio assessment. Candidates must be currently certified as a CHSE and meet other requirements before submitting a portfolio that includes video examples (Spain, Decker, & Kutzin, 2014).

Professional or personnel certification is a voluntary process. Participants who demonstrate that they meet these standards by successfully completing the assessment process are granted a time-limited credential. To retain the credential, the participant must maintain continued competence. The assessments are not designed to evaluate mastery of the intended learning outcomes of a specific class, course, or training program. The CHSE, CHSE-A, and CHSOS are the certification programs for simulation professionals. Table 54.1 shows an overview of several simulation programs.

Whereas certification leads to a recognized third-party credential that individuals can use to demonstrate meeting a minimum standard, certificates of attendance denote attendance and participation in education programs. These programs consist of lectures, group work, hands-on experiences, or a combination of these activities. Program length varies from a few hours to a week or more. Examples of simulation certificate programs are the Center for Medical Simulation's Institute for Medical Simulation, Drexel University's Certificate in Simulation, Institute for Simulation Educators (NLN), and Southern Indiana's Clinical Simulation Certificate Program.

There are also fellowships in simulation through which a group of people with interest in simulation come together to obtain understanding and skills within the field of health care simulation. Fellowships vary in length and purpose. Some allow an individual to acquire new knowledge and skills. Others focus on improving the participant's ability to create, operate, and facilitate simulations. Others focus on disseminating simulation information to stakeholders. Examples of these fellowships include the INACSL–Canadian Aviation Electronics (CAE) Healthcare Simulation Fellowship, which extends more than 6 months (INACSL, 2016), and the U.S. Veterans Health Administration's Interprofessional Fellowship in Advanced Clinical Simulation, which runs over 2 years. The purpose of the latter is to develop leaders with vision, knowledge, and commitment to advance, implement, teach, and evaluate simulation-based training strategies for the improvement of health care for veterans and the United States (Veterans Health Administration, 2016).

The INACSL–CAE fellowship is a three-part program consisting of webinars, face-to-face workshops, and mentoring. Each cohort consists of no more than 30 participants and three

Table 54.1 Certificate, Certifications, and Accreditation Programs

Name of Program	Certificate	Length	Principles Covered	Professional Organization Sponsor	Where?	Began	Accredited Program by Whom	Modalities
INACSL–CAE Healthcare Simulation Fellowship (academic and clinical)	Certificate of attendance	6–8 months 2 webinars, 22-day F2F sessions and a 4-month mentorship	Creating, developing, best practices, NCSBN Essentials	INACSL	Online and in various places throughout the world	2014	NLN	F2F Webinar Hands-on (Mixed)
Institute for Simulation Educators (academic)	2.4 CEUs or 24 contact hours, from NLN or International Association of Cont. Educ and Training	3.5 days	Debriefing based on NCSBN Essentials, foundation debrief practices, group-designed Sims, plan formulation	NLN Simulation Innovation Resource Center and University of Maryland at Baltimore	University of Maryland at Baltimore	Summer of 2015	NLN	Hands on F2F work sessions PreInstitute assignments
Veterans Health Administration–Interprofessional Fellowship in Advanced Clinical Simulation (clinical)	Certificate of attendance	One year Must make project in your health field	Two fellows per year	Must have master's degree (graduate degree) SimLEARN	Individual VA medical centers, Sim Centers, and SimLEARN Center	Approx. 2012 (in their fourth year)	Not accredited	F2F Reading Hands-on
Healthcare Simulation Certificate	Certificate Earn up to nine graduate academic credits	One class every 16 weeks			Boise State University College of Health Sciences Simulation Center	August 24, 2015	SSH-accredited program	

Program	Credential	Duration	Content	Sponsor	Location	Since	Accreditation	Delivery
Simulation educator training course		3 days	Curriculum and scenario deisgn; feedback and debriefing, evaluation	Royal College of Physicians and Surgeons of Canada	Montreal, QC, Canada			
Leadership in Simulation Instruction and Management (academic and sim center)	Graduate certificate program Post graduate certificate program	Three-course program	Standards, management, emotional intelligence, trends and innovations; licensure, etc	Not reported	Online Robert Morris University, PA		SSH accredited	Onine Product creation
Master's of Science in Healthcare Simulation (academic and sim center)	Master's degree, two certificates—one in instruction and one in leadership	31 credit hours	Foundations of simulations, financial set up of sim center, and developing simulations		University of San Francisco, CA		Not reported	Online, conference and clinical practicum in various sim centers
Keystones Certificate Program	Certificate	39 hours more than 2 academic years	Theoretical, teaching, skills, debriefing	SIM-one	Sim-one Network Toronto, ON, Canada		Accreditation in process	Hands-on F2F
Simulation instructor course (academic and clinical)	Certificate in simulation 38 AMA PRA from category 1 CME 38 PSNA contact hours	5-day experiential course Suggested reading prior to each class	Art of debriefing, interactive, sim learning vs. college learning components in simulation.	Not reported	Penn State Hershey Medical Center, Hershey, PA	Since 2007	Multi disciplinary faculty CHSE	Not reported

(continued)

Table 54.1 Table certificate, certifications, and accreditation programs *(continued)*

Name of Program	Certificate	Length	Principles Covered	Professional Organization Sponsor	Where?	Began	Accredited Program by Whom	Modalities
Master's of Science in Health-care Simulation (academic)	MSMS	Part-time, 2 years	Curriculum design, biostatis, assessment, and debriefing	Baccalaureate	Drexel University College of Medicine, Philadelphia, PA			Interprofessional, sync and async, online, 3 weeks of practicum
Simulation Education Graduate Certificate (academic and clinical)	Graduate level courses, certificate nine academic credit hours	10-week course	Online Hands-on Must add to the body of knowledge for simulation in education	Baccalaureate	Bryan College of Health Sciences, Lincoln, NE			Hands-on F2F
Simulation Fellowship and Visiting Scholars Program (nonclinical, academic)	Fellowship	Varies on student needs	Develop, manage, and implement simulation for health care practitioners	Baccalaureate for nurses and MD/ OD or advanced degrees for allied health and 2 yrs experience	Harvard University, Boston, MA		Accreditation Council for Continuing Medical Education	F2F Assignments No information available online
Clinical Simulation Certificate Program (clinical)	Certificate, continuing-education credit	4-week course = 32 hours	Intro and types of sims, outcomes measurement, strategies/ scenarios for clinical sim education		University of Southern Indiana, Evansville, IN		ANCC, California Board of Registered Nursing	Online, computer conferencing comprehensive exam at end

Accreditation of Simulation Programs	Accreditation body	N/A	Standards and process for accreditation of simulation programs (Canada)	Royal College of Physicians and Surgeons of Canada	Ottawa, ON, Canada	N/A	Biannual submission deadlines
Faculty Development Program	Certificate	N/A	Video-based debriefing, train the trainer, train the SP trainer, train the rater, curriculum development/ scenario design	Israel Centre for Medical Simulation	Ramat Gan, Israel		F2F

AMA, American Medical Association; CEU, continuing-education unit; CHSE, certified health care simulation educator; CME, continuing medical education; F2F, face to face; INACSL, International Association for Clinical Simulation and Learning; ISE, Institute for Simulation Educators; MSMS, master of science in medicine and healthcare simulation; NCSBN, National Council of State Boards of Nursing; NLN, National League for Nursing; OD, doctor of optometry; PRA, Physician's Recognition Award; PSNA, Pennsylvania State Nurses Association; SET, simulation educator training; SP, standardized patient; SSH, Society for Simulation in Healthcare.

Source: Information on accreditation and certifications came from multiple sources. See references listed for INACSL-CAE (2016), NLN and University of Maryland School of Nursing (2016), Veterans Health Administration (2016), Boise State Simulation (n.d.), Robert Morris University School of Nursing and Health Sciences (2016), Universit of San Francisco School of Nursing and Health Professions (2016), Keystones Certificate Program (2016) http://www.sim-one.ca/courses/certificate/keystones-certificate-program, Simulation Instructor Course (2016), Drexel University College of Medicine (2016). Simulation Education Graduate Certificate (2016), Simulation Fellowship and Visiting Scholars Program (2016), Clinical Simulation Certificate Program (2016), Royal College of Physicians and Surgeons of Canada (2016), Faculty Development Program (2016).

facilitators. Facilitators are simulation experts with 5 or more years of experience creating and delivering effective simulation education globally. The fellowship is designed for new simulation educators, existing simulation educators who need additional support, and directors overseeing a simulation center (INACSL, 2016).

Academic programs focused on simulation are becoming more popular. Many degree-granting institutions offer programs focused on a particular area of simulation, such as Leadership in Simulation Instruction and Management (Robert Morris University) or Modeling and Simulation of Behavioral Cybersecurity Certificate (University of Central Florida). Others are more general in nature; examples are the Simulation Education Graduate Certificate (Bryan College of Health Sciences), the Master's of Science in Healthcare Simulation (University of San Francisco), or the Master's in Medical and Healthcare Simulation (MSMS) at Drexel University College of Medicine.

Topping and colleagues (2015) said it best, "Nurse educators require a far broader range of competencies than those just associated with designing, running and debriefing. They need to draw on extensive knowledge, behaviors, skills and demonstrate comportment acquired from both nursing and education" (p. 1112). Choosing an educational program, whether it is a week-long certificate course, academic program, fellowship, or other continuing-education program, is the first step in demonstrating competence in simulation. Achieving a recognized credential, such as the certified health care simulation educator (CHSE), certified healthcare simulation educator—advanced (CHSE-A), or certified healthcare simulation operations specialist (CHSOS) is becoming the standard for many simulation professionals.

Certified Health Care Simulation Educator

A CHSE has mastered the content of the health care discipline in which he or she is enrolled. Mastery includes comprehension of the subject matter as well as how to apply the content in a simulated experience. Mastery of how to use instructional simulation to achieve participant objectives requires the CHSE to employ a variety of facilitation methods and strategies for this purpose.

Values and principles of simulation professionals that make certification a realistic career goal reflect a commitment to a diverse body of learners and a working knowledge of how learners master the discipline-specific content and apply that content in a simulation scenario. When developing instructional methods for a simulation experience, the CHSE takes into account the cultural and individual variations among participants, their development of self-confidence, and self-efficacy, and what motivates participants to achieve objectives. Respect for others, cultural competence, and confidentiality and privacy are ethical practices to be considered as well.

A significant contribution that a CHSE makes to a successful simulation experience is keeping participants focused, engaged, and motivated to achieve objectives. This is accomplished in many ways, two of which are instructional organization and maintaining a structured and safe learning environment. Through formative assessment, the CHSE assesses the participant's progress and can clearly communicate the participant's performance to others.

The CHSE is proficient in critical and creative thinking. By designing simulation scenarios, creative talents are demonstrated. The CHSE studies the literature and critically appraises research findings, staying abreast of international trends in simulation, its learning theories, and instructional methodologies. The CHSE is a thoughtful professional who examines his or her own best practices for the purposes of integrating new study findings, an expanded knowledge base, and an increased skill set into his or her own simulation practice.

The CHSE is a member of an active and stimulating community of professionals. Collaborative discourse and dissemination of research findings form the basis of a cooperative alliance among fellow CHSEs in an effort to improve participant performance during simulation. Simulation policies, curricular threads, staff development strategies, and allocation of resources are some of the topics that bring CHSEs together in collaboration.

The public can expect the process of certification for CHSEs to accomplish what certification of teachers has done: improve participant outcomes, enhance professional development, and develop effective instructional methods for future practitioners in a variety of health care disciplines.

KEY ASPECTS OF SIMULATION: THE PROCESS OF CERTIFICATION

The process of certification sets rigorous and high standards for planning, implementing, and evaluating simulation experiences. Knowledge of the key aspects of simulation is essential for the certification of health care simulation professionals. Achievement of certification status can be demonstrated by following best practices in simulation, such as establishing realistic participant objectives, ensuring standardized exposure of participants to simulation scenarios, accurate measurement of participant outcomes, competent debriefing strategies, facilitating research, using adequate staffing and resources, and managing simulation centers effectively. Examples of how the CHSE might exhibit best practices in key aspects of simulation are described in this section.

Establishing Participant Objectives

Fundamental to an effective simulation experience is the establishment of participant objectives that serve as a guide to the development and execution of the simulation. CHSE is familiar with driving forces influencing the need for instructional and evaluative simulation experiences. Patient safety may be the front-runner in this regard, as are health care curriculum outcomes and desired patient care outcomes. With these societal needs as a framework, and the purpose of the simulation identified as instructional or evaluative, participant objectives are created with consideration for the participant's knowledge level and clinical background. Because participant objectives are realistic and measurable, elements of the simulation scenario are predetermined accordingly.

High performance standards and rigor with respect to objectives are applied in the construction of participant objectives. Before the simulation experience, the CHSE provides unambiguous objectives to participants with respect to realistic time frames in which to meet the objectives. Objectives inform the participant of previously learned and newly acquired knowledge, skills, and attitudes required to complete the simulation experience.

For example, consider this part of a participant objective: "The participant will identify adventitious breath sounds." This statement requires the participant to auscultate the thorax and identify an abnormal auscultatory breath sound, such as crackles or rhonchi. Demonstration of this assessment skill by the participant presupposes adequate instruction and practice on the physical examination of lung sounds. Rigor is evident as the CHSE develops the simulation scenario with this skill in mind and observes the participant to verify that the thorax was indeed auscultated correctly, with proper stethoscope use and placement on the chest.

Standardized Exposure to the Simulation Experience

The CHSE strives to preserve the integrity of the simulation scenario by maintaining confidentiality. Simulation coordinators and participants are responsible for safeguarding the content of simulation experiences. Disclosure of any part of an instructional scenario detracts from the learning process, may compromise participant objectives, and deprives the participant of the full effect of the simulation for professional growth and development. If the scenario's purpose is summative evaluation, disclosure nullifies its validity.

Simulation educators have devised effective means of ensuring standardized exposure to evaluative simulation experiences. This can be accomplished with smaller groups of participants by simultaneously running the evaluation simulation for all participants. Of course, several simulation facilitators and labs are required when testing all participants at the same time. In contrast, larger numbers of participants may be required to sign confidentiality agreement forms. This method of providing confidentiality and standardized exposure to the simulation is more common and relies on an established and accepted honor system.

Measuring Participant Outcomes

Participant objectives drive the outcomes of a given simulation experience. Measurement of participant outcomes should follow a standardized procedure and format. The CHSE plans instruments, processes, and methods of measurement in advance. The effectiveness of the simulation experience is determined by evaluating participant outcomes.

Jeffries and Rogers (2007) describe participant outcomes as skill performance, acquisition of knowledge, development of critical thinking, and participant satisfaction and self-confidence. The CHSE ensures the valid and reliable measurement of these outcomes by using previously identified instruments that fit the summative assessment framework.

For example, participant self-confidence can be measured effectively by self-report. Questionnaires, journaling, and diary entries are valid methods used to assess self-confidence. Participant behaviors, such as psychomotor skills or communication techniques, have been assessed accurately using checklists, anecdotal notes, and direct observation. Attitudinal scales are instruments using a Likert-scale format and are useful for determining participant self-efficacy and participant satisfaction with an instructional strategy at a particular moment in time (Jeffries & Rogers, 2007). The CHSE remains accountable for the evaluation of participant outcomes by using accurate and dependable measurements.

Debriefing

Participant reflection enhances clinical judgment as part of the learning experience and is facilitated during the debriefing exercises that follow an instructional simulation. The CHSE is adept at identifying circumstances that encourage reflection, and therefore, intentionally incorporates reflection into the simulation's debriefing session in order to further participant outcomes.

The CHSE is competent in providing a safe environment for the debriefing process in which trust, confidentiality, and open dialogue are encouraged and protected. Practice with this competency is required for mastery. Providing a safe learning environment requires a command of complex instructional variables and their interactions. Fundamental to the success of the debriefing process is experience with instructional variables, such as group dynamics, seating configuration, and establishing an atmosphere of acceptance. Too many participants or insufficient time for debriefing can invalidate the outcomes of the simulation experience. Many advocates of simulation affirm that a satisfactory debriefing session is required for an effective simulation experience.

Conducting Research

Best practices in simulation are established through scientific inquiry. In addition to using evidence-based research findings, the CHSE facilitates, performs, and evaluates simulation research. Because certification confers status related to high-performance standards on the individual knowledgeable in simulation, the CHSE uses research findings that reflect best practices by incorporating rigorous standards into the planning, implementation, and evaluation of simulation experiences.

Facilitating research is accomplished by the CHSE in a variety of ways. The CHSE occupies a strategic position for the development of research questions expanding knowledge related to simulation experiences. Decker (2007) lists examples, such as, "What conditions promote reflection during a simulated learning experience?" or "Does the integration of reflection into a simulated learning experience affect learning outcomes?" (p. 82). The CHSE facilitates research efforts by grant writing, collecting data, participating in interrater reliability studies, and analyzing simulation study findings.

The CHSE carries out simulation research on a continuum. Discrete instructional strategies or evaluation techniques used during simulation have been investigated by CHSEs. Alternatively, the CHSE has been involved in comprehensive, complex, high-stakes, multisite scientific inquiries. In addition, the incorporation of technical staff into the simulation experience has been examined by CHSEs.

Evaluation research in simulation is a current focus in the literature. Valid and reliable instruments are needed to assess the effectiveness of simulation experiences. Once these instruments are developed, replication studies are required to establish validity and reliability. The CHSE is integral in testing the psychometrics of evaluation instruments. Regardless of the context or type of research, the CHSE is a leader in establishing simulation standards of best practice.

Managing Staff

The CHSE is an effective manager of personnel and resources necessary to carry out effective simulation experiences. The CHSE oversees support staff, often student workers, who stock the simulation lab and perform setup and cleanup activities. Additional support staff responsibilities managed by the CHSE include record keeping, ordering supplies, operating audiovisual and computer equipment, and peer tutoring of psychomotor skills. Graduate student staff are a good resource for participants who are new to the simulation experience. Student staff at the doctoral level are able to assist with research activities, such as data collection and analysis or evaluating study findings.

Professional staff assisting the CHSE may perform skills instruction or evaluate skills performance by participants. The CHSE may be responsible for professional and nonprofessional staff assisting in simulation activities for prelicensure students in addition to graduate students. Students enrolled in more than one health care discipline may be simulation lab consumers, and therefore under the supervision of the CHSEs.

Simulation Centers

Certified individuals may be the manager of a simulation center, a large simulation environment devoted entirely to simulated experiences. In this case, the certified individual must have a working knowledge of the planning, construction, and use of a complex physical structure or building serving several disciplines and curriculum levels. In a collaborative relationship, the CHSE may employ a newly evolving simulation professional—the simulation center architect. The value of this type of architect in the planning phase of a simulation center is significant.

The CHSE uses his or her knowledge of simulation experiences, required level of fidelity, health care courses, discipline-specific curricula, budgetary constraints, and dedicated physical space to assist in the planning and construction of the simulation center. The number of simulation labs with and without control rooms, classrooms, smaller debriefing rooms or conference rooms, skills testing areas, observation rooms, break rooms and areas for staff, and space for technologic infrastructure are all considered by the CHSE in setting up a simulation center. This is usually a collaborative effort with departmental or community partners as stakeholders. However, the CHSE takes the leadership role in the creation of the simulation center.

Certified Health Care Simulation Operations Specialist

A recent role in simulation has its origin in technology. The CHSOS is a specialized professional staff member who assists the CHSE with the technical operations of simulation scenarios. Some simulation educators are also simulation technicians, just as some simulation coordinators also function in this role. The CHSOS is acquainted with simulation content for courses, curricula, and health care programs, and is proficient in managing the environment needed to achieve participant outcomes. Although the CHSE and CHSOS are not mutually exclusive in larger simulation facilities, staff tend to become more highly specialized, thus leading them to choose one role or the other. However, in many simulation facilities staff function in multiple roles leading to many individuals obtaining both the CHSE and CHSOS credential to demonstrate their competence in both aspects of simulation.

Additional Considerations

The process of certification in simulation is rigorous and is designed to ensure that individuals achieving certification have met basic requirements as set forth by the certifying body. Although every key aspect of simulation cannot be accounted for in the certification process, many of the core knowledge areas are assessed, from the idea for a simulation scenario, to creating a simulation experience, to the evaluation of the effectiveness of a simulation, to the creation of multidisciplinary simulation centers. Experience and knowledge of simulation instructional and evaluation techniques are necessary to achieve the rigor characteristic of the status of certification. High standards of practice are required and are easily identified as the signature feature of the CHSE.

ACCREDITATION

General accreditation of simulation programs is conducted by the SSH. Both provisional accreditation and full accreditation are offered by SSH for simulation programs around the world. Provisional accreditation allows programs with established structure and processes but no outcomes to apply for this status. Full accreditation allows programs to be recognized for meeting the standards in a core set of criteria along with an additional specialty area, which includes assessment, research, teaching/education, or systems integration. To obtain full accreditation, simulation facilities must submit documentation and then also undergo a site visit to ensure they have met the standards (SSH, 2012). If successful, the simulation program is accredited for a term of 5 years, after which reaccreditation is required.

In addition to SSH, other organizations accredit simulation programs: the American College of Surgery (ACS), the American Society of Anesthesiologists (ASA), and the Veterans Health Administration (VHA) through its SimLEARN National Simulation Center initiative. The differences among these discipline-or agency-specific accreditations and the more general SSH accreditation is that the SSH accreditation program recognizes simulation expertise and is open to any agency conducting simulation-based training.

SIMULATION STANDARDS

INACSL set out to establish best practice standards for simulation early on in the evolution of healthcare simulation development. The INACSL is the only health care organization to date to create standards for simulation. It asserts that best practices in health care disciplines and curricula are reflected in standards of practice. According to INACSL, simulation standards are shared principles, beliefs, and values that provide the framework for decisions, policies, and procedures in academic or practice settings. INACSL standards are discussed in detail in Chapter 1.

The CHSE should have a working knowledge of these standards and how to apply them in educational and clinical environments. These standards for simulation experiences were designed not only for the purpose of establishing consensus among simulation experts with regard to the content of the standards, but also for meeting the needs of the health care providers using simulation. The standards can be applied to instruction, curriculum design, and participant evaluation in health care disciplines and curricula. In addition, the standards can be used as a framework for research development and testing. Regardless of the context within which these standards are used, they were developed to represent a best practice perspective, and hence are at the heart of all health care simulation certification efforts.

The CHSE follows Standard I: Standardized Terminology by being conversant in the terminology of simulation. Likewise, the CHSE enforces the second standard that addresses professional integrity. However, one of the best practice principles of this standard requires the CHSE to safeguard the emotional and psychologic safety of participants interacting within the simulation setting.

The importance of Standard III: Participant Objectives and its interaction with the fourth standard describing facilitation methods holds the key to the effectiveness of the simulation experience with regard to participant outcomes. The CHSE has mastered a repertoire of methods for facilitating the achievement of participant objectives.

The CHSE is aware that time to think and problem solve on the part of the participant is necessary in a safe learning environment, and highlights the fifth standard addressing attributes and qualities of the simulation facilitator. Role modeling of ethical and professional actions is a quality of effective simulation facilitators.

Some simulation experts believe that debriefing is the most important part of a simulation exercise. Debriefing is the topic of the sixth simulation standard. The CHSE is aware that during debriefing activities, the participant learns to apply critical thinking methods. The CHSE must be skillful in directing the tone and direction of debriefing activities in order to maintain confidentiality, a safe learning environment, and the integrity of the simulation scenario.

A challenge to the CHSE is adherence to the seventh standard, which deals with evaluation of outcomes. Because formative and summative evaluation occur in simulation experiences, the CHSE must be purposeful and focused in eliciting expected outcomes, especially during high-stakes evaluations. A high-stakes evaluation determines outcomes of a simulation activity that have significant consequences, such as a major grading decision or ranking of the participant.

Contemporary evidence-based health care is a team effort, which drove the development of Standard VIII. Institute of Medicine recommendations, such as collaboration, professional communication, and related interprofessional health care provider skill sets, form the foundation for mastering this standard's competencies. The nature of simulation-based experiences are effective approaches in meeting the outcomes of interprofessional education.

Design features are particular to the objectives of the simulation, as Standard IX states, thus maintaining the worth and value of the simulation-based experiences. A simulation developed with an instructional design has a purpose necessarily distinct from a simulation designed for testing and evaluation. Likewise, one can expect that instructional designs for different levels of learners should be different.

The CHSE who demonstrates expertise with these standards has invested time, effort, and commitment to the performance of best practices in simulation. Because the process of certification communicates to the public that the simulation educator has achieved a status defined by established standards of practice, adherence to these simulation standards is incorporated into the day-to-day work behaviors of the CHSE. Likewise, the accredited simulation center represents a cluster of best practice criteria fostering high-quality simulation-based experiences and staff. Consumers of health care education and its related disciplines should expect the highest level of performance when engaged in simulation-based experiences in accredited simulation centers hosted by CHSEs.

REFERENCES

Boise State Simulation. (n.d.). Healthcare simulation certificate. Retrieved from https://graduate college.boisestate.edu/programs2/healthcare-simulation

Bryan College of Health Sciences. (2017). Simulation education certificate. Retrieved from https://www.bryanhealthcollege.edu/bcohs/academic-programs/certificate-programs/simulation-certificate

Center for Medical Simulation. (2017). Simulation Fellowship and International Scholars Program. Retrieved from https://harvardmedsim.org/simulation-fellowship-and-international-scholars-program

Decker, S. (2007). *Simulation as an educational strategy in the development of critical and reflective thinking: A qualitative exploration.* Denton: Texas Woman's University.

Drexel University College of Medicine. (2016, July 13). Master of science in medical and health-care simulation. Retrieved from http://drexel.edu/medicine/Academics/Graduate-School/Medical-and-Healthcare-Simulation

Institute for Credentialing Excellence. (2010). *Defining features of quality certification and assessment-based certificate programs.* Washington, DC: Author. Retrieved from www.credentialingexcellence.org

International Association for Clinical Simulation and Learning. (2016). INACSL–CAE fellowship of healthcare in simulation. Retrieved from http://www.inacsl.org/i4a/pages/index.cfm?pageid=3476

Jeffries, P. R., & Rogers, K. (2007). Evaluating simulations. In P.R. Jeffries (Ed.) *Simulation in nursing education: From conceptualization to evaluation* (pp. 87–103). New York, NY: National League for Nursing.

Monash University. (2012). Graduate certificate in clinical simulation. Retrieved from http://www.monash.edu.au/pubs/handbooks/courses/3973.html

National Board for Professional Teaching Standards. (2017). The proven impact of board-certified teachers on student achievement. Retrieved from https://mea-mft.eventready.com/docs/download/Submission/Handouts/7941_3.pdf

National League for Nursing. (n.d.). Simulation Innovation Resource Center. Retrieved from http://sirc.nln.org

NLN and University of Maryland School of Nursing. (2016). Institute for simulation educators. Retrieved from https://www.nursing.umaryland.edu/academics/pe/simulation-institute

PennState Hershey Clinical Simulation Center. (2017). Teaching with simulation: An instructor course certificate program. Retrieved from http://www.pennstatehershey.org/documents/307082/10239962/04042014+B5439SpringFlyer.pdf/1187e29b-1a86-45e3-bd95-494b18ba949c

Robert Morris University School of Nursing and Health Sciences. (2016). Leadership in simulation instruction and management. Retrieved from https://www.usfca.edu/nursing/programs/non-degree/healthcare-simulation

Society for Simulation in Healthcare. (2012). Committees. Retrieved from https://ssih.org/committees/accreditation

Spain, A., Decker, S., & Kutzin, J. (2014). *Healthcare simulation certification.* Presented at the 13th Annual International Nursing Simulation/Learning Resource Centers Conference, Lake Buena Vista, FL.

Topping, A., Boje, R. B., Rekola, L., Hartvigsen, T., Prescott, S., Bland, A.,…Hannula, L. (2015). Towards identifying nurse educator competencies required for simulation-based learning: A systemized rapid review and synthesis. *Nurse Educator Today, 35*(11), 1108–1113. doi:10.1016/ j.nedt.2015.06.003

University of San Francisco School of Nursing and Health Professions. (2016, July). Master's of science in healthcare simulation. Retrieved from https://www.usfca.edu/nursing/programs/masters/healthcare-simulation/program-details

U.S. Department of Veterans Affairs. (2017). VA SimLEARN. Retrieved from https://www.simlearn.va.gov

Veterans Health Administration. (n.d.). Interprofessional fellowships in advanced clinical simulation (clinical). Retrieved from http://www.va.gov/oaa/specialfellows/default.asp

CHAPTER 55

Publishing Your Simulation Work

Suzan Kardong-Edgren

WHY WRITE?

Umberto Eco said that writing for publication and having children allow one to overcome death (Safire & Safir, 1992). (This may be true, but I recommend writing an article. It is much cheaper than having children.) If your manuscript is listed in a database, such as the Cumulative Index of Nursing and Allied Health (CINAHL) or PubMed, your work will still be there for others to find and read, long after you are gone. That is pretty powerful! An editor thought your manuscript was good enough to send out to your peers for review. Those reviewers critiqued your work and an editor published your manuscript as an article. You have made a contribution to the profession and perhaps even the world as a whole. One published article reaches many more people than a presentation at a conference ever will. You may receive emails from around the world as readers respond to your work. You may receive invitations to speak because publishing gives your thoughts legitimacy. People perceive you as an expert when you write and publish your work.

Publishing is an expectation in many academic roles. However, some of us work for academic programs in which publications are not an expectation. This does not mean you should not write, especially if you think you have something worthwhile to share with others. Some of the most creative simulation work today is being done in academic programs in which there is no expectation that faculty will publish. But they do it anyway. They feel compelled to write. What about you? Do you have something to say? How do you go about the task of writing a manuscript? *How* does one get published? This chapter reviews the steps of writing, writing in a team, submitting a manuscript for publication, and responding to reviewers.

To write well, it helps to be an avid reader. If you read your nursing journals, you will already know the literature and what is being published. If you are an avid reader, you will know what a sentence looks like and know when grammar is incorrect. (This seems simple but it is a big thing.) Many of us never write in full sentences anymore and do not know when we are mangling sentence structure. Many of us graduated before the American Psychological Association's publication manual (APA, 2010) was written, the most often used style manual for nursing journals. If you do not know what APA is, it is time to buy or borrow the manual and read it; it is actually interesting and tells you how to write a scientific manuscript. (It is also useful for nonscientific articles.) OK, so you are buying in, getting excited, and ready to write . . . something...but what? Be thinking; and here are some other things to know.

There are now four major journals devoted to simulation. They are *Advances in Simulation*, *BMJ Simulation*, *Clinical Simulation in Nursing*, and *Simulation in Healthcare*. Most nursing and medical education journals also publish simulation articles. This provides a wide selection of places to publish for novice and experienced writers. How do you decide where to send your manuscript? Always consider who the audience is, for your story or work. Who needs to read what you are writing? Select the journal that best targets this audience. Some authors are under pressure to publish in a high impact factor journal, however, many authors are not under such constraints. The larger simulation community is served by considering the audience first.

WHAT TO WRITE?

There is a symbiotic relationship between editors and writers; editors have pages to fill with new and interesting things for their readers, and you, the writer, are the provider of these new and interesting things. Editors are happy to answer a query letter or email about an idea for a manuscript, however, this is not common practice anymore. It used to be "good form" to query an editor about a potential manuscript through email, but it is most common today to just submit a manuscript to a journal, with no earlier contact with the editor.

If you have presented a peer-reviewed poster, you probably have an outline for a good manuscript waiting for you to build on. Alternately, think about what you have done that might be of interest to others. Did you open a simulation center, invent a solution to a human patient simulator (HPS) or simulation problem, invent a novel simulation or game, get interdisciplinary buy-in from an unusual source, partner with another school or hospital in simulation on a project? All of these are worthy ideas for publication. Other nonresearch ideas recently published include optimizing space in a simulation center or moving a simulation center, group study for simulation certification, and simulation use in large classrooms. How do you know you have a publishable idea? Share it with an acquaintance. If he or she seem interested, check the simulation journals to see whether someone else has published a similar article. If someone has, all is not lost. Think about a different "slant" or approach on the same topic to make it fresh. Be creative.

Remember, there is usually more leeway allowed with manuscripts describing experiences, thought pieces, and so on. This is both a blessing and a curse. As a nonresearch article is less structured, it allows both the writer and the reviewer a larger chance for creativity. Try to be thorough in developing and reporting your ideas, leading the reader through a logical progression of thought and idea development.

Remember that reviewers for a specific journal are looking for a recognizable pattern. They read the journal all the time and expect manuscripts to read in a certain way. So, thoroughly study articles in your selected journal that are similar to what you want to write. There are different format expectations for general-interest articles, qualitative articles, and so on. Study the format and sentence structure of similar articles. Outline the paragraphs in a published article that is similar to the one you are writing to get a good sense of how the authors put the manuscript together. You will be expected to make your sentence structure and writing style match this format. If you do not, the journal reviewers, who are experts at what the journal sentence structure and syntax look like, will more than likely perceive "that something is wrong with the manuscript" (Regan & Pietrobon, 2010, p. 439). Taking the time to study similar articles before writing could save you a lot of time and rewriting in the long run.

Read and follow the journal guidelines for authors. If there is a section in your article that does not fit the guidelines, remove it. Or make it conform to what is required for the manuscript format. Reviewers and editors catch on very quickly to the fact that an article has been submitted in its entirety without any editing done to its original format.

RESEARCH WRITING AND REPORTING

Every paper you write while in a master's or doctoral program should be considered a potential manuscript for publication somewhere. Your job is to tweak it to fit the requirements of the journal you choose to submit it to. Note, remove the professor's comments and the final grade. (An editor does not care what grade your professor gave you.) The extensive literature reviews one completes in preparation for a research study or a program evaluation can be published as a free-standing article before the completion of the study or evaluation. Literature reviews are the most cited type of article, and are helpful to others, if done well. Editors and your fellow researchers love them.

Use standardized definitions in your writing, based on either the new Simulation Dictionary (Lopreiato, 2016) published by the Society of Simulation in Healthcare or the glossary of the International Nursing Association for Clinical Simulation and Learning INACSL *Standards for Best Practice: Simulation*[SM] (2016). The use of standardized terminology in writing and reporting allows researchers to quickly understand each other and to share mental models more quickly.

One excellent resource for writing a research-based manuscript is the Enhancing the QUAlity and Transparency Of health Research (EQUATOR) website (www.equator-network.org); it provides resources for writing (reporting) guidelines for all kinds of research articles, including qualitative articles. A recent publication by Fey, Gloe, and Mariani (2015) provides a thorough research evaluation article rubric. One can use the rubric to double-check that one has covered all of the bits and pieces required for a simulation study manuscript and that one has put them in the right order. More recently, a large consortium group of simulation researchers published extensive reporting guidelines for simulation research, based on both the Consolidated Standards of Reporting Trials (CONSORT) and Strengthening the Reporting of Observational Studies in Epidemiology (STROBE) Statements (Cheng et al., 2016). An extended list of what to include in a study report is included in this article, which was published in the four leading simulation journals simultaneously in August 2016. The goal of jointly publishing this article was to widely disseminate the new guidelines to rapidly improve the planning and reporting of simulation research across all disciplines. Both the Fey et al. (2015) and the Cheng et al. (2016) articles should be on a researcher's desk at all times.

HOW TO WRITE

When you are just starting out, you do not really know what writing method will work best for you. Writing in long hand may be helpful for some, as it slows the thinking process down; others like to write at the computer. (This may be a function of one's age also!) I could not write at the computer for several years; it was a learned skill for me. Some people need a whole day to write, to immerse themselves in their thoughts. Others can write successfully by writing briefly each day. You will need to develop a style. Some writers outline the manuscript; others just start writing. Some write several paragraphs in long hand, then cut and paste these thoughts into some semblance of order and then start typing. Some writers start in the middle; some start in the beginning. The bottom line is … start. Get something on the page and build out from there.

Writing with partners can be immensely helpful and also fraught with peril. Clark (2014) provides an excellent review of collaborative writing, should you decide this is something you want to try. Early in the process, Clark suggests establishing writing team norms, including such things as free and open discussion about all things relevant to the manuscript, how missed deadlines will be handled, and author order and what this will be based on, early in the process. You could be working on the same manuscript or multiple manuscripts at the same time, with different author orders for each. Writing partners make you accountable for getting things done and give you convenient reviewers for your work. It is nice if one of the writing partners has published before; there is nothing like experience. However, this is not critical.

All journals publish author guidelines online or in the journal itself. Do *not* email an editor and ask him or her to send you the author guidelines. This makes for a bad start to an author–editor relationship. Be sure that you note the word limits for different manuscript types, the number of tables allowed, recommendations for photos or diagrams, margin settings, line numbering expectations, and so on. Follow the guidelines, because they are really rules!

AVOIDABLE ERRORS

Justice Brandeis said, "There is no great writing, only great rewriting" (Goodreads, n.d.). It is RARE that a manuscript does not go through one or two rewrites before publication. Expect this as the price of authorship. BUT, you do not need to give reviewers things to "fix." Let us discuss the most common errors in manuscripts and how to avoid them.

Conducting a thorough literature review before you begin writing is a must for any topic. Nothing is more embarrassing than your manuscript landing in the hands of an author (now one of your blinded reviewers) to whom you proclaim that "no one has written anything about..." (except for the fact that this reviewer is the expert on your topic and has published extensively on the topic). This actually happens quite often. Save yourself this exercise in humility by conducting a thorough literature review before beginning to draft a manuscript, so you can quote or cite what others have said, agree or disagree with them, but know the literature.

Most journals require line numbering in a manuscript, to make the reviewer's job easier, that is, "in line 345, note that you are negating the argument you previously made." A line numbering feature is included in any major writing program, such as Microsoft Word.

The most grievous and painful error a researcher or author can make is gathering participant data without institutional review board (IRB) approval. Even if you are doing a course or program evaluation, when you are using student data, you should seek IRB approval from your institution if you think you want to publish your findings. Many wonderful manuscripts stop abruptly and excellent data is never shared with anyone else but the research team because of this error. Rule of thumb—if you are considering presenting or publishing anything, seek IRB approval. If you are in a program that does not have an IRB, you must still seek permission from your dean or director for what you did and have documentation showing they approved of what you did.

Check all of your manuscript citations against your reference page before submitting it for review. Do not include reference you inadvertently cut out of the manuscript on your reference page. Do not have citations in your manuscript that you do not list on your reference page.

Be sure you are using the correct format for citations and references in your manuscript for the journal you are submitting to. Not all nursing journals use APA format. If you are rejected by a journal and resubmit your manuscript to another journal (always a good idea), check the reference formatting required by the new journal and change yours if needed.

Verbs frequently migrate from the past to the present to the future and back again in novice manuscripts, frequently within the same sentence and often in the same paragraphs. Pick a tense and stay there. Literature reviews are usually written in the past tense. Results and discussion are usually written in the present tense. When writing a "how we did it" article, write in the past tense until describing what is currently happening or what future plans include. Using passive voice is common, unbelievably boring, and frequently the "kiss of death" to even a good idea. Some examples: "A mistake was made"; "It was determined by the researchers that the treatment was ineffective." There is nothing more boring or aggravating than reading an entire manuscript written in this way.

THE ONLINE SUBMISSION PROCESS

Online submission is ubiquitous these days. It can be a very trying and tedious process on the best of systems and at the best of times. To save yourself time and aggravation, read the instructions for authors for online submission before starting this process. Some systems cannot take documents formatted in MS Word 2010. Some systems want all tables and figures in the actual manuscript sent at the end as attachments. Some systems want your figures and tables embedded where you think they should go in your manuscript. Some want all figures and tables uploaded as separate files. Many systems have special formatting requirements for figures or diagrams. Note that there is almost no way to get the number of pixels needed into a PowerPoint-drawn figure without converting it to a larger dots per inch (DPI) file using one of many free online figure-enhancing programs. This is something you may want your information technology (IT) department's help with. A tip: always look at your manuscript proof in the submission system before accepting it. Manuscripts look very different when turned into a PDF file. Mistakes and misspellings that you missed for months now jump off of the page at you. Remove the manuscript file from the system, fix it, and upload it again. Then read it yet again. Authors are frequently surprised when an editor sends their manuscript back to them with errant lingering "track changes" still visible in the manuscripts. This is evidence that the author did not proofread the submission before accepting all the changes. Very embarrassing!

THE PEER REVIEW PROCESS

Most journals use some kind of peer review process. The level of rigor the review depends on the journal itself and the type of article submitted. Some journals receive 500 manuscripts a month and triage heavily, rejecting the majority of manuscripts outright. This can be a gift in disguise, as a writer now knows that he or she can cross that journal off the list for this particular manuscript and move along to another journal. Of course, picking the right journal for a manuscript is an important skill. Asking a more experienced writer or your university librarian to help you match your manuscript to a journal is a good idea. Sending a query email to an editor is another good idea but is becoming uncommon.

You should be delighted if your manuscript is sent out for peer review; an editor thought what you wrote had some merit and might be of interest to others. Now expect that you will be asked to rewrite something in your manuscript...and you will probably not be disappointed. It is RARE that an author is not asked to rewrite parts and on occasion, all of a manuscript. It is not uncommon for three reviewers to write conflicting comments about the same manuscript. However, when all reviewers make the same comments or mention the same thing, you know there is something amiss and you need to address it. There are times you may not agree with a reviewer. It is okay to say this in your reply to reviewers if you state your case and supply the rationale for your decision not to change something. Some authors copy and paste each reviewer's comment into a two-column table format; the actual reviewer comment in the left column and the author response in the right column. A second way to address reviewer comments is to type in a different font or color directly below each reviewer's comment in the reviewed document. The important point, not to be missed here, is respond to each reviewer and every comment. If this is well done, an editor may not need to send your manuscript out for review again, which speeds up the acceptance and publication process. If you are thoroughly confused by reviewer comments, it is often a good idea to consult with the editor about what he or she would like you to do. Never send in a revised manuscript without a Reply to Reviewer's table. Build a table in which you have included every reviewer comment and how you addressed it, or chose not to address it. If your rewrite was so extensive that you have basically rewritten the manuscript entirely, then and only then, is it okay to write a blanket statement to the reviewers and editor. For anything less than a complete manuscript revision, expect that the editor will request that you complete an extensive reply to reviewers. There are times a manuscript may go through multiple revisions. This is not a bad thing, the manuscript is getting better and better with each revision. There are some manuscripts that have been through five or six major rewrites before publication. Writing can require fortitude and perseverance; however, this rewriting occurs more frequently for novice writers.

FINAL STEPS IN THE PUBLISHING PROCESS

After your manuscript is accepted, you will receive proofs of the manuscript containing copyeditor questions. You are required to review every word of the manuscript and approve it. If you are a sole author, this is an easy process. If you are the corresponding author, representing multiple authors, it is your responsibility to make sure every other author has seen and approved the manuscript before stating that you accept the proofs. Be sure you have discussed the author order early in the writing process and that everyone is in agreement. Some journals require that every author individually sign a copyright authorization form. Gathering all of these signatures can be much worse than writing the actual manuscript, especially if authors are in geographically disparate areas.

PARTING THOUGHTS

Expect that even with electronic publication, there can be a wait of several months or several years (depending on the journal) before your article comes out in print or in a formally paginated way in an online journal. Many journals have several years of manuscripts backed up and waiting for formal publication. However, many journals now make these accepted manuscripts available online in an *In press* or in a *Publication Ahead of Print* section on the journal website. Because of advances in technology, many cited articles are not formally published yet. A copy of the proof of your manuscript is often all you need for a tenure and promotion committee to demonstrate that you have a manuscript waiting to be published. All scholars know the manuscript backlog exists.

To hone your writing skills, it is helpful to become a journal reviewer for the type of journal you would most probably write for. An advantage to reviewing is that most online systems now let you see what other reviewers have written about the same manuscript after all the reviews are submitted. Your writing can improve dramatically by paying close attention to what other reviewers are alerting on in a manuscript. You will find yourself editing your own writing based on what you learn as a reviewer. Writing gets easier the more you do it; however, I do not know that it is ever "easy." It is a learned skill and one that is well worth the effort.

REFERENCES

American Psychological Association. (2010). *Publication manual of the American Psychological Association* (6th ed.). Washington, DC: Author.

Cheng, A., Kessler, D., Mackinnon, R., Chang, T. P., Nadkarni, V. M., Hunt, E. A.,...Auerbach, M.; International Network for Simulation-based Pediatric Innovation, Research, and Education (INSPIRE) Reporting Guidelines Investigators. (2016). Reporting guidelines for health care simulation research: Extensions to the CONSORT and STROBE statements. *Simulation in Healthcare, 11*(4), 238–248.

Clark, C. (2014). A formula for collaborative writing. *Journal of Nursing Education, 53*(3), 119–120.

Fey, M. K., Gloe, D., & Mariani, B. (2015). Assessing the quality of simulation-based research articles: A rating rubric. *Clinical Simulation in Nursing, 11*(12), 496–504.

Goodreads. (n.d.). Justice Brandeis. Retrieved from http://www.goodreads.com/quotes/6772530 -there-is-no-great-writing-only-great-rewriting

International Nursing Association for Clinical Simulation and Learning Standards Committee. (2016, December). Standards of best practice: Simulation: Simulation glossary. *Clinical Simulation in Nursing, 12*(S), S39–S47. doi:10.1016/j.ecns.2016.09.012

Lopreiato, J. O. (2016). Healthcare simulation dictionary. Retrieved from http://www.ssih.org/ Portals/48/Docs/Dictionary/simdictionary.pdf

Regan, M., & Pietrobon, R. (2010). A conceptual framework for scientific writing in nursing. *Journal of Nursing Education, 49*(8), 437–443.

Safire, W., & Safir, L. (1992). *Good advice on writing: Great quotations from writers past and present on how to write well.* New York, NY: Simon & Schuster.

CHAPTER 56

Final Words of Wisdom on Simulation

Suzanne Hetzel Campbell and Karen M. Daley

BACKGROUND TO THE THIRD EDITION

Since the writing of the first and second edition, as our simulation journey continues, we are stunned and amazed—never did we believe the book would be on the best seller list, translated into Korean, or become such an essential resource for so many. For this edition we reached out to our faithful readers through the International Nursing Association for Clinical Simulation and Learning (INACSL) and the national American Association of Colleges of Nursing (AACN) deans and directors list serves to contact national leaders in simulation and lab directors and coordinators for nursing education. With thanks to our SurveyMonkey® guru, Colleen Cox, at Western Connecticut State University (WCSU), we were able to assess the usefulness of the book in addition to this group's perception of the gaps that needed to be filled in the second edition. The national survey demonstrated that readers found the following most useful: ideas for building a lab, specialty scenarios, leveled scenarios, including increased complexity, objectives that matched National League for Nursing (NLN) and AACN categories, and details for running scenarios. Secondly, debriefing guidelines and evaluation checklists were most useful. The second question on the survey asked what areas would be most helpful—participants identified advanced practice scenarios with an emphasis on nurse practitioners (NPs), interprofessional team building scenarios, and identified that new scenarios were needed at all levels: undergraduate, graduate, and doctorate. We also found that participants identified the following types of scenarios as most needed: assessment, communication, interprofessional, competency evaluation, and cultural awareness as well as including patients of various ages, gender, and ethnicity.

Other areas of importance that we assessed included the use of web applications (iPhone, iPad, social media) and participants only showed interest in the iPad and in the incorporation of electronic health records. Similar to the National Council of State Boards of Nursing (NCSBN) surveys (Hayden, 2010; Kardong-Edgren, Willhaus, Bennett, & Hayden, 2012), our participants reported the importance of simulation, the integration into their curriculum, but participants classified only 50% of the faculty as champions. We feel that this "50%" is encouraging, given that 10 years ago most nursing faculty probably would have reported less than 10% as champions in the use of simulation. Participants believed that an expanded version of the book would assist faculty to become more comfortable with the use of simulation and with the integration of innovative educational pedagogy into their nursing programs. As we suspected, although survey participants identified using preprogrammed scenarios, it appears that faculty who have developed expertise in simulation prefer to develop their own scenarios. To that end, this book was revised to assist faculty to continue to do just that!

Much has changed in the last 5 years and research on simulation has proliferated not just in nursing. The NCSBN studies (Hayden, 2010; Kardong-Edgren et al., 2012) demonstrated that schools of nursing are using simulations in very different ways and there is no uniform methodology A study in Canada provided an inventory on the use of simulated clinical learning experiences and evaluation of their effectiveness (Garrett, Van der Wal, Tench, & Fretier, 2007). Conclusions were that the simulated clinical learning offered advantages, such as a safe environment, especially in high-risk procedures; exposure to rare but complicated events; the manipulation of opportunities for care; the provision of feedback in a timely manner; the ability to standardize, repeat, evaluate, and assess performances; and to organize and practice team behavior (Garrett et al., 2007, p. 2). A lack of standardization of terminology, issues of cost and access to equipment, and minimal actual replacement of clinical hours by simulation were part of key findings. In addition, cost-benefit analyses have not been done to demonstrate the effectiveness of particular approaches (Garrett et al., 2007).

INSIGHTS GLEANED

We learn so much about the creativity and innovation of simulation in nursing education as we work with authors nationally and internationally in various areas where simulation is being used. The authors who submitted chapters are truly engaging in the pedagogy of simulation, paving the path toward the future where simulation becomes a standard in the transformation of health care professional education. The introduction of the book sets the stage for all the changes that have occurred and the Framework for Simulation Learning has been moved to the second chapter to set the stage for descriptions of integrating simulation throughout the pedagogy (Chapter 4), innovative approaches to faculty development including international and interprofessional perspectives from teaching intensive and research intensive sites (Chapter 5), and the description of building a learning resource center has taken into consideration many changes that have occurred from when the coeditors began (Chapter 6). This third edition benefits from the updated version of our contributors Meakim and Rockstraw description in Chapter 7 of a detailed simulation center that incorporates the highest level of technology. We endeavored in the first edition to present basic scenarios with a focus on prelicensure nursing education, with only a few chapters offering multiple scenarios. In contrast, the second edition presented more complex undergraduate scenarios: and discipline-specific chapters as well as Home care blending cultural sensitivity and scenarios written according to Quality and Safety Education for Nurses (QSEN) competencies. This third edition continues the practice of significant additions in specialties, the advanced practice, master's, and doctoral level scenarios as well as the interdisciplinary and interprofessional scenarios. This continues to reflect the trends globally where undergraduate simulation has expanded to the graduate level. Because of increasing focus on interprofessional education, Part III of this new edition provides 16 interdisciplinary and interprofessional scenarios of varying complexity and from the United States and Canada. Finally, Part IV describes the continuing maturity level of simulation by providing insight to learning to write like a nurse during simulation, how to publish your simulation work, and how to assess your expertise by outlining certification and accreditation programs internationally.

TRENDS AND GAPS

Still a pervading issue is the configuration of simulation labs and the role of who staffs the labs and who oversees and has responsibility for simulation. In relationship to the configuration of the labs, learning resource centers, there is still a lot of variation nationally and internationally from distinct rooms to complete learning resource centers, which may consist of full floors or actual buildings to interdisciplinary regional resource centers. We are still challenged in defining the role of simulation directors. Although masters-prepared nurses as simulation lab managers are ideal, there still exist many spunky and resourceful baccalaureate-prepared nurses who manage the responsibilities of the lab, including equipment maintenance, setup and running of simulations, and scheduling day-to-day activities. For true integration and curricular development using simulation in nursing programs, doctorally prepared faculty in the role of directing and overseeing the learning resource center are ideal. In order for us to truly achieve a simulation-focused pedagogy throughout the curriculum, doctorally prepared faculty will need to be engaged in the work of the learning resource center. This role could include overseeing lab managers and staff for the day-to-day running of activities; curricular development and integration of simulation-focused pedagogy; faculty development and skill enhancement in the use and development of simulation scenarios; research on the effectiveness of simulation and innovative educational techniques to enhance health care professional education; outreach to the community to develop partnerships for the running of the center and its use for regional training; and competency-based continuing education for health care professionals.

Another trend is the increased rigor of "Simulation Based Research" (SBR) and quality to enhance moving forward the science of simulation within nursing and health care. Better research will be done when simulation scenarios are developed in a consistent manner using evidence-based best practice standards for the clinical situation as well as for the development of the scenario (INACSL, 2016). Increasing the use of theory-based research to study simulation is also a key factor to increasing the rigor and efficacy of nursing research in this area (Kaakinen & Arwood, 2009; Rourke, Schmidt, & Garga, 2010) as well as looking beyond self-efficacy (Kardong-Edgren, 2013) and faculty and student satisfaction. The next phase of research in simulation needs to demonstrate that knowledge transfer, retention, and behavior modification result as a direct outcome of simulation education, whether for prelicensure nursing students or interprofessional teams in situ, and that these changes result in increased patient safety and improved patient outcomes and quality of care. Part of rigorous research includes using valid and reliable tools. An evaluation of simulation tools was done (Kardong-Edgren, Adamson, & Fitzgerald, 2010) and presently INACSL provides a repository of instruments used in simulation research on their website (INACSL, 2015).

Faculty Buy-In, Professional Development, and Time Management

We were hoping that in the elapsed time between the editions of this book we would see more faculty buy-in and professional development and allotment of time for simulation integration, but these issues are still a challenge. Here we feel we should address the issue of the national crisis of faculty shortages, which impact faculty workload. Adamson (2010), DaRosa et al. (2011), and Schneider Sarver, Senczakowicz, and Slovensky (2010) discuss these issues as barriers to the full integration of simulation. Although there is no replacement for full administrative support for simulation, at the university level, such as exists at Davenport University, we still have to find ways to enable faculty to meet this goal. We still contend that simulation is a vehicle for the faculty to achieve the goal of working smarter, not harder, with good student outcomes and increased faculty and student self-efficacy and satisfaction. As we have suspected since the inception of simulation in nursing, research is now demonstrating the benefits in increased self-confidence, problem solving, and the importance of debriefing (Alfers, 2011; Reese, Jeffries, & Engum, 2010).

In addition to getting faculty buy-in, supporting new faculty in their role and the learning curve involved in taking on tenure track positions not to mention learning about the integration of innovative technology and experiential learning methods such as simulation. There is a difference in the level of respect for the Scholarship of Teaching and Learning, and although the U.S. Health Resources and Service Administration (HRSA) funds provide support for educational program development and research, similar resources are not easily available in Canada. One of the major shifts since the writing of the second edition has been the increased rigor in the science of simulation. The INACSL Best Practice Standards: Simulation[SM] (INACSL, 2016), the NCSBN Simulation Guidelines for Prelicensure Nursing Programs (Alexander et al., 2015) and the increase in integrative and systematic reviews of simulation research are providing more consistent and standardized ways to support the provision of the highest quality learning experiences possible.

We are pleased to see that work is being done on an interprofessional collaboration to match the Interprofessional Education Collaborative Expert Panel (IPEC, 2011a, 2011b). This is a tremendous use of simulation for the enhancement of collaborative teamwork in areas to increase patient safety and satisfaction and addresses the QSEN competencies (Gantt & Webb-Corbett, 2010; Ironside, Jeffries, & Martin, 2009; Morello et al., 2013; Reeves, Perrier, Goldman, Freeth, & Zwarenstein, 2013; Thomas & Galla, 2013), including medication safety (Berdot et al., 2016; Härkänen, Voutilainen, Turunen, & Vehviläinen-Julkunen, 2016; Sears, Goldsworthy, & Goodman, 2010). Other research has been done on enhanced interprofessional communication between nursing students and medical students (Reising, Carr, O'Shea, & King, 2011; Scherer, Myers, O'Connor, & Haskins, 2013), as well as between nursing students at various levels (Leonard, Shuhaibar, & Chen, 2010). Systematic reviews of interprofessional simulations include: emergency situations (Murphy, Curtis, & McCloughen, 2016), intensive care (O'Leary, Nash, & Lewis, 2015; Watts et al., 2014), and with standardized patients (Koo, Idzik, Hammersla, & Windemuth, 2013).

On the horizon, we see the use of simulation to educate nurses in the care of veterans (Anthony, Carter, Freundl, Nelson, & Wadlington, 2012) and publications documenting the experiences of veteran nurses (Scannell-Desch & Doherty, 2012). Schools of nursing are using simulation and other innovative technologies to teach students about posttraumatic stress disorder (PTSD) and traumatic brain injury (TBI) so they can better treat veterans who are coming home from war as part of the Joining Forces Initiative. Dr. Campbell was thrilled to present the first edition of this book to First Lady Michelle Obama in support of the Joining Forces Initiative.

We are pleased to see that additional work is being done in end-of-life care (Gillan, Jeong, & van der Riet, 2014; Leighton & Dubas, 2009) and simulation to enhance cultural awareness (Grossman, Mager, Opheim, & Torbjornsen, 2012; Haas, Seckman, & Rea, 2010; Ozkara San, 2015; Roberts, Warda, Garbutt, & Curry, 2014; Rock, Schaar, & Swenty, 2012), as prescribed in our Framework for Simulation Learning in Nursing Model (Daley & Campbell, 2009). We now have research documenting that simulation increases knowledge and skills at the graduate level, increases self-confidence in students and nurse educators, and the benefits of simulation as a method of teaching (Jeffries et al., 2011).

When academic metrics were used to measure psychomotor skills in students, no differences were found on standardized examinations between teaching using simulation or traditional methods (Sportsman, Schumacher, & Hamilton, 2011). The researchers felt that their study provided initial evidence of the impact of simulation on academic success. More studies are necessary in this area. Another study revealed documentation of gaps in critical thinking and problem recognition by students during simulation, for example not reporting essential information and a need for further research in this area (Fero, Witsberger, Wesmiller, Zullo, & Hoffman, 2009). This study demonstrates how essential the integration of simulation experiences are with traditional clinical experiences. As reflected in the Framework for Simulation Learning in Nursing Model (Daley & Campbell, 2009), through debriefing and concept mapping faculty can see how students develop in their thinking, acting, and reflecting like a nurse.

Setting the Priorities Increased Interest in Interdisciplinary Education, Team Building, Communication, and Safety—Knowledge Transfer, Retention, Behavior Change

As aptly stated by Brewer (2011) "HPS use has not yet developed to its fullest potential" (p. 317). There is much work to be done. We, the editors of this book, would like to challenge nurse educators (and nurse researchers) to continue to persevere and go beyond simple assessment of confidence and attitudes, and begin the work of metric-based assessment of outcomes to continue the work to make simulation measureable! We believe the priorities for simulation in nursing education should be to continue to work toward full integration of simulation throughout all levels of nursing education. Furthermore, we believe that simulation is a means for meeting the demand for interprofessional and interdisciplinary educational opportunities (Institute of Medicine [IOM], 2011) and is rich in research opportunities.

LOOKING TOWARD THE FUTURE

There are many changes on the horizon, which mean that nursing faculty need themselves to be constantly vigilant, creative, fearless, and passionate. With increasing faculty shortages and health care practitioner shortages, especially nurses, new ways of delivering nursing programs must be envisioned. Better collaboration between practice partners and educators needs to happen. Use of more technology for flipped classrooms, virtual simulation, and online clinics and learning opportunities will become a reality. More sensitive simulators providing sensory feedback to guide health professionals' assessment and skill in techniques already exist (e.g., pelvic, prostate, breast examination or catheter or intravenous insertions; Laufer et al., 2016). This text has provided a summary of the many advantages of using simulation to educate nurses, interprofessional teams, and has focused on both technical and nontechnical skills. The scenarios provided are written using the INACSL Best Practice Standards Simulation[SM] (INACSL, 2016) and the authors describe the integration in their curriculums, the effect on students, and the lessons they have learned. In addition, the scenarios outline objectives and essentials from AACN or the NCLEX-RN® Blueprint so that the faculty using the scenarios can decide where they best fit to meet the student competency needs and abilities. In addition, many of the scenarios describe ways to level the experiences such that they can be used with novice students or those more advanced. Many of the scenarios in the text are at a level that would be easily translated for use in clinical settings to maintain staff competency and allow for practice of team-building skills.

Overall, the authors of the chapters in this book recognize the barriers they face, especially when it comes to the use and research of simulation, for example the lack of time, workload, and fear of technology. Yet, similar to research findings, they felt enabled when they were provided professional development and training, felt that administration was supportive and had a dedicated simulation coordinator (Al-Ghareeb & Cooper, 2016). In conclusion, we look forward to a day when simulation in nursing education is a commonplace and "a given" as part of nursing education. We have already experienced great growth over the time that the third edition of this text has evolved and look back and say "Remember when simulation meant sticking an orange with a needle, and there were no human patient simulators?" Even more now we believe simulation will prove the key to the future of nursing education that is well-grounded in safety, excellence, and reflection.

REFERENCES

Adamson, K. (2010, May). Integrating human patient simulation into associate degree nursing curricula: Faculty experiences, barriers, and facilitators. *Clinical Simulation in Nursing, 6,* e75–e81.

Alexander, M., Durham, C. F., Hooper, J. I., Jeffries, P. R., Goldman, N., Kardong-Edgren, S. S., . . . Tillman, C. (2015). NCSBN simulation guidelines for prelicensure nursing programs. *Journal of Nursing Regulation, 6*(3), 39–42. doi:10.1016/S2155-8256(15)30783-3

Alfers, C. M. (2011). Evaluating the use of simulation with beginning nursing students. *Journal of Nursing Education, 50*(2), 89–93.

Al-Ghareeb, A. Z., & Cooper, S. J. (2016). Barriers and enablers to the use of high-fidelity patient simulation manikins in nurse education: An integrative review. *Nurse Education Today, 36,* 281–286.

Anthony, M., Carter, J., Freundl, M., Nelson, V., & Wadlington, L. (2012, April). Using simulation to teach veteran-centered care. *Clinical Simulation in Nursing, 8*(4), e145–e150.

Berdot, S., Roudot, M., Schramm, C., Katsahian, S., Durieux, P., & Sabatier, B. (2016). Interventions to reduce nurses' medication administration errors in inpatient settings: A systematic review and meta-analysis. *International Journal of Nursing Studies, 53,* 342–350.

Brewer, E. P. (2011). Successful techniques for using human patient simulation in nursing education. *Journal of Nursing Scholarship, 43*(3), 311–317.

Daley, K., & Campbell, S. H. (2009). Chapter 26 Framework for simulation learning in nursing educa-tion. In S. H. Campbell & K. Daley (Eds.), *Simulation scenarios for nurse educators: Making it REAL* (pp. 287–290). New York, NY: Springer Publishing.

DaRosa, D. A., Skeff, K., Friedland, J. A., Coburn, M., Cox, S., Pollart, S.,...Smith, S. (2011). Barriers to effective teaching. *Academic Medicine, 86*(4), 453–459.

Fero, L. J., Witsberger, C. M., Wesmiller, S. W., Zullo, T. G., & Hoffman, L. A. (2009). Critical thinking ability of new graduate and experienced nurses. *Journal of Advanced Nursing, 65*(1), 139–148.

Gantt, L. T., & Webb-Corbett, R. (2010). Using simulation to teach patient safety behaviors in under-graduate nursing education. *Journal of Nursing Education, 49*(1), 48–51.

Garrett, B. M., Van der Wal, R., Tench, E., & Fretier, P. (2007). Inventory on the use of simulated clin-ical learning experiences and evaluation of their effectiveness. Retrieved from http://casn.ca/vm/newvisual/attachments/856/Media/InventoryoftheUseofSimulated

Gillan, P. C., Jeong, S., & van der Riet, P. J. (2014). End of life care simulation: A review of the literature. *Nurse Education Today, 34*(5), 766–774.

Grossman, S., Mager, D. M., Opheim, H. M., & Torbjornsen, A. (2012). A bi-national simulation study to improve cultural awareness in nursing students. *Clinical Simulation in Nursing, 8*(8), e341–e346. doi:10.1016/j.ecns.2011.01.004

Haas, B., Seckman, C., & Rea, G. (2010). Incorporating cultural diversity and caring through simulation in a baccalaureate nursing program. *International Journal for Human Caring, 14*(2), 51–52.

Härkänen, M., Voutilainen, A., Turunen, E., & Vehviläinen-Julkunen, K. (2016). Systematic review and meta-analysis of educational interventions designed to improve medication administration skills and safety of registered nurses. *Nurse Education Today, 41*, 36–43.

Hayden, J. (2010). Use of simulation in nursing education: National survey results. *Journal of Nursing Regulation, 1*(3), 52–57.

Institute of Medicine. (2011). *The future of nursing: Leading change, advancing health.* Washington, DC: National Academies Press.

International Nursing Association for Clinical Simulation and Learning. (2015). *Repository of instruments used in simulation research.* Retrieved from http://www.inacsl.org/i4a/pages/index.cfm?pageID=3496

International Nursing Association for Clinical Simulation and Learning. (2016). Standards of best prac-tice: Simulation. *Clinical Simulation in Nursing, 12*, S48–S50. doi:10.1016/j.ecns.2016.10.001

Interprofessional Education Collaborative Expert Panel. (2011a). *Core competencies for interprofessional collabo-rative practice: Report of an expert panel.* Washington, DC: Author.

Interprofessional Education Collaborative Expert Panel. (2011b). *Core competencies for interprofes-sional collaborative practice.* Retrieved from http://www.aacn.nche.edu/education-resources/ipecreport.pdf

Ironside, P. M., Jeffries, P. R., & Martin, A. (2009). Fostering patient safety competencies using multiple-patient simulation experiences. *Nursing Outlook, 57*(6), 332–337.

Jeffries, P. R., Beach, M., Decker, S. I., Dlugasch, L., Groom, J., Settles, J., & O'Donnell, J. M. (2011). Multi-center development and testing of a simulation-based cardiovascular assessment curriculum for advanced practice nurses. *Nursing Education Perspectives, 12*(5), 116–322.

Kaakinen, J., & Arwood, E. (2009). Systematic review of nursing simulation literature for use of learning theory. *International Journal of Nursing Education Scholarship, 6*, Article 16. doi:10.2202/1548-923X.1688

Kardong-Edgren, S. (2013). Bandura's self-efficacy theory: Something is missing. *Clinical Simulation in Nursing, 9*(9), e327–e328. doi:10.1016/j.ecns.2013.07.001

Kardong-Edgren, S., Adamson, K. A., & Fitzgerald, C. (2010). A review of currently published eval-uation instruments for human patient simulation. *Clinical Simulation in Nursing, 6*(1), e25–e35. doi:10.1016/j.ecns.2009.08.0004

Kardong-Edgren, S., Willhaus, J., Bennett, D., & Hayden, J. (2012, April). Results of the National Council of State Boards of Nursing national simulation survey: Part II. *Clinical Simulation in Nursing, 8*(4), e117–e123.

Koo, L. W., Idzik, S. R., Hammersla, M. B., & Windemuth, B. F. (2013). Developing standardized patient clinical simulations to apply concepts of interdisciplinary collaboration. *Journal of Nursing Education, 52*(12), 705–708.

Laufer, S., D'Angelo, A. D., Kwan, C., Ray, R. D., Yudkowsky, R., Boulet, J. R.,...Pugh, C. M. (2016). Rescuing the clinical breast examination: Advances in classifying and asessing physician competency. *Annals of Surgery* [epub ahead of print]. doi:10.1097/SLA.0000000000002024

Leighton, K., & Dubas, J. (2009, November). Simulated death: An innovative approach to teaching end-of-life care. *Clinical Simulation in Nursing, 5*(6), e223–e230.

Leonard, B., Shuhaibar, E. L., & Chen, R. (2010). Nursing student perceptions of intraprofessional team education using high-fidelity simulation. *Journal of Nursing Education, 49*(11), 628–631.

Morello, R. T., Lowthian, J. A., Barker, A. L., McGinnes, R., Dunt, D., & Brand, C. (2013). Strategies for improving patient safety culture in hospitals: A systematic review. *British Medical Journal Quality & Safety, 22*(1), 11–18.

Murphy, M., Curtis, K., & McCloughen, A. (2016). What is the impact of multidisciplinary team simulation training on team performance and efficiency of patient care? An integrative review. *Australasian Emergency Nursing Journal, 19*(1), 44–53.

O'Leary, J. A., Nash, R., & Lewis, P. A. (2015). High fidelity patient simulation as an educational tool in paediatric intensive care: A systematic review. *Nurse Education Today, 35*(10), e8–e12.

Ozkara San, E. (2015). Using clinical simulation to enhance culturally competent nursing care: A review of the literature. *Clinical Simulation in Nursing, 11*(4), 228–243. doi:10.1016/j.ecns.2015.01.004

Reese, C. E., Jeffries, P. R., & Engum, S. A. (2010). Learning together: Using simulations to develop nursing and medical student collaboration. *Nursing Education Perspectives, 31*(1), 33–37.

Reeves, S., Perrier, L., Goldman, J., Freeth, D., & Zwarenstein, M. (2013). Interprofessional education: Effects on professional practice and healthcare outcomes (update). *Cochrane Database of Systematic Reviews,* (3). doi:10.1002/14651858.CD002213.pub3

Reising, D. L., Carr, D. E., Shea, R. A., & King, J. M. (2011). Comparison of communication outcomes in traditional versus simulation strategies in nursing and medical students. *Nursing Education Perspectives, 32*(5), 323–327.

Roberts, S. G., Warda, M., Garbutt, S., & Curry, K. (2014). The use of high-fidelity simulation to teach cultural competence in the nursing curriculum. *Journal of Professional Nursing, 30*(3), 259–265.

Rock, M. J., Schaar, G. L., & Swenty, C. F. (2012, April). The nurse attorney's role: Linking legal concepts to an obstetrical simulation. *Clinical Simulation in Nursing.* Advance Online Publication.

Rourke, L., Schmidt, M., & Garga, N. (2010). Theory-based research of high fidelity simulation use in nursing education: A review of the literature. *International Journal of Nursing Education Scholarship, 7,* Article 11. doi:10.2202/1548-923X.1965

Scannell-Desch, E., & Doherty, M. E. (2012) *Nurse in war: Voices from Iraq and Afghanistan.* New York, NY: Springer Publishing.

Scherer, Y. K., Myers, J., O'Connor, T. D., & Haskins, M. (2013). Interprofessional simulation to foster collaboration between nursing and medical students. *Clinical Simulation in Nursing, 9*(11), e497–e505. doi:10.1016/j.ecns.2013.03.001

Schneider Sarver, P. A., Senczakowicz, E. A., & Slovensky, B. M. (2010). Development of simulation scenarios for an adolescent patient with diabetic ketoacidosis. *Journal of Nursing Education, 49*(10), 578–586.

Sears, K., Goldsworthy, S., & Goodman, W. M. (2010). The relationship between simulation in nursing education and medication safety. *Journal of Nursing Education, 49*(1), 52–55.

Sportsman, S., Schumacker, R. E., & Hamilton, P. (2011). Evaluating the impact of scenario-based high-fidelity patient simulation on academic metrics of student success. *Nursing Education Perspectives, 32*(4), 259–265.

Thomas, L., & Galla, C. (2013). Building a culture of safety through team training and engagement. *BMJ Quality Safety, 22*(5), 425–434. doi:10.1136/bmjqs-2012-001011

Watts, P., Langston, S. B., Brown, M., Prince, C., Belle, A., Skipper, M. W., . . . Moss, J. (2014). Interprofessional education: A multi-patient, team-based intensive care unit simulation. *Clinical Simulation in Nursing, 10*(10), 521–528. doi:10.1016/j.ecns.2014.05.004

INDEX